Military Strategies for Sustainment of Nutrition and Immune Function in the Field

Committee on Military Nutrition Research

Food and Nutrition Board

Institute of Medicine

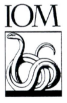

NATIONAL ACADEMY PRESS
Washington, D.C. 1999

NATIONAL ACADEMY PRESS • 2101 Constitution Avenue, N.W. • Washington, DC 20418

NOTICE: The project that is the subject of this report was approved by the Governing Board of the National Research Council, whose members are drawn from the councils of the National Academy of Sciences, the National Academy of Engineering, and the Institute of Medicine. The members of the committee responsible for the report were chosen for their special competences and with regard for appropriate balance.

The Institute of Medicine was established in 1970 by the National Academy of Sciences to enlist distinguished members of the appropriate professions in the examination of policy matters pertaining to the health of the public. In this, the Institute acts under both the Academy's 1863 congressional charter responsibility to be an adviser to the federal government and its own initiative in identifying issues of medical care, research, and education. Dr. Kenneth I. Shine is president of the Institute of Medicine.

This report was produced under grant DAMD17-94-J-4046 between the National Academy of Sciences and the U.S. Army Medical Research and Materiel Command. The views, opinions, and/or findings contained in chapters in Parts II through VI that are authored by U.S. Army personnel are those of the authors and should not be construed as official Department of the Army positions, policies, or decisions, unless so designated by other official documentation. Human subjects who participated in studies described in those chapters gave their free and informed voluntary consent. Investigators adhered to U.S. Army regulation 70-25 and United States Army Medical Research and Materiel Command regulation 70-25 on use of volunteers in research. Citations of commercial organizations and trade names in this report do not constitute an official Department of the Army endorsement or approval of the products or services of these organizations. The chapters are approved for public release; distribution is unlimited.

Library of Congress Catalog Card No. 98-89702

International Standard Book Number 0-309-06345-0

Additional copies of this report are available from:
National Academy Press, 2101 Constitution Avenue, N.W., Lock Box 285, Washington, D.C. 20055

Call (800) 624-6242 or (202) 334-3313 (in the Washington metropolitan area), or visit the NAP's on-line bookstore at *http://www.nap.edu.*

Printed in the United States of America

The serpent has been a symbol of long life, healing, and knowledge among almost all cultures and religions since the beginning of recorded history. The image adopted as a logotype by the Institute of Medicine is based on a relief carving from ancient Greece, now held by the Staatliche Museen in Berlin.

Cover: Resting monocyte/macrophage being activated to produce proinflammatory cytokines which form complexes with receptor binding proteins. Adapted from Figure 1-2.

FOOD AND NUTRITION BOARD

Preface

This publication, *Military Strategies for Sustainment of Nutrition and Immune Function in the Field,* is the latest in a series of reports based on workshops sponsored by the Committee on Military Nutrition Research (CMNR) of the Food and Nutrition Board (FNB), Institute of Medicine, National Academy of Sciences. Other workshops or symposia have included such topics as food components to enhance performance; nutritional needs in hot, cold, and high-altitude environments; body composition and physical performance; nutrition and physical performance; cognitive testing methodology; and fluid replacement and heat stress. These workshops form part of the response that the CMNR provides to the Commander, U.S. Army Medical Research and Materiel Command (USAMRMC), regarding issues brought to the committee through the Military Nutrition Division (currently the Military Nutrition and Biochemical Division) of the U.S. Army Research Institute of Environmental Medicine (USARIEM) at Natick, Massachusetts.

HISTORY OF THE COMMITTEE

The CMNR was established in October 1982 following a request by the Assistant Surgeon General of the Army that the Board on Military Supplies of the National Academy of Sciences set up a special committee. The purpose of this committee was to advise the U.S. Department of Defense on the need for and conduct of nutrition research and related issues. The CMNR was transferred to the FNB in 1983. The CMNR's current tasks are

- to identify nutritional factors that may critically influence the physical and mental performance of military personnel under all environmental extremes,
- to identify deficiencies in the existing database,
- to recommend research that would remedy these deficiencies as well as approaches for studying the relationship of diet to physical and mental performance, and
- to review and advise on standards for military feeding systems.

Within this context, the CMNR was asked to focus on nutrient requirements for performance during operational missions rather than requirements for military personnel in garrison (the latter were judged to be not significantly different from those of the civilian population).

Although the membership of the committee has changed periodically, the disciplines represented consistently have included human nutrition, nutritional biochemistry, performance physiology, food science, and psychology. For issues that require broader expertise than exists within the committee, the CMNR has convened workshops or utilized consultants. The workshops provide additional state-of-the-art scientific information and informed opinion for the consideration of the committee.

COMMITTEE TASKS AND PROCEDURES

The request for this review of nutrition and immune function and its application to military operations originated with Army scientists from USARIEM and USAMRMC. In December 1995, a committee subgroup of the CMNR participated in a series of conference calls with USARIEM, USAMRMC, and other CMNR members to identify the key areas that should be reviewed and to solicit suggestions for names of scientists who were active in the research fields of interest.

On May 20–21, 1996, the CMNR convened a workshop in response to a request from Army representatives to provide information on the impact of nutritional status on immune function. The purpose of the workshop was twofold: (1) to assess the current state of knowledge about immune function to ascertain how military stressors (including food deprivation) could impact unfavorably upon these functions and (2) to evaluate ongoing research efforts by USARIEM scientists to study immune status in special forces troops.

ORGANIZATION OF THE REPORT

The CMNR's background summary, responses to questions, conclusions, and recommendations constitute Part I of this volume; Parts II through VI include papers contributed by speakers at the workshop. Part I has been reviewed anonymously by an outside group with expertise in the topic areas and experience in military issues. For the most part, the authored papers in Parts II through VI appear in the order in which they were presented at the workshop (see the workshop agenda in Appendix E). These chapters have undergone limited editorial changes, have not been reviewed by the outside group, and represent the views of the individual authors. Selected questions directed toward the speakers and the speakers' responses are included when they provide a flavor of the workshop discussion. An overview of the immune system and other host defense mechanisms is presented in Appendix A and a glossary of immunological terms is provided in Appendix B. The invited speakers also were requested to submit a brief list of selected background papers prior to the workshop. These recommended readings, relevant citations collected by CMNR staff prior to the workshop, and selected citations from each chapter are included in the selected bibliography (see Appendix H).

ACKNOWLEDGMENTS

It is my pleasure as chairman of the CMNR to acknowledge the contributions of the FNB staff. Their involvement in the planning, organization, and publication of the proceedings of this workshop was essential in responding to the Army's request for this review. In particular, I wish to acknowledge the excellent efforts of Sydne J. Carlson-Newberry, staff officer for the CMNR. She successfully enlisted the participants and organized the proceedings in a timely manner. Rebecca B. Costello joined the FNB staff as project director for the CMNR in July 1996 and worked actively in organizing the summary and publication of the proceedings, and Mary I. Poos who brought the report to completion.

I also wish to commend the workshop speakers for their excellent contributions in preparing papers and participating through their presentations and discussions at the workshop. Without their willing cooperation, this review and report could not have been accomplished.

In addition, I wish to acknowledge the excellent editorial efforts and able assistance of technical editor Judy Grumstrup-Scott and research assistant Susan M. Knasiak-Raley, and project assistant Mariza Silva who also prepared the camera-ready copy for this report. The effort of Donna F. Allen, former senior project assistant to the CMNR, in coordinating the workshop arrangements is greatly appreciated.

I express my deepest appreciation to the members of the CMNR who participated extensively during the workshop and in the discussions and preparation of summaries and recommendations in this report. I wish to commend William R. Beisel for his preparation of the overview of the immune system (see Appendix A). I want to thank former committee member Dick Jansen for his contributions and faithful services to the CMNR. I would also like to express appreciation to Gilbert A. Leveille, who rotated off the committee prior to its preparation of this report, for his many years of service. I continue to be stimulated by the committee's dedication and willing contribution of their time and expertise to the activities of the CMNR. I thank all of you for your continuing contributions to this program.

This report has been reviewed by individuals chosen for their diverse perspectives and technical expertise, in accordance with procedures approved by the NRC's Report Review Committee. The purpose of this independent review is to provide candid and critical comments that will assisst the authors and the Institute of Medicine in making the published report as sound as possible and to ensure that the report meets institutional standards for objectivity, evidence, and responsiveness to the study charge. The review comments and draft manuscript remain confidential to protect the integrity of the deliberative process. The CMNR wishes to thank the following individuals for their participation in the review of this report: Kent L. Erickson, University of California, Davis; Arthur L. Hecker, Abbott Laboratories; Ronald B. Herberman, University of Pittsburg; John L. Ivy, University of Texas; Melvin M. Mathias, U.S. Department of Agriculture; Charles E. Putman, Duke University; David D. Schnakenberg (retired); Adria R. Sherman, Rutgers University; and Esther M. Sternberg, National Institute of Mental Health. While the individuals listed above have provided many constructive comments and suggestions, it must be emphasized that responsibility for the final content of this report rests entirely with the authoring committee and the IOM.

ROBERT O. NESHEIM,
Chair
Committee on Military
Nutrition Research

Contents

VI   HEALTH AND STRESS

APPENDIXES

Nutrition and Immune Function, 1999
Pp. 1–15. Washington, D.C.
National Academy Press

Executive Summary

This report, *Military Strategies for Sustainment of Nutrition and Immune Function in the Field*, is a review of nutrition and immune function and its application to military operational missions. It is the latest in a series of reports by the Institute of Medicine's Committee on Military Nutrition Research (CMNR) and was requested by Army scientists from the U.S. Army Medical Research and Materiel Command (USAMRMC) and the Military Nutrition Division (currently the Military Nutrition and Biochemical Division) of the U.S. Army Research Institute of Environmental Medicine (USARIEM).

COMMITTEE'S TASK

Specifically, the committee was charged with reviewing the current state of knowledge about immune function, assessing how it may be impacted unfavorably by military stresses (including food deprivation), and with evaluating ongoing research efforts by USARIEM scientists to study immune status in Special Forces troops.

In order to accomplish this task, the CMNR held a workshop, reviewed the literature, and deliberated on its findings to provide responses to the following task questions:

1. What are the significant military hazards or operational settings most likely to compromise immune function in soldiers?

2. What methods for assessment of immune function are most appropriate in military nutrition laboratory research, and what methods are most appropriate for field research?

3. The proinflammatory cytokines have been proposed to decrease lean body mass, mediate thermoregulatory mechanisms, and increase resistance to infectious disease by reducing metabolic activity in a way that is similar to the reduction seen in malnutrition and other catabolic conditions. Interventions to sustain immune function can alter the actions, nutritional costs, and potential changes in the levels of proinflammatory cytokines. What are the benefits and risks to soldiers of such interventions?

4. What are the important safety and regulatory considerations in the testing and use of nutrients or dietary supplements to sustain immune function under field conditions?

5. Are there areas of investigation for the military nutrition research program that are likely to be fruitful in the sustainment of immune function in stressful conditions? Specifically, is there likely to be enough value added to justify adding to operational rations or including an additional component?

This report focuses on the many stresses encountered by military personnel and the complexity of their immune responses.

OVERVIEW OF NUTRITIONAL STATUS AND IMMUNE FUNCTION

Immunity, if defined broadly, encompasses all mechanisms and responses used by the body to defend itself against foreign substances, microorganisms, toxins, and incompatible living cells. Such responses may be conferred by the immune system itself or by the protective role of other generalized host defensive mechanisms.

The immune system resides in no single organ but depends on the interactions and secretions of various organs and white blood cells. The physiologic function of the immune system may be viewed simplistically as a mechanism by which the human body responds to and eliminates an initiating antigen. This process is mediated by a myriad of specialized cells and depends on a pathway involving recognition, activation, differentiation, and response to lymphocytes. Thus, this simplistic view becomes significantly more complicated when one is examining the biological nature of these responses in greater detail.

Every aspect of immunity and host defense is dependent upon a proper supply and balance of nutrients (Chandra, 1988; Cunningham-Rundles, 1993; Forse, 1994; Gershwin et al., 1985; Watson, 1984). Severe protein-energy malnutrition can cause significant alterations in the immune response, but even subclinical deficits may be associated with a catabolic response, an impaired immune response, and an altered risk of infection (Beisel, 1982; Keusch and Farthing, 1986). Research using laboratory animals and work with human subjects has extended these observations to the recognition that nutritional deficiencies are associated with a large number of alterations in cell-mediated immunity and the cytokine-initiated acute-phase response. Fever and other hypermetabolic components of acute-phase reactions can deplete the body of essential nutrients. Deficiencies of many individual nutrients, including protein, essential fatty acids, vitamin A, vitamin B_6, folic acid, zinc, iron, copper, and selenium, have been associated with altered immune function. An overview of the nutrients that support immune function is presented in Table S-1, which is a summary of data presented in Chapter 1. Cytokine-induced changes in metabolism can become severe and lead to malnutrition, as seen clinically in many victims of trauma, infections, or other wasting illnesses.

Background

The stresses experienced by military personnel are numerous and varied, encompassing changes in temperature, altitude, humidity, and the availability of food and water; limited or nonrestful sleep; prolonged moderate-to-heavy physical activities; increased susceptibility to infection and injury; and other psychological stresses associated with training or battlefield combat. Military personnel frequently face simultaneous (and often varying) combinations of these diverse stresses for weeks or months at a time. Very little is currently known about the possible additive immunological consequences of these combined stresses. However, much has been learned about the immunological consequences of several of these stresses on an individual basis (for example, malnutrition, semistarvation, severe exercise, infection, and trauma). The primary goal of the Army Operational Medicine Program is to develop physiologic strategies to protect and sustain deployed soldiers, thereby enhancing readiness by maintaining their ability to accomplish assigned missions. One program with a critical need to enhance and maintain readiness is the U.S. Army Special Operations Training Program, which includes the U.S. Army Ranger Training Courses.

TABLE S-1 Overview of Nutrients Involved in Immune System Function

	Humoral Immunity	Surface Immunity	Cell-Mediated Immunity	Antioxidant Activity	Cytokine Release and Eicosenoid Production
Multiple nutrients for cellular synthesis	X	X	X		X
Multiple nutrients for protein synthesis	X		X		X
Vitamin A	X	X	X (−)		
Vitamins C and E				X	
Thiamine		X			
Vitamin B$_6$	X	X	X		X
Folate	X		X		
Iron	X		X (=)		X
Copper	X		X		X
Zinc	X	X	X (−)		X
Selenium	X		X	X	
PUFAs	X		X (−)		X
Arginine			X		
Glutamine		X	X		

NOTES: As components of the host's defense mechanisms, *humoral immunity* involves the antigen-specific immune response mediated by B- and plasma-cell production of circulating or secretory antibodies (immunoglobulins). *Surface immunity*, or passive defense measures, include anatomical barriers and pathways (e.g., skin and mucous membranes), exogenous body secretions (e.g., mucin, saliva, bronchial fluids), and a host of physiologic factors. *Cell-mediated immunity* is the antigen-specific and nonspecific immunity provided by the direct localized cellular activity of T-lymphocytes and natural killer cells. *Cytokines* play a role in cellular communication, function as intercellular signals and mediators, and are active participants in nonspecific immune responses such as acute-phase reactions. PUFAs, polyunsaturated fatty acids; (−), excessive amounts can sometimes be immunosuppressive; (=), excessive amounts can sometimes increase severity of infections.

At the conclusion of the 1990 U.S. Army Ranger Training Course (Moore et al., 1992), an unusually high incidence of infection was documented in the Rangers. This promoted an extensive investigation by a military epidemiology team. An increased incidence of upper respiratory infection, cellulitis, and pneumococcal pneumonia was reported. In addition to the increased infection rates noted in the Rangers, laboratory tests of immune function, showed decreased proliferative activity of both T- and B-lymphocytes in response to an applied mitogenic stimulus (phytohemagglutinin) in cultures of whole blood samples. Other significant findings included marked deficits in energy intake resulting in an average weight loss of 15.9 percent over the eight-week training period; significant losses in body fat from an average of 14.6 percent at entry to 6.9 percent at the end of training. Therefore, the team of epidemiologists recommended that further studies be conducted by military researchers to evaluate the effects of multiple stresses on host defense mechanisms.

After discussions between military research personnel and the Ranger Training School officials, it was decided to perform an additional field study, a nutritional intervention study using a modified ration (Long-Life Ration Packet, LLRP) containing approximately 15 percent more energy on a per-ration basis than the previously supplied Meal, Ready-to-Eat (MRE) ration.

The Ranger II study, which was conducted between the months of August and September 1992, was a collaborative effort among investigators and resources from USARIEM; the Walter Reed Army Institute of Research; the U.S. Department of Agriculture Human Nutrition Research Center in Beltsville, Maryland; and the Pennington Biomedical Research Center at Louisiana State University, Baton Rouge (Shippee et al., 1994). In Ranger II, two significant training stresses were changed after the Ranger I course: (1) the order of the geographically different testing phases was changed (military base field training, desert, mountain, and jungle, to military base field training, mountain, jungle, and desert) because significant immune depression was noted in the Ranger I training course at the end of the mountain and jungle phases; and (2) energy intake was increased by approximately 15 percent (220 kcal/d). In the first two training phases, the MRE was supplemented with a carbohydrate-containing drink and fruit, and in the last two training phases, the MRE was replaced with the LLRP.

A major finding from the Ranger II study was a less dramatic weight loss, which averaged 12.5 percent of initial body weight compared to 15.9 percent in Ranger I. This resulted in an average body fat content at the end of training of 8.4 percent compared to 6.9 percent in Ranger I. Researchers found that with the increased energy intake, there was less suppression of T-lymphocyte cell proliferation in response to an applied mitogenic stimulus, indicating an improvement in immune response. The depression in T-cell proliferative response that was demonstrated at the midpoint of the training phases of Ranger I was found to occur in the later testing phases of Ranger II. Although there was a reduction in the absolute number of circulating T-lymphocytes (CD3), T-helper lymphocytes (CD4), and T-suppressor lymphocytes (CD8) in response to stress during Ranger II, this reduction was less severe than that observed in Ranger I.

Although significant improvements were noted in the maintenance of normal nutritional status of the Ranger trainees with the Ranger II intervention study many questions remained regarding the impact and intensity of Ranger training with respect to body composition changes and host defense mechanisms. In order to delineate further some of the mechanisms and stresses contributing to these alterations, the CMNR conducted a focused review of current information pertaining to: (1) the combined effects of health, exercise, and stress on immune function; (2) the impact of nutritional status on immune function; (3) the role of nutritional supplements and biotechnology in enhancement of immune function; and (4) the assessment of immune status under field conditions. The CMNR then used this review to identify and recommend future research needs and directions for the military in the area of nutrition and immune function.

FINDINGS AND CONCLUSIONS

Many stressful conditions encountered by military personnel have immunological consequences. Undoubtedly, food deprivation is one of the most common and important of these stresses. Total energy intake appears to play the greatest role in nutritional modulation of immune function. Since it has been demonstrated that prolonged energy deficits resulting in significant weight loss have an adverse effect on immune function, emphasis should be placed on the importance of adequate ration intake during military operations to minimize weight loss.

The military's use of prophylactic immunization provides sufficient benefits beyond risk to warrant continued development. This is supported by a recent decision by the Secretary of Defense to begin systematic immunization of all U.S. military personnel against the biological warfare agent anthrax.

Pharmacologic agents such as aspirin, ibuprofen, and glucocorticoids, which modulate the effects of cytokines, can be used to minimize signs and symptoms of cytokine-induced acute-phase reactions and the nutrient losses that accompany them. Future investigations into the changing immunological status of troops in the field must obviously be based upon available current knowledge about the immunological impact of individual stresses. However, because multiple stresses (including food deprivation) are expected, these will have to be studied using experimental designs and methods that have been validated by pilot studies prior to their use in large field studies.

Evidence to suggest that the administration of recombinant cytokines can modulate immune function in a desirable manner is limited. Their effectiveness has not been demonstrated in healthy subjects.

Field studies must be based on the results of prior experiments conducted in controlled laboratory and clinical settings. Experimental designs and methods must be validated by pilot tests prior to use.

Nutritional Status

Total energy intake appears to play the greatest role in nutritional modulation of immune function. Since it has been demonstrated that prolonged energy deficits resulting in significant weight loss have an adverse effect on immune function, emphasis should be placed on the importance of adequate ration intake during military operations to minimize weight loss. Weight loss in the range of 10 percent in operations extending over 4 weeks raisee the concern of reduced physical and cognitive performance and has potential health consequences for some individuals (IOM, 1995).

The nutritional status of soldiers should be optimized prior to deployment, engagement in any exercise or training course, or even brief encounters with anything that would present a potential immune challenge (disease, toxic agent, or environmental stress). When consumed as recommended, operational rations provide adequate energy and macronutrients.

Nutrients that appear to play a role in immune function include protein, iron, zinc, copper, and selenium; the B-group vitamins, especially B_6, B_{12}, and folate; vitamin A and its precursor, β-carotene, vitamins C and E; the amino acids glutamine and arginine; and the polyunsaturated fatty acids. It is difficult, however, to consider the role of one nutrient in isolation. Evidence for a distinct role for vitamin C in immunomodulation remains controversial, and the role of vitamin E has been demonstrated chiefly in the elderly. There is no evidence at this time to indicate that the levels of vitamins A, C and E, or trace elements including zinc, copper, or selenium, are inadequate in operational rations. Increasing or decreasing the consumption of n-6 or n-3 PUFAs or altering their intake ratios may impact immunological function.

Nutritional Supplements

The effects of providing supplements of vitamins A, C and E, as well as certain polyunsaturated fatty acids and amino acids, prior to, during, or following infections are virtually unknown in young, healthy adult men. Many questions remain regarding the efficacy of these nutrients in amounts that exceed Military Recommended Dietary Allowance (MRDA) levels. However, during protracted infections, nutritional supplements (multivitamin and/or multimineral pills, antioxidants, and amino acids such as glutamine and arginine) may provide valuable immunological support. Further, the consumption of high-quality diets should be encouraged early in convalescence to restore body nutrient pools and lost weight.

Excess iron as well as iron deficiency may compromise immune status. The problem of compromised iron status in female personnel is a matter of concern because it may impact immune function, physical performance, and cognitive function. It is important to maintain adequate iron status in female soldiers and to do so without causing excess iron intake by males.

Glutamine has demonstrated potential for improving immune function in critical illness, but its usefulness in healthy populations is unknown. Parenteral and enteral administration of glutamine has been observed to improve recovery following gastrointestinal surgery. Thus far, the effect of glutamine has been observed only in supraphysiological amounts and only in patients undergoing bone marrow transplantation or major operations and those who sustain life-threatening sepsis. Studies to evaluate the effects of supplemental glutamine on the immune function of soldiers have shown no demonstrable effects. An effect of glutamine deficiency also has not been demonstrated.

Risks associated with excess consumption of supplements are much more likely for some nutrients than for others. Toxicity and the potential for nutrient–nutrient interactions must be considered individually. Excess vitamin A may be toxic, whereas vitamins C and E are relatively nontoxic and have been shown to enhance the immune response in some individuals. Trace elements are particularly problematic since requirements may be increased during periods of illness, but at the same time, excessive intakes of some trace elements may be immunosuppressive. Very little is yet known about the immunological effects of short-term food deprivation when accompanied by varying combinations of other military stresses.

RECOMMENDATIONS

Optimizing General Health Status

• **The CMNR recommends the use of medically appropriate and directed prophylactic medications and procedures to minimize the adverse effects of infectious agents. However, the CMNR sees no potential value at this time in administering cytokines or anti-cytokines to healthy military personnel.** It is generally assumed that the body's production of endogenous cytokines during stressful situations is beneficial to the host. However, if endogenous proinflammatory cytokines accumulate in large excesses or are given in large doses, they may have noxious or even dangerous consequences.

The military should remain cognizant of the very active civilian-sector research concerning cytokines, their complex control mechanisms, and their functions, and should apply any pertinent new findings to the management of militarily relevant infectious diseases, trauma, or other stresses.

• **In light of the importance of military immunization programs for achieving and maintaining immune status at optimal levels, the CMNR reiterates its previous recommendations (IOM, 1997) that vigorous research efforts be undertaken to create and evaluate militarily relevant oral vaccines.** These should include optimization of administration schedules and elucidation of the influence of nutritional status on vaccine efficacy. Immunological responses to vaccines may be altered by the stresses of mobilization and/or overseas deployments. Antibody responses to vaccines are known to be depressed by protein-energy malnutrition. The potential problem of reduced responsiveness to military vaccines given during periods of mobilization and deployment stresses (in comparison to normal responses, as measured in control studies) also deserves future study.

• **It is recommended that soldiers maintain good physical fitness via a regular, moderate exercise program as a means of sustaining optimum immune function.** Since the intensity and duration of physical activity can affect immune function, training regimens that achieve high levels of physical fitness without adverse effects on immune status should be established.

• **Additionally, the CMNR recommends the use of methods to minimize psychological stresses, including training, conditioning, and structured briefing and debriefing.**

Optimizing Nutritional Status

• **In view of the compromised immune function noted in studies of Ranger trainees, the CMNR recommends that, where possible, individuals who have lost significant lean body mass should not be redeployed until this lean mass is regained.** Although data showing an effect of weight loss on immune function may be limited, it is reasonable to suggest that the maintenance of body weight within 10 percent of ideal weight should increase the likelihood that adequate immune function will be maintained. Thus, the committee recommends that soldiers be advised to achieve an energy intake sufficient to maintain normal weight. The energy intakes required to maintain body weight will vary with the intensity and duration of physical activity; therefore, the best field guide for individual soldiers and commanders is to monitor body weight changes and to emphasize, through a "field-feeding doctrine," the importance of ration intake as the fuel for the soldier to maintain health and performance.

• **The CMNR recommends that nutritional anemias be treated prior to deployment and that individuals classified as anemic[1] and requiring iron supplements not be deployed.** With the reduced personnel in today's Army and the potential for frequent deployment, it is important that soldiers be in good nutritional health at the time of deployment and that an effort be made to correct any compromise in status that may have resulted from previous deployment. Some scientists believe that iron supplements, if given during the course of bacterial or parasitic infections, may increase the severity of these illnesses. Because this topic is a controversial one, it requires further investigation. Nevertheless, it is recommended that if supplemental iron is required (for prophylactic purposes), it should be in the form of an optional ration component, and the iron content of operational rations themselves should not exceed MRDA levels.

• **As a means of reducing the number of stresses encountered by military personnel, the committee encourages the development and implementation of nutrition education programs targeted at high-risk military groups, such as Special Forces troops and female soldiers**, to communicate information regarding healthy eating habits and supplement use.

Nutritional Supplement Use

Supplementation with certain nutrients may be of value for sustaining host defense mechanisms (including those conferred by the immune system) at normal levels during periods of extreme physiological and physical stress. It is unlikely, however, that nutritional supplements can produce a state of superimmunity in military personnel.

• **At this time, the CMNR cannot recommend general supplementation of military rations above MRDA levels for the purpose of enhancing immune function.** There are no definitive studies that demonstrate positive benefits to young, healthy, active individuals of nutrient supplements at levels significantly in excess of those recommended by the MRDAs and commonly provided by foods. Soldiers should be cautioned regarding the indiscriminate use of individual supplements.

• **The CMNR recommends that, when needed, the preferred method of providing supplemental nutrients is through a ration component.** This would reduce both the potential for excessive intake by those individuals whom do not need the nutrient and the misuse that may occur when supplemental nutrients are provided in single nutrient form. Because energy is one nutrient

---

[1] Iron deficiency anemia is defined as a serum ferritin concentration of less than 12 ng/ml in combination with a hemoglobin of less than 120 g/L.

that has been identified as playing a role in immune function, provision of supplemental energy in the form of a food bar would allow soldiers to increase their nutrient intake as needed according to activity levels.

• **The CMNR recommends that the military gain a better understanding of the prevalence of supplement use and abuse by personnel and make strong recommendations for their appropriate use or nonuse.** The emphasis should be on education and wise choices. A better understanding of supplement use will provide information on the prevalence and frequency of use, its impact on an individual's nutritional status, and the likelihood of reckless or dangerous nutrition practices. Such information will help provide for the delivery of targeted and focused nutritional education messages. As more information is gained on supplement use and misuse and the risks and benefits of supplements, the Army may want to consider formulating a "supplement doctrine" to address these concerns and add a component to nutrition education programs.

Research Methodology

• **The CMNR recommends that research be conducted to determine the appropriate field measures (see Table S-2) for monitoring nutritionally induced immune responses, particularly for determining the presence of acute-phase reactions and changes in immune function of the type and degree that are likely to occur as a result of the nutritional insults suffered by soldiers in typical deployment situations.** This will require basing field study design and methodology on appropriate clinical investigations, piloting experimental designs, and using a simple panel of standard tests that have been validated for the field. Particular attention must be paid to the timing of sample collection; the conditions under which samples are transported, stored and handled; and the use of proper controls.

A rapid assessment of immune functions for use in the field includes clinical evaluations of local lesions, sites of inflammation, and signs and symptoms of generalized infectious illness. The C-reactive protein (CRP), erythrocyte sedimentation rate (ESR), and white cell counts are the most rapid and least expensive lab tests.

TABLE S-2 Methods Adaptable to Field Assessment of Immune Function

Method	Advantages	Disadvantages	Cost (1–4, 4 = most expensive)
Clinical epidemiology	Determines the "true" incidence of infection	Need to develop appropriate assessment tool	2–3
Assay of CRP,* ESR*	Involves common laboratory procedures	None	1
Assay of acute-phase reactants	Helps define course of illness	Special reagents required	1–2
Measures of humoral immunity			
Serum immunoglobulins and antibody levels	•Measures response to immunization or infectious exposure •Requires only serum •Multiple stored samples can be determined later at a convenient time	Individuals with normal levels may be immunosuppressed	1
Measures of cell-mediated immunity			
Skin testing	Involves all phases of classic immune response, predictions of outcome	•48 hours required •Difficult to quantitate	2
Determination of cell number, populations, and subpopulations	Semiautomated techniques	•Some cell preparation necessary for blood sample •Special handling required*	2–3
Assay of circulating cytokines and soluble receptors	•ELISA allows batch processing •Urine is a possible sample source	•Need initial preparation step for blood sample; samples must be stored appropriately •Special handling required*	1–2

TABLE S-2 *Continued*

Whole-blood cytokine production assays	•ELISA allows batch processing •ELISA patterns of cytokine response are detectable; effects of stress hormones are quantifiable ex vivo	•Need initial preparation step for blood sample; samples must be stored appropriately •Special handling required[*]	1–2

NOTE: CRP, C-reactive protein; ESR, erythrocyte sedimentation rate; ELISA, enzyme-linked immunosorbent assay.

[*] Lab tests may require special sample transport, handling, preparation, and storage, plus skilled technicians, and expensive equipment and/or reagents. Sample size requirements may be limiting.

• **The CMNR emphasizes the need for carefully designed research protocols.** Efforts should be directed towards ensuring the control of as many environmental, behavioral, and treatment variables as possible, so that effects attributed to a deficiency of a particular nutrient are not in fact the result of some other operational stress. The military nutrition research program should attempt to differentiate between nutrition-induced immune dysfunction and that caused by other forms of operational stress.

• **The CMNR strongly encourages the military to increase its awareness of and consider the military applications of the findings within the civilian research community regarding nutrition and immune function.** The advice of civilian and military immunologists should be sought to identify the testing methods that have proven to be most useful and field applicable for monitoring immune status and function.

RECOMMENDATIONS FOR FUTURE RESEARCH

• **The CMNR reiterates its previous recommendations (IOM, 1997)** that *laboratory-based studies* be performed to determine if an interleukin-6 (IL-6)–creatinine ratio (or some comparable measure) can be measured in single "spot" urine samples as an index of the 24-h excretion of IL-6 and if 24-h IL-6 excretion is, in turn, a reliable indicator of acute stress response. Such a determination should be made before urinary IL-6 measurements are used in field studies, where 24-h urinary collections are virtually impossible to obtain.

• **The CMNR recommends the development and *field testing* of appropriate cytokine markers in urine and blood that are reflective of ongoing acute-phase reactions and of changes in immune status in**

multistress environments. Developmental efforts should be focused on one or two measurements that could be standardized with sufficient accuracy to serve as marker replacements for an entire (and complex) cytokine battery and would have some clinical correlate in immune function; some examples are skin test response or peak titer following vaccination. Civilian research efforts in this area should be followed carefully, and collaborative relationships should be formed.

• **The CMNR recommends that if research is conducted on the ability of nutrients to influence immune status, priority should be placed on the antioxidant nutrients β-carotene and vitamins C and E.** The committee acknowledges that insufficient data are available to identify any specific nutrient or combination of nutrients as having adequately demonstrated the ability to enhance immune function under the military operational conditions investigated. This would include vitamins C and E, as well as the amino acids glutamine and arginine.

• **It is recommended that the military keep apprised of research being conducted in the civilian sector on immune function in physically active women and consider conducting studies on military women in situations of deployment to augment the findings of civilian studies.** At present, there are few studies on immune function in women.

• **The influence of iron status on the risk of infection requires further investigation. This is also an area of interest to the civilian medical community.**

The Committee on Military Nutrition Research is pleased to participate with the Military Nutrition Division, U.S. Army Research Institute of Environmental Medicine, and the U.S. Army Medical Research and Materiel Command in progress relating to the nutrition, performance, and health of U.S. military personnel.

REFERENCES

Anderson, A.O. 1997. New Technologies for Producing Systemic and Mucosal Immunity by Oral Immunization: Immunoprophylaxis in Meals, Ready-to-Eat. Pp. 451–500 in Emerging Technologies for Nutrition Research, Potential for Assessing Military Performance Capability, S.J. Carson-Newberry and R.B. Costello, eds. A report of the Committee on Military Nutrition Research, Food and Nutrition Board, Institute of Medicine. Washington, D.C.: National Academy Press.

Beisel, W.R. 1982. Single nutrients and immunity. Am. J. Clin. Nutr. 35(suppl.):415–468.

Chandra, R.K., ed. 1988. Nutrition and Immunology. New York: Alan R. Liss, Inc.

Cunningham-Rundles, S., ed. 1993. Nutritional Modulation of the Immune Response. New York: Marcel Decker, Inc.

Forse, R.A., ed. 1994. Diet, Nutrition, and Immunity. Boca Raton, Fla.: CRC Press.

Gershwin, M.E., R.S. Beach, and L.S. Hurley, eds. 1985. Nutrition and Immunology. Orlando, Fla.: Academic Press.

IOM (Institute of Medicine). 1991. Fluid Replacement and Heat Stress, 3d printing., B.M. Marriott, ed. A report of the Committee on Military Nutrition Research, Food and Nutrition Board. Washington, D.C.: National Academy Press.

IOM (Institute of Medicine). 1993a. Nutrition Needs in Hot Environments, Applications for Military Personnel in Field Operations, B.M. Marriott, ed. A report of the Committee on Military Nutrition Research, Food and Nutrition Board. Washington, D.C.: National Academy Press.

IOM (Institute of Medicine). 1995a. Not Eating Enough, Overcoming Underconsumption of Military Operational Rations, B.M. Marriott, ed. A report of the Committee on Military Nutrition Research, Food and Nutrition Board. Washington, D.C.: National Academy Press.

IOM (Institute of Medicine). 1997. Emerging Technologies for Nutrition Research, Potential for Assessing Military Performance Capability, S.J. Calrson-Newberry and R.B. Costello, eds. A report of the Committee on Military Nutrition Research, Food and Nutrition Board. Washington, D.C.: National Academy Press.

Keusch, G.T., and M.J.G. Farthing. 1986. Nutrition and infection. Annu. Rev. Nutr. 6:131–154.

Moore, R.J., K.E. Friedl, T.R. Kramer, L.E. Martinez-Lopez, R.W. Hoyt, R.E. Tulley, J.P. DeLany, E.W. Askew, and J.A. Vogel. 1992. Changes in soldier nutritional status and immune function during the Ranger training course. Technical Report No. T13-92, AD-A257 437. Natick, Mass.: U.S. Army Research Institute of Environmental Medicine.

Shippee, R., K. Friedl, T. Kramer, M. Mays, K. Popp, E.W. Askew, B. Fairbrother, R. Hoyt, J. Vogel, L. Marchitelli, P. Frykman, L. Martinez-Lopez, E. Bernton, M. Kramer, R. Tulley, J. Rood, J. DeLany, D. Jezior, and J. Arsenault. 1994. Nutritional and immunological assessment of Ranger students with increased caloric intake. Report No. T95-5. Natick, Mass.: U.S. Army Research Institute of Environmental Medicine.

Watson, R.R., ed. 1984. Nutrition, Disease Resistance, and Immune Function. New York: Marcel Decker, Inc.

I

Committee Summary, Responses to Questions, Conclusions, and Recommendations

Part I outlines the task presented to the Committee on Military Nutrition Research (CMNR) by scientists at the Military Nutrition and Biochemical Division, U.S. Army Institute of Environmental Medicine (USARIEM). This task was to provide information on the impact of nutritional status on immune function, assess the current state of knowledge on how military stresses (including food deprivation) unfavorably influence immune status, and evaluate ongoing research efforts of USARIEM scientists to study immune status in Special Forces troops. As part of the charge to CMNR the Army posed the following five questions:

1. What are the significant military hazards or operational settings most likely to compromise immune function in soldiers?
2. What methods for assessment of immune function are most appropriate in military nutrition laboratory research, and what methods are most appropriate in field research?

3.   Interventions to sustain immune function can alter the actions, nutritional costs, and potential changes in levels of proinflammatory cytokines. The proinflammatory cytokines have been proposed to decrease lean body mass, mediate thermoregulatory mechanisms, and increase resistance to infectious disease by reducing metabolic activity in a way that is similar to the reduction seen in malnutrition and other catabolic conditions. What are the benefits and risks to soldiers of such interventions?

4. What are the important safety and regulatory considerations in the testing and use of nutrients or dietary supplements to sustain immune function under field conditions?

5. Are there areas of investigation for the military nutrition research program that are likely to be fruitful in the sustainment of immune function in stressful conditions? Specifically, is there likely to be enough value added to justify adding to operational rations or including an additional component?

In Chapter 1, the committee presents an overview of the project using relevant background materials and the proceedings of the workshop held on May 20–21, 1996. The committee then reviews the Army's Ranger studies as well as other Army Operational Training Program studies which have evaluated the effects of multiple physical, psychological, and nutritional stressors on immune system function, and provides a summary of the topics presented at the workshop.

The detailed answers to the five questions posed by the Army are in Chapter 2, and the committee's conclusions and recommendation, including recommendations for future research are in Chapter 3.

Nutrition and Immune Function, 1998
Pp. 19–97. Washington, D.C.
National Academy Press

1

A Review of the Role of Nutrition in Immune Function

The infectious disease threats facing soldiers are multiple and vary with geography. In fact, during major wars, infectious diseases usually have accounted for more noneffective days than combat wounds or nonbattle injuries. Combined stressors may reduce the normal ability of soldiers to resist pathogens, may increase their susceptibility to biological agents employed against them, and may reduce the effectiveness of vaccines intended to protect them. Military studies in multistressor environments have demonstrated that higher energy intakes will better sustain the indices of immune status. Troops must be supplied with foods of high biological quality that will enable them to sustain performance and that will counter an array of immunological impairments caused by a myriad of unknown stressors.

THE COMMITTEE'S TASK

As part of its responsibility to the Military Nutrition Division (currently the Military Nutrition and Biochemical Division) at the U.S. Army Research Institute of Environmental Medicine (USARIEM), the Committee on Military Nutrition Research (CMNR) has, on many occasions, evaluated both research plans and ongoing research efforts funded by U.S. Department of Defense appropriations. Examples include a 1996 review of research activities at the Louisiana State University's Pennington Biomedical Research Center, a 1995 review of issues related to the iron status of women enrolled in U.S. Army Basic Combat Training, and a review of the results of a nutrition intervention project conducted during a 1992 U.S. Army Ranger training class.

On May 20–21, 1996, the CMNR convened a workshop in response to a request from Army representatives to provide information on the impact of nutritional status on immune function (see Appendix E for agenda). The purpose of the workshop was to assess the current state of knowledge about how military stresses (including food deprivation) could unfavorably influence immune function and to evaluate ongoing research efforts by USARIEM scientists to study immune status in Special Forces troops. Army representatives asked the CMNR to include in its response the answers to the following five questions:

1. What methods for assessment of immune function are most appropriate in military nutrition laboratory research, and what methods are most appropriate for field research?

2. What are the significant military hazards or operational settings most likely to compromise immune function in soldiers?

3. The proinflammatory cytokines have been proposed to decrease lean body mass, mediate thermoregulatory mechanisms, and increase resistance to infectious disease by reducing metabolic activity in a way that is similar to the reduction seen in malnutrition and other catabolic conditions. Interventions to sustain immune function can alter the actions, nutritional costs, and potential changes in the levels of proinflammatory cytokines. What are the benefits and risks to soldiers of such interventions?

4. What are the important safety and regulatory considerations in the testing and use of nutrients or dietary supplements to sustain immune function under field conditions?

5. Are there areas of investigation for the military nutrition research program that are likely to be fruitful in the sustainment of immune function in stressful conditions? Specifically, is there likely to be enough value added to justify adding to operational rations or including an additional component?

To assist the CMNR in responding to these questions, the workshop included presentations from individuals with expertise in immune function. As a background to these presentations, an Army representative provided an overview of why the Army is interested in nutrition and immune function. In preparing their presentations, the invited speakers were asked to address the questions posed by the Army. The speakers discussed their presentations with committee members at the workshop and submitted written reports based on their verbal presentations. The committee met after the workshop on May 22, 1996, to discuss the proceedings and the information provided. Later, the CMNR reviewed the workshop presentations and drew on its collective expertise and the scientific literature to summarize the information pertinent to nutrition and immune function, and to evaluate the potential contribution of military nutrition research to the maintenance or enhancement of the ability of the immune system to protect soldiers engaged in military operations. The committee's responses to the five questions posed by the Army appear in Chapter 2; while its conclusions and recommendations are contained in Chapter 3. The final report was reviewed and approved by the entire committee.

STAGE SETTING: THE MILITARY SITUATION

The opportunities to study the effects of multiple stressors on the immune system occur infrequently, intermittently, and largely in uncontrolled environments. As described by LTC Karl E. Friedl in Chapter 4, studies in multistressor environments, such as basic training and the Special Forces' Assessment and Selection Course (SFAS), demonstrated that higher energy intakes were better able to sustain the indices of immune status. As nutritional studies conducted with Ranger trainees (Ranger I: Moore et al., 1992; Ranger II: Shippee et al., 1994) demonstrated, troops must be supplied with high-quality foods that will enable them to sustain performance and counter an array of immunological impairments caused by a myriad of unknown stressors.

Studies of immunocompetence conducted under field conditions, where inadequate energy intake, strenuous exercise, adverse environmental and physical conditions, and psychological stress interact to create an extremely complex stimulus, are markedly different from those conducted in the laboratory. Under laboratory conditions, confounding variables can be controlled and only the variables of interest investigated. In Chapters 5 and 6 respectively, LTC Ronald L. Shippee and Pål Wiik present data describing the effect on the immune system of various training regimens imposed on elite military troops.

The Army's Interest in Nutrition and Immune Function

The primary goal of the Army Operational Medicine Program is to develop physiological strategies (including nutritional, pharmacological, and diagnostic strategies) to protect and sustain deployed soldiers, thereby enhancing readiness by maintaining their ability to accomplish assigned missions. One program with a critical need to enhance and maintain readiness is the U.S. Army Special Operations Training Program. Both the U.S. Army Ranger Training and the SFAS are physically and psychologically demanding programs used by the U.S. Army to screen male officers and enlisted soldiers for entry into Special Operations units. Since the summer of 1992, a number of studies have been conducted with these Special Operations schools through collaborative research between the U.S. Army Medical Research and Materiel Command (USAMRMC), the Soldier System Command (SSCOM), the U.S. Department of Agriculture, and industry. Currently, U.S. Ranger training consists of three 3-week phases conducted at widely varying sites with differing physical demands: military base training, mountain training, and swamp training. A desert phase originally was included in Ranger training but recently was omitted from the training program. The last 10 d of each phase were conducted entirely in stressful field situations. An overview of studies conducted by the Army Operational Medicine Program with Special Operations training courses and clinical assessment procedures employed during these studies is presented in Table 1-1.

Ranger I, the first joint USAMRMC–SSCOM study (Moore et al., 1992), was conducted from July 1991 through October 1991. Baseline assessments were performed on 190 soldiers, and this group was followed throughout the course, although attrition from the course left a final sample size of 55.

Ranger II (a nutritional intervention study; Shippee et al., 1994) was conducted from August through October 1992, and provided for increased rations to mitigate the weight loss and immune dysfunctions that occurred in Ranger I. The primary objective of the Ranger II study was to test the effect of increasing the daily caloric intake by approximately 15 percent (above that documented in the Ranger I study) on body weight loss and on the status indicators for body composition and immune function. It was hoped that the number of infections documented during previous U.S. Ranger studies would be decreased by nutritional intervention. In Ranger II, there was an overall decrease in the incidence of infections (for example, cellulitis, conjunctivitis, acute gastroenteritis, otitis, upper respiratory tract infection, and sore throat) documented in the medical records. Reports of abrasions, injuries, and knee problems also were more common during the earlier training classes. Baseline and periodic assessments were performed on 175 soldiers. Attrition during Ranger II left a final sample size of 53. The Ranger II training course was composed of four phases that included training exercises in different environmental conditions at four geographically diverse locations. In the summer of 1993, the first nutritional and immune study of SFAS entrants was conducted using a research design and methodology similar to that in the Ranger studies. The SFAS is a physically and psychologically demanding 21-day course. In this course, unlike the Ranger studies, food deprivation was not used as an overt training stressor.

Research conducted at the U.S. Army Medical Research Institute of Infectious Diseases by William R. Beisel demonstrated that febrile infections induce a state of hypermetabolism with subsequent losses of protein, minerals, and vitamins, leading to a wasting of muscle mass (Beisel, 1977; Beisel and Sobocinski, 1980; Beisel et al., 1967). These effects were later found to be mediated through the cytokines. Current military research focuses on the effects of nutrition on the sustainment and enhancement of immune status in healthy individuals, rather than on the nutritional consequences of infection and their causal relationship to cytokine responses.

During World War II, diseases such as the diarrheal disease encountered by Rommel's troops in North Africa and the malaria suffered by units such as Merrill's Marauders in the China–Burma theater were of major concern to the military. Today, these diseases are still part of the military's high-priority research because of their common and widespread occurrence and the Army's limited ability to provide specific protections. In Chapter 4, LTC Karl E. Friedl hypothesizes that the soldier's defense against biological threat agents may depend on physiological enhancement of the immune system, possibly through various nutritional strategies.

Knowledge arising from civilian (that is, academic, governmental, private, and industrial) medical research may not be applicable to troops who are exposed to the stress of a variety of combat–work conditions. This lack of relationship between military immunological data and data from civilian hospital records exists because of the differences in the two populations. Members of the military are initially normal, nutritionally intact, physically fit, and relatively young. In contrast, nonmilitary medical patients are generally older, often demonstrate altered nutritional status (obesity, undernutrition), are rarely physically fit, and often have chronic confounding disease processes (for example, diabetes, atherosclerosis, and cancer) or undesirable life-style habits (for example, drugs, alcohol, and tobacco) that greatly modify their immunological baseline and limit their ability to respond to subsequent stimuli. The stressors faced by military personnel include altered environments (heat or cold, varying altitudes and terrains), excessive work loads, alterations in nutrient intake, and possible exposure to new pathogens and/or chemical toxins. The stress experienced by the military patient may include an emergency or elective

TABLE 1-1 Overview of Army Operational Medicine Program Studies with Special Forces Training Courses: Demographics and Clinical Assessments

	Ranger I Class 91-11	Ranger II Class 92-11	Fort Jackson BCT	SFAS-1 Class 07-93
Dates	7/91–10/91	8/92–10/92	5/93–6/93	6/93
Days in training	63	63	63	21
No. of subjects at start	190 (male)	175 (male)	174 (female)	100 (male)
No. of subjects to finish	55	50	158	37
Procedures				
Dietary assessment				
Energy intakes	X (estimation of food provided)	X (estimation of food provided)	X (visual estimation)	X (diet logs, visual estimation)
Energy expenditure (DLW)	X	X	–	X
Survey of food knowledge and attitudes	–	–	X	–
Activity monitor				
TDEE	–	X	–	X
Body composition				
Circumference and skinfolds	X	X	X	X
Body fat (DXA)	X	X (and BIA)	X (and BIA)	X
Bone mineral	X	X	X	–

TABLE 1-1 *Continued*

	Ranger I Class 91-11	Ranger II Class 92-11	Fort Jackson BCT	SFAS-1 Class 07-93
Strength testing	X	X	X	X
Biochemistry				
Clinical	X	X	X	X
Nutritional*	X	X	X (no copper, zinc)	X
Hormones	X†	X	X‡	–
Immune assessment (*N*)	49	41	48	37
Leukocytes§	X	X	X	X
Lymphocyte pro-liferation studies	X	X	X	X
Cytokines‖				
IL-2 cellular production	X	X	X	X
IL-2 receptor	X	X	X	X
IL-6 cellular production and plasma	X	X	X	X
DTH	X	–	–	–
CD	–	3,4,8,19, 4/8	–	–
Throat and nasal cultures	X	–	–	–

Continued

TABLE 1-1 *Continued*

	Ranger I Class 91-11	Ranger II Class 92-11	Fort Jackson BCT	SFAS-1 Class 07-93
Clinical (No. of cases)				
Injuries	17	10	110	–
Infections	42	22	94	–
Cognitive function	–	X	–	X

NOTE: X, measured; –, not measured; BCT, basic combat training; BIA, bioelectrical impedance; CD, cell determinant factors; DLW, doubly labeled water; DTH, delayed-type hypersensitivity; DXA, dual-energy x-ray absorptiometry; IL, interleukin; TDEE, total daily energy expenditure.

* Nutritional battery: iron status; vitamins A, D, B_6, B_{12}, thiamine, riboflavin, folate, ascorbic acid; minerals, calcium, phosphorus, magnesium, sodium, potassium, and chloride.

† Hormone battery for Ranger Studies: triiodothyronine, thyroxine, thyroid binding globulin, testosterone, cortisol, insulin-like growth factor; luteinizing hormone, growth hormone.

‡ Hormone battery for BCT included only serum estradiol, progesterone, 17 α-hydroxyprogesterone, sex hormone binding globulin, and osteocalcin.

§ Laboratory tests done at local facilities.

∥ All done in U.S. Department of Agriculture Laboratories by T. R. Kramer.

SOURCE: Ranger I: Moore et al. (1992); Ranger II: Shippee et al. (1994); Fort Jackson BCT: Westphal et al. (1995); SFAS-I: Fairbrother et al. (1993).

operation, severe infection, or possibly acute hemorrhage. Thus, it may be difficult to compare the immune defects described in civilian patients with those observed in military personnel under combat conditions.

The ability to carry out research on the impact of these operational stressors presents many challenges. Ethical considerations limit the ability to design experiments that incorporate many of these stressors and employ human experimental models. Therefore, many experiments have evolved as opportunistic field studies in which investigators do not impose the stressors but are able to study the consequences. From these field studies, recommendations often are made to correct the problem associated with the stressors evaluated, which in turn limits the ability to study this problem further through the field model. For example, the increase in food intake recommended to Ranger II program participants appeared to reduce the high incidence of infections that had been observed in Ranger I (Shippee et al., 1994). The Ranger training studies have provided a unique opportunity to evaluate some of these stressors because of the rigors of the program and the duration of the course, permitting the investigator an evaluation period beyond what may be the manifestation of an initial acute-phase response. A number of investigations have grown out of the use of the Ranger training model. These studies established a relationship between energy deficit (as rate of weight loss) and the suppression of lymphocyte response (see Table 1-2, which is taken from Friedl, Chapter 4).

The most important feature of Table 1-2 is the relationship it shows between increasing energy deficit (as a rate of weight loss) and suppression of the lymphocyte response. The lowest levels of interleukin-6 (IL-6) were found in soldiers with the highest stress conditions. Additionally, the very lowest level of IL-6 was demonstrated in the individual soldier with the greatest relative weight loss.

Since soldiers do not maintain adequate energy intakes while participating in various simulated combat programs, the intake of protein, vitamins, minerals, and trace elements may be reduced proportionally, thus limiting the supply of cofactors necessary for optimal host defense. Moreover, stress could hypothetically increase the need for antioxidant vitamins and minerals that also serve as cofactors to enhance immunological functions. If this is the case, immunological responses could be attenuated by the lack of adequate nutrients. The potential of specific dietary supplements (pills, foods, or liquid formulas given, in addition to meals, to increase nutrient intakes above the RDA [Recommended Dietary Allowance] to sustain immune function, or even offer superimmunity (a state of enhanced function of the immune system), has not been evaluated fully. There are currently few military studies evaluating the potential for nutritional supplements or whole foods to provide sustained benefits. One such pilot study (Kramer et al., 1997) did report a markedly enhanced mitogen-stimulated lymphocyte proliferation response (a measure of

TABLE 1-2 Energy Deficit and Its Relation to Stress Indices and PHA-Stimulated T-Lymphocyte Proliferation

Study	N	Weeks	% BW	% FFM	% IL-6	% PHA-T	% T
RGR-I	49	4	−9.2	—	−17	−52	−69
		8	−15.9	−6.9	−63	−21	−74
RGR-II	41	4	−7.0	—	+15	−32	−60
		8	−12.8	−6.1	−84	−5	−83
SFAS	37	3	−4.0	−1.0	−46	−20	−15
BCT	48	4	0.8	2.0	−37	+165	—
		8	−1.4	+5.0	+220	+144	—

NOTE: Values represent percent change from baseline measurements. BW, body weight; FFM, fat-free mass; IL-6, interleukin-6; PHA-T, phytohemagglutinin-stimulated T-cell proliferation; T, testosterone.

SOURCE: Adapted from RGR-I, 1991 Ranger course (Kramer et al., 1997); RGR-II, 1992 Ranger course (Kramer et al., 1997); SFAS, 1993 Special Forces Assessment and Selection Course (B. Fairbrother and T.R. Kramer, Unpublished data, USARIEM, Natick, Mass., 1993); BCT, 1993 Army Basic Combat Training (Westphal et al., 1995).

T-cell activity) in unstressed individuals given a whole-food supplement that consisted of kale, sweet potato, and tomato juice and thus was high in antioxidants.

There is a concern with the inappropriate use of dietary supplements by individual soldiers, particularly in elite units. These soldiers are susceptible to the claims of many manufacturers regarding enhanced performance following use of such products. Since these products are readily available in post exchanges and commissaries, there is, in the view of many, an implied military endorsement of their use. However, the use of these supplements may carry some risk (Herbert, 1997; Rock et al., 1996) and may impair rather than enhance readiness, because enhanced responsiveness of the immune system may not always be desirable. An example of a large-scale epidemic of severe inflammatory illness and mortality associated with a food supplement was the l-tryptophan eosinophilia myalgia syndrome epidemic of 1989 (Crofford et al., 1990; Silver et al., 1990). At that time, l-tryptophan was freely available over the counter and was taken for insomnia, muscle building, depression, and premenstrual syndrome. Although the major etiologic factor in the cause of the epidemic was impure l-tryptophan manufactured by a Japanese petrochemical company (Showa Denko K.K.), further testing in animals showed that pure l-tryptophan in doses comparable to the large doses consumed by the patients was associated with related deleterious risks, such as pancreatic acinar hyperplasia (Love et al., 1993). Thus, without adequate research, it cannot be assumed that "natural products" are safe, even if manufactured according to Good Manufacturing Practices. Clearly there is a need for studies to evaluate the benefits, risks, and safety limits, if any, associated with intakes of dietary supplements.

U.S. Army Training Courses

In Chapter 5, Shippee describes four years of studies with the U.S. Army Ranger Training Brigade and SFAS. These studies were designed to test proposed guidelines for sleep deprivation, food restriction, and environmental exposure, with immune response as one of the variables of concern. Shippee points out that in modern warfare, nonbattle injury and infection account for more casualties than actual military action.

Currently, U.S. Ranger training consists of three 3-week phases conducted at widely varying sites with differing physical demands: military base field training, mountain training, and swamp training. The last 10 d of each 21-day phase involve a field training period. Changes to the training course have occurred over the years in response to infections, accidents, and death (Consolazio et al., 1966; Johnson et al., 1976), as well as in response to findings from independent research studies (IOM, 1993; Moore et al., 1992; Shippee et al., 1994) that evaluated the effects of training and possible strategies for improved outcome. Typically, data collection occurred pre-course and at the end of each phase *before* refeeding, sleep, or hygiene (except for dual-energy x-ray absorptiometry determinations, measurement of muscle strength, and particular anthropometric assessments, samples were collected in a fasted state [IOM, 1992]). Blood samples were obtained 3–6 h after individuals returned to the training camp site.

Energy was provided initially in these studies by one Meal, Ready-to-Eat (MRE) per day, and in Ranger I, a negative energy balance was reported (– 1,203 kcal/d [Moore et al., 1992]). Consequently, mean weight loss over the 62 d of training was significant (15.9 percent), with a large proportion of this loss resulting from the depletion of fat stores, from 14.6 to 5.8 percent. Changes in endocrine function (especially decreases in blood testosterone and triiodothyronine [T_3] concentrations) compromised the individual's ability to adapt to environmental stress. Assessment of immune function using an in vitro T-lymphocyte proliferation assay showed that the immune system was significantly suppressed by training. These results explain, in part, the high infection rates observed among the troops (8, 25, and 24 percent at the end of the desert, jungle, and swamp phases [Moore et al., 1992] respectively) during the latter phases of Ranger training.

The CMNR (IOM, 1993) recommended increasing food intake by use of a Long-Life Ration Packet (LLRP) in place of the MRE in Ranger II (Shippee et al., 1994). The resultant energy balance was less negative (–847 kcal), with a weight loss of only 12 percent (a decrease from 14.7 to 8.4 percent body fat) (Shippee et al., 1994). Under these circumstances, immune function was somewhat improved (infection rates were reduced in Ranger II to 8, 12, and 2 percent during the mountain, desert, and swamp phases, respectively [Shippee et al., 1994]); however, responses to mitogens that stimulate lymphocyte proliferation were still significantly depressed in Ranger II subjects (see Table 1-3). The persistent problem of inadequate energy and nutrient intake by soldiers in the field was the focus of a 1995 CMNR report entitled *Not Eating Enough* (IOM, 1995a). As discussed in that report and subsequently in the report of the Subcommittee on Body Composition, Nutrition, and Health of Military Women, *Assessing Readiness in Military Women* (IOM, 1998), the Army Natick Research Laboratory, in conjunction with USARIEM, continually reevaluates and modifies the MRE and other operational rations to improve palatability, acceptability, portability, nutrient delivery, and nutritional labeling.

Additional studies have been performed with the SFAS to address the efficacy of various supplement in improving immune function. Evaluation of the effect of a carbohydrate–electrolyte beverage on performance showed no significant effect on lymphocyte proliferation; however, the study involved more-than-adequate energy intakes (4,890–7,846 kcal/d) and was probably not directly applicable to the field situation (Montain et al., 1995). A study employing a drink that supplied 15 g of glutamine and 200 kcal/d, showed no effect on in vitro lymphocyte proliferation but did improve delayed-type hypersensitivity (DTH) responses to tetanus toxoid compared to a control group (see Shippee, Chapter 5). In comparison, three MREs per day contain between 4.2 and 10.8 g of glutamine. Another study, involving a beverage supplying 200 kcal, as well as the antioxidant vitamins A (as β–carotene, 30 mg), E (400 IU RRR-α-tocopherol), and C (1 g); and selenium (200 µg), produced only a slight decrease in lymphocyte proliferation in the treated group and an improved booster response to tetanus toxoid (see Shippee, Chapter 5).

An additional stressor during the Ranger I and II studies was the lack of restful and uninterrupted sleep. The average sleep period for both studies was identical at 3.6 h/d. The longest sleep periods (averaging approximately 4.25 h/d) were experienced in Ranger II during the swamp phase, and this sleep was of poor quality as measured by indices of movement during sleep and of sleep fragmentation. Similarly, sleep periods during the desert phase of Ranger II averaged approximately 3.4 h/d and were of poor quality (Shippee et al., 1994).

In summary, it has been shown that the multistressor components of rigorous military training induce weight loss, alterations in immunological indices and, at times, increases in the incidence of infectious illnesses. In contrast, higher energy intakes appear to preserve immune functions. Based on the results of Ranger I, the focus of Ranger II in terms of immune function was to determine the effect of increased energy intake on T-lymphocyte function and IL-6 levels. Data indicated that there was slightly less suppression of T-lymphocyte function during Ranger II compared to Ranger I; however, plasma IL-6 continued to be reduced. At an earlier presentation to the CMNR (Moldawer, 1997), the urinary excretion of IL-6 was suggested as a diagnostic measure of an acute-phase response. However, care must be taken in interpretating lymphocyte proliferation tests to evaluate immune function because they yield measures that are relatively insensitive and nonspecific. They are less responsive to stress hormones than are cytokine response patterns, which may explain, in part, the apparently improved immune function and lower infection rates demonstrated in Ranger II. Results of micronutrient intervention studies may offer potential benefits of military significance.

Norwegian Ranger Training

In Chapter 6, Wiik describes the Norwegian Ranger Training program undertaken by cadets in the Norwegian Military Academy. This training program was designed to stress individuals to their limits, both physiologically and psychologically, over a short period of seven days. During this time, cadets were engaged in continuous military activities of average work intensity (32 percent $Vo_{2\ max}$ for 24 h/d). Using heart rate monitoring as an indicator of hydration status, total energy expenditure was estimated in one study to be 8,500 kcal/d (although Wiik admits that this value may have been an overestimate). Energy intake in this training regimen was very low. In one study, energy intake averaged 420 kcal/d, with no food intake at all during 4 out of 7 days. Intakes in another study averaged 1,620 kcal/d when a supplement of 1,200 kcal/d was provided with the daily ration. Additionally, cadets averaged 3 hours of sleep per day (Wiik et al., 1996).

No significant increase in infectious disease was observed in cadets participating in these studies. Changes in specific immune parameters documented during these training periods show a general decline in immune function, similar to that seen in response to strenuous exercise (see Table 1-3). In these troops, an increase in energy intake of 1,200 kcal/d appeared to have little effect on modulating the overall immune response to exercise.

TABLE 1-3 Combined Data on Immunological Status During Military Training Exercises

Immunological Parameter	U.S. Ranger I (N=49) Early (4 weeks)	U.S. Ranger I (N=49) Late (8 weeks)	U.S. Ranger II (N=41) Early (4 weeks)	U.S. Ranger II (N=41) Late (8 weeks)	Norwegian Ranger (N=20) Days 1–3	Norwegian Ranger (N=20) Days 4–7	BCT (N=48) 4 Weeks	BCT (N=48) 8 Weeks	SFAS (N=37) 3 Weeks
White blood cell studies									
Granulocyte number*	↑	—	↑	↑	↑	↑			
Granulocyte function†					↑	↓			
Monocyte number*			↓	↓↓	↑	↑			
Monocyte function†					↓	↑			
Eosinophils			↓		↓	↓			
Lymphocyte count	↓	—	↓	↓					
CD4+ helper lymphocytes			↑	↑	↓	↓			
CD8+ suppressor			↓	↓	↓	↓			
CD4+:CD8+			↑	↑					
NK-cells					↓	↓			
B-lymphocyte count					↓	↓			
Lymphocyte response to mitogens	↓			↓	↑↓	↑↓	↑	↑	↓
T-cell		↓		↓↓					
B-cell		↓		↓↓					

TABLE 1-3 *Continued*

Immunological Parameter	U.S. Ranger I (n = 49) Early (4 weeks)	U.S. Ranger I (n = 49) Late (8 weeks)	U.S. Ranger II (n = 41) Early (4 weeks)	U.S. Ranger II (n = 41) Late (8 weeks)	Norwegian Ranger (n = 20) Days 1–3	Norwegian Ranger (n = 20) Days 4–7	BCT (n = 48) 4 weeks	BCT (n = 48) 8 weeks	SFAS (n = 37) 3 weeks
Immunoglobulin measurements									
IgG					↓	↓			
IgA					↓	↓			
IgM					↓	↓			
Cytokine measurements									
TNF*					—	—			
IL-1*		↑			—	—			
IL-2 cellular	↓		↓	↓	—	—			
IL-4					—	—			
IL-6* cellular and	—	↓	↑	↓	↓	↓	↓	↑	↓
plasma	—	↓							
GMCSF					↑	↑			

NOTE: ↑, increase; ↓, decrease; →, no change; BCT, basic combat training; GMCSF, granulocyte-macrophage colony-stimulating factor; Ig, immunoglobulin; IL, interleukin; NK, natural killer; SFAS, Special Forces Assessment and Selection Course; TNF, tumor necrosis factor.

* Participates in acute-phase response.

† As detected by chemiluminescence methodology.

In an attempt to provide a plausible explanation for the training-induced changes in immune parameters, Wiik presents data on blood concentrations of the hormone vasoactive intestinal polypeptide (VIP). VIP and other neuropeptides play a role in immune regulation at the local level, for example in the spleen, lymph nodes, and Peyer's patches in the gut which are innervated by the autonomic nervous system and at local sites of inflammation. VIP is known to inhibit lymphocyte mitogenic responses and the monocyte production of oxygen free radicals. Additionally, VIP stimulates resident central nervous system (CNS) glial cell production of a wide range of cytokines. Within the CNS, such cytokine production plays a role in neuronal cell death and survival. Wiik reports that blood concentrations of VIP increased during the Norwegian Ranger training, and VIP-receptor activity was upregulated, resulting in the observed inhibition of monocyte activity. In contrast, catecholamine receptor activity was found to be downregulated in Norwegian Ranger trainees. It is important to note that all of these neuropeptides and neurotransmitter systems are components of stress-responsive neuronal systems that contribute to immune changes in stress situations. Changes in any neuropeptide or altered neuroendocrine autonomic responses are important when considering immune changes in stress situations (Sternberg, 1997b).

Additionally, studies of the combined effects of glucocorticoids and fasting on immune function in rats support the hypothesis that the interaction of these two factors may result in greater diminution of immune activity than either alone (Wiik, 1995).

The immune response seen in U.S. Ranger studies is similar in most respects to that observed in the Norwegian training. The exception is that cytokine-mediated immunity, as evaluated by plasma or cellular levels of IL-1, IL-12, and IL-4, did not change in the Norwegian study, whereas in the U.S. Ranger studies, the response increased or decreased depending on the cytokine evaluated (IL-2 or IL-4). Differences in immune response among participants in the two programs may be explained by (1) the more intense nature of the Norwegian program, (2) differences in the duration of training, and especially, (3) differences in assessment methodologies (cell-adjusted in Norwegian versus. whole-blood preparations in U.S. studies, as described by Tim R. Kramer in Chapter 10. It has also been reported that relative increases or decreases of different cytokines are important because glucocorticoids (released during stress) differentially suppress some cytokines and stimulate others (DeRijk et al., 1997).

Clearly, the various training courses reviewed, differ in many respects, and interpretation of these findings is difficult. Nevertheless, several conclusions can be drawn from these studies:

• Longer-term strenuous training is more debilitating in general (increase in incidence of upper respiratory infection [URI], cellulitis, and pneumococcal pneumonia as seen in U.S. Ranger trainees) than short, intense training situations.

• Partial restoration of energy balance over the short run *may not* have a significant impact on immune function (any potential improvement in terms of positive gains may be overridden by physical and psychological stresses).

• Restoration of energy requirements over the long run can improve the composition of weight loss dramatically, influencing immune function less severely.

• Nonspecific granulocyte function seems to be stimulated during the first days of training and then suppressed, which is consistent with the effects of glucocorticoids.

• Stressful military training of up to 1-week duration may be well tolerated in healthy individuals; however, training of longer duration may be associated with a decline in immune and other physiological functions.

INTRODUCTION TO IMMUNE FUNCTION

In Chapter 7, Ranjit K. Chandra reviews what is known about the stress exerted by compromised nutrition on the immune system and elucidates several additional factors that come into play in the military setting, thus providing an immunological background for this report. Stephen S. Morse (see Appendix D) provides insights into the impact of emerging infections and the movement of soldiers around the globe.

As William R. Beisel mentions in the overview in Appendix A, knowledge about the cytokines is now of key importance in the practice of medicine and surgery and in understanding many aspects of disease progression. Jeffrey L. Rossio (see Chapter 8) describes the roles of many families of cytokines, including the interleukins, interferons, various hematopoietic growth and differentiation factors, and cytotoxic–cytostatic inducers and effectors. Many actions of the immune system are initiated and controlled by cytokines. Although immune system cells often interact by direct, histocompatibility-requiring contact, they also employ cytokines as their principal agents for humoral communication and cellular proliferation, activation, and maturation to effector cell function. Many fundamental texts containing a more detailed review of immunology are available (for example, Abbas et al., 1991; Kuby, 1997) to the reader, as well as reviews of the immune system and its dysfunction in immunodeficiency disorders (Keusch, 1994; Myrvik, 1994; Roitt and Brostoff, 1991).

Current State of Knowledge of the Field

Chandra (see Chapter 7) summarizes much of the state of current knowledge regarding the interaction of nutrition and the immune response. This area of investigation is relatively new, with much of the available information having emerged in the past 25 years. The 1968 World Health Organization (WHO) monograph *Interactions of Nutrition and Infection* (Scrimshaw et al., 1968) suggested for the first time that the relationship between infection and malnutrition is a synergistic one. Three factors have provided the impetus to study the immune system in states of compromised nutrition: (1) the compilation of an epidemiologic database; (2) the development of new disease concepts and assessment techniques in immunology; and (3) the emergence of dramatic human interest cases, emanating largely from studies of protein-energy malnutrition (PEM) in young children, which stimulated the interest of researchers and the concerned public.

Severe PEM can cause significant alterations in the immune response. Research using laboratory animals and work with human subjects extended these observations to the recognition that nutritional deficiencies are associated with a large number of alterations in cell-mediated immunity, decreased lymphocyte stimulation response to mitogens and antigens, altered production of cytokines, lower secretory immunoglobulin A (IgA) antibody response on mucosal surfaces, decreased antibody affinity, and phagocyte dysfunction. Deficiencies of many individual nutrients, including protein, essential fatty acids, vitamin A, pyridoxine, folic acid, zinc, iron, copper, and selenium, have been associated with altered immune function (Figure 1-1).

Based on the scientific literature (Beisel, 1982; Chandra 1988; Cunningham-Rundles, 1993; Forse, 1994; Gershwin et al., 1985; Keusch and Farthing, 1986; Watson and Retro, 1984) highlighting the integral relationship between nutrition and immunity, Chandra proposes the following general principles, which are developed throughout this chapter:

- PEM and deficiencies of individual nutrients, even subclinical deficits, may be associated with a catabolic response, an impaired immune response, and an altered risk of infection (Beisel, 1982; Keusch and Farthing, 1986).
- Excessive intakes of some nutrients may result in reduced immune responses.
- Dose–response curves should form the basis of recommendations for optimal nutrient intake.
- Immune responses provide sensitive and functional indices of nutritional status and can aid in assessing prognosis in medical and surgical patients.
- Many factors other than nutrition can modulate immune competence.

• Basic knowledge of nutrition–immune interactions can be utilized to formulate nutritional recommendations and interventions that may be expected to reduce illness and improve chances for survival.

As mentioned by Chandra and discussed later in this chapter, many nonnutritional factors may also influence the immune response; these include genetics, physical and thermal trauma, environmental and body temperature, infection, emotional stress, and physical activity. For example, the reduced immunologic response in elderly subjects pre- and postbereavement is an example of emotional stress that may interact with nutritional or other factors to reduce immune responses. Moderate, graded exercise in elderly subjects has been shown to enhance immune responses and decrease the incidence of infection. However, strenuous exercise, both severe and prolonged, reduces immunity and increases the incidence of infection in the short term (see Chandra, Chapter 7). A J-curve of risk has been proposed (see Chapter 17 by David C. Nieman), which states that at moderate activity, the risk to the individual of developing a URI is lower than in a sedentary or strenuously active situation.

Emerging Infections, Nutritional Status, and Immunity

Emerging infections, discussed by Morse (see Appendix D), are those that suddenly appear in the population, or in some new geographic range, or that rapidly increase in prevalence. The Ebola outbreak that occurred in Africa and the Ebola–Reston virus are two recent emerging infections that have been in the news (Breman et al., 1997). Another of the more surprising infections to emerge in recent years has been the human immunodeficiency virus (HIV) infection that leads to AIDS. Finally, one of the most common of the emerging infections throughout the world is dengue hemorrhagic fever (Gubler and Trent, 1993), a severe manifestation of dengue infection in children.

The military has a long-standing interest in the threat of emerging infections. Soldiers serve as efficient sentinels for these infections, intentionally or unintentionally, as observed during the Korean War in 1951 when thousands of U.S. and UN troops began to develop Korean hemorrhagic fever, a severe infection previously unknown to U.S. physicians, although similar illnesses had been recognized (but not widely reported) in Manchuria, Northern Russia, and Scandinavia. Morse describes in detail how a common field mouse that lives in the rice fields throughout Korea (and now China) introduced the *Hantavirus* responsible for Korean hemorrhagic fever. A similar situation is occurring in North America, but the vector is a deer mouse, and the virus causes *Hantavirus* pulmonary syndrome.

38

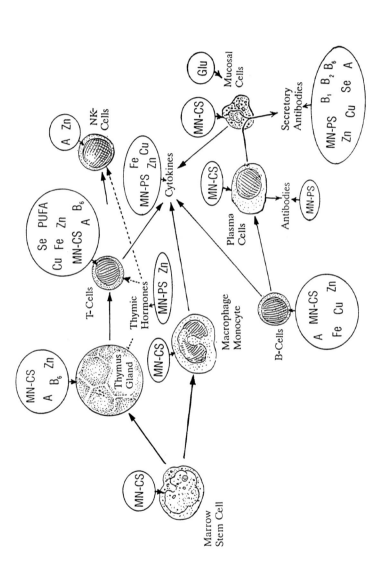

FIGURE 1-1 Nutrients known to be involved with immune system function. A, vitamin A; B₁, vitamin B₁; B₂, vitamin B₂; B₆, vitamin B₆; Cu, copper; Fe, iron; Glu, glutamine; MN-CS, multiple nutrients for cellular synthesis; MN-PS, multiple nutrients for protein synthesis; NK, natural killer; PUFA, polyunsaturated fatty acid; Se, selenium; Zn, zinc. SOURCE: Beisel (1982); Chandra (1988).

The process of infectious disease emergence occurs in two steps: introduction and dissemination. Many infections that are introduced into humans are not disseminated successfully. Factors that affect the introduction of an infectious disease include ecological changes, land-use changes, human demographics, and behavior. Human behavior, including the high rates of international travel and commerce that move people and goods across continents, also plays a very important role in the second step of dissemination as experienced with HIV.

There is concern not only about the movement of people, but also about biological products and foodstuffs, which may harbor pathogens (for example, a toxic and deadly form of *Escherichia coli* [0157H7] that can produce hemolytic uremic syndrome [Griffin and Tauxe, 1991]; cyclospora, a parasite that causes diarrheal disease [Pieniazek and Herwaldt, 1997]; or the agent responsible for bovine spongiform encephalopathy [Dealler and Lacey, 1990; Almond and Pattison, 1997]). Also important is the highly adaptive nature of microbes, as evidenced by the rise of new antibiotic-resistant organisms. Reemerging diseases such as diphtheria are often present and a continual threat to military troops, and outbreaks of salmonellosis are not uncommon.

Both macro- and micronutrient status must be considered among relevant host factors. Nutrition and nutritional practices can be additive or synergistic with the biologic factors noted above and can have indirect effects. Many important infectious diseases are food- or waterborne. Relatively little is known about the role of nutrition or malnutrition in affecting cytokine balance or the many factors involved in producing resistance to viral infections in humans.

The Cytokine System

Rossio (see Chapter 8) enumerates the most significant characteristics of cytokines: multiple biologic activities (pleiotropy; for example, IL-1 exhibits more than 50 unique and separate functions), redundancy of actions (for example, IL-1, IL-6, and tumor necrosis factor [TNF] can all induce fever), and synergistic activity.

Like hormone activities, cytokine activities are controlled partially by biological checks and balances; these control measures are much more complex for the cytokines than those that regulate endocrine functions. Target cells can shed their cytokine receptors into the plasma to inactivate circulating cytokines; receptor-blocking proteins can be produced; hormones can blunt the actions of proinflammatory cytokines; and certain cytokines can inhibit the production of others.

Although concentrations of individual plasma cytokines can now be measured, interpretation of these measurements is confounded by the need also to know the interacting effects of circulating receptors, receptor antagonists, and inhibitory cytokines. Interpretation of plasma cytokine values also is complicated by their sporadic production and by the fact that accumulations of large amounts of cytokines in specific tissues or in pathologic lesions may not be reflected by increases in their plasma values.

As noted earlier, cytokines have multiple and overlapping roles and can function as two-edged swords. Cytokines that control the growth and differentiation of T- and B-lymphocytes initiate many "beneficial" immunological responses, such as cell killing and antibody production. On the other hand, excess production of the proinflammatory cytokines (IL-1, IL-6, IL-8, IL-17, γ-interferon, and TNF) during sepsis can initiate lethal hypotensive shock (Moldawer, 1997). Stress and glucocorticoid responses during stress are important regulators of cytokine production, tending to shift immune responses from T-helper 1 (Th1) to Th2-type responses (cellular to humoral), and are immunosuppressive overall (DeRijk et al., 1997; Sternberg, 1997a). Fever and other hypermetabolic components of acute-phase reactions can deplete the body of essential nutrients. Losses include muscle protein and amino acids, vitamins, minerals, and essential trace elements. In Chapter 8. Rossio points out that immunological dysfunctions observed during various forms of malnutrition may include a reduced ability of the body to synthesize cytokines, as broadly depicted in Figure 1-2.

Cytokine-induced malnutrition can become extremely severe, as seen clinically in many victims of trauma, infections, or other wasting illnesses. The pathogenesis of cytokine-induced malnutrition differs drastically from malnutrition due to starvation alone (see Table 1-4) (Beisel, 1995), but because cytokine-induced acute-phase reactions often include (and induce) severe anorexia, these two forms of malnutrition can coexist in a synergistic relationship during generalized febrile infections or other severe medical and surgical illnesses.

The importance of the cytokines for intercellular communications within the immune system and for the multiple host responses (immunological, physiological, and nutritional, as depicted in Figure 1-3) during inflammatory and infectious stress is emphasized by numerous references to cytokine functions by authors throughout this report. Additional viewpoints are provided in Chapter 19 by Leonard P. Kapcala and are discussed later in this chapter.

ASSESSMENT OF IMMUNE FUNCTION

A review of techniques for the assessment of immune function, as well as a discussion of assessment in the context of nutritional deprivation and

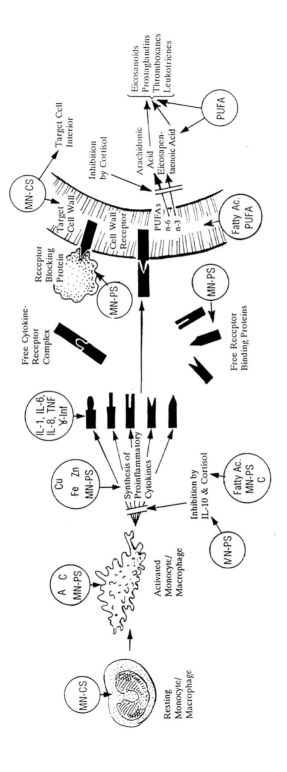

FIGURE 1-2 Macrophage/monocyte production of cytokines is representative of all body cells that produce proinflammatory cytokines. Nutrients needed for the synthesis, action, and control of proinflammatory cytokines (IL–1, IL–6, IL–8, TNF, and γ-interferon [γ-Inf]): A, vitamin A; C, vitamin C; Cu, copper; Fatty Ac., fatty acid; Fe, iron; MN-CS, multiple nutrients for cellular synthesis; MN-PS, multiple nutrients for protein synthesis; PUFA, polyunsaturated fatty acid; Zn, zinc.

42

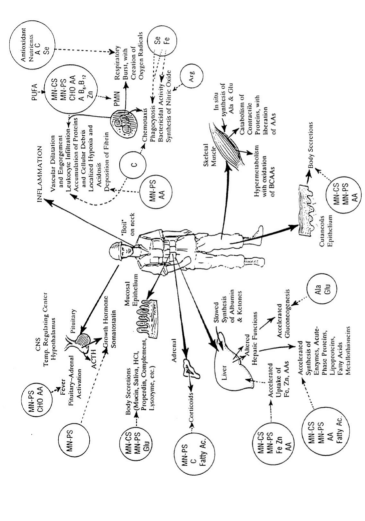

FIGURE 1-3 Nutrients needed for maintenance and function of other neuroendocrine or other endogenous mechanisms of host defense: A, vitamin A; AA, amino acid; Ala, alanine; Arg, arginine; B6, vitamin B6; B12, vitamin B12; BCAA, branch chain amino acid; C, vitamin C; CHO, carbohydrate; CNS, central nervous system; Cu, copper; Fatty Ac, fatty acid; Fe, iron; Glu, glutamine; HCl, hydrochloric acid; MN-CS, multiple nutrients for cellular synthesis; MN-PS, multiple nutrients for protein synthesis; PMN, polymorphonuclear (leukocyte); PUFA, polyunsaturated fatty acid; Se, selenium.

TABLE 1-4 Differences in the Pathogenesis of Malnutrition

	Starvation Induced	Cytokine Induced
Basal metabolic rate	Decreased	Increased
Body nitrogen	Conserved	Lost quickly
Body water	Lost	Retained
Body sodium	Lost	Retained
Glucose synthesis	Inhibited	Stimulated
Ketone synthesis	Stimulated	Inhibited
Urea synthesis	Reduced	Increased
Muscle BCAA oxidation	Minimized	Increased
Acute-phase plasma proteins	Unchanged	Produced rapidly
Antimicrobial defenses	Unchanged or weakened	Activated

NOTE: BCAA, branched-chain amino acid.
SOURCE: Beisel (1995).

military field operations, is presented by Susanna Cunningham-Rundles in Chapter 9; in Chapter 10, Tim R. Kramer presents a description of the use of one particular technique for the assessment of several parameters of immune function in cultures of whole blood.

Assessment Techniques

There is no criterion test for immune deficiency. Many existing indicators such as lymphocyte proliferation assays tend to be poor predictors of disease attributable to immune deficiency (Straight et al., 1994). However, assays of whole-blood cytokine production (De Rijk et al., 1996, 1997) may provide a more sensitive method than was available previously to measure immune changes associated with exercise and stress. The choice of techniques will depend on the investigator's resources and the availability and accessibility of tissue, blood, or biological fluid to be assayed.

A number of examples exist of test panels that are in use or have been recommended by government agencies and private-sector scientists involved in immunologic field assessment (Beisel and Talbot, 1985; Taylor, 1993). One such group, the Agency for Toxic Substances and Disease Registry (ATSDR) of the Department of Health and Human Services convened a workshop in 1992 to refine panels of standardized immune tests previously recommended by the Centers for Disease Control and Prevention for use in environmental health field studies (Straight et al., 1994). The outcomes of this workshop included recommendations for a panel of tests for assessment of immune deficiency as well as factors that must be considered in the design of field studies. The test panel recommended by the ATSDR is two tiered: the first tier consists of basic tests of immune status; the second tier consists of more focused tests to be used for individuals with suspected immune deficiency. To provide an example, the tests comprising this panel are described in Appendix C.

Considerations in Study Design

The desire to measure the influence of any stimulus on immune function, in this case the stresses of training and field operations, is based on two underlying assumptions presented by Cunningham-Rundles (see Chapter 9):

1. Measurement of immune function, either in vitro or ex vivo (following removal of cells from the body and placement in culture), reflects the internal status of the immune system;
2. These measures may be interpreted to predict future immune system response.

Among the problems cited are that relationships observed under various (artificial) conditions (for example, in previous experiments on nutritional status and immune function conducted in a clinical or laboratory setting) may not parallel those seen in training or deployment situations, particularly when clinical subjects were exposed to only one type (Cunningham-Rundles, Chapter 9). For example, the experimental conditions may involve the use of endocrine (cortisol and/or epinephrine) or bacterial endotoxin injections, for which the metabolic and immunologic responses in normal volunteers have been studied. Many, but not all, of these observed responses are similar to those described in injured or infected patients (Bessey et al., 1984; Michie et al., 1988; Watters et al., 1986).

An additional problem is that recovery (defined by Cunningham-Rundles as the ability to recover from a threat to the immune system) may be the most critical parameter for assessing the likely response to future immune exposure but may not be predictable based on the magnitude of the immune response in a test situation.

Other problems include the fact that the response of an individual to a pathogen at any given time is influenced by a multitude of independent as well as interdependent factors. In addition to nutritional status, these factors include general health status, genetic predisposition, pharmacologic effects, presence of immunosuppressive diseases, neuroendocrine stress, and prior exposure. Therefore, it may be impossible to isolate the effect of a single nutrient or even nutritional status as a whole. In addition, the nutritional effects may be those of a single nutrient as well as the effects of nutrient interactions, and each may manifest with a complicated time course (which influences whether immune function assessments performed at isolated times will detect any effects). Cunningham-Rundles' recommendations include the need to document the type and range of alterations in immune function expected under typical training conditions, followed by careful design of studies allowing assessment at several levels of immune response.

One of the primary challenges of performing immune function assessments in field settings is that the necessity for the subjects to continue to perform physically challenging work significantly limits the amount of blood that can be sampled. Kramer (see Chapter 10) describes the ongoing efforts of his laboratory to modify techniques for the assessment of immune indices in samples of whole blood. According to Kramer, assaying whole blood samples, rather than isolating peripheral blood mononuclear cells (PBMCs) as is customarily done, has several advantages. First, additional indices of immune function can be assayed using smaller samples. Second, more samples can be processed in less time (using less equipment and fewer technical staff) because the requirement to purify cells has been eliminated. Kramer shows that the coefficients of variation for measurement of mitogen-stimulated proliferation of cells compared favorably with those in PBMCs in a study of zinc-deficient women in Thailand (Kramer et al., 1990). Shephard and coworkers (1994b), in reviewing studies of the impact of exercise on the immune system, describe the finding of Shinkai et al. (1993) that washing of PBMCs tends to lead to incomplete recovery but if care is taken, the results can agree well with those from whole blood. In contrast, Shephard et al. (1994b) report a study (Radomski et al., 1980) showing that whole-blood responses may be modified by soluble factors found in the blood. A study by Bocchieri and coworkers (1995), comparing mitogen-induced proliferation in both whole-blood cultures and PBMCs to actual disease state and T-cell phenotype in HIV-seropositive individuals and controls, found stronger correlations between proliferation in whole-blood cultures and other disease indicators than between the same indicators and proliferation in PBMCs. According to Cunningham-Rundles (Chapter 9), the whole-blood method has the advantage of reflecting the number of cells actually circulating as well as all plasma proteins and nutrients present in vivo. Whole blood is also a better medium for measurement of cytokine stimulation and glucocorticoid sensitivity ex vivo (DeRijk et al., 1996, 1997). If an observed defect must be shown to be intrinsic to cell function, then isolation and study in a standardized test is needed. However, whole blood is a physiological medium that is well suited to testing under field conditions. Whole blood also is currently preferred for phenotypic analysis of cellular subsets; it is advantageous for field studies to use both functional and phenotypic analysis.

In summary, the design of an immune function assessment study is a significant challenge. According to Cunningham-Rundles and others, population research must move in the direction of identifying correlations among changes in individual parameters of immune function and patterns of immune responses, imposition of specific stressors, and disease outcome. Table 1-5 provides an outline of assessment methods for immune function.

NUTRITION

Most nondeployed military personnel live at home or in nonbarracked conditions, consuming a diet ad libitum. Depending on food preferences and the use of vitamin or mineral supplements, there may be great variations in the quantities of nutrients ingested. As these individuals are deployed and move from their self-selected diets to a constant ration, there may be profound alterations in nutrient intake, and these changes may result in altered host defense.

Part V of this report (see Douglas W. Wilmore, Chapter 11; Richard D. Semba, Chapter 12; Laura C. Rall and Simin Nikbin Meydani, Chapter 13; Darshan S. Kelley, Chapter 14; Gerald T. Keusch, Chapter 15; and Melinda A. Beck, Chapter 16) discusses essential individual nutrients known to be important for sustaining immune system functions. However, it must not be forgotten that, worldwide, the most significant adverse impact of nutritional status on the immune system results from PEM. Its adverse effects on the immune system may be magnified by the deficiencies of essential single nutrients that almost always accompany PEM. These poorly defined nutritional interrelationships were undoubtedly of importance during the short-term effects of PEM associated with the sizable losses of weight and muscle mass experienced during Ranger I training and may have been major contributing factors in the immunological dysfunctions detected in these Rangers (Beisel, 1991).

Given the evidence that deficits in energy, protein, and certain fatty acids adversely affect immune function, it is also important to consider other nutrients such as vitamins and minerals more explicitly. Finally, it must be emphasized that in many cases, an "overdose" of a nutrient, as well as a deficiency, can lead to negative consequences.

Nutrients with Roles Implicated in Immune Function

Evidence demonstrates that severe protein or calorie malnutrition in humans results in impairment of both humoral and cell-mediated immune functions (Bistrian et al., 1975; McMurray et al., 1981; Neumann et al., 1975; Watson and Retro, 1984). There is also evidence that moderate energy restriction, such as that experienced by overweight individuals on weight loss diets, interferes with normal immune function (Kelley et al., 1994; Nieman et al., 1996; Stallone et al., 1994).

Protein and Amino Acids

Protein deficiency is consistently observed to interfere with maintaining resistance to infection because most immune mechanisms are dependent on cell replication or the production of active protein compounds. As might be expected, deficiencies of essential amino acids can result in an altered humoral response, whereas deficiencies of single nonessential amino acids may have little effect on the immune system, although there are some exceptions.

Certain amino acids have been shown to play a direct role in immunity. Glutamine and arginine are two amino acids that have been shown to have immunoregulatory functions (Kirk and Barbul, 1992; Reynolds et al., 1988).

Glutamine. Glutamine is an abundantly available, nonessential (or "conditionally essential") amino acid that functions in the regulation of both energy and nitrogen balance. Most glutamine in the body is synthesized in skeletal muscle, from which it is released into the circulation and supplied to the visceral organs (Souba et al., 1985). Glutamine appears to have numerous important functions within the body: in the liver, it plays an important role in gluconeogenesis, amino acid synthesis, and the production of urea and glutathione; in the kidneys, it functions to promote ammonia excretion and thus neutralize acid loads; and in cells such as intestinal enterocytes, colonocytes, lymphocytes, and macrophages, it functions as a major source of carbohydrate skeletons for fuel and promotes cell proliferation.

In catabolic states such as stress, surgery, and disease, both synthesis and release of muscle glutamine increase (Muhlbacher et al., 1984) simultaneously with demand. The competition for glutamine increases among the visceral organs, the major consumers being the liver, gastrointestinal mucosa, kidney, and immunological tissues. Under such conditions, glutamine may become a conditionally essential amino acid, because the supply can no longer keep up with the demand. In such cases, the diet may become an important source, although at present the extent to which dietary glutamine might supply the additional glutamine required is unknown.

TABLE 1-5 Assessment of Immune Function

Method	Advantages	Disadvantages	Cost (1–4, 4 = most expensive)	Applicability (F, field; E, experimental)
Clinical epidemiology	Determines the "true" incidence of infection	•Need to develop appropriate assessment tool. •May be labor intensive.	2–3	F
Assay of CRP,* ESR*	Common lab procedures	None	1	F,E
Assay of acute-phase reactants	Helps define course of illness	Special reagents required	1–2	F,E
Measures of humoral immunity				
Serum immunoglobulins and antibody levels	•Measures response to immunization or infectious exposure •Requires only serum •Multiple stored samples can be determined later at a convenient time	Individuals with normal levels may be immunosuppressed	1	F, E
In vitro humoral immune responses	None	Consistent differences cannot be detected with present methods	3–4	E
Measures of cell-mediated immunity				
Skin testing	Involves all phases of classic immune response, predictions of outcome	48 h needed Difficult to quantitate	2	F, E

TABLE 1-5 *Continued*

Method	Advantages	Disadvantages	Cost (1–4, 4 = most expensive)	Applicability (F, field; E, experimental)
Determination of cell number, populations, and subpopulations	Semiautomated techniques	Some cell preparation necessary for blood sample Special handling required*	2–3	E, F
Assay of circulating cytokines and soluble receptors (whole-blood cytokine production assays)	•ELISA assays allow batch processing •ELISA patterns of cytokine responses detectable, effect of stress hormones quantifiable ex vivo •Urine a possible sample source	•Need initial sample preparation step for blood sample, and samples must be stored appropriately •Special handling required*	1–2	F, E
Assessment of in vitro lymphocyte function	Evaluate DNA synthesis or IL-2 release following a mitogenic stimulus	•In vitro culture techniques difficult to perform in the field •Special handling required*	3–4	E
Functional assays of specific cells	Only method used to determine NK-cell activity and cytotoxicity	•In vitro studies difficult to perform in the field •Special handling required*	3–4	E
Phagocytic cell assays	Only method used to note phagocytosis or respiratory burst	•Studies difficult to perform in the field •Special handling required*	3–4	E

NOTE: CRP, C-reactive protein; ELISA, enzyme-linked immunosorbent assay; ESR, erythrocyte sedimentation rate; IL-2, Interleukin-2; NK, natural killer.   * Lab tests may require special sample transport, handling, preparation, and storage, plus skilled technicians, and expensive equipment and/or reagents. Sample size requirements may be limiting.

Wilmore (see Chapter 11) focuses his discussion of glutamine on its role in immune function. Over the past decade, glutamine has been studied for its ability to promote immune cell proliferation and enhance immune function. Glutamine appears to promote lymphocyte proliferation and macrophage phagocytosis (Parry-Billings et al., 1990), the bactericidal activity of neutrophils (Ogle et al., 1994), the generation of lymphokine-activated killer cells (Juretic et al., 1994), and monocyte surveillance (Roth et al., 1982). Because of these effects, the amino acid has been studied for its potential use in reducing infection in patients undergoing surgical, chemotherapeutic, and cancer treatment procedures, where endogenous glutamine availability may become insufficient to supply increased metabolic needs. In several trials, some evidence has been obtained that glutamine administration can reduce infection and promote recovery (see MacBurney et al., 1994; Ziegler et al., 1992). Castell et al. (1996) found that the provision of glutamine in a sports drink decreased the incidence of infections (self-reported cold, cough, sore throat, or influenza) in marathon runners during the week following participation in various types of exhaustive, prolonged exercise. This effect is not uniformly positive, suggesting that glutamine may be efficacious in some, but not all, infectious conditions.

The gastrointestinal tract also has been the focus of study relating to the use of glutamine to improve host defenses and immune function. Under conditions of stress, infection, and injury, the permeability of the bowel to pathogens and toxic molecules increases, making the body more susceptible to disease. Glutamine is known to enhance intestinal mucosal growth and integrity and has been found to improve intestinal function in surgical patients (Van der Hulst et al., 1993) and patients with diseases of the large intestine (Zoli et al., 1995). Such findings suggest that glutamine ultimately may be found useful in promoting the recovery of patients from surgical treatments and disease states in which immune function may be compromised. In a controlled clinical trial, the administration of glutamine to previously immune-suppressed bone marrow transplant patients was found to reduce the length of hospital stay significantly, primarily due to reductions in clinical infections (Ziegler et al., 1992). A reduction in mortality was observed in patients with intra-abdominal sepsis who received glutamine (Griffiths et al., 1997). Unfortunately, studies that have reported beneficial effects of glutamine have used a parenteral or enteral (gastric tube) route of administration. This factor may explain the inability of Shippee and coworkers (see Chapter 5) to observe any effect of oral glutamine supplements.

In summary, the administration of exogenous glutamine appears to improve immune functions in patients, whose glutamine demands may not be met by endogenous production or dietary supply. Such effects may derive from one or more of the amino acid's many metabolic and cell proliferative effects in the body. If additional work continues to show a positive effect of glutamine in reducing infection and disease, the amino acid ultimately may prove to be of value prophylactically in reducing sickness and speeding the recovery of soldiers from illness, although the adequacy of normal dietary glutamine will have to be assessed as well.

Arginine. The nonessential amino acid arginine, in addition to glutamine, should also be considered as a possible immune-enhancing nutrient. Arginine has multiple biological effects that are beneficial in a variety of situations, such as trauma, tumors, infections, and depressed immunity. l-Arginine supplementation in healthy human subjects has been shown to increase blood lymphocyte proliferation and suppressor T-cell numbers (Barbul et al., 1981) and to enhance phagocytic activity of alveolar macrophages in rats bearing tumor transplants (Tachibana et al., 1985). Arginine is the sole precursor of nitric oxide, a newly recognized but important microbicidal molecule (Koshland, 1992) that appears to be involved in macrophage killer function and in regulating interactions between macrophages and lymphocyte adhesion and activation (Denham and Rowland, 1992; Kirk et al., 1992; Kubes et al., 1991; Liew et al., 1990).

Vitamins

Vitamin A and Carotenoids. The effects of vitamin A deficiency on immune function are significant, and there is convincing evidence for a role of vitamin A in resistance to infection, although the mechanism is not known (Kjolhede and Beisel, 1995). Epidemiologic studies, clinical trials, and experimental studies in animal models have firmly established that vitamin A deficiency is a nutritionally acquired immunodeficiency disorder that is characterized by widespread immune alterations and increased infectious disease and mortality (Semba, 1994). Infections are known to accelerate the metabolic degradation of vitamin A and to increase its urinary excretion. Evidence has accrued from many types of laboratory studies and some clinical studies (reviewed in Ross and Hämmerling, 1994) that vitamin A deficiency affects immunocompetence through several processes. A hallmark of vitamin A deficiency is depressed antibody responses to T-cell-dependent and independent antigens, which may be mediated by alterations in the production of some cytokines. However, some viral infections do not reduce and may increase immunoglobulin G response, which may reduce or otherwise alter other immune responses (Ross and Stephenson, 1996). It should be noted, however, that most of the data available are from children because vitamin A deficiency is relatively rare in adults (especially in the United States) and quite difficult to induce experimentally. Trauma, or sterile inflammation, may cause a significant decrease in some plasma nutrients by reducing the biosynthesis of their transport proteins in liver, including retinol-binding protein and prealbumin, the transport proteins for retinol (Aldred and Schreiber, 1993). A reduction in plasma retinol, into the range considered marginally vitamin A deficient, has been produced in well-nourished rats following induction of acute inflammation (Rosales et al., 1996), and low plasma retinol has been reported during infections in children and adults (reviewed in Ross and Stephensen, 1996).

Reviews of randomized, controlled epidemiological studies as well as clinical trials have led to the conclusion that although the incidence of infectious disease does not appear to be greatly increased by vitamin A deficiency, vitamin A supplementation (to correct a deficiency) can reduce the severity of some infections, including diarrheal diseases (Beaton, 1996; Kirkwood, 1996). Because excess vitamin A can be toxic and is a suspected teratogen, no case can be made for supplementation of nondeficient individuals with amounts of preformed vitamin A significantly beyond the RDA level. Provitamin A carotenoids (vitamin A precursors from plant sources), however, are more limited in their toxicity and may have some effects on the immune system that are not seen with preformed vitamin A. Semba (see Chapter 12) discusses the varying bioavailability of carotenoids from dietary fruits and vegetables.

Vitamin E. The predominant physiologic function of vitamin E is in its role as an antioxidant required for the protection of cellular as well as membrane polyunsaturated fatty acids. Vitamin E also protects membrane-bound nucleic acids and thiol-rich proteins from oxidative damage. It is also known that antioxidants such as vitamin E are important for controlling signal transduction and genetic expression of the various cytokines and ultimately proliferation of the cells that synthesize them. This is particularly important for cells of the immune system because their membranes contain a high level of PUFAs that are exposed to high concentrations of free-radical products. So, not only are the levels of antioxidants reduced during normal cellular processes, but they also can be reduced by the presence of a pathogen itself. Because of the rare occurrence of symptomatic vitamin E deficiency in humans, most studies related to immunity have been conducted in either nondeficient subjects or laboratory animals, and in fact, animal studies have demonstrated improvements in immune function expressed through changes in cell proliferation (Meydani and Hayek, 1992).

Rall and Meydani (see Chapter 13) describe a number of controlled clinical trials performed in Meydani's laboratory demonstrating that vitamin E supplementation of elderly subjects as well as healthy young subjects may enhance immune function (Meydani et al., 1990, 1994). Meydani found that supplementation with 400 mg RRR-α-tocopherol (natural form) or placebo for 6 months resulted in an increased DTH response in both young and elderly subjects.

Rall and Meydani also present some data interrelating the role of vitamin E to prostaglandins and immune function. Prostaglandins have a regulatory role in maintaining the function of T-cells as well as inhibiting lymphocyte proliferation, NK cell cytotoxicity, antibodies, and certain cytokines (Meydani et al., 1990). For example, prostaglandin E_2 (PGE_2) can downregulate the function of Th1 cells and also upregulate the function of Th2 cells. Meydani hypothesized and later demonstrated in aged mice that vitamin E, acting as an antioxidant, would inhibit PGE_2 production (by altering the cyclooxygenase pathway) and would thus be effective in enhancing the immune response as monitored by T-cell-mediated functions (Kramer et al., 1991; Meydani et al., 1986). Meydani and coworkers (1990) have also demonstrated enhanced cell-mediated immune indices of DTH, lymphocyte proliferation to concanavalin A (ConA), and IL-2 production in a group of healthy elderly subjects receiving 800 IU of vitamin E daily for 30 days. The authors therefore believe that vitamin E supplements act to improve the immune response by decreasing the production of PGE_2, which in turn moderates cyclooxygenase activity. Thus, benefits may be conferred on the elderly in the face of PGE_2 levels and oxidative tissue damage that tend to rise with age.

Vitamin C. Despite widespread coverage by the popular press of the influence of vitamin C on the common cold, its role in modulating immune function remains controversial. Based on epidemiological studies of individuals consuming diets deficient in vitamin C and on administration of vitamin C supplements to injured and surgical patients, several mechanisms have been proposed for the apparent immunomodulatory effect, but none have been confirmed definitively.

Vitamin C is known to function as an antioxidant and in this capacity may serve to protect the integrity of plasma, other extracellular fluids, plasma membranes, and intracellular spaces. Neutrophil activity (but not number) is attributed to the high levels of vitamin C in these cells (Khaw et al., 1995; Myrvik, 1994). A recent study in rats has shown that the antioxidant effect of vitamin C also serves to protect the level of cell energetics in burned tissues (Lalonde and Boetz-Marquard, 1997).

Other proposed mechanisms of vitamin C's role in immune function include stimulation of lymphocyte blastogenesis and synthesis of other immune modulators such as prostaglandins, prostacyclins, histamine (Myrvik, 1994), and IL-1. Vitamin C is also essential for the locomotion of neutrophils and other phagocytic cells (Beisel, 1982). Because the decrease in vitamin C status noted with smoking is associated with increased plasma values of IL-6 and TNF soluble receptors (Borelli et al., 1996), and vitamin C status is also inversely associated with levels of C-reactive protein (CRP) and other acute-phase proteins (Khaw et al., 1995), the effects of vitamin C on immune function have been proposed to be mediated through these changes. However, in the latter studies, cause and effect were not determined.

Attempts to show a relationship among dietary vitamin C intake or vitamin C supplementation, vitamin C status, and incidence of infection or cancer have provided controversial and often contradictory results, raising questions in the minds of some scientists regarding how requirements for the vitamin should be determined (Levine et al., 1996). Several types of surgical procedures as well as burn injuries, physical overtraining, and smoking are associated with decreased vitamin C status (Ballmer and Staehlin, 1994; Lalonde and Boetz-Marquard, 1997; Peters et al., 1993; Tappia et al., 1995), which has been proposed to be responsible for the increased incidence of infection in these individuals. However, attempts to show that normalization of vitamin C status by dietary supplementation decreases the incidence of infection have resulted in contradictory observations. Although one study observed enhanced resistance to URIs in supplemented (versus unsupplemented) marathon runners (Peters et al., 1993), a meta-analysis of the largest supplementation studies involving humans concluded that vitamin C supplementation influences susceptibility to URIs (colds) only in those individuals with the lowest initial dietary intakes of vitamin C (Hemila, 1997).

A significant amount of attention has recently focused on whether antioxidant nutrients, particularly vitamins E and C, may help to reduce oxidative stress and damage during exercise (Cannon et al., 1991; Kanter et al., 1993; Meydani et al., 1993; Witt et al., 1992). Although antioxidant supplementation may attenuate oxidative stress following prolonged and strenuous exertion, the effect of this attenuation on the exercise-induced immune response is uncertain (see David C. Nieman, Chapter 17).

In summary, the effects of vitamin A deficiency on immune function are significant, and infections can accelerate its loss of vitamin A. Vitamin A supplements have been shown to reduce the severity of some infections if a deficiency is present; however, an excess can be toxic. The carotenoids are less toxic and may have some effects on the immune system that are not seen with preformed vitamin A. Vitamins C and E are both powerful antioxidants, have been shown to enhance the immune response, and are relatively nontoxic. There is considerable evidence regarding the possible benefits of vitamin E and C supplementation in terms of reducing oxidative stress and/or damage during exercise. However, data remain incomplete, particularly in terms of the optimal amount of supplementation that should be recommended to achieve these benefits.

B-Vitamins. The B vitamins are involved in a broad spectrum of cellular metabolic reactions and, as a group, have been shown to have an effect on cellular disease resistance and the immune response (Bendich and Chandra, 1990). Vitamins B_6, B_{12}, and folate are particularly important for cell-meditated immunity (CMI) functions, and thiamine, is necessary for the synthesis of antibodies or the expression of humoral immunity (Beisel, 1991, 1992). Experimental vitamin B_6 deficiency in humans results in only slight impairment of antibody formation in response to a challenge by tetanus toxoid or typhoid (Hodges et al., 1962). Vitamin B_6 deficiency is not uncommon in humans, although when present, it is usually found in combination with PEM and a deficiency of other B vitamins such as riboflavin. Lymphocyte differentiation and maturation are altered by a deficiency of vitamin B_6, DTH responses are reduced, and antibody production may be directly impaired (Chandra, 1991; Rall and Meydani, 1993). Although repletion of vitamin B_6 restores these functions, megadoses do not produce benefits beyond those observed with moderate supplementation (Rall and Meydani, 1993). Folate deficiency can lead to decreased responses of T-cells to phytohemagglutinin (PHA) as well as to decreased cytotoxic T-cell function (Gross and Newberne, 1976; Hollingsworth and Carr, 1973). CMI is depressed in individuals with anemia due to folate deficiency (Gross et al., 1975). Folate and vitamin B_{12} are both essential to cellular replication, and experimental deficiencies interfere with antibody formation and replication of stimulated leukocytes. In humans, neither phagocytosis nor the bactericidal capacity of neutrophils toward *Staphyloccus aureus* is altered by folate deficiency (Gershwin et al., 1985), but responses are reduced by vitamin B_{12} deficiency.

Fatty Acids

Among the fatty acids present in the diets of humans, the PUFAs are immunologically the most important. The PUFAs are substrates for the synthesis of two families of immunologically important products: the eicosanoids (i.e., prostaglandins, prostacyclins, and thomboxanes) through the cyclooxygenase pathway, and the leukotrienes and lipoxins through the lipoxygenase pathway. These compounds affect many physiological functions (including immunity and inflammation) to varying degrees, depending on structure, amounts, and ratios. Fatty acids affect immune function not only by the total amount of fat present, but also by the amounts of and ratio between the n-6 and n-3 types of PUFA that act primarily through prostaglandins and leukotriene production and activity, as depicted in Figure 1-4. For example, linoleic acid (18:2n-6) occurs in particularly high concentration in sunflower, safflower, corn, and soybean oils. On the other hand, soybean, linseed, and canola oils have a high concentration of linolenic acid (18:3n-3). Animal tissues are unable to synthesize linoleic and α-linolenic acids, so these "essential" fatty acids must be consumed in the diet. Typical North American diets provide 7 percent of energy as linoleic acid, much more than is needed to prevent deficiency (Lands, 1991). The n-6 and n-3

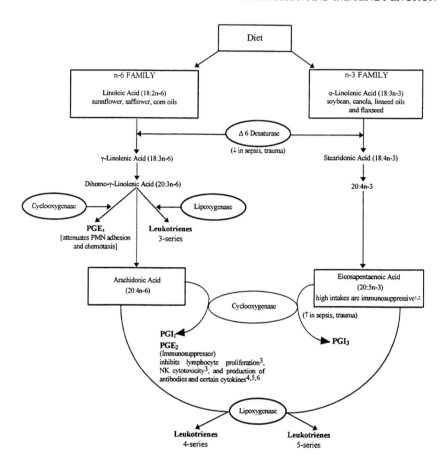

FIGURE 1-4 Metabolic pathways for conversion of dietary PUFAs to eicosanoids. Depending on their concentration and type, prostaglandins and leukotrienes stimulate or inhibit the activity of immune cells. Other 20-carbon fatty acids compete with arachidonic acid for the lipoxygenase and cyclooxygenase enzymes and reduce the products formed from arachidonic acid, including eicosanoids of the 2-series and leukotriene B_4, which are potent modulators of the immune cell: PGE_1, PGI_2, PGI_3, and PGE_2, prostaglandins E_1, I_2, I_3, and E_2, respectively. PMN, polymorphonuclear (leukocyte).

NOTE: For a more detailed review of dietary fatty acids and the Immune system, the reader is referred to Calder (1998).

SOURCE: Pathway adapted from Palombo et al. (1997); [1]Meydani (1993); [2]Hughes (1996); [3]Wasserman et al. (1987); [4]Meydani (1990); [5]Dinarello (1983); [6]Chouarh and Fradeliz (1982).

families of PUFAs are not metabolically interconvertible in mammals. High intakes of 18:2n-6 with low intakes of 18:3n-3 (because of hydrogenation of polyunsaturated oils) and relatively low intakes of other oils (fish oils) could result in competitive pressure against n-3 fatty acids. As noted earlier in this chapter, increasing amounts of PUFAs in the diet increase the vitamin E requirement because of the propensity of PUFAs to undergo lipid peroxidation. The richest sources of vitamin E in the U.S. diet are vegetable oils. Clinical and experimental studies have demonstrated that the structural and functional properties of immune cells can be modified by dietary supplementation with n-3 PUFAs from fish oil or linolenic acid, and in vivo tests are the most appropriate approach for determining the effect of different dietary fatty acids on immune function and inflammation, but few studies have been reported in humans (Calder, 1998).

Amount of Fatty Acid Intake

The effect on immune function of reducing total fat intake has been studied in healthy men (Kelley et al., 1989). In this study, the baseline diet supplied PUFA at 6 percent of energy, and the experimental diets supplied PUFA at either 3.5 percent (four subjects) or 12.9 percent (four subjects) of energy. In both groups, immune function improved as measured by such indices as the numbers of circulating T- and B-lymphocytes and their proliferation in response to specific mitogens. Neutrophils and serum complement C3 decreased, and leukocyte counts and plasma concentrations of all major classes of immunoglobulins remained unchanged.

In another study cited, Kelley and colleagues (1992a) measured the immune status of seven healthy women fed diets reduced in total fat with higher or lower levels of PUFA than the stabilization diet containing 5.2 percent of energy as PUFA and 40 percent of energy as total fat. The experimental diets contained either 3.2 percent of energy as PUFA and 26.1 percent as total fat, or 9.1 percent of energy as PUFA and 31.1 percent total fat. In this study, a number of parameters reflecting immune status improved on the lower-fat diets. In contrast, no differences in these indices were observed between individuals consuming diets containing 9.1 percent of energy as PUFA or 3.2 percent as PUFA. The authors suggested but did not conclude that immune function may have improved in response to the reduction of total fat intake.

Amount of n-6 PUFA

In the two studies cited above, changing the level of linoleic acid (LA) from 3 to 13 percent of energy but reducing total fat intake did not adversely affect the indices of immune function. In another study cited (Barone et al., 1989), results were more equivocal, with adverse effects sometimes being observed when dietary n-6 PUFA increased along with an increase in total fat. Inconsistencies apparent among studies measuring the effect of PUFA on immune function may be due to differences in total fat intake, antioxidants, duration of feeding, and the immune indices measured. Another obvious factor is the ratio of n-6 to n-3 PUFA in the diets. To evaluate this more fully, Kelley et al. (1996) used a crossover study design in which healthy men were fed a baseline diet containing 30 percent of energy as fat (with equal amounts of saturated fatty acids, monounsaturated fatty acids, and PUFAs) and containing 200 mg of arachidonic acid, which was subsequently increased to 1.5 g. This moderate level of arachidonic acid (that is, the intake of additional PUFA) had no adverse effect on various indices of immune function, including DTH response, NK-cell activity, lymphocyte proliferation in response to the mitogens ConA and PHA, and in vitro secretion of IL-1, IL-2, and TNF. It appears that n-6 PUFAs have little effect, if any, on immune function, independent of fat and n-3 PUFA intake.

Amount of n-3 PUFA

A number of studies have been carried out to evaluate the effect of n-3 PUFAs derived from plant sources (Bjerve et al., 1989; Caughey et al., 1996; Kelley et al., 1991), as well as those derived from marine oils (Caughey et al., 1996; Endres et al., 1989, 1993; Kelley et al., 1992b; Kramer et al., 1991; Lee et al., 1985; Madden et al., 1991; Molvig et al., 1991; Payan et al., 1986; Virella et al., 1989), on immune function. These studies have suggested that consumption of n-3 PUFA reduces a number of indices of immune function and, because of this, has been reported to be beneficial in the management of autoimmune diseases such as arthritis in humans.

Kelley et al. (1991) added flaxseed oil (to provide 6 percent of energy as α-linolenic acid [ALA]) to a baseline diet containing 23 percent of energy as total fat, and fed this diet to healthy, young, adult male volunteers for 8 weeks. The addition of flaxseed oil inhibited the proliferation of PBMCs in response to T- and B-cell-specific mitogens because of either the added n-3 PUFA or the higher fat level (a control group receiving 30 percent of energy as total fat was not included).

In a study by Meydani et al. (1993) utilizing fish oil supplements, 22 healthy adults were fed a baseline diet for 6 weeks, followed by a 24-week test diet. The low-fish-oil test diet, low in marine n-3 PUFA (0.13 percent EPA + DHA), increased the response to T-cell mitogens and had no effect on DTH, IL-6, granulocyte macrophage colony stimulating factor (GMCSF), or PGE$_2$

production. In contrast, the high-fish-oil diet, high in marine n-3 PUFA (0.54 percent EPA + DHA), decreased the percentage of CD4+ cells and increased the percentage of CD8+ cells. In addition, this diet decreased responses to T-cell mitogens, the hypersensitivity skin response, and the production of cytokines IL-1β, TNF, and IL-6 by mononuclear cells. In another study, Kelley et al. (1992b) observed that the immune response of healthy young men (25–40 years old) was not inhibited by consumption of 500 g/d of salmon that supplied 2.1 percent of energy as marine oil-derived n-3 PUFA. In a recent study not previously cited, Hughes et al. (1996) reported that fish oil supplementation inhibited the expression of major histocompatibility complex Class II molecules and adhesion molecules on human monocytes. Since these surface molecules are involved in the immune response to presenting antigens, the authors suggested that this is a potential mechanism by which n-3 PUFA may suppress the immune response.

A series of studies has examined the effects of fish oil medium-chain triglycerides (so-called structured lipids) on the incidence of postoperative infection and other indicators of renal, hepatic, and immune function. Bistrian and coworkers (Swails et al., 1997) report significant decreases in infection and improved clinical indices in patients fed enteral diets containing these structured lipids in the immediate postoperative period following surgery for gastrointestinal malignancies.

Mixtures of fish oils and arginine, with or without nucleic acids, have also been administered in the immediate postoperative period with mixed results. Two large clinical trials, one in the United States and the other in Germany, have demonstrated significant decreases in postoperative infection and length of hospitalization following immediate postsurgical feeding with an enteral supplement (Trade name: Impact, manufactured by Sandoz) (Bower et al., 1995; Senkal et al., 1997). In a more recent study, patients given a mixture of n-3-fatty acids (contained in fish oils) and arginine in the immediate postoperative period experienced no beneficial effects on immune function.

Calder (1997) has suggested that diets enriched in fish oil n-3 PUFAs may be of use in the therapy of acute and chronic inflammation and disorders involving inappropriately active immune responses (such as autoimmune disorders). High-fat diets also have the potential to affect immune function adversely as evidenced by the fact that such diets were once used to delay or prevent transplant rejection (Beisel, 1992).

In summary, limited data suggest that moderate reductions in total fat calories (i.e., 26 percent versus 30 percent) may have some beneficial effects in enhancing immune function. To interpret data in this area, a number of caveats are important. Many variables (including total fat, n-6 PUFA, n-3 PUFA, and antioxidants among others) were changed simultaneously in all of these studies. These variables significantly interact with each other, and in human studies, the

possible number of subjects does not allow for the kind of statistical analysis
necessary to sort through all variables and interactions. The most important
caveat may be that in all of these studies, surrogates of immune function were
measured, rather than immune function itself (that is, immunity to disease and
resistance to infection). Finally, it should be noted that although increasing the
consumption of marine oils that supply eicosapentaenoic acid (EPA) and DHA
may reduce the risk of heart disease and be useful in treating autoimmune
disease and inflammation, such diets may well reduce immune function.

Minerals

Iron

In Chapter 15, Keusch provides an overview of iron metabolism and the
role of iron in both host defense and the virulence of the invading pathogen. As
with many other aspects of the immune system, iron has both positive and
negative effects, promoting host defense or microbial virulence under differing
circumstances. Iron is highly reactive, with considerable ability to generate free
radicals that are toxic to both host and microbial cells. The host and the invading
organism both require the biological mechanisms to acquire and detoxify iron.
The battle between host and pathogen is partly a battle of binding affinity in
which the chelator protein that binds iron with greater affinity is able to strip it
from the protein that binds it with less affinity.

In the mammalian host, iron is bound primarily to protein complexes,
including iron transport (transferrin or lactoferrin) and storage proteins (ferritin),
enzymes (cytochrome c), and oxygen transport systems (heme) (Griffiths,
1987). The mammalian iron acquisition system is very efficient, having the
ability to compete for ferric iron even from insoluble ferric hydroxide. Because
most iron is present in the bound form, the free iron pool is very small. Free
radicals that are formed are destroyed by iron-containing enzymes such as
catalase. Synthesis of the transferrin receptor and synthesis of ferritin (for iron
transport and storage) are regulated reciprocally by iron concentration via a
posttranscriptional mechanism (Klausner et al., 1993). Iron influences immune
functions via cytokines and nitric oxide (Weiss et al., 1995), and iron-containing
enzymes play a key role in the bactericidal activities of phagocytic cells.
Morikawa et al. (1995) reported that ferritin directly suppresses the
differentiation and maturation of human B-lymphocytes into antibody-
producing cells. Lactoferrin, the milk protein, has a direct transcriptional role
that may help explain the direct transmission of passive immunity from mother
to child (Fleet, 1995).

Iron also is required for microbial growth; hence, microorganisms compete
with the host for iron by using analogous systems of acquisition, transport, and

detoxification. Many microbes make siderophores (iron-binding chelators), which are high-affinity binding molecules for the ferric ion that have the ability to remove iron from host iron-binding proteins including ferritin (Neilands, 1995). In response to low iron availability, *E. coli*, for example, depresses transcription of genes involving iron acquisition and transport, including iron chelators, outer membrane siderophores, and inner membrane transport proteins. Under anaerobic conditions, ferrous iron is more available because of its increased solubility. In addition, a ferrous iron transport gene has been demonstrated in *E. coli*. It is clear that pathogenic microorganisms adapt to low iron availability through the regulation of gene transcription and translation by iron. In Keusch's view, this raises doubts about enhancing immunity by withholding iron.

Iron Deficiency. Iron is needed by both pathogens and their hosts and is required for host immune function. Transferrin iron is required for the clonal expansion of lymphocytes via ribonucleotide reductase, and iron uptake also must precede DNA synthesis (Kay and Benzie, 1986; Phillips and Azari, 1975). In humans with iron deficiency anemia, decreases in CD3+ and CD4+ B-lymphocytes, and killer-cell activity have been reported (Santos and Falcao, 1990). In addition, iron deficiency is associated with a decrease in delayed-type skin test reactivity to antigens and with impaired mitogen-stimulated lymphocyte proliferation in vitro (Krantman et al., 1982). Data from animal studies suggest that antibody production and CMI are likely to be impaired by iron deficiency because of the role of iron metalloenzymes in DNA synthesis and cell proliferation. Whether iron deficiency affects the host–pathogen relationship at the clinical level remains to be demonstrated conclusively. However, as discussed below, it is clear that iron deficiency does not and will not enhance immune responses.

Iron Excess. Because invading microorganisms require iron and compete for it, it has been hypothesized that withholding therapeutic iron during infection will protect the host, and excess iron will enhance infection (Weinberg, 1984). It has been reported that iron overload states such as β-thalassemia, sickle cell anemia with multiple transfusions, or idiopathic hemochromatoses result in iron-saturated transferrin. Any excess iron then can form loose complexes with albumin, thereby increasing the availability of iron to microorganisms (Hershko and Peto, 1987). Increased infections and fatal outcomes have been associated with these conditions (Barrett-Conner, 1971; Buchanan, 1971) and also have been observed in animal models of hemochromatosis. However, it is difficult to attribute these adverse effects completely to free iron-related microbial growth and infection rather than to damage occurring to the reticuloendothelial system and disrupted cellular function resulting from iron-mediated oxidation or peroxidation effects (Hershko et al., 1988). For example, although 20 percent of β-thalassemia deaths result from infection, nearly all occur in splenectomized patients. Nevertheless, free iron does increase oxidative damage to cells, and iron excess is, in fact, likely to impair immune function. A number of defects in immune mechanisms have been demonstrated in thalassemia patients. The addition of increasing amounts of iron to T-lymphocytes diminishes clearing efficiency and reduces the proliferative response to mitogens (Good et al., 1988; Munn, 1981). Reductions in the number and function of CD4+ cells and decreases in NK-cell activity have been reported in iron-overload patients (Akbar et al., 1986).

Clinical Studies. To clarify the conditions under which iron deficiency or iron excess is harmful, data obtained from well-controlled clinical studies are essential. In reviewing published clinical studies dealing with the effects of iron deficiency or overload on susceptibility to infection, Keusch (1994) concludes that most studies are flawed in design for one reason or another. The most frequently cited studies showing a benefit of iron fortification are those that involve a comparison of infant formula with and without added iron (Andelman and Sered, 1966). Unfortunately, in these studies, the morbidity data involving respiratory and intestinal disease were obtained by maternal recall rather than observation by trained personnel. Thus, the clinical consequences of iron deficiency with respect to immune function remain uncertain.

Several clinical studies, however, have reported that iron overload can sometimes increase the severity of infections. These typically occur under conditions where the host does not compete well with the invading pathogen for protein-bound iron; thus the pathogen benefits from the increase in free iron that results from iron overload. For example, life-threatening infections from low-virulence strains such as *Yersinia enterocolitica* have occurred in patients on iron chelation therapy or with iron overload following massive ingestion of iron (Carniel et al., 1987, 1989). High plasma iron values (following nutritional therapy) have also induced lethal cerebral malaria in asymptomatic, parasitemic, malnourished African children (Murray et al., 1978). Clearly iron in relation to infection has both positive and negative effects.

Iron Status of Military Personnel. In December 1995, the CMNR responded to a request by USARIEM and the Commander, USAMRMC to examine data pertaining to the iron status of women in basic combat training (BCT) and to make recommendations on the extent of the problem, how to treat it, and any additional research necessary. According to data presented (Friedl et al., 1990; Klicka et al., 1993; Westphal et al., 1995), when the criterion for iron deficiency was defined as a serum ferritin concentration of less than 12 µg/L and the criteria for iron deficiency anemia were defined as a combination of low serum ferritin and a hemoglobin concentration of less than 120 g/L, 17 percent of new female recruits who were tested at entry to BCT fit the criteria for iron deficiency while 8 percent could be classified as having iron deficiency anemia. A survey of a similar (but not the same) population of women at the end of BCT showed that by the end of training, 33 percent were iron deficient and 26 percent were anemic. When iron deficiency is defined as a serum ferritin concentration of less than 12 μg/L, the sensitivity for detecting iron deficiency is 61 percent and the specificity is 100 percent (Hallberg et al., 1993).

Iron deficiency anemia can be expected to have adverse effects on military performance of both men and women depending in part on its severity. Performance deficits in both men and women due to compromised iron status have been demonstrated most clearly during exercise of prolonged duration such as long-distance running (Newhouse and Clement, 1988). Iron deficiency anemia may also have an adverse impact on recovery from trauma, especially trauma involving significant blood loss. However, data to support deficits in physical performance in iron-compromised individuals have not been systematically collected by the military. Some preliminary evidence suggests that iron supplementation of nonanemic women can improve aerobic capacity (J. Haas, Cornell University, personal communication, 1997).

After reviewing the data, the CMNR recommended to the Army that personnel with iron deficiency or iron deficiency anemia should receive appropriate medical treatment and monitoring until laboratory results show a return to normal values; a delay in deployment was also recommended for personnel with iron deficiency anemia. Current guidelines for treatment of nonpregnant women of childbearing age recommend an oral dose of 60–120 mg/d of iron with nutritional counseling. If, after 4 weeks, the anemia does not respond to iron treatment despite compliance with supplementation and the absence of illness, further evaluation is warranted using other laboratory tests (CDC, 1998).

In summary, mechanistic data exist to suggest strongly that both iron deficiency and iron excess can increase susceptibility to infection, albeit by different mechanisms. It is important to note, however, that there is a fairly large range of iron intakes over which the immune system can function normally. Although the evidence for iron excess may be compelling, it is likely that for the military, the potential reduction in immune function due to iron deficiency is of more immediate and consequential importance than iron overload. The negative consequences of low iron status are especially dire for women in the military.

Zinc

Zinc is clearly the most important trace element with respect to immune function. Many animal studies have shown that zinc deficiency leads to decreased T-cell function, impaired antibody response, reduced thymus size, and depletion of macrophages and lymphocytes in the spleen (Beisel, 1982). The inherited defect in intestinal zinc absorption, acrodermatitis enteropathica, causes a severe (but treatable) zinc deficiency state in afflicted infants, resulting in similar widespread immunological dysfunctions. There also is evidence that zinc deficiency in elderly persons can result in heightened susceptibility to infectious disease (Chandra, 1988). Conversely, excess intakes of zinc also have been reported to be immunosuppressive so that both excess and deficient zinc status can have adverse effects on immune function (Chandra, 1982). Given that zinc is a vital cofactor for many different enzymes, regulates some immune-related genes, influences cytokine effects in some situations, and may play a key role as a component of thymic hormones that help regulate all T-cell functions, it is not surprising that deficiency of this essential trace element results in numerous immunological impairments, but its precise role in proper immune system functioning has yet to be clarified fully.

Clinically, zinc deficiency is almost impossible to prove in individual patients, in contrast to groups, by any current, clinically available, diagnostic methods. However, zinc deficiency almost always coexists with severe PEM, and it is difficult to separate the overlapping effects of these two states on immune system function. Animal data show that unifactorial, experimental zinc deficiency leads to a greatly heightened susceptibility to infection and immune system dysfunctions similar to those seen in PEM (Fraker, 1993). Zinc deficiency also impairs the body's ability to mobilize its stores of vitamin A (Udomkesmalee et al., 1992).

In contrast, excess intakes of zinc can have an adverse impact on the immune system (Chandra, 1982). Long-term clinical studies (Tang et al., 1996) showed that HIV patients with zinc intakes greater than 20.2 mg/d had decreased survival rates beginning at about 1,000 d and worsening through a 2,500-d period of observation, compared to HIV patients whose zinc intake was less than 14.2 mg/d. Furthermore, excess zinc intake can interfere with intestinal absorption of copper (Kramer et al., 1993). Imbalances between zinc and copper may occur because of either deficient or excessive copper intake, or excessive zinc intake relative to copper. There is some evidence to suggest that the interactive effects of zinc and copper on the immune response may involve differential cytokine stimulation (Scuderi, 1990). In studies with children, zinc has been shown to reduce the morbidity associated with secretory diarrhea (Rosado et al., 1997; Sazawal et al., 1995). This effect of supplemental zinc is of unknown mechanistic basis but could be related to enhanced immune function of the intestine. An effect on diarrheal disease in the field is possible.

Copper

Copper, like zinc, is a necessary constituent of numerous metalloenzymes, and deficiency of this essential trace element results in an increased susceptibility of animals to a wide range of infectious agents. Copper deficiency in a variety of animal models has caused a decreased antibody response to a number of antigens, decreased T-cell proliferative response, decreased NK-cell activity, and thymic atrophy (Bala, 1991; Blakley and Hamilton, 1987; Prohaska et al., 1983; Lukasewycz and Prohaska, 1990). Copper deficiency is rare in human adults and, if present, is characterized by leukopenia and anemia (Prasad et al., 1978). Moreover, children suffering from Menkes disease, an inborn error that results in failure to absorb copper, normally die of infectious bronchopneumonia. A well-controlled human metabolic feeding study showed that lymphoproliferative responses to mitogens were markedly impaired in healthy adult men fed a low-copper diet for 66 d (Hopkins and Failla, 1997). Despite compelling evidence that copper is required for a normal immune system, more research is needed to clarify its role in proper immune function.

Selenium

Selenium is now known to be a part of several mammalian enzymes including four glutathione peroxidases (Burk, 1997), three deiodinases (Arthur and Beckett, 1994; Berry and Larsen, 1992; Croteau et al., 1995), and thioredoxin reductase, as well as a variety of microbial enzymes (Chaudiere et al., 1984). Selenium also is found in a number of selenoproteins (selenoprotein P, selenoprotein W) whose enzymatic activities have yet to be determined. Many of selenium's effects can be explained most simply on the basis that it is a required constituent of the glutathione peroxidase family of enzymes. Selenium deficiency has been associated with an increased susceptibility to certain infectious pathogens, perhaps because of decreased antibody production and impaired lymphoproliferative responses in the deficient state (Kiremidjian-Schumacher and Stotzky, 1987). In China, selenium deficiency also has been associated with an endemic juvenile cardiomyopathy (known as Keshan disease). This association has led to the discovery that the selenium status of the host may have an effect on the genetic makeup of a pathogen. Because of pronounced seasonal and annual variations in the incidence of Keshan disease, an infectious component may be involved in its etiology. In fact, a number of enteroviruses were isolated from Keshan disease patients, and one of these, a coxsackievirus B4, was tested by the Chinese for its cardiotoxic effects in mice fed diets of varying selenium content (Bai et al., 1980).

Beck (see Chapter 16) and Orville A. Levander confirmed the Chinese results by showing that feeding mice a selenium-deficient diet increased damage to the heart caused by a myocarditic viral strain, coxsackievirus B3/20 (CVB3/20). Subsequently, they showed that a normally amyocarditic strain, coxsackievirus B3/0 (CVB3/0) (that is, a strain that normally does not cause heart damage) became myocarditic when inoculated into selenium-deficient mice. Similar changes in Coxsackievirus virulence (i.e., the myocarditic strain became more so and the amyocarditic strain became myocarditic) have been demonstrated in vitamin E-deficient, fish oil-fed mice. All of these dietary effects (selenium deficiency, vitamin E deficiency, fish oil supplementation) can be explained most readily on the basis of an increased oxidative stress imposed on the host by the diet.

The biochemical mechanisms responsible for these dietary effects on viral virulence in mice are not known, but defects in certain host immune functions were observed (impaired mitogen- and antigen-stimulated T-cell proliferation). Other immune parameters (antibody production, NK-cell function) were not affected by selenium or vitamin E deficiency.

Isolation of the CVB3/0 that exhibited virulence in selenium-deficient mice (now called CVB3/0Se), followed by passage through cell culture and reinoculation into a normal mouse, revealed that this virus had undergone a genomic alteration that was stable for at least one such passage. This observation appears to be the first report that the nutritional status of the host might affect the genetic makeup of a pathogen.

If these results are generally applicable to other viruses (or perhaps even other microbial pathogens) and/or other nutritional deficiencies, the implications for public health in general and military health in particular could be profound. As pointed out by Morse (see Appendix D), soldiers often must perform in crowded and unsanitary environments, which increases their vulnerability to infection by a variety of pathogenic agents. If, for any reason, the nutritional well-being of military personnel is compromised, they could become unwitting incubators of novel viruses with unpredictable properties.

In summary, dietary deficiencies of a variety of nutritionally essential trace elements (zinc, copper, selenium) have all been shown to have an adverse impact on a number of immune functions in laboratory animals. Moreover, deficiencies of zinc and/or copper have resulted in increased susceptibility of humans to certain infections. However, excessive intake of some trace elements (for example, zinc) may lead to immunosuppressive effects; so there clearly exists an optimal range of nutritional status for proper immune function.

Other Factors

Alcohol

Excessive alcohol consumption is a major health problem in the United States, and high rates of excessive consumption have been observed among military personnel (Bray et al., 1995). Although data were not presented at the workshop, it is important to discuss the various mechanisms by which alcohol interferes with the complex mechanisms of nutritional immunomodulation. Alcohol acts directly on mechanical barriers in the gastrointestinal tract and increases the permeability of the intestinal wall, which results in a greater absorption of immunogenic material in the intestine. Alcohol further affects granulocytopoiesis and suppresses various immune functions (Watzl and Watson, 1992).

Indirect effects on immune response also can be caused by alcohol-induced malnutrition. Heavy alcohol intake (abuse) is associated with a high percentage of total energy intake being contributed by alcohol and sometimes with an inadequate intake of protein, vitamins, and minerals. In addition, alcohol abuse impairs absorption, utilization, storage, and excretion of nutrients, which in combination with inadequate nutrient intake results in nutritional immunosuppression. The nutrients most likely at risk of becoming depleted are folate, thiamine, vitamins A and B_6, and zinc.

Alcohol in vivo causes abnormalities in the function and/or structure of a broad array of cells involved in humoral and cellular immunity--including lymphocytes, Kupffer cells (mononuclear phagocytes found on the luminal surface of liver), and other macrophages—and cytokines, namely, TNF, IL-1, and IL-6 (Martinez et al., 1992).

HEALTH AND STRESS

In Chapter 17, David C. Nieman discusses how the immune system responds to chronic exercise of varying intensity and duration, both in health and during periods of compromised health. In Chapters 18 and 19, respectively, Seymour Reichlin and Leonard P. Kapcala review the role of the neuroendocrine system in moderating immune function. Reichlin describes the hypothalamic–pituitary–adrenal, thyroid, and gonadal system interrelationships and responses to inflammatory disease conditions, whereas Kapcala discusses the involvement of individual cytokines in stimulating the hypothalamic–pituitary–adrenal axis. Superimposed on the demands of exercise and neurohormonal or neuroimmunological activation, an individual's innate biologic rhythms also may affect changes in the body's immune response, as described by Erhard Haus in Chapter 20.

Exercise, Infection, and Immunity

The interaction of exercise and immunity has two facets: the first is the effect of exercise on various elements of the immune system; the second is the effect of infection on exercise performance and the ability to recover. In Chapter 17, Nieman addresses both of these issues.

The effect of exercise on the immune system depends on a variety of factors, the most important of which seem to be the intensity and duration of exercise and the immune component being discussed. The acute response (within 1–2.5 h) to strenuous exercise (> 65 percent $Vo_{2\ max}$) includes neutrophilia and lymphocytopenia. This response is probably due to an exercise-induced increase in stress hormones (especially cortisol) and increased cytokine concentrations. Increased levels of cortisol are associated with neutrophilia, eosinophilia, lymphocytopenia, and a suppression of NK- and T-cell activity (Cupps and Fauci, 1982). Mitogen-induced lymphocyte proliferation (Eskola et al., 1978; Nieman et al., 1995b), upper airway neutrophil phagocytosis, and neutrophil oxidative burst (Macha et al., 1990; Müns, 1993) have been shown to be suppressed for several hours after strenuous activity, leading to the idea that exercise creates a window of opportunity for infection (see Nieman, Chapter 17). Other stresses such as chronic mental stress and anxiety have been associated with similar suppression of immune function, probably through the same hormonal mechanism.

Highly trained endurance athletes, both young and old, appear to have enhanced NK-cell activity and decreased neutrophil function in comparison to age- and sex-matched sedentary controls (Nieman et al., 1993b, 1995; Pedersen et al., 1989; Tvede et al., 1991). However, measurements taken after 8–15 weeks of moderate exercise show that this exercise does not seem to affect either parameter. Mitogen-induced lymphocyte proliferative response (a measure of T-cell activity) does not appear to be changed by moderate physical activity, although strenuous activity may negatively affect the immune system in the young. Swedish studies indicated that moderate physical training stimulates the immune system, whereas exhaustive and long-lasting exercise is followed by a temporary immunodeficiency and an increased susceptibility to respiratory tract infections (Friman et al., 1997).

In the elderly, intense physical training is associated with an increase in NK- and T-cell activity (Shinkai et al., 1995) and PHA-induced lymphocyte proliferation (Nieman et al., 1993b), compared to individuals having a sedentary life-style. However, moderate activity does not seem to have the same effect, and training may have to be sufficient to induce changes in body weight and fitness to be effective in stimulating the immune system in the elderly as well as the young.

A J-curve of risk has been proposed by Nieman, which means that at moderate activity, the risk to the individual of developing a URI is lower than in a sedentary or strenuously active situation (Nieman, 1994). In addition, the symptoms associated with any URI are diminished in those who are moderately active regardless of age; however, he points out the dearth of well-controlled studies of this phenomenon. Infection does decrease various measures of performance. Nieman suggests that mild exercise during infection with localized symptoms is not contraindicated, but exercise should be curtailed for 2 to 4 weeks after severe infections with systemic involvement.

The military relevance of the interaction between nutrition and physical activity and the effect of this interaction on the immune system are pointed out by Nieman (see Chapter 17). Low energy intake, weight reduction, and increased levels of circulating glucocorticoids often associated with field maneuvers (see Shippee and Wiik, Chapters 5 and 6, respectively) may suppress the immune system independently, and superimposing physical activity may increase vulnerability. The use of flu shots to minimize risk in exercising troops is recommended by Nieman. In addition, the use of immunomodulator drugs, such as indomethacin, aspirin, and ibuprofen, could be considered; however, studies on these compounds are ongoing, and no clear conclusions are available at present. Studies of glutamine (see Wilmore, Chapter 11), vitamin C (see Rall and Meydani, Chapter 13), n-acetylcysteine, and carbohydrate-containing beverages (by way of their ability to decrease cortisol levels) suggest that these may be candidates for prophylactic agents.

Two final conclusions regarding exercise and immunity can be drawn:

1. Low- to moderate-intensity exercise (< 60 percent $Vo_{2\ max}$, such as that performed by most troops in daily life) of reasonable duration (< 60 min) may exert less stress on the immune system than more strenuous or longer exercise, with little change in immune function being documented under conditions of moderate exercise.

2. Repeated bouts of strenuous activity may put individuals at risk for infection (especially URIs) because of suppression of neutrophil activity. Risk of illness is particularly high during the first 2 weeks following a bout of prolonged strenuous exercise.

Hormonal Responses to Stress

The anterior pituitary gland secretes a number of hormones vital for normal physiological processes, including those that are involved in the regulation of other endocrine glands. Secretion of hormones from the anterior pituitary is regulated by neurohormones produced in the hypothalamus and delivered to the pituitary gland through a portal circulation system that directly connects the hypothalamus to the anterior pituitary (Rang et al., 1995).

The Stress Response Model

The body responds to bouts of moderate–severe exercise, changes in environmental exposure (heat, cold), or hypovolemia (due to excess sweating, decreased intake, or diarrhea) in a rather stereotypic manner by elaborating "stress hormones." All of the hormones that regulate carbohydrate metabolism participate in host responses to infection. Among these are the glucocorticoids from the adrenal cortex, the catecholamines from the adrenal medulla and sympathetic nervous system, and glucagon, a pancreatic hormone. These three families of stress hormones have been infused into normal volunteers, and the metabolic and immunologic responses monitored. Many, if not all, of the changes observed are similar to those described in injured and infected humans (Bessey et al., 1984; Watters et al., 1986). The glucocorticoid cortisol, when infused into healthy volunteers, has major immunological effects; lymphocyte counts increase, while the proportions of T3-, T4-, and T11-lymphocytes decrease (Barber et al., 1993; Calvano et al., 1987). When epinephrine was added to the infusion, the marginating pool of circulating neutrophils was mobilized, but chemotaxis measured after 6 h of infusion was reduced (Davis et al., 1991). When cortisol alone was administered for 6 h before an endotoxin challenge, the immunological response was greatly reduced compared to the response in volunteers receiving endotoxin alone (Barber et al., 1993). When the three stress hormones were administered together to volunteers, NK-cell activity was suppressed (Blazar et al., 1986). Different cytokines show differential sensitivity to suppression after administration of glucocorticoids in vivo and ex vivo, with IL-6 relatively resistant to suppression by glucocorticoids (DeRijk et al., 1997).

Neuroendocrine Consequences of Systemic Inflammation

In Chapter 18, Reichlin focuses on the manner in which infection and inflammatory disease alter the secretion of hypothalamic and pituitary hormones and the subsequent functioning of their target tissues.

Hypothalamic–Pituitary–Adrenal System

The hypothalamic–pituitary–adrenal system is altered significantly by inflammatory disease. Infections or injections of bacterial toxins stimulate the release of a number of cytokines including IL-1, IL-2, IL-6, and TNF. Within the hypothalamus, these cytokines directly stimulate the synthesis and secretion of corticotropin-releasing hormone (CRH) and vasopressin (VP) (Kapcala, 1997; Reichlin, 1993). Acting in concert, these hormones increase the release of adrenocorticotrophic hormone (ACTH) from the anterior pituitary, which in turn augments the secretion of cortisol from the adrenal gland. Additionally, in the hypothalamus, CRH activates the peripheral autonomic nervous system, enhancing the release of epinephrine from the adrenal medulla. Epinephrine acts synergistically with CRH and VP to stimulate the secretion of ACTH, thereby regulating the circulating concentrations of cortisol. Since almost all components of the immune response are inhibited by cortisol and other glucocorticoids, pituitary–adrenal activation is accompanied by a reduction in the intensity of the immune response (Kapcala, 1997; Reichlin 1993) (Figure 1-5).

The pituitary–adrenal response to stress, which is characterized by intense mobilization of cytokines and related inflammatory mediators that can compromise healing, has been proposed to have a suppressive effect on excessive inflammatory reactions (Munck et al., 1984), and this has been supported by several animal models (Sternberg et al., 1992).

Humans with adrenal insufficiency are affected more detrimentally by sepsis than are individuals with normal adrenal function. However, clinical studies indicate that the treatment of sepsis with glucocorticoids does not improve survival in patients with normal adrenal function (Reichlin, 1993).

Hypothalamic–Pituitary–Thyroid System

A variety of acute and chronic illnesses can lead to abnormalities in the hypothalamic–pituitary–thyroid system, characterized by low circulating levels of triiodothyronine, low or normal blood levels of thyroxine (T_4), and depressed thyroid-binding proteins (Wartofsky and Burman, 1982). Additionally, the depressed plasma concentrations of thyroid hormones fail to stimulate the secretion of thyroid-stimulating hormone (TSH), thus indicating an impairment in the pituitary–thyroid feedback system (Beisel, 1991, 1992; Reichlin, 1993; Shambaugh-Beisel, 1966). These abnormalities are the result of cytokine-induced alterations at all levels of this system (Reichlin, 1993, 1994). Within the hypothalamus, cytokines suppress the synthesis and secretion of thyrotropin-releasing hormone (TRH) (Kakuscska et al., 1994) and increase the secretion of somatostatin. Within the pituitary, cytokines inhibit secretion and reduce the biological potency of TRH. Finally, responsiveness to TRH is reduced in the thyroid, and circulating concentrations of thyroid hormones are low (Reichlin, 1993). Starvation can exacerbate the effects of inflammation on thyroid functioning, as noted by decreased T_4 to T_3 conversion. Whether these inflammation-induced changes in the hypothalamic–pituitary–thyroid are beneficial, remains open to question.

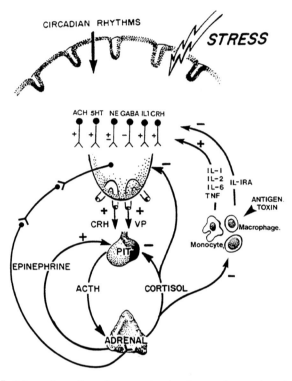

FIGURE 1-5 Schematic outline of neuroendocrine factors that regulate the secretion of the adrenal cortex. ACTH release from the pituitary is stimulated by corticotropin-releasing hormone (CRH) and vasopressin (VP) acting synergistically. Circulating epinephrine (the response of the activated sympathetic nervous system) is also synergistic for ACTH release. Secretion of ACTH is inhibited at the pituitary level by circulating glucocorticoids, and at the hypothalamic level, CRH and VP are also under negative feedback control by glucocorticoids. VP, CRH neurons are in turn subject to a wide range of influences— circulating cytokines, prostaglandins, and many neurotransmitters. Some, such as acetylcholine (ACH), are stimulatory; others, such as gama-aminobutyric acid (GABA), are inhibitory. Interacting with the hypothalamic–pituitary–adrenal axis is the peripheral immune system (as well as endothelia and other structures), which releases cytokines into the blood that then can activate the adrenals. Each of the major inflammatory cytokines, IL-1 (α or ß), IL-2, IL-6 and TNF-α, is capable of activating ACTH release. The peripheral immune system provides a chemosensory system by which the presence of foreign molecules can be communicated to the brain and induce an appropriate response, a model of "bidirectional communication between the brain and the immune system" (Blalock, 1989).

SOURCE: Blalock, 1989.

NOTE: 5HT, 5-hydroxy tryptamine; NE, norephrine.

Pituitary–Gonadal System

Gonadal function also is reduced in severe inflammatory disease. Burns, sepsis, and severe trauma are associated with a reduction in plasma concentrations of sex steroids in both males and females. The reductions in steroid values are related in part to the direct actions of cytokines on the testes and ovaries. Normally, low circulating levels of estrogens or testosterone stimulate the secretion of gonadotropin-releasing hormone (GnRH) from the hypothalamus. However, in inflammatory disease, IL-1 inhibits the pulsatile release of GnRH from the hypothalamus, which in turn inhibits the release of gonadotropins from the pituitary and thus contributes to the low plasma concentrations of circulating gonadal steroids (Reichlin, 1993). Although a decreased availability of testosterone might be hypothesized to be associated with muscle wasting, the functional role of gonadal hormone suppression in inflammatory disease is unknown at present.

Growth Hormone

Inflammatory disease often is accompanied by increases in plasma growth hormone (GH) concentrations (Beisel et al., 1968; Reichlin, 1993). However, circulating levels of GH may not be representative of the effects of this hormone on the tissues themselves. GH-directed protein metabolism is mediated by insulin-like growth factor-I (IGF-I, somatomedin C), a protein derived from the liver whose secretion is regulated by GH and the availability of metabolic substrate. In sepsis and severe burns, plasma GH concentrations are elevated, while IGF-I values are low, suggesting that in these conditions, there may be resistance to GH at the tissue level. Because administration of GH to individuals with severe burns can improve graft healing and survival (Knox et al., 1995), the burn-induced increase in GH may be positive but suboptimal. Reichlin suggests that administration of IGF-I to sepsis or burn patients might thus be preferable to administration of GH. IGF-I infusion has been shown to lower protein oxidation and to stimulate glucose uptake in a small study of burn patients (Cioffi et al., 1994), and IGF-I enhances the immune response in rats (Hinton et al., 1995).

In summary, a variety of changes in the hypothalamic–pituitary system occur via activation of inflammatory responses (and cytokine release) through products of cell injury or toxins affecting pituitary–endocrine end organ functioning. Some of these changes in neuroendocrine function are valuable because they help to promote healing and survival. However, others may potentiate the detrimental consequences of inflammation. Reichlin concludes that interactions between cytokine-mediated changes in neuroendocrine activity and poor nutrition could detrimentally affect immunological activity and resistance to stress in military personnel.

Inflammatory Stress and the Immune System

In Chapter 19, Kapcala deals principally with how cytokines act through the brain to induce glucocorticoid and epinephrine secretion. As previously mentioned by Reichlin, the cytokines most involved in the stimulation of the hypothalamic–pituitary–adrenal axis (HPAA) are IL-1 and IL-6, which are the most potent, and TNF (Chrousos, 1995). Kapcala reiterates the effect of IL-1 on the CRH–ACTH–cortisol axis and discusses data indicating that cytokines might act at all levels of the HPAA to induce glucocorticoid release, but he concludes that the dominant effect is mediated through the brain and that the CRH neurons are probably the most important site. Since peptides, including IL-1, normally do not cross the blood–brain barrier in appreciable amounts (Coceani et al., 1988), one or more specialized mechanisms must exist for giving circulating cytokines access to brain if they are to influence central CRH neurons.

Under conditions of infection and/or inflammation, and even in the absence of infection or inflammation, cytokines may permeate the brain through specialized regions termed circumventricular organs (CVOs) to influence CRH (see Kapcala, Chapter 19). This communication also may occur via circulating cytokines that can activate peripheral sensory neurons, relaying input to the brain, which ultimately stimulates CRH neurons (Wan et al., 1994; Watkins et al., 1995). Also, cytokines may signal the brain through binding to receptors on cerebral blood vessel endothelial cells and activating synthesis of second messengers, prostaglandins, and nitric oxide (Sternberg, 1997b). Regardless of the mechanism, stimulation of central IL-1 receptors by peripheral and central IL-1 is thought to promote CRH release and ultimately ACTH and glucocorticoid secretion (Chrousos, 1995).

The importance of glucocorticoid release in limiting the toxic effects of cytokine overexpression also is of concern. The lethality of an infectious agent in animals with a compromised glucocorticoid response has been documented (Bertini et al., 1988; Fan et al., 1994; Kapcala et al., 1995; Nakano et al., 1987), and the administration of glucocorticoid protects against these effects (Bertini et al., 1988; Butler et al., 1989; Kapcala et al., 1995; MacPhee et al., 1989; Nakano et al., 1987). Moreover, compromised adrenal function is associated with a prolonged elevation in circulating concentrations of IL-1 and TNF, providing further evidence that the adrenal responses normally limit widespread cytokine effects (Butler et al., 1989; Zuckerman et al., 1989). One such mechanism by which increased glucocorticoid secretion would counterbalance the toxic effects of excessive cytokine actions in the body involves inhibition by glucocorticoids of the production of a variety of cytokines and other mediators (for example, prostaglandins and leukotrienes) of the inflammatory response (Munck et al., 1984; Williams and Yarwood, 1990).

CRH neurons in the brain also influence sympathetic output, and their activation by cytokines (IL-1) leads to a clear rise in sympathetic firing and immune suppression. This could be tied pharmacologically to intact sympathetic functioning (Sundar et al., 1990).

In summary, infection leads to a host response that includes the release of cytokines, which promote and amplify cytotoxic actions to kill the infectious agent. Many such cytotoxic actions are not specific to the pathogen and, left unchecked, can damage the host. The additional ability of several cytokines to activate the HPAA and thus to raise levels of circulating glucocorticoids (which have immune-suppressive functions) via direct and indirect actions on central neurons is seen as one mechanism by which the initial immune reaction to infection is contained and toxic effects on the host are limited.

Biologic Rhythms in the Immune System and Nutrition

In Chapter 20 of this volume, Haus reviews the effects of biological rhythms on the functioning of the immune system. Alterations in the immune system are observed across the 24-hour day (circadian rhythm), 7-day week (circaseptan rhythm), and year (circannual rhythm).

Circadian rhythms are observed at all points in the development of the immune response, including the generation of immunoreactive molecules, immunoglobulin synthesis, and proliferation of immunocompetent cells. These rhythms result in differences in the immune response across the circadian cycle and are important for the response to both a primary antigenic stimulation and some extraneous challenge to the immunized subject. Alterations of the normal circadian (temporal) pattern of functioning of the cells in the immune system can have detrimental consequences.

Circaseptan rhythms also have been observed in immune responses. For example, the response of the body after kidney damage or exposure to an antigen (DeVecchi et al., 1981) or treatment with immunosuppressive compounds (Hrushesky and Marz, 1994) varies across an approximately 7 day period.

Immune responses vary across the year. These circannual rhythms may reflect variations in environmental variables, such as daily light levels, temperature, and differences in exposure to antigens, and may be mediated by seasonal changes in the function of the pineal or thyroid gland (Arendt, 1994; Nicolau and Haus, 1994). Circannual rhythms also have been observed in animals kept for generations under controlled environmental conditions and thus in some cases may be endogenous and genetically fixed.

Biologic Rhythms in the Number and Function of White Blood Cells

The number of white blood cells (WBCs) found in the circulation varies across the 24-h day. Several factors, including influx from storage sites, proliferation of cells, release of newly formed cells into the circulation, and cell destruction and removal, may contribute to the circadian variation in leukocyte number. Although circadian alterations in WBC number are relatively consistent within an individual, there is substantial interindividual variation in circadian patterns. Determinations of WBC number in 150 healthy individuals revealed that peaks or troughs in the values could occur at any hour of the day (Haus et al., 1983). Additionally, different cell types (such as lymphocytes, neutrophil leukocytes, monocytes, and eosinophils) display different rhythmic patterns. In most individuals, the number of lymphocytes peaks during the night, with the highest values between midnight and 1:00 a.m.

Lymphocyte function also varies across the day. Circadian variations in responses to external stimuli are reflected in changes in the number of cells in the peripheral blood and bone marrow. For example, the T-cell response to PHA and B-cell activation with pokeweed mitogen has been found to vary across the 24-h cycle (Haus et al., 1983). As another example, NK-cell activity in the blood of healthy adults is highest in the early morning and reaches a nadir during the night (Gatti et al., 1988).

Haus (see Chapter 20) discusses a number of factors, including alterations in the sleep–wake cycle, lymphoid tumors, and infection with lymphotrophic human HIV that can alter the circadian rhythms of circulating lymphocytes. For example, in HIV-infected patients, circadian rhythm disturbances in WBC numbers occur as an early consequence of the disease (Haus, 1996). Cytokine ratios also have been shown to vary in relation to circadian changes in glucocorticoid levels (DeRijk et al., 1997).

Biologic Rhythms in Cytokines and Their Inhibitors

Circadian variations in cytokines and their soluble receptors (for example, IL-1, IL-2, and IL-6) are found in the serum of healthy individuals. For example, serum concentrations of IL-6, which plays an important role in host defense mechanisms, inflammation, and immune responses, are highest during the night and lowest at midmorning (10:00 a.m.) (Sothern et al., 1995). Circadian rhythms in soluble IL-2 receptors have been found in healthy subjects, and rhythms in IL-6 (Arvidson et al., 1994; Suteanu et al., 1995) and neopterin (Suteanu et al., 1995) have been observed in patients with rheumatoid arthritis. Monocyte IL-1β and IL-1rα secretion and urinary IL-1rα excretion are significantly increased during the follicular phase of the menstrual cycle in premenopausal women relative to the luteal phase and significantly greater than those of men at all times (Lynch et al., 1994). The time at which cytokines reach the hypothalamus may in part determine the response to cytokines within the CNS and the subsequent activity of the endocrine system.

Biologic Rhythmicity of the Humoral Immune Response

In both animals and humans, there are circadian variations in the response of immunocompetent cells to an antigen and in the response of the immunized organism to secondary challenge following reintroduction of the antigen. For example, in mice injected with sheep red blood cells (commonly used in rodent studies), the fewest plaque-forming cells were found when the animals were injected at the beginning of the dark portion of the daily cycle (Fernandes et al., 1977). In humans, the concentrations of immunoglobulins and other components of serum proteins critical for immune function vary in a circadian manner. In healthy subjects, maximal concentrations of the three major types of immunoglobulins are detected in the early to late afternoon. Alterations in the circadian rhythms of these immunoglobulins have been noted in clinical conditions such as allergic asthma and allergic rhinitis.

Other rhythmic variations in humoral immune responses have been reported. Haus notes that circaseptan rhythms in antibody formation occur in a large number of animal species. Moreover, circannual rhythms in serum immunoglobulins, with peak concentrations during mid–summer to mid–autumn, have been reported in healthy human subjects.

Potential Clinical Relevance of Biologic Rhythms in Immune Function

Human immune responses to inoculation may vary as a function of the time of day at which an antigen is introduced. However, this variation may occur only with some antigens (for example, hepatitis B antigen) and may depend on other factors such as seasonal variations. Available data indicate that although all subjects achieve some level of immunity irrespective of the time of vaccination, higher antibody titers result when inoculations are given at midday (Pöllman and Pöllman, 1988). However, circadian variations in antibody responses to inoculations may be particularly relevant for the success of vaccinations in subjects with poor antibody formation.

Human immune responses to common antigens also vary in a circadian manner. For example, the greatest sensitivity to antigens of ragweed, house dust, and grass pollen is observed approximately 6 h preceding the middle of the patient's sleep cycle (see, for example, Lee et al., 1977). Similar rhythms have been reported for the hyperreactivity of the bronchial tree to histamine. The times of greatest cutaneous sensitivity to antigens and greatest susceptibility to asthmatic attacks correspond to the low point in the 24-h cycle of adrenocorticosteroid secretion and plasma catecholamine concentration. Haus suggests that these alterations in adrenocorticosteroids and catecholamines could contribute to the differences in day–night sensitivity to allergens and frequency of asthma attacks.

Factors That Interact with Circadian Rhythms in Immune Function

A number of factors, including patterns of sleep, the menstrual cycle, exercise, and the timing of food intake, can alter circadian rhythms associated with the functioning of the immune system. For example, sleep deprivation leads to alterations in biological rhythms and decrements in immune function and, if severe enough, can result in death (Everson, 1993). Impairments in immune function also have been noted in shift workers and individuals suffering from "jet lag." However, because shift work and jet lag are frequently associated with some degree of sleep deprivation, it is not known whether the alterations in immune function observed in these situations are primarily a consequence of sleep deprivation or of circadian desynchronization.

Circadian rhythms in immune function also are influenced by levels of physical activity and patterns of food intake. The effects of exercise on the immune system depend on the intensity of the activity, as described by Nieman in Chapter 17. Moderate exercise appears to improve certain immune functions, whereas extreme or exhaustive activities serve as immunosuppressants. Restricting food intake to a certain time of day (for example, all food eaten in the morning or at night) is associated with alterations in the circadian rhythms in digestive and metabolic functions, including endocrine and exocrine secretions from the pancreas and the secretion of liver enzymes (Fuller and Snoddy, 1968). These alterations could affect the timing of certain immune system responses, although critical evidence for such a relationship is not yet available.

Chronopharmacology and Chronotherapeutics

Knowledge of rhythmic changes in the immune system is important for treating of immune-related disorders and reducing the toxic effects of chemotherapeutic agents (see Haus, Chapter 20). Haus suggests that the timing of treatment relative to the critical periods of a cycle may permit optimal therapeutic effects with a minimal drug dose. Additionally, in the case of chemotherapy for cancer, understanding both circadian and seasonal rhythms may make it possible to obtain the desired treatment benefits with minimal toxicity (Levi, 1994).

In summary, these rhythms are important in mediating the body's responses to external stimuli such as pain, bacterial and viral infections, toxins, other antigens, and pharmacological agents. Many of these rhythms are inherited; however, others are adjusted in response to environmental variables such as light–dark cycles, environmental temperature, social situation, exercise, and food intake. Because military personnel may encounter infectious agents during field operations and can be subjected to extremes of environmental factors (for example, extreme heat or cold, intense physical exercise, sleep deprivation, and limited times for food consumption), it is important to consider biological rhythms in immune function. Additionally, knowledge of these time-related variations in immune function could be useful in determining the optimum timing of treatment for immune-related disorders.

Effects of Other Stressors on Immune Function

In addition to nutritional deficiency, physical exertion, and alterations in circadian rhythms, a number of other factors have been examined with respect to their influence on immune function or susceptibility to infection. These include temperature extremes, high altitude, sleep deprivation, emotional stress, smoking, and exposure to other environmental pollutants.

Extremes of Temperature

Attempts to examine the effects of cold temperature on immune function of laboratory animals have shown immune suppression in cold-exposed animals; however, the exposure of animals to cold temperatures is an established method of inducing stress. In addition, cold exposure influences sleep patterns for a period of time prior to acclimation (Pozos, 1996). Thus, it is not possible to conclude from this literature whether cold temperature exposures have effects on the immune system that are independent from those of a generalized stress response or sleep disturbance. Hot environments have been hypothesized to stimulate an increase in oxidative stress that could indirectly influence immune function (Young, 1990). As discussed by Morse in his presentation in Appendix D and others (Russell, 1998), attempts to study the effects of climate change on human health and immune function are also confounded by the altered pattern of infectious agents present in various climates.

Exposure to High Altitude

The influence of high-altitude exposure on immune function has been examined by several groups of investigators. Simon-Schnass (IOM, 1996) suggests that the increase in oxidative stress that appears to be induced at high altitude may be due to hypoxia, UV exposure, and other effects on the tricarboxylic acid cycle. However it is difficult to separate these effects from those of the anorexia that is induced by high altitude, the generally increased levels of physical exertion of people in field exercises at high altitude, and the extremes of temperature experienced at high altitude. Japanese investigators studying the mechanism of high-altitude pulmonary edema (HAPE) report significant elevations in many parameters of immune function, including IL-1β, IL-6 and 8, TNF-α, IL-1 receptor agonist, total WBC count, neutrophils, macrophages, lymphocytes, and a number of proteins (Kubo et al., 1998). These changes are believed to be associated with the early stage of HAPE and possibly with pulmonary hypertension; however it is not clear how the ability of the immune system to respond to infectious agents is affected.

Sleep Deprivation

The influence of sleep deprivation on immune function was mentioned earlier as a factor in the decreased immune response observed in the Ranger studies. Dinges and coworkers (1995) have reviewed studies of the influence of sleep deprivation on immune function. No consistent alterations in immune parameters have been reported across studies, suggesting that sleep deprivation has no consistently immunosuppresive effects that can be separated from the effects of other (simultaneously imposed) stressors. For example, the work of Haus (see Chapter 20) suggests that the effects of sleep deprivation would not be separable from those of changes in diurnal rhythms.

Emotional Stress

Deployed soldiers experience high levels of both chronic and acute emotional stress. As mentioned by Chandra (see Chapter 7), the stress of grieving for a bereaved spouse has been associated with depressed immune function in elderly individuals. Other studies by the same group have revealed that mucosal wound healing is slowed by the stress induced by final exams (Marucha et al., 1998), that immune response to vaccination and to HSV-1 exposure is inhibited by chronic stress (Glaser et al., 1998; Glaser and Kiecolt-Glaser, 1997), and that response to acute stress is influenced by the presence of chronic stress (Cacioppo et al., 1998). These researchers have proposed a model (the reactivity hypothesis) in which stress-related changes in HPA A activation are responsible for decreased immune response (Cacioppo et al., 1998).

Smoking and Environmental Pollutants

The effects of smoking on immune function are well known and are reviewed briefly in the discussion of vitamin C and immune function. Because the proportion of active-duty military personnel who smoke is higher than that of the general population, the effects of smoking on immune function are often superimposed on other stressors. Similarly, deployed troops may be exposed to a number of environmental pollutants (such as oil smoke) whose effects on the immune system must be determined. An upcoming CMNR workshop will examine these effects and their ability to be remedied by antioxidant administration.

Effects of Combined Stressors

It should be clear from the foregoing discussion that in the field, exposure to single stressors is not typical and the sources of stress may not always be immediately identifiable. Only well-controlled studies in clinical laboratory settings can assess the effects of single and combined stressors on immune function.

SUMMARY

The Ranger studies as well as other Army Operational Training Program studies have provided an opportunity to evaluate the effects of multiple physical, psychosocial, and nutritional stressors on immune system function. In this report, information is provided regarding the assessment of immune status under field conditions; the impact of compromised nutrition status on immune function; the interaction of health, exercise, and stress (both physical and psychological) in immune function; and the role of nutritional supplements and newer biotechnology methods reported to enhance immune function. The advantages and disadvantages of vitamin and mineral supplementation have been considered not only for their effects on immune system function, but for overall health in general. Finally, the physiologic and immune responses to alterations in neuroendocrine function are examined in depth. Included also is a thorough review of the interrelationship of biologic rhythms and immune system function.

During the workshop, a number of additional questions arose regarding the role of nutrition in immune function, and these are discussed at the conclusion of each author's chapter. These questions focused on assessment methodologies and individual stressors that could possibly alter nutrient requirements, which might in turn affect performance and immune function.

The CMNR's summary of the workshop and selected review of the nutrition and immunology literature set the stage for responding to the questions posed by the Army. The committee's responses, as well as its conclusions and recommendations, are presented in the next two chapters.

REFERENCES

Abbas, A.K., A.H. Lichtman, and J.S. Prober. 1991. Cellular and Molecular Immunology. Philadelphia, Pa.: W.B. Saunders Co.

Akbar, A.N., P.A. Fitzgerald-Bacarsly, M. deSousa, P.J. Giardina, M.W. Hilgartner, and R.W. Grady. 1986. Decreased natural killer activity in thalassemia major: A possible consequence of iron overload. J. Immunol. 136:1635–1640.

Aldred, A.R., and G. Schreiber. 1993. The negative acute phase proteins. Pp. 21–37 in Acute Phase Proteins: Molecular Biology, Biochemistry, and Clinical Applications, A. Mackiewicz, I. Kushner, and H. Bauman, eds. Boca Raton, Fla.: CRC Press.

Almond, J., and J. Pattison. 1997. Human BSE. Nature 389:437–438.

Andelman, M.B., and B.R. Sered. 1966. Utilization of dietary iron by term infants: A study of 1,048 infants from a low socioeconomic population. Am. J. Dis. Child. 111:45–55.

Arendt, J. 1994. The pineal. Pp. 348–362. In Biologic Rhythms in Clinical and Laboratory Medicine, Y. Touitou and E. Haus, editors. 2nd ed. Heidelberg: Springer-Verlag.

Arthur, J.R., and G.J. Beckett. 1994. Roles of selenium in type I iodothyronine 5'-deiodinase and in thyroid hormone and iodine metabolism. Pp. 93–115 in Selenium in Biology and Human Health, R.F. Burk, ed. New York: Springer-Verlag.

Arvidson, N.G., B. Gudbjornson, L. Elfman, and A.C. Ryden. 1994. Circadian rhythm of serum interleukin 6 in rheumatoid arthritis. Ann. Rheumat. Dis. 53(8):521–524.

Bai, J., S. Wu, K. Ge, X. Deng, and C. Su. 1980. The combined effect of selenium deficiency and viral infection on the myocardium of mice. Acta Acad. Med. Sci. Sin. 2:29–31.

Bala, S., M.L. Failla and J.K. Lunney. 1991. Alterations in splenic lymphoid cell subsets and activation antigens in copper-deficient rats. J. Nutr. 121(5):745–753.

Ballmer, P.E., and H.B. Staehlin. 1994. Beta carotene, vitamin E, and lung cancer. N. Engl. J. Med. 330(15):1029–1035.

Barber, A.E., S.M. Coyle, M.A. Marano, E. Fischer, S.E. Calvano, Y. Fong, L.L. Moldawer, and S.F. Lowry. 1993. Glucocorticoid therapy alters hormonal and cytokine responses to endotoxin in man. J. Immunol. 150:1999–2006.

Barbul, A., D.A. Sisto, H.L. Wasserkrug, and G. Efron. 1981. Arginine stimulates lymphocyte immune response in healthy human beings. Surgery 90(2):244–251.

Barone, J., J.R. Herbert, and M.M. Reddy. 1989. Dietary fat and natural-killer-cell activity. Am. J. Clin. Nutr. 50(4):861–867.

Barret-Connor, E. 1971. Bacterial infection and sickle cell anaemia. An analysis of 250 infections in 166 patients and a review of the literature. Medicine 50:97–112.

Beaton, G.H. 1996. Basic biology and biology of interventions: A synthesis view. In Beyond Nutritional Recommendations: Implementing Science for Healthier Populations, C. Garza, J.D. Haas, J-P. Habicht, and D.L. Pelletier, eds. Proceedings from the 14th Annual Bristol-Myers Squibb/Mead Johnson Nutrition Research Symposium, June 5–7, 1995. Ithaca, N.Y.: Cornell University.

Beisel, W.R. 1977. Symposium on impact of infection on nutritional status of the host. Am. J. Clin. Nutr. 30:1203–1371, 1439–1566.

Beisel, W.R. 1982. Single nutrients and immunity. Am. J. Clin. Nutr. 35(suppl.):415–468.

Beisel, W.R. 1991. Nutrition and infection. Pp. 507–542 in Nutritional Biochemistry and Metabolism, 2nd ed., M.C. Linder, ed. New York: Elsevier.

Beisel, W.R. 1992 Metabolic responses of the host to infections. Pp. 1–13 in Textbook of Pediatric Infectious Diseases, 3d ed., R.D. Feigin and J.D. Cherry, eds. Philadelphia: W.B. Saunders Co.

Beisel, W.R. 1995. Herman Award Lecture, 1995: Infection-induced malnutrition—From cholera to cytokines. Am. J. Clin. Nutr. 62:813–819.

Beisel, W.R., and P.Z. Sobocinski. 1980. Metabolic Aspects of Fever. Pp. 39–48 in Fever, J.M. Lipton, ed. New York: Raven Press.

Beisel, W.R., and J.M. Talbot, eds. 1985. Research Opportunities on Immunocompetence in Space. Report of the Life Science Research Office, FASEB. Prepared for the Life Science Division, Office of Space Science and Applications, NASA, Washington, D.C. Bethesda, Md.: Life Science Research Office, FASEB.

Beisel, W.R., W.D. Sawyer, E.D. Ryll, and D. Crozier. 1967. Metabolic effects of intracellular infections in man. Ann. Int. Med. 67:744–779.

Beisel, W.R., K.A. Woeber, P.J. Bartelloni, and S.H. Ingbar. 1968. Growth hormone response during sandfly fever. J. Clin. Endocrinol. Metab. 28(8):1220–1223.

Bendich, A., and R.K. Chandra, ed. 1990. Micronutrients and immune functions. New York, N.Y.: New York Academy of Sciences.

Berry, M.J., and P.R. Larsen. 1992. The role of selenium in thyroid hormone action. Endocr. Rev. 13:207–219.

Bertini, R., M. Bianchi, and P. Ghezzi. 1988. Adrenalectomy sensitizes mice to the lethal effects of interleukin 1 and tumor necrosis factor. J. Exp. Med. 167:1708–1712.

Bessey, P.Q., J.M. Watters, T.T. Aoki, and D.W. Wilmore. 1984. Combined hormonal infusion simulates the metabolic response to injury. Ann. Surg. 200:264–281.

Bistrian, B.R., G.L. Blackburn, N.S. Scrimshaw, J.P. Flatt. 1975. Cellular immunity in semistarved states in hospitalized adults. Am. J. Clin. Nutr. 28:1148–1155.

Bjerve, K.S., S. Fischer, F. Wammer, and T. England. 1989. α-linolenic acid and longchain omega-3 fatty acid supplementation in three patients with omega-3 fatty acid deficiency. Am. J. Clin. Nutr. 49:290–300.

Blakley, B.R., and D.L. Hamilton. 1987. The effect of copper deficiency on the immune response in mice. Drug Nutr. Interact. 5:103–111.

Blalock, J.F. 1989. A molecular basis for bidirectional communication between the immune and neuroendocrine systems. Physiol. Rev. 69:1–32.

Blazar, B.A., M.L. Rodrick, J.B. O'Mahoney, J.J. Wood, P.Q. Bessey, D.W. Wilmore, and J.A. Mannick. 1986. Suppression of natural killer-cell function in humans following thermal and traumatic injury. J. Clin. Immunol. 6:26–36.

Bocchieri, M.H., M.A. Talle, L.M. Maltese, I.R. Ragucci, C.C. Hwang, and G. Goldstein. 1995. Whole blood culture for measuring mitogen induced T cell proliferation provides superior correlations with disease state and T cell phenotype in asymptomatic HIV-infected subjects. J. Immunol. Meth. 181:233–243.

Borelli, M.I., F.E Estivariz, and J.J. Gagliardino. 1996. Evidence for the paracrine action of islet-derived corticotrophin-like peptides on the regulation of insulin release. Metabolism 45(5):565–570.

Bower, R.H., F.B. Cerra, B. Bershadksy, J.J. Licari, D.B. Hoyt, G.L. Jensen, C.T. Van Buren, M.M. Rothkopf, J.M. Daly and B.R. Adelsberg. 1995. Early enteral administration of a formula (Impact) supplemented with arginine, nucleotides, and fish oil in intensive care unit patients: results of a multicenter, prospective, randomized, clinical trial. Crit. Care Med. 23(3):436-449.

Bray, R.M., L.A. Kroutil, S.C. Wheeless, M.E. Marsden, S.L. Bailey, J.A. Fairbank, and T.C. Harford. 1995. Health behavior and health promotion. Department of Defense Survey of Health-Related Behaviors among Military Personnel. Report No. RTI/6019/06-FR. Research Triangle Park, N.C.: Research Triangle Institute.

Breman, J.G., G. van der Groen, C.J. Peters, and D.L. Heymann. 1997. International colloquium on Ebola virus research: summary report. J. Infect. Dis. 176(4):1058–1063.

Buchanan, W.M. 1971. Shock in bantu siderosis. Am. J. Clin. Pathol. 55:401–406.

Burk, R.F. 1997. Selenium-dependent gluthathione peroxidases. In Comprehensive Toxicology, vol. 3, Biotransformation, F.P. Guengerich, ed. Oxford: Pergamon.

Butler, L.D., N.K. Layman, P.E. Riedl, R.L. Cain, and J. Shellhaas. 1989. Neuroendocrine regulation of in vivo cytokine production and effects: I. In vivo regulatory networks involving the neuroendocrine system, interleukin-1 and tumor necrosis factor-α. J. Neuroimmunol. 24:143–153.

Cacioppo, J.T., G.G. Berntson, W.B. Malarkey, J.K. Kiecolt-Glaser, J.F. Sheridan, K.M. Poehlmann, M.H. Burleson, J.M. Ernst, L.C. Hawkley, and R. Glaser. 1998. Autonomic, neuroendocrine, and immune responses to psychological stress: the reactivity hypothesis. Ann. NY Acad. Sci. 840:664–673.

Calder, P.C. 1997. n-3 polyunsaturated fatty acids and cytokine production in health and disease. Ann. Nutr. Metab. 41:203-34.

Calder, P.C. 1998. Dietary fatty acids and the immune system. Nutr. Rev. 56:S70–83.

Calvano, S.E., J.D. Albert, A. Legaspi, B.C. Organ, K.J. Tracey, S.F. Lowry, G.T. Shires, and A.C. Antonacci. 1987. Comparison of numerical and phenotypic leukocyte changes during constant hydrocortisone infusion in normal humans with those in thermally injured patients. Surg. Gynecol. Obstet. 164:509–520.

Cannon, J.G., S.N. Meydani, R.A. Fielding, M.A. Fiatarone, M. Meydani, M. Farhangmehr, S.F. Orencole, J.B. Blumberg, and W.J. Evans. 1991. The acute-phase response in exercise. II. Associations between vitamin E, cytokines and muscle proteolysis. Am. J. Physiol. 260:R1235–R1240.

Carniel, E., D. Mazigh, and H.H. Mollaret. 1987. Expression of iron-regulated proteins in Yersinia species and their relation to virulence. Infect. Immun. 55:277–280.

Carniel, E., O. Mercereau-Puijalon, and S. Bonnefoy. 1989. The gene coding for the 190,000-dalton iron-regulated protein of Yersinia species is present only in the highly pathogenic strains. Infect. Immun. 57:1211–1217.

Castell, L.M., J.R. Poortmans, and E.A. Newsholme. 1996. Does glutamine have a role in reducing infections in athletes? Eur. J. Appl. Physiol. 73:488–490.

Caughey, G.E., E. Montzioris, R.A. Gibson, L.G. Cleland, and M.J. James. 1996. The effect on human tumor necrosis factor α and interleukin 1β production of diets enriched in n-3 fatty acids from vegetable oil or from fish oil. Am. J. Clin. Nutr. 63:116–122.

CDC (Centers for Disease Control and Prevention). 1998. Recommendations to Prevent and Control Iron Deficiency in the United States. MMWR 47(RR-3):1–36.

Chandra, R.K. 1982. Excessive intake of zinc impairs immune response. J. Am. Med. Assoc. 252:1443–1446.

Chandra, R.K., ed. 1988. Nutrition and Immunology. New York: Alan R. Liss, Inc.

Chandra, R.K. 1991. 1990 McCollum award lecture. Nutrition and immunity: Lessons from the past and new insights into the future. 53:1087–1101.

Chaudiere, J., E.C. Wilhelmsen, and A.L. Tappel. 1984. Mechanism of selenium-glutathione peroxidase and its inhibition by mercaptocarboxylic acids and other mercaptans. J. Biol. Chem. 259:1043–1050.

Chrousos, G.P. 1995. The hypothalamic–pituitary–adrenal axis and immune-mediated inflammation. New Engl. J. Med. 332:1351–1362.

Cioffi, W.G., D.C. Gore, L.W. Rue III, G. Carrougher, H.P. Guler, W.F. McManus, and B.A. Pruitt Jr. 1994. Insulin-like growth factor-1 lowers protein oxidation in patients with thermal injury. Ann. Surg. 220:310–316.

Coceani, F., J. Lees, and C.A. Dinarello. 1988. Occurrence of interleukin-1 in cerebrospinal fluid of the conscious cat. Brain Res. 446:245–250.

Consolazio, C.F., L.O. Matoush, R.A. Nelson, R.S. Harding, and J.E. Canham. 1966. Nutritional survey: Ranger Department, Fort Benning, Georgia. Laboratory Report No. 291. Denver, Colo.: U.S. Army Medical Research and Nutrition Laboratory, Fitzimons General Hospital.

Crofford, L.J., J.I. Rader, M.C. Dalakas, R.H. Hill Jr., S.W. Page, L.L. Needham, L.S. Brady, M.P. Heyes, R.L. Wilder, P.W. Gold, et al. 1990. l-tryptophan implicated in human eosinophilia-myalgia syndrome causes fascitis and perimyositis in the Lewis rat. J. Clin. Invest. 86:1757–1763.

Croteau, W., S.L. Whittemore, M.J. Schneider, and D.L. St. Germain. 1995. Cloning and expression of a cDNA for a mammalian type III iodothyronine deiodinase. J. Biol. Chem. 270:16569–16575.

Cunningham-Rundles, S., ed. 1993. Nutritional Modulation of the Immune Response. New York: Marcel Decker, Inc.

Cupps, T.R., and A.S. Fauci. 1982. Corticosteroid-mediated immunoregulation in man. Immunol. Rev. 65:133–155.

Davis, J.M., J.D. Albert, K.J. Tracy, S.E. Calvano, S.F. Lowry, G.T. Shires, and R.W. Yurt. 1991. Increased neutrophil mobilization and decreased chemotaxis during cortisol and epinephrine infusions. J. Trauma 31:725–731.

Dealler, S., and R.W. Lacey. 1990. Beef and bovine spongiform encephalopathy: the risk persists. Nutr. Health 7(3)117–133.

Denham, S., and I.J. Rowland. 1992. Inhibition of the reactive proliferation of lymphocytes by activated macrophages: The role of nitric oxide. Clin. Exp. Immunol. 87:157–162.

DeRijk, R., D. Michelson, D. Karp, J. Petrides, E. Galliven, P. Deuster, G. Paciotti, P.W. Gold, and E.M. Sternberg. 1997. Exercise and circadian rhythm-induced variations in plasma cortisol differentially regulate interleukin-1 β (IL-1 β), Il-6, and tumor necrosis factor-α (TNF α) production in humans: High sensitivity of TNF α and resistance of IL-6. J. Clin. Endocrinol. Metab. 82(7):2182–2191.

DeRijk, R.H., J. Petrides, P. Deuster, P.W. Gold, and E.M. Sternberg. 1996. Changes in corticosteroid sensitivity of peripheral blood lymphocytes after strenuous exercise in humans. J. Clin. Endocrinol. Metab. 81(1):228–235.

DeVecchi, A., F. Halberg, R.B. Sothern, A. Cantaluppi, and C. Ponticelli. 1981. Circaseptan rhythmic aspects of rejection in treated patients with kidney transplant. Pp. 339–353 in Chronopharmacology and Chemotherapeutics, C.A. Walker, C.M. Winget, and K.F.A. Soliman, eds. Tallahasse, FL: A and M University Foundation.

Dinges, D.F., S.D. Douglas, S. Hamarman, L. Zaugg, and S. Kapoor. 1995. Sleep deprivation and human immune function. Adv. Neuroimmunol. 5:97–110.

Endres, S., R. Ghorhani, V.E. Kelley, K. Georgilis, G. Lonnemann, J.W.M. van der Meer, J.G. Cannon, T.S. Rogers, M.S. Klempner, P.C. Weber, E.J. Schaefer, S.M. Wolff, and C.A. Dinarello. 1989. The effect of dietary supplementation with n-3 polyunsaturated fatty acids on the synthesis of interleukin-1 and tumor necrosis factor by mononuclear cells. N. Eng. J. Med. 320:265–271.

Endres, S., S.N. Madden, R. Ghorbani, R. Schindler, and C.A. Dinarello. 1993. Dietary supplementation with n-3 fatty acids suppresses interleukin-2 production and mononuclear cell proliferation. J. Leukocyte Biol. 54:599–603.

Eskola J., O. Ruuskanen, E. Soppi, M.K. Viljanen, M. Järvinen, H. Toivonen, and K. Kouvalainen. 1978. Effect of sport stress on lymphocyte transformation and antibody formation. Clin. Exp. Immunol. 32:339–345.

Everson, C.A. 1993. Sustained sleep deprivation impairs host defense. Am. J. Physiol. 265:R1148–R1154.

Fairbrother, B., E.W. Askew, M.Z. Mays, R. Shippee, K.E. Friedl, R.W. Hoyt, M. Kramer, T.R. Kramer, and K. Popp. 1993. Nutritional assessment of soldiers during the special forces assessment and selection course. USARIEM Study Protocol, May 1993. Natick, Mass.: U.S. Army Research Institute of Environmental Medicine.

Fan, J., X. Gong, J. Wu, Y. Zhang, and R. Xu. 1994. Effect of glucocorticoid receptor (GR) blockade on endotoxemia in rats. Circul. Shock 42:76–82.

Fernandes, G., E.J. Yunis, and F. Halberg. 1977. Circadian aspect of immune response in the mouse. Pp. 233–249 in Chronobiology in Allergy and Immunology, J.P. McGovern, M.H. Smolensky, and A. Reinberg, eds. Chicago, Ill.: Charles C Thomas.

Fleet, J.C. 1995. A new role for lactoferrin: DNA binding and transcription activation. Nutr. Rev. 53:226–227.

Forse, R.A., ed. 1994. Diet, Nutrition, and Immunity. Boca Raton, Fla.: CRC Press.

Fraker, P.J., L.E. King, B.A. Garry, and C.A. Medina. 1993. The immunopathology of zinc deficiency in humans and rodents. Pp. 267–283 in Human Nutrition—A Comprehensive Treatise, D.M. Klurfeld, ed., vol. 8: Nutrition and Immunology. New York: Plenum Press.

Friedl, K.E., L.J. Marchitelli, D.E. Sherman, and R. Tulle. 1990. Nutritional assessment of cadets at the U.S. Military Academy: Part 1. Anthropometric and biochemical measures. Technical Report No. T4-91. Natick, Mass.: U.S. Army Research Institute of Environmental Medicine.

Friman, G., E. Larsson, and C. Rolf. 1997. Interaction between infection and exercise with special reference to myocarditis and the increased frequency of sudden deaths among young Swedish orienteers 1979–1992. Scand. J. Infect. Dis. Supp. 104:41–49.

Fuller, R., and H. Snoddy. 1968. Feeding schedule alteration of daily rhythm in tyrosine α-ketoglutaride transaminase in rat liver. Science 159:738

Gatti, G., R. Cavallo, M.L. Sartori, R. Carignola, R. Masera, D. Delponte, A. Salvadori, and A. Angeli. 1988. Circadian variations of interferon-induced enhancement of human natural killer (NK) cell activity. Cancer Detec. 12:431–438.

Gershwin, M.E., R.S. Beach, and L.S. Hurley, eds. 1985. Nutrition and Immunology. Orlando, Fla.: Academic Press.

Glaser, R., and J.K. Kiecolt-Glaser, 1997. Chronic stress modulates the virus-specific immune response to latent herpes simplex virus type 1. Ann. Behav. Med. 19:78–82.

Glaser, R., J.K. Kiecolt-Glaser, W.B. Malarkey, and J.F. Sheridan. 1998. The influence of psychological stress on the immune response to vaccines. Ann. NY Acad. Sci. 840:649–655.

Good, M.F., L.W. Powell, and J.W. Halliday. 1988. Iron status and cellular immune competence. Blood Rev. 2:43–49.

Griffin, P.M., and R.V. Tauxe. 1991. The epidemiology of infections caused by *Escherichia coli* O157:H7, other enterohemorrhagic *E. coli*, and the associated hemolytic uremic syndrome. Epidemiol. Rev.

Griffiths, E. 1987. Iron in biological systems. Pp. 1–25 in Iron and Infection, J.J. Bullen and E. Griffiths, eds. London: John Wiley & Sons.

Griffiths, R.D., C. Jones, and T.E. Palmer. 1997. Six month outcome of critically ill patients given glutamine-supplemental parenteral nutrition. Nutrition 13:295–302.

Gross, R.L., and P.M. Newberne. 1976. Malnutrition, the thymolymphatic system and immunocompetence. Adv. Exp. Med. Biol. 73:179–187.

Gross, R.L., J.V.O. Reid, P.M. Newberne, B. Burgess, R. Marston, and W. Hift. 1975. Depressed cell-mediated immunity in megaloblastic anemia due to folic acid deficiency. Am. J. Clin. Nutr. 28:225–232.

Gubler, D.J., and D.W. Trent. 1993. Emergence of epidemic dengue/dengue hemorrhagic fever as a public health problem in the Americas. Infect. Agents Dis. 2:383–393.

Hallberg, L., C. Bengtsson, L. Lapidus, G. Lindstedt, P.A. Lundberg and L. Hulten. 1993. Screening for iron deficiency: an analysis based on bone-marrow examinations and serum ferritin determinations in a population sample of women. Br. J. Haematol. 85(4):787–798.

Haus, E. 1996. Biologic rhythms in hematology. Path. Biol. 44(6):618–630.

Haus, E., D.J. Lakatua, J. Swoyer, and L. Sackett-Lundeen. 1983. Chronobiology in hematology and immunology. Am. J. of Anatomy 168:467–517.

Hemila, H. 1997. Vitamin C intake and susceptibility to the common cold. Br. J. Nutr. 77(1):59–72.

Herbert, V. 1997. Destroying immune homeostasis in normal adults with antioxidant supplements. Am. J. Clin. Nutr. 65(6):1901–1903.

Hershko, C., and T.E.A. Peto. 1987. Non-transferrin plasma iron. Brit. J. Haematology 66:149–151.

Hershko, C., T.E.A. Peto, and D.J. Weatherall. 1988. Iron and infection. Br. Med. J. 296:660–664.

Hinton, P.S., C.A. Peterson, H.C. Lo, H. Yang, D. McCarthy, and D.M. Ney. 1995. Insulin-like growth factor-I enhances immune response in dexamethasone-treated or surgically stressed rats maintained with total parenteral nutrition. JPEN J. Parenter. Enter. Nutr. 19:444–452.

Hodges, R.E., W.B. Bean, M.A. Ohlson, and R.E. Bleiler. 1962. Factors affecting human antibody response. IV. Pyridoxine deficiency. Am. J. Clin. Nutr. 11:180–186.

Hollingsworth, J.W., and J. Carr. 1973. 3H-uridine incorporation as a T lymphocyte indicator in the rat. Cell Immunol. 8(2):270–279.

Hopkins, R.G., and M.L. Failla. 1997. Copper deficiency reduces interleukin-2 (IL-2) production and IL-2 mRNA in human T-lymphocytes. J. Nutr. 127(2):257–262.

Hrushesky, W.J.M., and W.J. Marz. 1994. Chronochemotherapy of malignant tumors: Temporal aspects of antineoplastic drug toxicity. Pp. 611–634 in Biologic Rhythms in Clinical and Laboratory Medicine, 2nd ed., Y.Touitou and E.Haus, eds. Heidelberg: Springer-Verlag.

Hughes D.A., A.C. Pinder, Z. Piper, I.T. Johnson, and E.K. Lund. 1996. Fish oil supplementation inhibits the expression of major histocompatibility complex class II molecules and adhesion molecules on human monocytes. Am. J. Clin. Nutr. 63:267–272.

IOM (Institute of Medicine). 1992. A Nutritional Assessment of U.S. Army Ranger Training Class 11/91. A brief report of the Committee on Military Nutrition Research, Food and Nutrition Board. March 23. Washington, D.C.: National Academy Press.

IOM (Institute of Medicine). 1993b. Review of the Results of Nutritional Intervention, Ranger Training Class 11/92 (Ranger II), B.M. Marriott, ed. A report of the Committee on Military Nutrition Research, Food and Nutrition Board. Washington, D.C.: National Academy Press.

IOM (Institute of Medicine). 1995a. Not Eating Enough, Overcoming Underconsumption of Military Operational Rations, B.M. Marriott, ed. A report of the Committee on Military Nutrition Research, Food and Nutrition Board. Washington, D.C.: National Academy Press.

Johnson, H.L., H.J. Krzywicki, J.E. Canham, J.H. Skala, T.A. Daws, R.A. Nelson, C.F. Consolazio, and P.P. Waring. 1976. Evaluation of calorie requirements for Ranger training at Fort Benning, Georgia. Technical Report No. 34. Presidio of San Francisco, Calif.: Letterman Army Institute of Research.

Juretic, A., G.C. Spagnoli, H. Hörig, R. Babst, K. von Bremen, F. Harder, and M. Heberer. 1994. Glutamine requirements in the generation of lymphokine-activated killer cells. Clin. Nutr. 13:42–49.

Kakucska, I., L.I. Romero, B.D. Clark, J.M. Rondeel, Y. Qi, S. Alex, C.H. Emerson, and R.M. Lechan. 1994. Suppression of thyrotropin-releasing hormone gene expression by interleukin-1β in the rat: Implications for nonthyroidal illness. Neuroendocrinology 59(2):129–137.

Kanter, M.M., L.A. Nolte, and J.O. Holloszy. 1993. Effects of an antioxidant vitamin mixture on lipid peroxidation at rest and postexercise. J. Appl. Physiol. 74:965–969.

Kapcala, L.P., T. Chautard, and R.L. Eskay. 1995. The protective role of the hypothalamic–pituitary–adrenal axis against lethality produced by immune, infectious, and inflammatory stress. Ann. N.Y. Acad. Sci. 771:419–437.

Kay, J.E., and C.R. Benzie. 1986. The role of the transferrin receptor in lymphocyte activation. Immunol. Lett. 12:55–58.

Kelley, D.S., D.B. Branch, and J.M. Iacono. 1989. Nutritional modulation of human status. Nutr. Res. 9:965–975.

Kelley, D.S., L.B. Branch, J.E. Love, P.C. Taylor, Y.M. Rivera, and J.M. Iacono. 1991. Dietary α-linolenic acid and immunocompetence in humans. Am. J. Clin. Nutr. 53:40–46.

Kelley, D.S., P.A. Dauda, L.B. Branch, H.L. Johnson, P.C. Taylor, and B. Mackey. 1994. Energy restriction decreases number of circulating natural killer cells and serum levels of immunoglobulins in overweight women. Eur. J. Clin. Nutr. 48(1):9–18.

Kelley, D.S., R.M. Dougherthy, L.B. Branch, P.C. Taylor, and J.M. Iacono. 1992a. Concentration of dietary n-6 polyunsaturated fatty acids and human status. Clin. Immunol. Immunopath. 62:240–244.

Kelley, D.S., G.J. Nelson, L.B. Branch, P.C. Taylor, U.M. Rivera, and P.C. Schmidt. 1992b. Salmon diet and human immune status. Eur. J. Clin. Nutr. 46:397–404.

Kelley, D.S., P.C. Taylor, G.J. Nelson, P.C. Schmidt, and B.E. Mackey. 1996. Effects of dietary arachidonic acid on human response. FASEB J. 10:A557.

Keusch, G.T. 1994. Nutrition and infection. Pp. 1241–1258 in Modern Nutrition in Health and Disease, 8th ed., M.E. Shils, J.A. Olson, and M. Shike, eds. Malvern, Pa.: Lea and Febiger.

Keusch, G.T., and M.J.G. Farthing. 1986. Nutrition and infection. Annu. Rev. Nutr. 6:131–154.

Khaw, K.T., P. Woodhouse. 1995. Interrelation of vitamin C, infection, haemostatic factors, and cardiovascular disease. BMJ 310(6994):1559–1563.

Kiremidjian-Schumacher, L.O., and G. Stotzky. 1987. Selenium and immune responses. Environ. Res. 42:277–303.

Kirk, S.J., and A. Barbul. 1992. Arginine and immunity. Pp. 160–161 in Encyclopedia of Immunology, Book I, I.M. Roitt and P.J. Delves, eds. London: Academic Press.

Kirk, S.J., M.C. Regan, H.L. Wasserkrug, M Sodeyama, and A. Barbul. 1992. Arginine enhances T-cell responses in athymic nude mice. J. Parenter. Enter. Nutr. 16:429–432.

Kirkwood, B.J. 1996. Epidemiology of interventions to improve vitamin A status in order to reduce child mortality and morbidity. In Beyond Nutritional Recommendations: Implementing Science for Healthier Populations, C. Garza, J.D. Haas, J-P. Habicht, and D.L. Pelletier, eds. Proceedings from the 14th Annual Bristol-Myers Squibb/Mead Johnson Nutrition Research Symposium, June 5–7, 1995. Ithaca, N.Y.: Cornell University.

Kjolhede, C., and W.R. Beisel. 1995. Vitamin A and the immune function: A symposium. J. Nutr. Immunol. 4:xv–143.

Klausner, R. D., T.A. Roualt, and J.B. Harford. 1993. Regulating the fate of mRNA: The control of cellular iron metabolism. Cell 72:19–28.

Klicka, M.V., D.E. Sherman, N. King, K.E. Friedl, and E.W. Askew. 1993. Nutritional assessment of cadets at the U.S. Military Academy: Part 2. Assessment of nutritional intake. Technical Report No. T94-1. Natick, Mass.: U.S. Army Research Institute of Environmental Medicine.

Knox, J.R. Demling, D. Wilmore, P. Sarraf, and A. Santos. 1995. Increased survival after major thermal injury: The effect of growth hormone therapy in adults. J. Trauma 39:526–530.

Koshland Jr., D.E. 1992. Science's 1992 molecule of the year [editorial]. Science 258:1861.

Kramer, T.R., R.J. Moore, R.L. Shippee, K.E. Friedl, L. Martinez-Lopez, M.M. Chan, and E.W. Askew. 1997. Effects of food restriction in military training on T-lymphocyte responses. Int. J. Sports Med. 18:S84–S90.

Kramer, T.R., K. Praputpittaya, Y. Yuttabootr, R. Singkamani, and M. Trakultivakorn. 1990. The relationship between plasma zinc and cellular immunity to Candida albicans in young females of northern Thailand. Ann. N.Y. Acad. Sci. 587:300–302.

Kramer, T.R., N. Schoene, L.W. Douglass, J.T. Judd, R. Ballard-Barbash, P.R. Taylor, H.N. Bhagavan, and P.P. Nair. 1991. Increased vitamin E intake restores fish-oil-induced suppressed blastogenesis of mitogen-simulated T-lymphocytes. Am. J. Clin. Nutr. 54:896–902.

Kramer, T.R., E. Udomkesmalee, S. Dhanamitta, S. Sirisinha, S. Charoenkiatkul, S. Tuntipopipat, O. Banjong, N. Rojroongwasinkul, and J.C. Smith Jr. 1993.

Lymphocyte responsiveness of children supplemented with vitamin A and zinc. Am. J. Clin. Nutr. 58:566–570.

Krantman, H.J., S.R. Young, B.J. Ank, C.M. O'Donnell, G.S. Rachelefsky, and G.S.Stiehm. 1982. Immune function in pure iron deficiency. Am. J. Dis. Child. 136:840–844.

Kubes, P., M. Suzuki, and D.N. Granger. 1991. Nitric oxide: An endogenous modulator of leukocyte adhesion. Proc. Natl. Acad. Sci. U.S.A. 88:4651–4655.

Kubo, K., M. Hanaoka, T. Hayano, T. Miyahara, T. Hachiya, M. Hayasaka, T. Koizumi, K. Fujimoto, T. Kobayashi, and T. Honda. 1998. Inflammatory cytokines in BAL fluid and pulmonary hemodynamics in high-altitude pulmonary edema. Respir. Physiol. 111:301–310.

Kuby, J. 1997. Immunology, 3d ed. New York: W.H. Freeman and Company.

Lalonde, R., and T. Boetz-Marquard. 1997. The neurobiological basis of movement initiation. Rev. Neurosci. 8(1):35–54.

Lands, W.E. 1991. Biosynthesis of prostaglandins. Annu. Rev. Nutr. 11:41–60.

Lee, R.E., M.H. Smolensky, C.S. Leach, and J.P. McGovern. 1977. Circadian rhythms in the cutaneous reactivity to histamine and selected antigens, including phase relationship to urinary cortisol excretion. Ann. Allergy 38(4):231–236.

Lee, T.H., R.L. Hoover, J.D. Williams, R.I. Sperling, J. Ravalese, B.W. Spur, D.R. Robinson, E.J. Corey, R.A. Lewis, and K.F. Austen. 1985. Effect of dietary enrichment with eicosapentaenoic acid and docosahexaenoic acids on in vitro neutrophil and monocyte leukotriene generation and neutrophil function. N. Engl. J. Med. 312:1217–1224.

Levi, F.A., R. Zidani, J.M. Vannetzel, B. Perpoint, C. Focan, R. Faggiuolo, P. Chollet, C. Garufi, M. Itzhaki, and L. Dogliotti. 1994. Chronomodulated versus fixed-infusion-rate delivery of ambulatory chemotherapy with oxaliplatin, fluorouracil, and folinic acid (leucovorin) in patients with colorectal cancer metastases: a randomized multi-institutional trial. J. Natl. Cancer Inst. 86(21):1608–1617.

Levine, M., C. Conry-Cantilena, Y. Wang, R.W. Welch, P.W. Washko, K.R. Dhariwal, J.B. Park, A. Lazarev, J.F. Graumlich, J. King, and L.R. Cantilena. 1996. Vitamin C pharmacokinetics in healthy volunteers: evidence for a recommended dietary allowance. Proc. Natl. Acad. Sci. 93(8):3704–3709.

Liew, F.Y., S. Millott, C. Parkinson et al. 1990. Macrophage killing of Leishmania parasite in vivo is medicated by nitric oxide from L-arginine. J. Immunol. 144:4794–4797.

Love, L.A., J.L. Rader, L.J. Crofford, R.B. Raybourne, M.A. Principato, S.W. Page, M.W. Trucksess, M.J. Smith, E.M. Dugan, and M.L. Turner. 1993. Pathological and immunological effects of ingesting L-tryptophan and 1,1'-ethylidenebis (L-tryptophan) in Lewis rats. J. Clin. Invest. 91:804–811.

Lukasewycz, O.A., and J.R. Prohaska. 1990. Immune response in copper deficiency. Ann. N.Y. Acad. Sci. 587:147–159.

Lynch, E.A., C.A. Dinarello, and J.G. Cannon. 1994. Gender differences in IL-1 alpha, IL-1 beta, and IL-1 receptor antagonist secretion from mononuclear cells and urinary excretion. J. Immunol. 153(1):300–306.

MacBurney, M., L.S. Young, T.R. Ziegler, and D.W. Wilmore. 1994. A cost-evaluation of glutamine-supplemented parenteral nutrition in adult bone marrow transplant patients. J. Am. Diet. Assoc. 94:1263–1266.

Macha, M., M. Shlafer, and M.J. Kluger. 1990. Human neutrophil hydrogen peroxide generation following physical exercise. J. Sports Med. Phys. Fit. 30:412–419.

MacPhee, I.A., F.A. Antoni, and D.W. Mason. 1989. Spontaneous recovery of rats from experimental allergic encephalomyelitis is dependent on regulation of the immune system by endogenous adrenal corticosteroids. J. Exp. Med. 169:431–445.

Madden, S.N., S. Endres, M.N. Woods, B.R. Goldin, C. Soo, A. Morrill-Labrode, C.A. Dinarello, and S.L. Gorbach. 1991. Oral n-3 fatty acid supplementation suppresses cytokine production and lymphocyte proliferation: Comparision between young and old women. J. Nutr. 121:547–555.

Martinez, F, E.R. Abril, D.L. Earnest, and R. R. Watson. 1992. Alcohol and cytokine secretion. Alcohol 9(6):455–458.

Marucha, P.T., J.K. Kiecolt-Glaser, and M. Favagehi. 1998. Mucosal wound healing is impaired by examination stress. Psychosom. Med. 60:362–365.

McMurray, D.N., S.A. Loomis, L.J. Casazza, H. Rey, and R. Miranda. 1981. Development of impaired cell-mediated immunity in mild and moderate malnutrition. Am. J. Clin. Nutr. 34(1):68–77.

Meydani, S.N., and M. Hayek. 1992. Vitamin E and immune response. Pp. 105–128 in Nutrition and Immunology, R.K. Chandra, ed. St. John's, Newfoundland: ARTS Biomedical.

Meydani, S.N., M.P. Barklund, S. Liu, M. Meydani, R.A. Miller, J.G. Cannon, F.D. Morrow, R. Rocklin, and J.B. Blumberg. 1990. Vitamin E supplementation enhances cell-mediated immunity in healthy elderly subjects. Am. J. Clin. Nutr. 52(3):557–563.

Meydani, S.N., A.H. Lichtenstein, S. Cornwall, M. Meydani, B.R. Goldin, H. Rasmussen, C.A. Dinarello, and E.J. Schaefer. 1993b. Immunologic effects of national cholesterol education panel step-2 diets with and without fish-derived n-3 fatty acid enrichment. J. Clin. Invest. 92:105–113.

Meydani, S.N., M. Meydani, L.C. Rall, F. Morrow, and J.B. Blumberg. 1994. Assessment of the safety of high-dose, short-term supplementation with vitamin E in healthy older adults. Am. J. Clin. Nutr. 60(5):704–709.

Meydani, S.N., M. Meydani, C.P. Verdon, A.C. Shapiro, J.B. Blumberg, and K.C. Hayes. 1986. Vitamin E supplementation suppresses prostaglandin E2 synthesis and enhances the immune response of aged mice. Mech. Aging Dev. 34:191–201.

Michie, H.R., K.R. Manogue, D.R. Spriggs, A. Revhaug, S.T. O'Dwyer, C.A. Dinnarello, A. Cerami, S.M. Wolff, and D.W. Wilmore. 1988. Detection of circulating tumor necrosis factor after endotoxin administration. N. Engl. J. Med. 318:1481–1486.

Moldawer, L.L. 1997. The validity of blood and urinary cytokine measurements for detecting the presence of inflammation. In Emerging Technologies for Nutrition Research: Potential for Assessing Military Performance Capability, S.J. Carlson-Newberry and R.B. Costello, eds. Committee on Military Nutrition Research, Food and Nutrition Board. Washington, D.C.: National Academy Press.

Molvig, J., F. Pociot., H. Worssaae, L.D. Wogensen, L. Baek, P. Christensen, T. Mandrup-Poulsen, K. Anderson, P. Madsen, J. Dyerberg, and J. Nerup. 1991. Dietary supplementation with omega-3-polyunsaturated fatty acids decreases mononuclear cell proliferation and interleukin-1β content but not monokine secretion in healthy and insulin-dependent diabetic individuals. Scan. J. Immunol. 34:399–410.

Montain, S.J., R.L. Shippee, W.J. Tharion, and T.R. Kramer. 1995. Carbohydrate-electrolyte solution during military training: Effects of physical performance, mood state and immune function. Technical Report No. T95-13, AD-A297 258. Natick, Mass.: U.S. Army Research Institute of Environmental Medicine.

Moore, R.J., K.E. Friedl, T.R. Kramer, L.E. Martinez-Lopez, R.W. Hoyt, R.E. Tulley, J.P. DeLany, E.W. Askew, and J.A. Vogel. 1992. Changes in soldier nutritional status and immune function during the Ranger training course. Technical Report No. T13-92 AD-A257 437. Natick, Mass.: U.S. Army Research Institute of Environmental Medicine.

Morikawa, K., F. Oseko, and S. Morikawa. 1995. A role for ferritin in hematopoiesis and the immune system [review]. Leuk. Lymphoma Res. 18:429–433.

Muhlbacher, F., C.R. Kapadia, M.F. Colpoys, R.J. Smith, and D.W. Wilmore. 1984. Effects of glucocorticoids on glutamine metabolism in skeletal muscle. Am. J. Physiol. 247:E75–E83.

Munck, A. P.M. Guyre, and N.J. Holbrook. 1984. Physiological functions of glucocorticoids in stress and their relation to pharmacological actions. Endocrinol. Rev. 5:25–44.

Munn, C.G., A.L. Markenson, A. Kapadia, and M. deSousa. 1981. Impaired T cell mitogen responses in some patients with thalassemia intermedia. Thymus 3:119–128.

Müns, G. 1993. Effect of long-distance running on polymorphonuclear neutrophil phagocytic function of the upper airways. Int. J. Sports Med. 15:96–99.

Murray, M.J., A.B. Murray, N.J. Murray, and M.B. Murray. 1978. Diet and cerebral malaria: The effects of famine and refeeding. Am. J. Clin. Nutr. 31:57–61.

Myrvik, Q.N. 1994. Immunology and nutrition. Pp. 623–662 in Modern Nutrition in Health and Disease, 8th ed., M.E. Shils, J.A. Olson, and M. Shike, eds. Malvern, Pa.: Lea and Febiger.

Nakano, K., S. Suzuki, and C. Oh. 1987. Significance of increased secretion of glucocorticoids in mice and rats injected with bacterial endotoxin. Brain Behav. Immun. 1:159–172.

Neilands, J.B. 1995. Siderophores: Structure and function of microbial iron transport compounds. J. Biol. Chem. 270:26723–26726.

Neumann, C.G., G.J. Lawlor Jr., E.R. Stiehm, M.E. Swenseid, C. Newton, J. Herbert, A.J. Ammann, and M. Jacob. 1975. Immunologic responses in malnourished children. Am. J. Clin. Nutr. 28:89–104.

Nicolau, G.Y. and E. Haus. 1994. Chronobiology of the hypothalamic–pituitary–thyroid axis. Pp. 330–347 in Biologic Rhythms in Clinical and Laboratory Medicine, 2nd ed., Y. Touitou and E. Haus, ed. Heidelberg: Springer-Verlag.

Nieman, D.C. 1994. Exercise, upper respiratory tract infection, and the immune system. Med. Sci. Sports Exerc. 26:128–139.

Nieman, D.C., K.S. Buckley, D.A. Henson, B.J. Warren, J. Suttles, J.C. Ahle, S. Simandle, O.R. Fagoaga, and S.L. Nehlsen-Cannarella. 1995c. Immune function in marathon runners versus sedentary controls. Med. Sci. Sports Exerc. 27:986–992.

Nieman, D.C., D.A. Henson, G. Gusewitch, B.J. Warren, R.C. Dotson, D.E. Butterworth, and S.L. Nehlsen-Cannarella. 1993a. Physical activity and immune function in elderly women. Med. Sci. Sports Exerc. 25:823–831.

Nieman, D.C., A.R. Miller, D.A. Henson, B.J. Warren, G. Gusewitch, R.L. Johnson, J.M. Davis, D.E. Butterworth, J.L. Herring, and S.L. Nehlsen-Cannarella. 1994. Effects of high- versus moderate-intensity exercise on lymphocyte subpopulations and proliferative response. Int. J. Sports Med. 15:199–206.

Nieman, D.C., A.R. Miller, D.A. Henson, B.J. Warren, G. Gusewitch, R.L. Johnson, J.M. Davis, D.E. Butterworth, and S.L. Nehlsen-Cannarella. 1993b. The effects of high- versus moderate-intensity exercise on natural killer cell cytotoxic activity. Med. Sci. Sports Exerc. 25:1126–1134.

Nieman, D.C., S.I. Nelson-Cannarella, D.A. Henson, D.E. Butterworth, O.R. Fagoaga, B.J. Warren, and M.K. Rainwater. 1996. Immune response to obesity and moderate weight loss. Int. J. Obes. Relat. Metab. Disord. 20(4):353–360.

Ogle, C.K., J.D. Ogle, J-X. Mao, J. Simon, J.G. Noel, B-G. Li, and J.W. Alexander. 1994. Effect of glutamine on phagocytosis and bacterial killing by normal and pediatric burn patient neutrophils. JPEN 18:128–133.

Palombo, J.D., S.J. DeMichele, E. Lydon, and B.R. Bistrian. 1997. Cyclic vs continuous enteral feeding with omega-3 and gamma-linolenic fatty acids: effects on modulation of phospholipid fatty acids in rat lung and liver immune cells. JPEN J. Parenter. Enteral Nutr. 21(3):123–132.

Parry-Billings, M., J. Evans, P.C. Calder, and E.A. Newsholme. 1990. Does glutamine contribute to immunosuppression after major burns? Lancet 336:523–525.

Payan, D.G., M.Y.S. Wong, T. Chernov-Rogan, F.H. Valone, W.C. Pickett, V.A. Blake, and W.M. Gold. 1986. Alteration in human leukocyte function induced by ingestion of eicosapentaenoic acid. J. Clin. Immunol. 6:402–410.

Pedersen, B.K., N. Tvede, L.D. Christensen, K. Klarlund, S. Kragbak, and J. Halkjaer-Kristensen. 1989. Natural killer cell activity in peripheral blood of highly trained and untrained persons. Int. J. Sports Med. 10:129–131.

Peters, E.M, J.M. Goetzsche, B. Grobbelaar, and T.D. Noakes. 1993. Vitamin C supplementation reduces the incidence of postrace symptoms of upper-respiratory-tract infection in ultramarathon runners. Am. J. Clin. Nutr. 57(2):170–174.

Philips, J.L., and P. Azari. 1975. Effect of iron transferrin on nucleic acid synthesis in phytohaemagglutinin-stimulated human lymphocytes. Cell Immunol. 15:94–99.

Pieniazek, N.J. and B.L. Herwaldt. 1997. Reevaluating the molecular taxonomy: is human-associated Cyclospora a mammalian Eimeria species? Emerg. Infect. Dis. 3(3):381–383.

Pöllman, L., and B. Pöllman. 1988. Variations of the efficiency of hepatitis B vaccination. Annual Rev. Chronopharmacol. 5:45–48.

Pozos, R.S., D.E. Roberts, A.C. Hackney, and S.J. Feith. 1996. Military Schedules vs. Biological Clocks. Pp. 149–160 in Nutritional Needs in Cold and in High-Altitude Environments, Applications for Military Personnel in Field Operations, B.M. Marriott and S.J. Carlson, eds. A report of the Committee on Military Nutrition Research, Food and Nutrition Board, Institute of Medicine. Washington, D.C.: National Academy Press.

Prasad, A.S., G.J. Brewer, E.B. Schoomaker, and P. Rabbani. 1978. Hypocupremia induced by zinc therapy in adults. J. Am. Med. Assoc. 240:2166–2168.

Prohaska, J.R., S.W. Downing, O.A. Lukasewycz. 1983. Chronic dietary copper deficiency alters biochemical and morphological properties of mouse lymphoid tissues. J. Nutr. 113(8):1583–1590.

Radomski, M.W., B.H. Sabiston, and P. Isoard. 1980. Development of "sport anemia" in physically fit men after daily sustained submaximal exercise. Aviat. Space Environ. Med. 51(1):41–45.

Rall, L.C., and S.N. Meydani. 1993. Vitamin B6 and immune competence. Nutr. Rev. 51:217–225.

Rang, H.P., M.M. Dale, J.M. Ritter, and P. Gardner. 1995. Pharmacology. New York: Churchill Livingstone.

Reichlin, S. 1993. Neuroendocrine–immune interactions [review article]. New Engl. J. Med. 329(17):1246–1253.

Reichlin, S. 1994. Neuroendocrine consequences of systemic inflammation. Pp. 83–96 in Advances in Endocrinology and Metabolism, E.L. Mazzaferri, R.S. Bar, and R.A. Kreisberg, eds. St. Louis: Mosby.

Reynolds, J.V., J.M. Daly, S. Zhang, E. Evantash, J. Shou, R. Sigal, and M.M. Ziegler. 1988. Immunomodulatory mechanisms of arginine. Surgery 104(2):142–151.

Rock, C.L., R.A. Jacob, and P.E. Bowen. 1996. Update on the biological characteristics of the antioxidant micronutrients: vitamin C, vitamin E, and the carotenoids. J. Am. Diet. Assoc. 96(7):693–702.

Roitt, I.M., and J. Brostoff. 1991. Immunology. London: Gower.

Rosado, J.L., P. Lopez, E. Munoz, H. Martinez, and L.H. Allen. 1997. Zinc supplementation reduced morbidity, but neither zinc nor iron supplementation affected growth or body composition of Mexican preschoolers. Am. J. Clin. Nutr. 1997. 65:13–29.

Rosales, F.J., S.J. Ritter, R. Zolfaghari, J.E. Smith, and A.C. Ross. 1996. Effects of acute inflammation on plasma retinol, retinol-binding protein, and its mRNA in the liver and kidneys of vitamin A-sufficient rats. J. Lipid Res. 37:962–971.

Ross, A.C., and U.G. Hammerling. 1994. Retinoids and the immune system. Pp. 521–543 in The Retinoids: Biology, Chemistry, and Medicine, 2nd ed., M.B. Sporn, A.B. Roberts, and D.S. Goodman, eds. New York: Raven Press.

Ross, A.C., and C.B. Stephensen. 1996. Vitamin A and retinoids in antiviral responses. FASEB J. 10:979–985.

Roth, E., J. Funovics, F. Muhlbacher, P. Sporn, W. Mauritz, and A. Fritsch. 1982. Metabolic disorders in severe abdominal sepsis: Glutamine deficiency in skeletal muscle. Clin. Nutr. 1:25.

Russell, R.C. 1998. Mosquito-borne arboviruses in Australia: the current scene and implications of climate change for human health. Int. J. Parasitol. 28:955–169.

Santos, P.C., and R.P. Falcao. 1990. Decreased lymphocyte subsets and K-cell activity in iron deficiency anemia. Acta Haemtologica 84:118–121.

Sazawal, S., R. E. Black, M.K. Bhan, N. Bhandari, A. Sinha, and S. Jalla. 1995. Zinc supplementation in young children with acute diarrhea in India. N. Engl. J. Med. 333:839–844.

Scrimshaw, N.S., C.E. Taylor, and J.E. Gordon. 1968. Interactions of nutrition and infection. Monograph. Geneva: World Health Organization.

Scuderi, P. 1990. Differential effects of copper and zinc on human peripheral blood monocyte cytokine secretion. Cell Immunol. 126:391–405.

Semba, R.D. 1994. Vitamin A, immunity, and infection. Clin. Infect. Dis. 19:489–499.

Senkal, M., A. Mumme, U. Eickhoff, B. Geier, G. Spath, D. Wulfert, U. Joosten, A. Frei, M. Kemen. 1997. Early postoperative enteral immunonutrition: clinical outcome and cost-comparison analysis in surgical patients. Crit. Care Med. 25:1489–96.

Shambaugh, G.E., and W.R. Beisel. 1966. Alterations in thyroid physiology during pneumococcal septicemia in the rat. Endocrinology. 79(3):511–523.

Shephard, D.S., J.A. Walsh, E. Kleinau, S. Stansfield, and S. Bhalotra. 1995a. Setting priorities for the Children's Vaccine Initiative: a cost-effectiveness approach. Vaccine 13(8):707–714.

Shephard, R.J., S. Rhind, and P.N. Shek. 1994b. Exercise and training: Influences on cytotoxicity, interleukin-1, interleukin-2 and receptor structures. Int. J. Sports Med. 15(suppl. 3):S154–S166.

Shinkai, S., H. Kohno, K. Kimura, T. Komura, H. Asai, R. Inai, K. Oka, Y. Kurokawa, and R.J. Shephard. 1995. Physical activity and immunosenescence in elderly men. Med. Sci. Sports Exerc. 27:1516–1526.

Shippee, R., K. Friedl, T. Kramer, M. Mays, K. Popp, E.W. Askew, B. Fairbrother, R. Hoyt, J. Vogel, L. Marchitelli, P. Frykman, L. Martinez-Lopez, E. Bernton, M. Kramer, R. Tulley, J. Rood, J. DeLany, D. Jezior, and J. Arsenault. 1994. Nutritional and immunological assessment of Ranger students with increased caloric intake. Report No. T95-5. Natick, Mass.: U.S. Army Research Institute of Environmental Medicine.

Silver, R.M., M.P. Heyes, J.C. Maize, B. Quearry, M. Vionnet-Fuasset, and E.M. Sternberg. 1990. Scleroderma, fascitis, and eosinophilia associated with the ingestion of tryptophan [see comments]. N. Engl. J. Med. 322(13):874–881.

Simon-Schnass, I. 1996. Oxidative Stress at High Altitudes and Effects of Vitamin E. Pp. 393–418 in Nutritional Needs in Cold and in High-Altitude Environments, Applications for Military Personnel in Field Operations, B.M. Marriott and S.J. Carlson, eds. A report of the Committee on Military Nutrition Research, Food and Nutrition Board, Institute of Medicine. Washington, D.C.: National Academy Press.

Sothern, R.B., B. Roitman-Johnson, E.L. Kanabrocki, J.G. Yager, M.M. Roodell, J.A. Weatherbee, M.R. Young, B.M. Nemchausky, and L.E. Scheving. 1995. Circadian characteristics of circulating interleukin-6 in men. J. Allergy Clin. Immunol. 95:1029–1035.

Souba, W.W., R.J. Smith, and D.W. Wilmore. 1985. Glutamine metabolism by the intestinal tract. J. Parenter. Enteral Nutr. 9:608–617.

Stallone, D.D., A.J. Stunkard, B. Zweiman, T.A. Wadden, and G.D. Foster. 1994. Decline in delayed-type hypersensitivity response in obese women following weight reduction. Clin. Diagn. Lab. Immunol. 1(2):202–205.

Sternberg, E.M. 1997a. Emotions and disease: From balance of humors to balance of molecules. Nat. Med. 3(3):264–267.

Sternberg, E.M. 1997b. Perspectives Series: Cytokines and the brain: Neural-Immune interactions in health and diseases. J. Clin. Invest. 100(11):107.

Sternberg, E.M., G.P. Chrousos, R.L. Wilder, and P.W. Gold. 1992. The stress response and the regulation of inflammatory disease. Ann. Intern. Med. 11:854–866.

Straight, J.M., H.M. Kipen, R.F. Vogt, and R.W. Amler. 1994. Immune Function Test Batteries for Use in Environmental Health Studies. U.S. Department of Health and Human Services, Public Health Service. Publication Number: PB94-204328.

Sundar, S.K., M.A. Cierpial, C. Kilts, J.C. Ritchie, and J.M. Weiss. 1990. Brain IL-1-induced immunosuppression occurs through activation of both pituitary–adrenal axis and sympathetic nervous system by corticotropin-releasing factor. J. Neurosci. 10:3701–3706.

Suteanu, S., E. Haus, L. Dumitriu, G.Y. Nicolau, E. Petrescu, H. Berg, L. Sackett-Lundeen, I. Ionescu, R. Reilly. 1995. Circadian rhythm of pro- and anti-inflammatory factors in patients with rheumatoid arthritis- No. 226 [abstract]. Biological Rhythm Research 26(4):446.

Swails, W.S., A.S. Kenler, D.F. Driscoll, S.J. DeMichele, T.J. Babineau, T. Utsunamiya, S. Chavali, R.A. Forse, and B.R. Bistrian. 1997. Effect of a fish oil structured lipid-based diet on prostaglandin release from mononuclear cells in cancer patients after surgery. J. Parenter. Enteral. Nutr. 21:266–274.

Tachibana, K., K. Mukai, I. Haraoka, S. Moriguchi, S. Takama, and Y. Kishino. 1985. Evaluation of the effects of arginine-enriched amino acid solution on tumor growth. J. Parenter. Enter. Nutr. 9:428–434.

Tang, A.M., N.M.H. Graham, and P. Saah. 1996. Effects of micronutrient intake on survival in human immunodeficiency virus 1 infection. Am. J. Epidemiol. 143:1244–1256.

Tappia, P.S., K.L. Troughton, S.C. Langley-Evans, and R.F. Grimble. 1995. Cigarette smoking influences cytokine production and antioxidant defences. Clin Sci (Colch) 88(4):485–489.

Taylor, G.R. 1993. Overview of spaceflight immunology studies. J. Leukocyte Biol. 54:179–188.

Tvede, N., J. Steensberg, B. Baslund, J. Halkjaer-Kristensen, and B.K. Pedersen. 1991. Cellular immunity in highly-trained elite racing cyclists and controls during periods of training with high and low intensity. Scand. J. Sports Med. 1:163–166.

Udomkesmalee, E., S. Dhanamitta, S. Sirisinha, S. Charoenkiatkul, S. Tantipopipat, O. Banjong, N. Rojroongwasinkul, T.R. Kramer, and J.C. Smith Jr. 1992. Effect of vitamin A and zinc supplementation on the nutriture of children in Northeast Thailand. Am. J. Clin. Nutr. 56:50–57.

Van der Hulst, R.R., B.K. van Kreel, M.F. von Meyenfeldt, R.J. Brummer, J.W. Arends, N.E. Deutz, and P.B. Soeters. 1993. Glutamine and the preservation of gut integrity. Lancet 334:1363–1365.

Virella, G., J.M. Kilpatrick, M.R. Rugeles, B. Hayman, and R. Russell. 1989. Depression of humoral responses and phagocytic functions in vivo and in vitro by fish oil and eicosapentaenoic acid. Clin. Immunol. Immunopathol. 52:257–270.

Wan, W., L. Wetmore, C.M. Sorensen, A.H. Greenberg, and D.M. Nance. 1994. Neural and biochemical mediators of endotoxin and stress-induced c-fos expression in the rat brain. Brain Res. Bull. 34:7–14.

Wartofsky, L., and K.D. Burman. 1982. Alterations in thyroid function in patients with systemic illness: the "euthyroid sick syndrome." Endocr. Rev. 3(2):164–217.

Watkins, L.R., L.E. Goehler, J.K. Relton, N. Tartaglia, L. Silbert, D. Martin, and S.F. Maier. 1995a. Blockade of interleukin-1 induced hyperthermia by subdiaphragmatic vagotomy: Evidence for vagal mediation of immune–brain communication. Neuroscience Lett. 183:27–31.

Watson, R.R., and T.M. Retro. 1984. Resistance to bacterial and parasitic infections in the nutritionally compromised host. CRC Crit. Rev. Microbiol. 10:297–315.

Watters, J.M., P.Q. Bessey, C.A. Dinarello, S.M. Wolff, and D.W. Wilmore. 1986. Both inflammatory and endocrine mediators stimulate host responses to sepsis. Arch. Surg. 121:179–190.

Watzl, B., and R.R. Watson. 1992. Role of alcohol abuse in nutritional immunosuppression. J. Nutr. 122 (3 suppl.):733–737.

Weinberg, E.D. 1984. Iron withholding: A defense against infection and neoplasia. Physiol. Rev. 64:65–102.

Weiss, G., H. Wachter, and D. Fuchs. 1995. Linkage of cell-mediated immunity to iron metabolism [review]. Immunol. Today 16:495–500.

Westphal, K.A., K.E. Friedl, M.A. Sharp, N. King, T.R. Kramer, K.L. Reynolds, and L.J. Marchitelli. 1995a. Health, performance, and nutritional status of U.S. Army women during basic combat training. Technical Report No. T96-2. Natick, Mass.: U.S. Army Research Institute of Environmental Medicine.

Wiik P., P.K. Opstad and A. Bøyum. 1996. Granulocyte chemiluminescence response to serum opsonized particles ex vivo during long-term strenuous exercise, energy, and sleep deprivation in humans. Eur. J. Appl. Physiol. 73:251–258.

Wiik, P., K.K. Skrede, S. Knardahl, A.H. Haugen, C.E. Ærø, P.K. Opstad, A. Bøyum. 1995. Effect of in vivo corticosterone and acute food deprivation on rat resident peritoneal cell chemiluminescence after activation ex vivo. Acta Physiol Scand 154(3):407–416.

Williams, T.J., and H. Yarwood. 1990. Effect of glucocorticosteroids on microvascular permeability. Am. Rev. Resp. Dis. 141:S39–S43.

Witt, E.H., A.Z. Reznick, C.a. Viguie, P. Starke-Reed, and L. Packer. 1992. Exercise, oxidative damage, and effects of antioxidant manipulation. J. Nutr. 122 (suppl. 3):766–773.

Ziegler, T.R., L.S. Young, K. Benfell, M. Scheltinga, K. Hortos, R. Bye, F.D. Morrow, D.O. Jacobs, R.J. Smith, J.H. Antin, and D.W. Wilmore. 1992. Clinical and metabolic efficacy of glutamine-supplemented parenteral nutrition after bone marrow transplantation. A randomized, double-blind, controlled study. Ann. Intern. Med. 116:821–828.

Zoli, M., M. Carè, C. Falco, R. Spanò, G. Bernardi, and I. Gasbarrini. 1995. Effect of oral glutamine on intestinal permeability and nutritional status in Crohn's disease. Gastroenterology 108:A766.

Zuckerman, S.H., J. Shellhaas, and L.D. Butler. 1989. Differential regulation of lipopolysaccharide-induced interleukin-1 and tumor necrosis factor synthesis: Effects of endogenous and exogenous glucocorticoids and the role of the pituitary–adrenal axis. Eur. J Immunol. 19:301–305.

Nutrition and Immune Function, 1999
Pp. 99–124. Washington, D.C.
National Academy Press

2

Committee Responses to Questions

As summarized in Chapter 1, the Committee on Military Nutrition Research (CMNR) was asked to provide information on the impact of nutritional status on immune function. The purpose of the committee's workshop was to assess the current state of knowledge about the impact of environmental stressors and physiological changes on immune function. In addition, the committee was asked to evaluate the ongoing research efforts by scientists at the U.S. Army Research Institute of Environmental Medicine (USARIEM) to study immune status in Special Forces troops.

In this chapter, the CMNR provides answers to the five specific questions posed by the Army, basing its conclusions on information from presentations and the scientific literature, with a focus on the current assessment techniques and methodologies applicable to the military setting. More specifically, the committee evaluated the effects of alterations in nutrition on immune status and function during conditions of stress unique to the military environment. The responses, conclusions, and recommendations were developed and prepared in executive session of the CMNR. Some areas of consideration were augmented by limited literature searches to ensure adequate coverage of each area.

RESPONSES TO QUESTIONS POSED BY THE ARMY

Below are the committee's answers to the five questions posed by the Army regarding nutrition and sustainment of immune function in the field.

1. What are the significant military hazards or operational settings most likely to compromise immune function in soldiers?

As described previously and outlined below, many conditions or stressors have been associated with compromised immune function during Ranger training and basic combat training, as well as during arctic training and in deployments to locations such as Somalia, Haiti, Panama, and the Persian Gulf.

• *Reduced ration consumption.* Intakes less than 60 percent of the total energy needed, particularly during exposure to harsh environments and/or dehydration, were shown to be a significant stressor. In U.S. Ranger II, the increase in energy intake from that in Ranger I (2,780 to 3,250 calories or approximately 470 kcal/d), which tempered weight loss to only 12.8 percent of initial body weight, appeared to minimize the adverse effects on immune function. Thus, weight loss, particularly that involving lean body mass, appears to be a major factor in inducing immune system dysfunction.

The effects of dehydration on immune function are not reviewed in this report. However, weight losses of as little as 3–5 percent in 24–48 h, which are primarily due to dehydration, have a significant impact on performance. Weight losses of 6–10 percent in a similar period may affect health adversely. Thus, the effects of dehydration must be separated from those of underconsumption of rations (see IOM, 1995a).

• *Prolonged moderate-to-heavy physical activity.* The week-long Norwegian Ranger training studies with heavy exercise and limited sleep did not demonstrate significant weight loss or alterations in immune function, whereas the U.S. Ranger I study of 8- to 9-week duration demonstrated a greater weight loss (14 percent of body weight) and an altered immune response. Low- to moderate-intensity exercise (<60 percent $Vo_{2\,max}$), such as that performed in most troop activity of a duration of 60 minutes or less, appears to exert less stress on the immune system than activity that is more strenuous (>60 percent $Vo_{2\,max}$) performed for longer than 1 h. Repeated bouts of strenuous activity may increase the risk of infection, particularly of the upper respiratory tract.

• *Limited, interrupted or nonrestful sleep.* Limited or nonrestful sleep over a prolonged period (as little as 3 hours or less was noted in the Norwegian Ranger studies), particularly when coupled with stressful physical activity, may result in some compromise of the immune system. Short periods of severe caloric and sleep deprivation appear to have less adverse effect on immune function than a more prolonged period with greater weight loss (caloric deficit).

• *Increased infection and injury.* This category includes infections associated with trauma and burns, such as cellulitis, osteomyelitis, wound abscesses, and sepsis, as well as naturally occurring infections and diseases such as conjunctivitis, otitis, upper and lower respiratory tract infections, urinary tract infections, and gastroenteritis. Diarrhea is commonly experienced by soldiers in military operations, most likely due to exposure to infectious organisms from strange environments (dust, water, local foods). Influenza also is common, and in some environments, other diseases occur that are rare in the United States.

• *Increased exposure to extremes of temperature and humidity.* Increased exposures in areas such as the tropics or desert, as well as with operations in the arctic areas of North America or northern Europe during winter conditions, can adversely affect food intake and sleep. Heavy activity or environmental extremes may increase energy requirements by as much as 15 percent after acclimatization without compensatory ration intake. For example, hypohydration may lead to temporary anorexia and a worsening cycle of lowered water and food intake. The factors that influence ration consumption may be even more significant for operations in the cold and at high altitudes.

• *Increased psychological stresses.* Stresses such as those imposed by deployment, separation from family, imminence of combat, threat of biological agents, and long periods of vigilance with interrupted sleep and inadequate rest, may also be significant and often result in field training- or combat-induced anorexia. All of these factors may impinge on immunological health.

• *Prolonged exposure during training or battlefield combat to environmental assaults.* Environmental exposure (for example, to smoke or fumes from fuels or chemicals, dust, dirt, and blast overpressure) may induce oxidative stress on protective systems.

2. What methods for assessment of immune function are most appropriate in military nutrition laboratory research, and what methods are most appropriate for field research?

It is important first to identify a number of methodologic issues that must be be considered when assessing immune function.

Technical Issues

In addition to the choice of assay, a large number of issues must be considered in the design of studies to assess immune function. The first consideration in a study of immune challenge is the choice of antigen, described previously for tests of primary and secondary antibody response (Straight et al., 1994; see Cunningham-Rundles, Chapter 9).

The second consideration is the timing of sample collection. As described by Erhard Haus in Chapter 20, the immune system is significantly influenced by biological rhythms; thus, samples must be drawn on an established schedule (Straight et al., 1994). Additionally, it is important to standardize collections in relation to physical activity because differential cell counts can change acutely during and immediately after exercise (DeRijk et al., 1996, 1997).

The third, and possibly most critical consideration, is the protocol for storage and transportation of samples. According to G. Sonnenfeld (University of Kentucky, Louisville, personal communication, 1997), human blood samples must be shipped at room temperature in Styrofoam containers, and for most status indicators, must be assayed within 24 h. If necessary, some preparatory steps, such as harvesting cells from blood, may be performed in rudimentary makeshift labs and the samples sent under controlled conditions to a central facility for completion of analysis.

A fourth but related consideration is the choice of laboratory for sample analysis. The Agency for Toxic Substances and Disease Registry (ATSDR) of the Department of Health and Human Services recommends the use of a central or core reference facility for all analyses to avoid small differences in protocols and solutions used. Some methods, such as the measurement of mitogen-induced lymphocyte proliferation by [^{3}H]thymidine incorporation are extremely sensitive to such factors (see Cunningham-Rundles, Chapter 9). Thymidine incorporation is also a variable, relatively nonspecific measure not easily standardized and not well applicable to field studies. Because some procedures must be performed within a short period of time, the number of samples that can be processed is thus limited.

Finally, the use of controls is extremely critical both in the collection and assessment of samples and in the interpretation of data. It is recommended that each time samples are drawn and an assay is performed, a standard is drawn and included for the assay, consisting of the blood (or cells) of one individual, to correct for intraindividual and interassay variability. Whenever possible, subjects should be used as their own baselines, and longitudinal studies should be performed (Straight et al., 1994). Of major concern are the lack of population-based normative reference ranges for most immune function parameters and the need to obtain complete health histories (including such factors as smoking, use of other drugs, and pregnancy) from subjects to rule out possible confounding factors.

Methodologic Issues

Immunologic function can be related to nutritional status by utilizing two distinct methodological approaches. First, under *controlled* conditions, normal healthy individuals can be studied; after an appropriate baseline period, a nutritional perturbation can be imposed and the changes in immune responses from baseline determined. This approach allows single nutrient or environmental perturbations to be studied while many other factors that also cause immune dysfunction are controlled. In addition, appropriate controls (with adequate sample size) can be included, and a period of refeeding (or second control period) can be included at the end of the experiment. Highly sophisticated immune tests can be performed on subjects enlisted in such studies as presented in Table 1-1.

Second, in *field* studies, the conditions are quite different, and other variables, in addition to altered nutritional intake, affect individuals. Immune dysfunction due to both nutritional and other operational stressors may be present. Under these conditions, it is possible to study the incidence of infection using epidemiologic techniques, while food intake and nutritional status are determined. Appropriate ambulatory tests of immunologic function can be validated and compared to results obtained in more controlled settings.

A longitudinal study of immune function in simulated combat conditions in the field could be performed that would have the ability to detect accurately over time the subjects' nutritional state and the incidence of infection. When clinical signs are clearly defined and documented, and symptoms indicate the occurrence of infectious illnesses, studies to determine etiology and therapy can be initiated, along with serial studies of C-reactive protein (CRP), erythrocyte sedimentation rate (ESR), acute-phase reactants, whole blood, plasma, cytokines, and their receptors. The longitudinal course of illness can then be correlated with nutritional parameters.

Prior to pursuing field investigations, researchers must undertake appropriate studies in a controlled clinical setting to answer some of the more basic questions about the impact of altered nutritional status on immune function. These studies must precede those that attempt to confer a state of enhanced immune function or to study the response to a specific nutrient. For example, limited studies of subjects placed under conditions of reduced caloric intake could be undertaken. Attempts could also be made to see if supplementation with one or more essential single nutrients could maintain normal immunological competence in the face of generalized dietary deprivation. Before extensive field evaluations of the influence of nutrition on immune response are undertaken, carefully controlled laboratory studies should be performed and data collected from more fundamental research studies. To hypothesize which of the nutrients may enhance immune response, it may be helpful first to determine under controlled conditions which nutrients, by their deficiency or exclusion from the diet, impact the immune response negatively; however, this will not provide a complete picture.

The CMNR confirms the need to determine appropriate field measures for monitoring the immune response, particularly for determining the presence and magnitude of an acute-phase reaction, which may be adversely influenced by nutritional status in stressed individuals. Based on standardized test panels recommended by government agencies or private-sector scientists, the committee suggests the following. If clinical signs of infection are present or there has been significant weight loss induced by nutritional stress, a simple-to-use basic screening panel of immune function tests such as CRP protein, ESR, a baseline battery (testing six or more antibody titers for several previously administered military vaccines, immunoglobulins G, A, and M; and complete blood count with CD4 lymphocyte count and CD4:CD8 ratio should be employed initially. In the event that these basic tests of immune response indicate the existence of immune compromise of an unusual nature or unusually great incidence, the CMNR suggests a second tier of immune function tests. These would include natural killer (NK) cell numbers and activities; lymphocyte mitogenesis assays; thymosin measurements; and estimations of phagocytic cell chemotaxis and microbicidal activities (for example, *Listeria monocytogenes*-killing assay). However, these tests must first be validated for field use. A standardized battery of delayed dermal hypersensitivity tests may be employed at baseline and again if stress-induced weight loss exceeds 10 percent.

If validated, these tests would be valuable in research studies for rapid field assessment of immune status and might suggest steps that could be taken to improve resistance to potential exposures and thus improve unit effectiveness. As previously noted by the CMNR (IOM, 1997), tests based on cytokine assays, especially of the proinflammatory cytokines and related molecules excreted in urine and whole-blood cytokine production assays, have great potential for adding important new diagnostic measures at a relatively low cost–benefit ratio. Differential changes in production patterns of specific cytokines (that is, shifts from T-helper 1 [Th1] to Th2-type patterns) may be the most sensitive way to determine whether changes in immune responses are stress related. Such tests currently are being evaluated in many civilian research studies and may have very real potential value for suggesting the presence of cytokine-induced malnutrition in military personnel who are being exposed to the stresses of rigorous training exercises or ongoing operational missions. Additionally, in the development and validation of more precise readout measures, attention should be paid to the development of microassays that can be applied in field settings to minimize stress and blood loss during sampling.

3. The proinflammatory cytokines have been proposed to decrease lean body mass, mediate thermoregulatory mechanisms, and increase resistance to infectious disease by reducing metabolic activity in a way that is similar to the reduction seen in malnutrition and other catabolic conditions. Interventions to sustain immune function can alter the actions, nutritional costs, and potential changes in the levels of proinflammatory cytokines. What are the benefits and risks to soldiers of such interventions?

One of the most fundamental needs is to sustain the functional competence of the immune system in military personnel who must experience the stresses of rigorous training and operational assignments and who face the risks of infectious illnesses as well as diverse forms of trauma. Cytokine effects in the body can be influenced by a variety of factors as outlined below.

• *Nutritional interventions.* It is well known that in the course of infection, proinflammatory cytokines mediate the loss of specific nutrients, which must be repleted or redistributed. In turn, growing evidence suggests that a number of nutrients may influence immune function by affecting synthesis of specific cytokines, their soluble receptors, or inhibitory factors. For example, research on the antioxidant vitamins A, E, and C, as well as certain polyunsaturated fatty acids (PUFAs) and amino acids (AAs), has shown that their apparent ability to modulate immune status may be mediated by their effects on cytokines, at least under some conditions, but many questions remain regarding the efficacy of these nutrients in amounts that exceed Military Recommended Dietary Allowance (MRDA) levels. Research is also needed on whether nutritional intervention during stress is effective or whether it must be combined with agents that suppress inflammation.

• *Pharmacological interventions (including immunizations).* Research has demonstrated that a number of pharmacological agents including aspirin, ibuprofen, and glucocorticoids modulate the effects of cytokines and can be used to minimize signs and symptoms of cytokine-induced acute-phase reactions and the nutrient losses that accompany them. Glucocorticoids can block fever and reduce many of the metabolic consequences of acute-phase responses caused when proinflammatory cytokines are released by cells, but the adverse consequences of prolonged systemic administration of glucocorticoids have long been recognized. On the other hand, drugs such as aspirin and ibuprofen can block the intracellular formation of many of the eicosanoids (prostaglandins, prostacyclins, leukotrienes, thromboxanes) and thereby reduce the fevers, myalgias, and headaches that accompany cytokine-induced acute-phase reactions. Because losses of body nutrients during these reactions are often proportional to the magnitude and duration of fevers, the use of such generally safe and effective anti-inflammatory drugs serves indirectly to maintain the body's nutritional status and immune system functions. Further, the use of anti-inflammatory drugs for the management of minor traumas or infections (for example, upper respiratory tract infections) is well recognized and provides for sustained military performance during severe training exercises and operational missions. The immune system can be "educated" in advance by the prophylactic administration of immunizations against all possible foreign agents. Such immunization procedures do carry some risks, depending on the vaccine being administered, but the ultimate military benefits of such immunization practices far outweigh the risks. Furthermore, the risks of immunization can be reduced and the benefits increased (that is, improved vaccine effectiveness) by the use of oral vaccines, whose development by the military was recommended in an earlier CMNR report (IOM, 1997).

• *Administration of products of biotechnology.* Biotechnological methods have allowed the production of many individual cytokines and their receptors. At the present time, their use is limited to the administration of granulocyte macrophage colony stimulating factor for the treatment of bone marrow recipients and those undergoing a limited number of other experimental procedures, and their effectiveness has not been demonstrated in healthy subjects or in clinical trials. A recent review by Mackowiak and colleagues (1997) discusses the therapeutic use of pyrogenic cytokines and the use of their inhibitors. The authors comment on the failure, or even the harm, associated with their therapeutic use in humans (in contrast to rodents). The administration of exogenous cytokines and the modulation of cytokines in vivo are areas of active research in the civilian sector; the use of cytokines to enhance resistance to infections, however, should be carefully studied in animals before application to clinical situations.

4. What are the important safety and regulatory considerations in the testing and use of nutrients or dietary supplements to sustain immune function under field conditions?

The basic considerations in the testing and fielding of nutrients or dietary supplements to sustain immune function are to ensure, first, that the nutrients are in fact safe under the conditions of intended use and, second, that they are effective. Since the levels of some of the nutrients that must be fed to achieve potential effects are much higher than levels usually ingested in foods, further safety testing is warranted. Such testing involves attempts to delineate the upper limits of safety (see Table 2-1, which summarizes some of the considerations for nutrients discussed in this report).

For any substance, there are a number of major considerations relevant to the question posed. These include the following:

- the intake levels that are suggested and referenced by the Recommended Dietary Allowance (RDA)/MRDA;
- the customary range of intake;
- the tolerable upper level;
- the safety and efficacy of the substance at the level of intended use; and
- special groups or circumstances that deserve attention.

Generally accepted tolerable upper intake limit values have not yet been established for individual nutrients, but the Food and Nutrition Board's (FNB's) Subcommittee on Upper Reference Levels of Nutrients is now considering these levels. For purposes of planning further military research on individual nutrients, there is already evidence that safety problems associated with excess consumption are much more likely for some nutrients than for others. In clinical practice, the general rule of thumb is that it is generally unwise to exceed three to four times the traditional RDA for most fat-soluble vitamins; however, margins of safety may be lower for vitamins A and D in some groups. In general, water-soluble vitamins tend to be less toxic and can be consumed in larger multiples of the traditional RDA than can fat-soluble vitamins.

Trace minerals are difficult to discuss in general terms. It is important to remember that supplements of a single nutrient cannot be considered in isolation. The World Health Organization (WHO, 1996) Expert Consultation examined upper safe levels for trace minerals and concluded that the toxicity and the potential for nutrient–nutrient interactions must be considered individually. Risks of pathology resulting from such interactions are higher when intakes of other essential nutrients with which they interact are low or

TABLE 2-1 Reported Doses and Toxicities of Nutrients Proposed to Sustain Immune Function

Nutrient	RDA, MRDA, ESADDI	Reported Concerns Regarding Possible Toxicity of Large Doses	Possible Role in Sustaining Immune Function	Special Concerns in Military Situations
Vitamin B1 (thiamin)	RDA: 1–1.5 mg/d (0.5 mg/1,000 kcal) MRDA: 1.2–1.6 mg/d	Quite safe; excess excreted	Needed for antibody synthesis (Beisel, 1991, 1992)	Requirements increase with energy demands
Vitamin B6 (pyridoxine)	RDA: 1.6–2.0 mg/d MRDA: 2.0–2.2 mg/d	Neurotoxicity and photosensitivity have been noted with large doses (>500 mg/d) on a chronic basis (Bernstein and Lobitz, 1988; Schaumburg et al., 1983). Estimated daily adult oral minimum toxic dose is 2,000 mg (NRC, 1989)	Highly important for CMI functions (Beisel, 1991, 1992; Meydani et al., 1991)	Requirements increase with protein intake
Vitamin B12 (cobalamine)	RDA: 2.0 μg/d MRDA: 3.0 μg/d:	Some are allergic to large doses (>0.5 mg/d)	Important for CMI functions (Beisel, 1991, 1992)	No known concerns
Folate	RDA: 180–200 μg/d MRDA: 400 μg/d CDC: 400 μg/d	Supplements can mask anemia or B12 deficiency. Estimated daily adult oral minimum toxic dose is 400 mg (NRC, 1989)	Important for CMI functions (Beisel, 1991, 1992)	Military women have been shown to have compromised status
Vitamin C (ascorbic acid)	RDA: 60 mg/d MRDA: 60 mg/d	Has little frank toxicity. Estimated daily adult oral minimum toxic dose is	Needed for WBC movement; also an important antioxidant	Infected or traumatized patients may need >RDA amounts

TABLE 2-1 *Continued*

Nutrient	RDA, MRDA, ESADDI	Reported Concerns Regarding Possible Toxicity of Large Doses	Possible Role in Sustaining Immune Function	Special Concerns in Military Situations
Vitamin C *continued*		1,000–5,000 mg (NRC, 1989). Diarrhea, abdominal bloating with gram doses (Levine et al., 1995). Incidents of acute scurvy have been reported if megadoses are suddenly stopped. Possible formation of renal stones (Urivetzky et al., 1992). May alter B$_{12}$ availability (Herbert, 1979)		
Vitamin A and related retinoids	RDA: males, 1,000 µg/d females, 800 µg/d pregnancy, 800 µg/d lactation: 1,200–1,300 µg/d MRDA: males, 1,000 µg females, 800 µg	Three levels of toxicities exist: acute (documented at >110 × RDA [Rothman et al., 1995]), chronic (≤10 × RDA), and teratogenicity, which has been reported in pregnancy at much lower levels (Rothman et al., 1995). Estimated daily adult oral minimum toxic dose is 25,000–50,000 IU (NRC, 1989). Excess intakes of vitamin A may be toxic* and result in immunosuppression. Carotenoids, even in very large amounts, do not appear	β-Carotene may have small added immunopotentiating effects in elderly men (Santos et al., 1996). Also an important antioxidant	Infections cause loss of body vitamin A stores, and supplementation can reduce the severity of some infections and diarrheal diseases

Continued

TABLE 2-1 *Continued*

Nutrient	RDA, MRDA, ESADDI	Reported Concerns Regarding Possible Toxicity of Large Doses	Possible Role in Sustaining Immune Function	Special Concerns in Military Situations
Vitamin A *continued*		to be toxic (Brubacher and Weiser, 1985; Miller et al., 1987)		
Vitamin D (calciferols)	RDA: 5–10 µg/d MRDA: 5–10 µg/d	Toxicity is rare, but doses > 100 µg/d cause toxicity†	Only slight effects recognized	No known concerns
Vitamin E (tocopherols)	RDA: 8–10 mg TE/d MRDA: 8–10 mg TE/d	Relatively nontoxic. Estimated daily adult oral minimum toxic dose is 1,200 IU (NRC, 1989). Decreased platelet function and increased bleeding are a concern if taken in high doses (>1,200 mg TE/d); may interact with aspirin or anticoagulants (Bendich, 1992).	Serves as an antioxidant with vitamin C and selenium to enhance selected immune responses in the elderly (Meydani et al., 1990, 1997b)	Those at risk of trauma, or those taking anticoagulants or PUFA supplements‡. Potential for increased oxidative stress at high altitudes may increase need (IOM, 1996)
Protein	RDA: 0.6–0.08 g/kg/d MRDA: 80–100 g/d (0.8 g/kg/d desirable body weight)	Quite safe in absence of renal failure	Essential for all aspects of immune function. PEM is the most common cause of NAIDS (Chandra, 1992a; Chandra and Kumari, 1994)	Needs increase with trauma, infection, exercise, etc. Intake should have a balance of AAs
Glutamine (Glu)	No RDA Glu = 3–7% of ingested protein	No toxicities reported with intakes as high as 43 g × 5 d (Ziegler et al., 1990)	Supplements help to sustain immune function in traumatized patients	No known benefits of supplementation apart from critical care situations

TABLE 2-1 *Continued*

Nutrient	RDA, MRDA, ESADDI	Reported Concerns Regarding Possible Toxicity of Large Doses	Possible Role in Sustaining Immune Function	Special Concerns in Military Situations
Glutamine *continued*			(Alexander, 1993; Griffith et al., 1997; Kudsk et al., 1996)	
Arginine (Arg)	No RDA Arg = 4–9% of ingested protein.	No toxicities reported	Arginine is the only precursor of nitric oxide, is a key bactericidal agent (*in some infectious diseases*), and may enhance selected CMI responses. (Kirk and Barbul, 1992)	Arginine becomes a semiessential AA with trauma, infection, malnutrition, etc.
Polyunsaturated Fatty Acids (PUFAs)	No RDA WHO = 3–5% dietary energy (WHO, 1993) with essential fatty acids (linoleic and/or linolenic) at 1–2% total calories	PUFAs and all other lipids become immunosuppressive nutrients (Endres et al., 1993) since increased intakes of fish oils (EPA and or DHA 4–20 g/d) have been found to inhibit aspects of neutrophil, monocyte, and lymphocyte functions for variable periods of time (Fisher et al., 1990; Schmidt et al., 1992). Alteration in blood coagulation may occur	PUFAs are precursors of prostaglandins, leukotrienes, and other eicosanoids	Some immune functions can be modified by altering dietary n-3/n-6 PUFA ratio. Increased PUFAs may increase vitamin E needs. ~0.4 mg of α-tocopherol for each gram of PUFA equivalent is thought to be adequate for adults (Sokol, 1996)

Continued

TABLE 2-1 *Continued*

Nutrient	RDA, MRDA, ESADDI	Reported Concerns Regarding Possible Toxicity of Large Doses	Possible Role in Sustaining Immune Function	Special Concerns in Military Situations
Iron	RDA: 10–15 mg/d MRDA: 10–18 mg/d	Estimated daily adult oral minimum toxic dose is 100 mg (NRC, 1989). Possibly increases susceptibility to certain infections. Chronic excessive intake can cause hemochromatosis in genetically susceptible individuals.§ Acute toxicity is rare in adults but can lead to organ damage and death; iv doses can be anaphylactic	Vital for bactericidal functions. Studies are mixed with respect to the effect of iron deficiency on increasing infection, chronic candidiasis, recurrent herpes simplex, and increased numbers of upper respiratory and GI tract infections (Andelman and Sered, 1996; Hershko, 1992; Hussein et al., 1988; Murray et al., 1978a).	Deficiency is quite common in women. Iron excess can exacerbate uncontrolled infections. Iron deficiency should be controlled, but the relationship between iron and infection remains unclear
Zinc	RDA: 12–15 mg/d MRDA: 15 mg/d	Acute toxicity is uncommon.# Supplementation in doses exceeding 15 mg/d plus usual food sources is not recommended without medical supervision (FNB, 1989). Estimated daily adult oral minimum toxic dose is 500 mg (NRC, 1989); >60 mg/d may be immunosuppressive (Chandra, 1984, 1988). Excesses may reduce copper	A major requirement for all immunological functions. Key component of thymic hormones. Enhances selected immune responses (Cunningham-Rundles et al., 1990a)	Deficiency generally coexists with PEM. Trauma, infections, illness can cause excess loss of body zinc

TABLE 2-1 *Continued*

Nutrient	RDA, MRDA, ESADDI	Reported Concerns Regarding Possible Toxicity of Large Doses	Possible Role in Sustaining Immune Function	Special Concerns in Military Situations
Zinc *continued*		absorption (Prasad et al., 1978)		
Copper (Cu)	ESADDI: 1.5–3.0 mg/d	Relatively nontoxic but acute toxicity may occurll. Estimated daily adult oral minimum toxic dose is 100 mg (NRC, 1989). Most toxic effects probably result from the production of free radicals by Cu$^+$ chelates (Kadiiska et al., 1993; Shah et al., 1992). Gastrointestinal effects (nausea, vomiting, diarrhea, epigastric pain) generally limit oral exposure. Chronic excess causes cirrhosis	Limited data exist. Appears to play a role in both CMI and humoral immunity, and IL-2 metabolism (Hopkins and Failla, 1997; Sullivan and Ochs, 1978)	Deficiency is rare, but may occur during chronic TPN
Selenium (Se)	RDA: 55–70 μg/d	Lack of a specific and sensitive biochemical marker of Se overexposure makes it difficult to establish a safe upper limit. ** Estimated daily adult oral minimum toxic dose is 1 mg (NRC, 1989). EPA has established a reference dose (RfD) of 5 μg/kg/d or 350	Contributes to immune functions as the antioxidant component of glutathione peroxidases and may enhance selected immune responses, although data from humans are lacking	Serves as an antioxidant with vitamins C and E

Continued

TABLE 2-1 *Continued*

Nutrient	RDA, MRDA, ESADDI	Reported Concerns Regarding Possible Toxicity of Large Doses	Possible Role in Sustaining Immune Function	Special Concerns in Military Situations
Selenium *continued*		μg/d for a 70-kg individual (Poirier, 1994). No signs of toxicity were seen in North Americans consuming as much as 724 μg/d (Longnecker et al., 1991), but chronic selenosis occurred in Chinese individuals ingesting about 853 μg/d (Yang et al., 1989)		

NOTE: AAs, amino acids; CDC, Centers for Disease Control; CMI, cell-mediated immunity; CNS, central nervous system; DHA, docosahexaenoic acid; EPA, eicosapentaenoic acid; ESADDI, Estimated Safe and Adequate Daily Dietary Intake; GI, gastrointestinal; IL, interleukins; MRDA, Military Recommended Dietary Allowance; NAIDS, nutritionally-acquired immune dysfunction syndromes; PEM, protein/energy malnutrition; PUFA, poly unsaturated fatty acids; RDA, Recommended Dietary Allowance; TE, tocopherol equivalents; TPN, total parenteral nutrition; WBC, white blood cell.

* Vitamin A toxicity includes headaches, nausea and vomiting, hepatomegaly, diplopia, alopecia, dermal lesions, and dry mucous membranes (Baurenfreund, 1980). In addition, slight excesses of vitamin A are of concern in periconceptional females (during organogenesis) (Miller et al., 1987; Pinnock and Alderman, 1992).

† Vitamin D toxicity includes hypercalcemia, calcification of soft tissues, and renal stone formation (Baurenfreund, 1980; Olson, 1983; Rothman et al., 1995), as well as anorexia, nausea, vomiting, polyuria, and muscular weakness.

‡ Vitamin E interferes with platelet function at pharmacologic levels, modulating platelet adherence and aggregation (Farrell and Bieri, 1975).

§ Individuals who are genetically at risk of iron overload: recent estimates of the prevalence of the hemochromatosis gene defect in the United States is that 4.5 persons per 1,000 are homozygous and ~12.5 persons per 1,000 are heterozygous (Beard, 1993). Males are 10 times more likely to suffer from hemochromatosis than females.

Zinc doses >2,000 mg may cause acute toxicity, including nausea, vomiting, colic, and diarrhea (Prasad, 1976).

‖ Acute copper toxicity involves hemolysis and cellular damage to the liver and brain. (Davis and Mertz, 1987)

** 27.3 mg selenium produced nausea, abdominal pain, diarrhea, nail and hair changes, peripheral neuropathy, fatigue, and irritability (Helzlsouer et al., 1985).

marginal, accentuating the nutrient imbalance. Therefore, conservatism is warranted in the consumption of trace minerals in excess of traditional RDA or suggested safe and adequate levels. However, requirements may change during an episode of illness, and requirements for some minerals may substantially increase (for example, zinc during diarrhea). The FNB's Dietary Reference Intakes (DRIs) Subcommittee on Upper Safe Levels is now considering the issue more fully.

Dietary deficiencies of a variety of nutritionally essential trace elements (zinc, copper, selenium) have been demonstrated to have an adverse impact on immune function in laboratory animals and elderly humans, and deficiencies of zinc and copper have resulted in increased susceptibility to certain infections in humans. Excessive intakes of some trace elements have led to immunosuppressive effects. Therefore, care must be exercised in the use of single-nutrient supplements until the optimal range of intakes for these trace elements is determined.

Iron. Both iron deficiency and iron excess appear to have the potential to increase susceptibility to infection. In a military situation, it is likely that the potential reduction in immune function due to iron deficiency is of more significance than any effects of iron overload. Because of their higher iron requirement and lower intake of operational rations, the iron intake of female soldiers may be lower than recommended in the MRDA, increasing their risk for iron deficiency anemia. Utilizing as the criterion for iron deficiency a serum ferritin concentration of less than 12 µg/L, and a combination of low serum ferritin and a hemoglobin of less than 120 g/L as the criteria for iron deficiency anemia, it was shown that 17 percent of new female recruits entering basic combat training (BCT) fit these criteria for iron deficiency, while 8 percent could be classified as having iron deficiency anemias. A survey of a similar (but not the same) population of women at the end of BCT showed that by the end of training, 33 percent were iron deficient and 26 percent were anemic (Westphal et al., 1994, 1995b).

Iron deficiency anemia can be expected to have adverse effects on the military performance of both men and women depending in part on its severity. Performance deficits in both men and women due to compromised iron status have been demonstrated most clearly during exercise of prolonged duration, such as long-distance running (Newhouse and Clement, 1988). Iron deficiency anemia may also have an adverse impact on recovery from serious wounds or injuries, especially those that involve large amounts of blood loss. However, data to support deficits in physical performance in iron-compromised individuals have not been systematically collected by the military. Some preliminary evidence suggests that iron supplementation of nonanemic women can improve aerobic capacity (J. Haas, Cornell University, personal communication, 1977). Male soldiers consuming operational rations appear to meet iron needs, as judged from current levels in the MRDA.

Glutamine. Glutamine is an amino acid that constitutes approximately 5 percent of most proteins. The CMNR recognizes that glutamine is a potential candidate for addition to operational rations to optimize immunity. It has demonstrated potential for promoting immune cell proliferation and improving immune function, especially under the stress of surgery, infection, or bowel disease. However, before it would be appropriate to consider providing supplemental glutamine to soldiers in training or deployment situations, it will first be necessary to demonstrate in a healthy population the benefits of providing glutamine at levels significantly greater than those normally obtained in the diet. The results of one military study presented at the workshop showed no beneficial effects of glutamine supplementation on immune function parameters. The CMNR recently hosted a workshop (The Role of Protein and Amino Acids in Sustaining and Enhancing Performance) that addressed more fully the safety and efficacy issues for this and other amino acids.

Vitamin A and Antioxidants. Vitamin A intakes beyond the MRDA do not appear to be beneficial; in fact, excess intakes can be toxic. Healthy adult men and women of military age represent the lowest-risk group for the development of vitamin A deficiency; however, under certain conditions, such as chronic infection or prolonged dietary deprivation, the risk of vitamin A deficiency and associated immune abnormalities may be significant (as described by Richard Semba, in Chapter 12). Carotenoids as supplied from fruits and vegetables may be important as modulators or stimulators of immune function.

Vitamins C and E are immunopotentiating agents most likely because of their function as antioxidants. Both of these vitamins are relatively nontoxic. However, it has not been demonstrated whether there is a functional benefit of increased intakes in protection against cancer, pathogenic viruses, or bacteria. Investigation of the role of these vitamins in protecting against or modulating the effects of infection is an active area of research. Toxicities of high-dose vitamin C supplements also have been difficult to demonstrate. Some evidence suggests that doses of 500 mg or more may result in increased excretion of oxalate (a precursor to one form of renal stone), but this observation has been limited to individuals who have an increased risk of forming stones (Urivetsky et al., 1992). A primary cause for concern among military personnel, who may be deployed on short notice, has been the risk of rebound scurvy due to sudden vitamin C withdrawal (Schrauzer and Rhead, 1973); however, clear evidence for this phenomenon is lacking. Likewise, the potential value of consumption from food sources rather than single-nutrient supplement intake requires greater study. However, the most prudent approach seems to be to increase fruit and vegetable consumption in the diet, thereby maximizing the potential benefits of antioxidant nutrients.

A factor that must be considered in recommending an increase in vitamin E intake is the level of PUFAs concomitantly being consumed in the diet. Increasing amounts of polyunsaturated fatty acids increase the vitamin E requirement because of the propensity of PUFAs to undergo lipid peroxidation. Approximately 0.4 mg of α-tocopherol equivalent for each gram of PUFA consumed has been suggested to be adequate in adult humans (Sokol, 1996).

Fatty Acids. Limited data suggest that moderate reductions in total fat calories (that is, 26 percent versus 30 percent) may have some beneficial effects in enhancing immune function. Increasing or decreasing the consumption of n-6 or n-3 PUFAs, or altering their intake ratios, may impact on immunological function. Although increased consumption of fish oils that supply eicosapentaenoic acid (EPA) and docosahexaenoic acid (DHA) may reduce the risk of heart disease and be beneficial in treating autoimmune diseases, their increased intake may reduce immune function, raise the dietary requirement for vitamin E, and affect blood clotting mechanisms (especially n-3 fatty acids).

Final Cautionary Notes. It is important to recognize that although modification of operational rations could potentially benefit the immune function of a large segment of the military population, a small but significant portion of the population could be harmed by such modifications because of genetic predisposition or other unknown factors. Also, it is possible that an elevated intake of a nutrient would result in a modification of immune function that is safe for a limited period but would diminish in safety or efficacy with prolonged use. Such a situation will necessitate a risk–benefit decision or the identification of a means by which to provide the supplemental nutrients in an additional ration component. Despite claims made by industry, some athletes, and sports coaches, most of the nutrients discussed in this report have failed thus far to demonstrate both safety and efficacy in modifying immune function, and further research is needed. Systematic studies should assess the extent to which subjects self-medicate with over-the-counter dietary food supplements, and such products should be evaluated carefully before their use is recommended.

5. Are there areas of investigation for the military nutrition research program that are likely to be fruitful in the sustainment of immune function in stressful conditions? Specifically, is there likely to be enough value added to justify adding to operational rations or including an additional component?

It is important to conduct research aimed at defining more specific nutrient–immune system interactions in order to elucidate the levels of key nutrients that are necessary to maintain proper immune function. Since these data also would be important for the general population, it is not necessary that this research be supported solely by the military; it could be conducted by other agencies. However, special studies of unique groups or circumstances (such as Ranger training) applying chiefly to the military might be warranted.

For some aspects of immune function, both beneficial and adverse effects related to nutrient intake may be encountered (some examples are vitamin A and iron). With this in mind, the CMNR suggests that the following areas are worthy of further investigation by the military nutrition research program:

• *Supplement use.* The military needs to gain a better understanding of supplement use by its personnel. Little information is available regarding the real benefits or potential toxic effects of nutritional supplements in supranormal amounts to warrant their further study for widespread use in the military at present. Indeed, some data indicate frank adverse effects of consuming one or more of these nutrients (such as copper and zinc) in pharmacologic amounts. Although there seems to be relatively little risk associated with the use of vitamins C and E, and there may be relatively little risk associated with the use of β-carotene, major differences in potential benefits may exist between dietary exposure to such antioxidants and the use of supplements. Excessive supplementation with vitamin A, zinc, or selenium could prove toxic. The basis for this discrepancy and its impact on how such supplements are used should be addressed. In addition, the use of botanical and herbal supplements may be associated with risks that require further study.

• *Cytokines as an index of immune function.* As previously recommended by the CMNR (IOM, 1997), further research will be needed to determine if stress-related changes in cytokines can be detected reliably in spot urine samples collected during military field operations. Proinflammatory cytokines and their receptors and antagonists are all excreted in the urine. The magnitude of stress-related increases in the production of proinflammatory cytokines can be determined in whole-blood stimulation assays and possibly in 24-h urinary samples obtained during periods of stress, infectious illness, and/or trauma; however, the practicality and validity of urinary cytokine measures for field research studies must be determined.

Studies are necessary to determine if cytokine-related measurements have greater value, greater sensitivity, or greater stimulus-related specificity than the standard measurements of red blood cell sedimentation rates and CRP protein as indicators of systemic disease and/or as models of stress-induced release or suppression of proinflammatory cytokines.

• *Disease conditions and long-term host defense.* Ensuring prompt etiologic diagnosis of infectious illness and early therapy with effective antimicrobial agents will spare the loss of body nutrients by minimizing disease severity and duration. The severity and duration of fever are in proportion to measurable losses of nutrients from the body and/or their accelerated consumption. Accordingly, the control of high fevers (but not necessarily their total elimination) by specific drugs (ibuprofen, and to a lesser extent, aspirin) that prevent the conversion of arachidonic acid to fever-related eicosanoids (for example, the prostaglandins) will conserve body weight and nutrient stores. During protracted infections, nutritional supplements (multivitamin and/or multimineral pills, antioxidants, and amino acids such as glutamine and arginine) may provide valuable immunological support. The potential value of similar combinations of supplements, given as a possible prophylactic measure during periods of severe military stress, is currently unknown but warrants future study. Further, the consumption of high-quality diets should be encouraged early in convalescence to restore body nutrient pools and lost weight.

One important disease condition as yet unstudied is diarrhea. This condition should be examined to evaluate its effect on immune status indicators, both as a single variable and in combination with other important variables such as immunization, exercise, and reduced food intake. The major losses during diarrhea are those of water, sodium, potassium, and bicarbonate. None of these are known to have a direct effect on immune system functions; nonetheless, the resultant acidosis affects a variety of cell functions.

A key question involving the immune status of Special Forces troops is how acute nutrient deprivation during training may influence host defense on a long-term basis, and whether temporary nutritional and immune deficits incurred during training may produce long-term vulnerability (see recommendation in the CMNR's report of Ranger I studies [IOM, 1992]). Research also will be needed to determine if cytokine-induced losses of essential body nutrients are important concerns in military personnel exposed to other nonnutritional stresses.

• *Immune function in women.* Most studies to date have focused largely on male soldiers. Therefore, there is a paucity of information about the immune response of energy- and sleep-deprived female personnel who participate in training activities. Research is needed to evaluate the interrelationships among sleep, nutrition, physical activity, female sex hormone responses, menstrual cycle, and immune function in women in the military. An emerging area of interest is the evaluation of the effects of endogenous and exogenous (phyto- and xeno-) estrogens on immune function. Of particular importance are the deficiency of iron in many military women and the immunological consequences of iron deficiency.

REFERENCES

Alexander, J.W. 1993. Immunoenhancement via enteral nutrition. Arch. Surg. 128(11):1242–1245.

Andelman, M.B., and B.R. Sered. 1966. Utilization of dietary iron by term infants: A study of 1,048 infants from a low socioeconomic population. Am. J. Dis. Child. 111:45–55.

Baurenfreund, J.C. 1980. The Safest Use of Vitamin A. International Vitamin A Consultative Group. Washington, D.C.: The Nutrition Foundation.

Beard, J. 1993. Iron dependent pathologies. Pp. 99–111 in Iron Deficiency Anemia, Recommended Guidelines for the Prevention, Detection, and Management Among U.S. Children and Women of Childbearing Age, R. Earl and C.E. Woteki, eds. A report of the Committee on the Prevention, Detection, and Management of Iron Deficiency Anemia Among U.S. Children and Women of Childbearing Age, Food and Nutrition Board, Institute of Medicine. Washington, D.C.: National Academy Press.

Beisel, W.R. 1991. Nutrition and infection. Pp. 507–542 in Nutritional Biochemistry and Metabolism, 2nd ed., M.C. Linder, ed. New York: Elsevier.

Beisel, W.R. 1992 Metabolic responses of the host to infections. Pp. 1–13 in Textbook of Pediatric Infectious Diseases, 3d ed., R.D. Feigin and J.D. Cherry, eds. Philadelphia: W.B. Saunders Co.

Bendich, A. 1992. Safety issues regarding the use of vitamin supplements. Ann. N.Y. Acad. Sci. 669:300–310.

Bernstein, A.L., and L.S. Lobitz. 1988. A clinical and electro-physiologic study of the treatment of painful diabetic neuropathies with pyridoxine. Pp. 415–423 in Clinical and Physiological Applications and Vitamin B-6, J.E. Leklem and R.E. Reynolds, eds. New York: Alan R. Liss.

Brubacher, G.B., and H. Weiser. 1985. The vitamin A activity of β carotene. J. Vit. Nutr. Res. 55:5–15.

Chandra, R.K. 1984. Excessive intake of zinc impairs immune responses. J. Am. Med. Assoc. 252:1443–1446.

Chandra, R.K., ed. 1988. Nutrition and Immunology. New York: Alan R. Liss.

Chandra, R.K. 1992a. Effect of vitamin and trace-element supplementation on immune responses and infection in elderly subjects. Lancet 340:1124–1127.

Chandra, R.K., and S. Kumari. 1994. Nutrition and immunity: an overview. J. Nutr. 124(8 Suppl):1433S–1435S.

Cunningham-Rundles, S., R.S. Bockman, A. Lin, P.V. Giardina, M.W. Hilgartner, D. Caldwell-Brown, and D.M. Carter. 1990a. Physiological and pharmacological effects of zinc on immune response. Ann. N.Y. Acad. Sci. 587:113–112.

Davis, G.K., and W. Mertz. 1987. Copper. Pp. 301–364 in Trace Elements in Human and Animal Nutrition, W. Mertz, ed. San Diego: Academic Press.

DeRijk, R., D. Michelson, B. Karp, J. Petrides, E. Galliven, P. Deuster, G. Paciotti, P.W. Gold, and E.M. Sternberg. 1997. Exercise and circadian rhythm-induced variations in plasma cortisol differentially regulate interleukin-1β (IL-1β), Il-6, and tumor necrosis factor-α (TNFα) production in humans: High sensitivity of TNFα and resistance of IL-6. J. Clin. Endocrinol. Metab. 82(7):2182–2191.

DeRijk, R.H., J. Petrides, P. Deuster, P.W. Gold, and E.M. Sternberg. 1996. Changes in corticosteroid sensitivity of peripheral blood lymphocytes after strenuous exercise in humans. J. Clin. Endocrinol. Metab. 81(1):228–235.

Endres, S., S.N. Madden, R. Ghorbani, R. Schindler, and C.A. Dinarello. 1993. Dietary supplementation with n-3 fatty acids suppresses interleukin-2 production and mononuclear cell proliferation. J. Leukocyte Biol. 54:599–603.

Hopkins, R.G., and M.L. Failla. 1997. Copper deficiency reduces interleukin-2 (IL-2) production and IL-2 mRNA in human T-lymphocytes. J. Nutr. 127(2):257–262.

Farrell, P.M., and J.G. Bieri. 1975. Megavitamin E supplementation in man. Am. J. Clin. Nutr. 28:1381–1386.

Fisher, M., P.H. Levine, B.H. Weiner, M.H. Johnson, E.M. Doyle, P.A. Ellis, J.J. Hoogasian. 1990. Dietary n-3 fatty acid supplementation reduces superoxide production and chemiluminescence in a monocyte-enriched preparation of leukocytes. Am. J. Clin. Nutr. 51(5):804–808.

Griffith, R.D., C. Jones, and T.E.A. Palmer. 1997. Six month outcome of critically ill patients given glutamine supplemental parenteral nutrition. Nutrition 13:295–302.

Helzlsouer, C.K., R. Jacobs, and S. Morris. 1985. Acute selenium intoxication in the United States. Fed. Proc. 44:1670.

Herbert, V. 1979. Ascorbic acid and vitamin B12. JAMA 242(21):2285.

Hershko, C. 1992. Iron and infection. Pp. 53–64 in Nutritional Anemias, Nestle Nutrition Workshop Series, vol. 30, S.J. Fomon and S. Zlotkin, eds. New York: Nestec Ltd. Vevey Raven Press Ltd.

Hussein, M.A., H.A. Hassan, A.A. Abdel-Ghaffar and S. Salem. 1988. Effect of iron supplements on occurrence of diarrhea among children in rural Egypt. Food Nutr. Bull. 10(2):35–49.

IOM (Institute of Medicine). 1992. A Nutritional Assessment of U.S. Army Ranger Training Class 11/91. A brief report of the Committee on Military Nutrition Research, Food and Nutrition Board. March 23, 1992. Washington, D.C.

IOM (Institute of Medicine). 1995a. Not Eating Enough, Overcoming Underconsumption of Military Operational Rations, B.M. Marriott, ed. A report of the Committee on Military Nutrition Research, Food and Nutrition Board. Washington, D.C.: National Academy Press.

IOM (Institute of Medicine). 1996. Nutritional Needs in Cold and in High-Altitude Environments, Applications for Military Personnel in Field Operations, B.M. Marriott and S.J. Carlson, eds. A report of the Committee on Military Nutrition Research, Food and Nutrition Board. Washington, D.C.: National Academy Press.

IOM (Institute of Medicine). 1997. Emerging Technologies for Nutrition Research: Potential for Assessing Military Performance Capability, S.J. Carlson-Newberry and R.B. Costello, eds. A report of the Committee on Military Nutrition Research, Food and Nutrition Board. Washington, D.C.: National Academy Press.

Kadiiska, M.A., P.M. Hanna, S.J. Jordan, and R.P. Mason. 1993. Electron spin resonance evidence for free radical generation in copper-treated vitamin E- and selenium-deficient rats: In vivo spin-trapping investigation. Molec. Pharmacol. 44:222–227.

Kirk, S.J., and A. Barbul. 1992. Arginine and immunity. Pp. 160–161 in Encyclopedia of Immunology, Book I, I.M. Roitt and P.J. Delves, eds. London: Academic Press.

Kudsk, K.A., G. Minard, M.A. Croce, R.O. Brown, T.S. Lowrey, F.E. Pritchard, R.N. Dickerson, and T.C. Fabian. 1996. A randomized trial of isonitrogenous enteral diets after severe trauma. An immune-enhancing diet reduces septic complications. Ann. Surg. 224(4):531-40; discussion 540–543.

Levine, M., K.R. Dhariwal, R.W. Welch, Y. Wang, J.B. Park. 1995. Determination of optimal vitamin C requirements in humans. Am. J. Clin. Nutr. 62(suppl.):S1347–S1356.

Longnecker, M.P., P.R. Taylor, O.A. Levander, M. Howe, C. Veillon, P.A. McAdam, K.Y. Patterson, J.M. Holden, M.J. Stampfer, J.S. Morris, et al. 1991. Selenium in diet, blood, and toenails in relation to human health in a seleniferous area. Am. J. Clin. Nutr. 53:1288–1294.

Mackowiak, P.A., J.G. Bartlett, E.C. Borden, S.E. Goldblum, J.D. Hasday, R.S. Munford, S.A. Nasraway, P.D. Stolley, and T.E. Woodward. 1997. Concepts of fever: Recent advances and lingering dogma. Clin. Infect. Dis. 25:119–138.

Meydani, S.N., M.P. Barklund, S. Liu, M. Meydani et al. 1990. Vitamin E supplementation enhances cell-mediated immunity in healthy elderly subjects. Am. J. Clin. Nutr. 52:557–563.

Meydani, S.N., M. Meydani, J.B. Blumberg, L.S. Leka, G. Siber, R. Loszewski, C. Thompson, M.C. Pedrosa, R.D. Diamond, and B.D. Stollar. 1997b. Vitamin E supplementation and in vivo immune response in healthy elderly subjects. A randomized controlled trial. JAMA 277(17):1380–1386.

Meydani, S.N., J.D. Ribaya-Mercado, R.M. Russell, N. Sahyoun, F.D. Morrow, and S.N. Gershoff. 1991. Vitamin B-6 deficiency impairs interleukin 2 production and lymphocyte proliferation in elderly adults. Am. J. Clin. Nutr. 53(5):1275–1280.

Miller, R.K., J. Brown, D. Cordero, B. Dayton, B. Hardin, and M. Greene. 1987. Teratology Society position paper: recommendations for vitamin A use during pregnancy. Teratology 35(2):269–275.

Murray, M.J., A.B. Murray, M.B. Murray, and C.J. Murray. 1978a. The adverse effect of iron repletion on the course of certain infections. Br. Med. J. 2(6145):1113–1115.

Newhouse, I.J., and D.B. Clement. 1988. Iron status in athletes. An update. Sports Med. 5:337–352.

NRC (National Research Council). 1989. Recommended Dietary Allowances, 10th ed. Subcommittee on the Tenth Edition of the RDAs, Food and Nutrition Board, Commission on Life Sciences. Washington, D.C.: National Academy Press.

Olson, J.A. 1983. Formation and function of vitamin A. Pp. 371–412 in Polyisopenoid Synthesis, vol. II, J.Q Porter, ed. New York: John Wiley & Sons.

Pinnock, C.B., and C.P. Alderman. 1992. The potential for teratogenicity of Vitamin A and its congeners. Med. J. Aust. 157:805.

Poirier, K.A. 1994. Summary of the derivation of the reference dose for selenium. Pp. 157–166 in Risk Assessment of Essential Elements, W. Mertz, C.O. Abernathy and S.S. Olin, eds. Washington, DC: ILSI Press.

Prasad, A.S., ed. 1976. Deficiency of zinc in man and its toxicity. Pp. 1–20 in Trace Elements in Health and Disease, vol. 1: Zinc and Copper. New York: Academic Press.

Prasad, A.S., G.J. Brewer, E.B. Schoomaker, and P. Rabbani. 1978. Hypocupremia induced by zinc therapy in adults. J. Am. Med. Assoc. 240:2166–2168.

Rothman, K.J., L.L. Moore, M.R. Singer, U.S. Nguyen, S. Mannino, and A. Milunsky. 1995. Teratogenicity of high vitamin A intake. N. Engl. J. Med. 333:1369.

Santos, M.S., S.N. Meydani, L. Leka, D. Wu, N. Fotouhi, M. Meydani, C.H. Hennekens, and J.M. Gaziano. 1996. Natural killer cell activity in elderly men is enhanced by beta-carotene supplementation. Am. J. Clin. Nutr. 64(5):772–777.

Schaumburg, H., J. Kaplan, A. Windebank, N. Vick, S. Rasmus, D. Pleasure, and M.J. Brown. 1983. Sensory neuropathy from pyridoxine abuse: A new megavitamin syndrome. N. Engl. J. Med. 309:445–448.

Schmidt, E.B., K. Varming, J.O. Pedersen, H.H. Lervang, N. Grunnet, C. Jersild, and J. Dyerberg. 1992. Long-term supplementation with n-3 fatty acids, II: Effect on neutrophil and monocyte chemotaxis. Scand. J. Clin. Lab. Invest. 52(3):229–236.

Schrauzer, G.N., and W.J. Rhead. 1973. Ascorbic acid abuse: effects on long term ingestion of excessive amounts on blood levels and urinary excretion. Int. J. Vitam. Nutr. Res. 43(2):201–211.

Shah, M.A., P.R. Bergethon, A.M. Boak, P.M. Gallop, and H.M. Kagan. 1992. Oxidation of peptidyl lysine by copper complexes of pyrroloquinoline quinone and other quinones: A model for oxidative pathochemistry. Biochem. Biophys. Acta. 1159(3):311–318.

Sokol, R.J. 1996. Vitamin E. Pp. 130–136 in Present Knowledge in Nutrition, 7th ed., E. Khard, E. Ziegler, and L.J. Filer, eds. Washington, D.C.: ILSI Press.

Straight, J.M., H.M. Kipen, R.F. Vogt, and R.W. Amler. 1994. Immune Function Test Batteries for Use in Environmental Health Studies. U.S. Department of Health and Human Services, Public Health Service. Publication Number: PB94-204328.

Sullivan, J.L., and H.D. Ochs. 1978. Copper deficiency and the immune system. Lancet 2(8091):686.

Urivetzky, M. D. Kessaris, and A.D. Smith. 1992. Ascorbic acid overdosing: A risk factor for calcium oxalate nephrolithiasis. J. Urol. 147:1215–1218.

U.S. Departments of the Army, the Navy, and the Air Force. 1985. Army Regulation 40-25/Navy Command Medical Instruction 10110.1/Air Force Regulation 160-95. "Nutritional Allowances, Standards, and Education." Washington, D.C.

Viteri, F.E. Prevention of iron deficiency. 1998. Pp. 45–102 in Prevention of Micronutrient Deficiencies: Tools for Policymakers and Public Health Workers. Institute of Medicine. Washington, D.C.: National Academy Press.

Westphal, K.A., L.J. Marchitelli, K.E. Friedl, and M.A. Sharp. 1995b. Relationship between iron status and physical performance in female soldiers during U.S. Army basic combat training. Fed. Am. Soc. Exp. Biol. J. 9(3):A361[abstract].

Westphal K.A., A.E. Pusateri, and T.R. Kramer. 1994. Prevalence of negative iron nutriture and relationship with folate nutriture, immunocompetence, and fitness level in U.S. Army servicewomen. USARIEM Approved Protocol OPD94002-AP024-H016. Defense Women's Health Research Program 1994, Log No. W4168016. Natick, Mass.: U.S. Army Research Institute of Environmental Medicine.

WHO (World Health Organization). 1993. FAO/WHO Recommendations on Fats and Oils in Human Nutrition. Geneva: WHO.

WHO (World Health Organization). 1996. Trace Elements in Human Nutrition and Health. Geneva: WHO.

Yang, G., S. Yin, R. Zhou, L. Gu, B. Yan, Y. Liu, and Y. Liu. 1989. Studies of safe maximal daily dietary Se intake in a seleniferous area in China. Part II. Relation between Se intake and the manifestation of clinical signs and certain biochemical alterations in blood and urine. J. Trace Elem. Electrolytes Health Dis. 3(3):123–130.

Ziegler, T.R., K. Benfell, R.J. Smith, L.S. Young, E. Brown, E. Ferrari-Baliviera, D.K. Lowe, D.W. Wilmore. 1990. Safety and metabolic effects of L-glutamine administration in humans. JPEN J. Parenter. Enteral Nutr. 14(4 Suppl):137S–146S.

Nutrition and Immune Function, 1999
Pp. 125–135. Washington, D.C.
National Academy Press

3

Committee Conclusions and Recommendations

As stated in Chapter 1, the Committee on Military Nutrition Research (CMNR) was asked to respond to five specific questions dealing with the impact of nutritional status on immune function as it pertains to soldiers deployed for military operations and Special Forces troops. The conclusions and recommendations that follow are based on the discussion of these questions appearing in Chapter 2. Recommendations for areas of future development for the U.S. Army nutrition research programs are also included in this chapter.

CONCLUSIONS

The study of the interaction of nutrition and immune function is an exceptionally active area of research in both the military and the civilian (academic and commercial) sectors.

General Health Status

A considerable number of conditions encountered by the military act as immune stressors. These stressors include operationally induced undernutrition and dehydration; alterations in biological rhythms; atmospheric conditions such as temperature, humidity, and altitude; and environmental pollutants such as dust, smoke, and chemical fumes, as well as injuries and infectious agents themselves. As a result, studies of immune function in field situations contain many uncontrollable variables, and it is often difficult to attribute observed effects to one variable such as nutritional status.

The military's use of prophylactic immunization provides sufficient benefit beyond risk to warrant continued development. Recommendations concerning research on militarily relevant vaccines are contained in an earlier CMNR report (IOM, 1997). This is supported by a recent decision of the Secretary of Defense to begin systematic immunization of all U.S. military personnel angainst the biological warfare agent anthrax.

Pharmacologic agents such as aspirin, ibuprofen, and glucocorticoids modulate the effects of cytokines and can be used to minimize signs and symptoms of cytokine-induced acute-phase reactions and the nutrient losses that accompany them. Their use in military operations for the management of minor traumas and infections is well recognized and has been shown to sustain military performance during severe training exercises and operational missions.

Evidence to suggest that the administration of recombinant cytokines can modulate immune function in a desirable manner is limited at the present time to a small number of disease states. Their effectiveness has not been demonstrated in healthy subjects.

Field studies must be based on the results of prior experiments conducted in controlled laboratory and clinical settings. Experimental designs and methods must be validated by pilot tests prior to use. Because of the effects of circadian rhythms on immune function, samples must be collected at precisely defined times. In addition, because of the sensitivity and low levels of the molecules of interest, biological samples must be handled, transported, and stored according to recommendations for the materials in question, and appropriate controls must be included.

Nutritional Status

Total energy intake appears to play the greatest role in nutritional modulation of immune function. Since it has been demonstrated that prolonged energy deficits resulting in significant weight loss have an adverse effect on immune function, emphasis should be placed on the importance of adequate ration intake during military operations to minimize weight loss.

Weight loss in the range of 10 percent in operations extending over 4 weeks raisee the concern of reduced physical and cognitive performance and has potential health consequences for some individuals (IOM, 1995).

The nutritional status of soldiers should be optimized prior to deployment or engagement in any exercise or training course or even brief encounters with anything that would present a potential immune challenge (disease, toxic agent, or environmental stress). When consumed as recommended, operational rations provide adequate energy and macronutrients.

In addition to energy intake, nutrients that appear to play a role in immune function include protein, iron, zinc, copper, and selenium; the antioxidants β-carotene and vitamins C and E; vitamin A and the B-group vitamins, especially B_6, B_{12}, and folate; the amino acids glutamine and arginine; and the polyunsaturated fatty acids (PUFAs). It is difficult to consider the role of one nutrient in isolation. Evidence for a role for vitamin C in immunomodulation remains controversial, and the role of vitamin E has been demonstrated chiefly in the elderly. There is no evidence at this time to indicate that the levels of vitamins A, E, and C, or trace elements including zinc, copper, or selenium are inadequate in operational rations. Increasing or decreasing the consumption of n-6 or n-3 polyunsaturated fatty acids (PUFAs), or altering their intake ratios, may impact on immunological functions. Available data also suggest that altered dietary intakes of essential polyunsaturated fatty acids (PUFAs), either the n-6 or the n-3 PUFAs, may influence immune functions. Iron deficiency impairs immune system competence and depresses the bactericidal functions of phagocytic cells. Excess iron as well as iron deficiency may also compromise immune status. Selenium deficiency is associated with increased susceptibility to particular infectious pathogens and may modify the virulence of a coxsackie virus that causes heart muscle damage. The latter observation may explain the apparent prevalence of Keshan disease, an endemic juvenile cardiomyopathy thought to be caused by a coxsackie virus, in areas of China experiencing periodic selenium deficiency. Glutamine has demonstrated potential for improving immune function in critical illness, and parenteral and enteral administration of glutamine has been observed to improve recovery following gastrointestinal surgery, but its usefulness in healthy populations must yet has not been determined. Studies to evaluate the effects of supplemental glutamine on the immune function of soldiers have shown no demonstrable effects. The amounts of vitamins and trace elements (including zinc, copper, and selenium), contained in operational rations, meet all MRDAs (Military Recommended Dietary Allowances) if the diet is fully consumed. However, varying combinations of military stresses may increase the need for certain essential nutrients to values greater than the MRDA to maintain immunological competence.

Nutritional Supplements

The effects of providing supplements of vitamins A, C and E, as well as certain polyunsaturated fatty acids and amino acids, prior to, during, or following infections are virtually unknown in young, healthy adult men. Many questions remain regarding the efficacy of these nutrients in amounts that exceed Military Recommended Dietary Allowance (MRDA) levels. However, during protracted infections, nutritional supplements (multivitamin and/or multimineral pills, antioxidants, and amino acids such as glutamine and arginine) may provide valuable immunological support. Further, the consumption of high-quality diets should be encouraged early in convalescence to restore body nutrient pools and lost weight. *The most prudent approach seems to be one of increasing fruit and vegetable consumption in the diet, thus maximizing the potential benefits of antioxidant nutrients.*

Safety problems associated with excess consumption of supplements are much more likely for some nutrients than for others. Toxicity and the potential for nutrient–nutrient interactions must be considered individually. Excess intakes of vitamin A may be toxic, whereas vitamins C and E are relatively nontoxic and have been shown to enhance the immune response. Trace minerals are particularly problematic because requirements may be altered during periods of illness (increased), while at the same time, excessive intakes of some trace elements may be immunosuppressive.

Excess iron as well as iron deficiency may compromise immune status. The problem of compromised iron status in female personnel is a matter of concern because it may impact immune function, physical performance, and cognitive function. It is important to maintain adequate iron status in female soldiers and to do so without causing excess iron intake by males.

Glutamine has demonstrated potential for improving immune function in critical illness, but its usefulness in healthy populations is unknown. Parenteral and enteral administration of glutamine has been observed to improve recovery following gastrointestinal surgery. Thus far, the effect of glutamine has been observed only in supraphysiological amounts and only in patients undergoing bone marrow transplantation or major operations and those who sustain life-threatening sepsis. Studies to evaluate the effects of supplemental glutamine on the immune function of soldiers have shown no demonstrable effects. An effect of glutamine deficiency also has not been demonstrated.

Although none of the major body nutrients lost during severe diarrheal episodes (sodium, potassium, and bicarbonate) are known to influence immune function, rehydration strategies (and in some situations, supplementation with glutamine) may be of use in the treatment of diarrhea.

Finally, it must be emphasized that the results of studies performed in deficient animals or individuals are different from those done on adequately nourished ones and that, in many cases, an "overdose" of a nutrient, as well as a deficiency, leads to negative consequences.

RECOMMENDATIONS

Optimizing General Health Status

• **The CMNR recommends the use of medically appropriate and directed prophylactic medications and procedures to minimize the adverse effects of infectious agents. However, the CMNR sees no potential value at this time administering cytokines or anti-cytokines to healthy military personnel.**

It is generally assumed that the body's production of endogenous cytokines during stressful situations is beneficial to the host. However, if endogenous proinflammatory cytokines accumulate in large excesses or are given in large doses, they may have noxious or even dangerous consequences. The military should remain cognizant of the very active civilian-sector research concerning cytokines, their complex control mechanisms, and their functions, and should apply any pertinent new findings to the management of militarily relevant infectious diseases, trauma, or other stresses. The military should also keep apprised of advances (in the form of proven treatments) that emerge from this research.

• **In light of the importance of military immunization programs for achieving and maintaining immune status at optimal levels, the CMNR reiterates its previous recommendations (IOM, 1997) that vigorous research efforts be undertaken to create and evaluate militarily relevant oral vaccines.**

These should include optimization of administration schedules and elucidation of the influence of nutritional status on vaccine efficacy. Immunological responses to vaccines may be altered by the stresses of mobilization and/or overseas deployments. Antibody responses to vaccines are known to be depressed by protein-energy malnutrition. The potential problem of reduced responsiveness to military vaccines given during periods of mobilization and deployment stresses (in comparison to normal responses, as measured in control studies) also deserves future study.

• **It is recommended that soldiers maintain good physical fitness via a regular, moderate exercise program as a means of sustaining optimum immune function.** Since the intensity and duration of physical activity can affect immune function, training regimens that achieve high levels of physical fitness without adverse effects on immune status should be established.

• Additionally, the CMNR recommends the use of methods to minimize psychological stresses, including training, conditioning, and structured briefing and debriefing.

Optimizing Nutritional Status

• **In view of the compromised immune function noted in studies of Ranger trainees, the CMNR recommends that, where possible, individuals who have lost significant lean body mass should not be redeployed until this lean mass is regained.**

Although data showing an effect of weight loss on immune function may be limited, it is reasonable to suggest that the maintenance of body weight within 10 percent of ideal weight should increase the likelihood that adequate immune function will be maintained. Thus, the committee recommends that soldiers be advised to achieve an energy intake sufficient to maintain normal weight. The energy intakes required to maintain body weight will vary with the intensity and duration of physical activity; therefore, the best field guide for individual soldiers and commanders is to monitor body weight changes and to emphasize, through a "field-feeding doctrine," the importance of ration intake as the fuel for the soldier to maintain health and performance.

• **The CMNR recommends that nutritional anemia be treated prior to deployment and that individuals classified as anemic[1] and requiring iron supplements not be deployed.**

With the reduced personnel in today's Army and the potential for frequent deployment, it is important that soldiers be in good nutritional health at the time of deployment and that an effort be made to correct any compromise in status that may have resulted from previous deployment. Some scientists believe that iron supplements, if given during the course of bacterial or parasitic infections, may increase the severity of these illnesses. Because this topic is a controversial one, it requires further investigation. Nevertheless, it is recommended that if additional iron is required (for prophylactic purposes), it should be in the form of an optional ration supplement, and the iron content of operational rations themselves should not exceed MRDA levels.

• **As a means of reducing the number of stresses encountered by military personnel, the committee encourages the development and implementation of nutrition education programs targeted at high-risk military groups, such as Special Forces troops and female soldiers.**

---

[1] Iron deficiency anemia is defined as a serum ferritin concentration of less than 12 µg/ml in combination with a hemoglobin of less than 120 g/L.

[2] Iron deficiency anemia is defined as a serum ferritin concentration of less than 12 µg/ml in combination with a hemoglobin of less than 120 g/L.

The military should increase efforts to communicate information regarding healthy eating habits and supplement use to all personnel. Since dehydration and energy deficit have a great potential for compromising immune function, soldiers should also be educated regarding compliance with the "water doctrine."

Nutritional Supplement Use

Supplementation with certain nutrients may be of value for sustaining host defense mechanisms (including those conferred by the immune system) at normal levels during periods of extreme physiological and physical stress. Carefully controlled pilot and more extensive field studies will be necessary to investigate this possibility. It is unlikely, however, that nutritional supplements can produce a state of superimmunity in normal subjects or military personnel.

- **At this time, the CMNR cannot recommend general supplementation of military rations above the MRDAs for the purpose of enhancing immune function.**

There are no definitive studies that demonstrate positive benefits to young, healthy, active individuals of nutrient supplements at levels significantly in excess of those recommended by the MRDAs and commonly provided by foods. Encouraging ration intake to sustain nutrient levels as described in the MRDAs appears to be the best recommendation until further research clearly can define the likely benefits of specific nutrient supplementation under defined operational conditions. Soldiers should be cautioned regarding the indiscriminate use of individual supplements and the potential effects of inadequate nutrient intake, as well as the use of single or combined supplements, since their effects on immune status are not known.

- **The CMNR recommends that, when needed, the preferred method of providing supplemental nutrients is through a ration component.**

This would reduce both the potential for excessive intake by those individuals who do not need the nutrient and the potential misuse that exists when supplemental nutrients are provided in individual nutrient form. Because energy is one nutrient that has been identified as playing a role in immune function, provision of supplemental energy in the form of a food bar would allow soldiers to increase their nutrient intake as needed according to activity levels.

- **The CMNR recommends that the military gain a better understanding of supplement use as well as supplement abuse by personnel and make strong recommendations for the appropriate use or nonuse of nutritional supplements.**

The emphasis should be on education and wise choices. In the past, the CMNR has suggested the development of a "field-feeding doctrine" (IOM, 1995a), with the guiding principle that the energy intakes of military personnel during training and combat operations should be adequate to meet their energy expenditures and to maintain body weight and lean body mass. This field-feeding doctrine would accompany the successful "water doctrine" that resulted from a recommendation in the report *Fluid Replacement in Heat Stress,* (IOM, 1991; and 1993a). 4). The guiding principle of the water doctrine was to ensure that adequate fluid intake is maintained to avoid dehydration and subsequent decreased food intake. As more information is gained on supplement use and misuse and on the risks and benefits of supplements, the Army may want to consider formulateing a "supplement doctrine" similar to the water and food doctrines to address these concerns and add a component to nutrition education programs. A better understanding of supplement use will provide information on the prevalence and frequency of use, its impact on an individual's nutritional status, and the likelihood of reckless or dangerous nutrition practices. Such information will help provide for the delivery of targeted and focused nutritional education messages. The committee is aware that some information on supplement use will be obtained by the Army Food and Nutrition Survey and suggests that additional information on supplement use can best be obtained by including appropriate questions in ongoing military health surveys, such as the Survey of Health-Related Behaviors Among Military Personnel.

Research Methodology

The CMNR strongly encourages the military to keep apprised of relevant civilian research and consider the application of selected findings and protocols to the military situation.

• **The CMNR recommends that research be conducted to determine the appropriate field measures for monitoring nutritionally induced immune responses, particularly for determining the presence of acute-phase reactions and changes in immune function of the type and degree that are likely to occur as a result of the nutritional insults suffered by soldiers in typical deployment situations.**

This will require basing field studies on appropriate clinical investigations, piloting experimental designs, and using a simple panel of standard tests (such as those described in Chapter 2) that have been validated for the field. Particular attention must be paid to the timing of sample collection; the conditions under which samples are transported, stored, and handled; and the use of proper controls.

A rapid assessment of immune functions for use in the field includes clinical evaluations of local lesions, sites of inflammation, and signs and symptoms of generalized infectious illness. The C-reactive protein (CRP), erythrocyte sedimentation rate (ESR), and white cell counts are the most rapid and least expensive lab tests. Skin tests are highly valuable markers of cell-mediated immunity but require 48 hours before they can be read. Other tests can be valuable if time and facilities permit. On the other hand, preliminary clinical trials may employ additional kinds of sophisticated immunological studies, along with those listed for field investigations.

• **In addition, the CMNR recommends careful design of research protocols.**

Efforts should be directed towards ensuring the control of as many environmental, behavioral, and treatment variables as possible so that the effects attributed to a deficiency of a particular nutrient are not in fact the result of some other operational stress. The military nutrition research program should attempt to differentiate between nutrition-induced immune dysfunction and that caused by other forms of operational stress.

• **The CMNR strongly encourages the military to increase its awareness of and consider the military applications of the findings within the civilian research community regarding nutrition and immune function.** The advice of civilian and military immunologists should be sought to identify the testing methods that have proven to be most useful and field applicable for monitoring immune status and function.

RECOMMENDATIONS FOR FUTURE RESEARCH

Very little is yet known about the immunological effects of short-term food deprivation when accompanied by varying combinations of other military stresses. Future investigations into the changing immunological status of troops in the field must obviously be based upon available current knowledge about the immunological impact of individual stresses. However, because multiple stresses (including food deprivation) are to be expected, these will have to be studied using experimental designs and methods that have been validated by pilot studies prior to their use in large field studies

• **The CMNR reiterates its previous recommendations (IOM, 1997) that *laboratory-based studies* be performed to determine if an interleukin-6 (IL-6)–creatinine ratio (or some comparable measure) can be measured in single "spot" urine samples as an index of the 24-h excretion of IL-6 and if 24-h IL-6 excretion is, in turn, a reliable indicator of acute stress response.**

Such determinations should be made before urinary IL-6 measurements are used in field studies, where 24-h urinary collections are virtually impossible to obtain.

• **The CMNR recommends the development and *field testing* of appropriate measurements of cytokines or their various markers in urine and blood that are reflective of ongoing acute-phase reactions and of changes in immune status in multistress environments.**

Developmental efforts should focus on one or two measurements that could be standardized with sufficient accuracy to serve as marker replacements for an entire (and complex) cytokine battery and would have some clinical correlate in immune function, such as skin test response and peak titer following vaccination. These may be useful in studies of the effects of nutritional status on immune function. Civilian research efforts in this area should be followed carefully, and collaborative relationships should be formed.

• **The CMNR recommends that if research is conducted on the ability of nutrients to influence immune status, priority at this time should be placed on the antioxidants β-carotene and vitamins C and E.**

The committee acknowledges that insufficient data are available to identify any specific nutrient or combination of nutrients as having adequately demonstrated the ability to enhance immune function under the military operational conditions investigated. This would include vitamins C and E, as well as the amino acids glutamine and arginine.

• **The influence of iron status on the risk of infection requires further investigation. This is also an area of interest to the civilian medical community.**

• **It is recommended that the military keep apprised of research being conducted in the civilian sector on immune function in physically active women and consider conducting studies on military women in situations of deployment to augment the findings of civilian studies.**

At present, there are very few studies on the immune function of healthy women or women in high stress situations.

The Committee on Military Nutrition Research is pleased to participate with the Military Nutrition Division, U.S. Army Research Institute of Environmental Medicine, and the U.S. Army Medical Research and Materiel Command in progress relating to the nutrition, performance, and health of U.S. military personnel.

REFERENCES

Anderson, A.O. 1997. New Technologies for Producing Systemic and Mucosal Immunity by Oral Immunization: Immunoprophylaxis in Meals, Ready-to-Eat. Pp. 451–500 in Emerging Technologies for Nutrition Research, Potential for Assessing Military

Performance Capability, S.J. Carlson-Newberry and R.B. Costello, eds. A report of the Committee on Military Nutrition Research, Food and Nutrition Board, Institute of Medicine. Washington, D.C.: National Academy Press.

IOM (Institute of Medicine). 1991. Fluid Replacement and Heat Stress, 3d printing., B.M. Marriott, ed. A report of the Committee on Military Nutrition Research, Food and Nutrition Board. Washington, D.C.: National Academy Press.

IOM (Institute of Medicine). 1993a. Nutritional Needs in Hot Environments, Applications for Military Personnel in Field Operations, B.M. Marriott, ed. A report of the Committee on Military Nutrition Research, Food and Nutrition Board, Washington, D.C.: National Academy Press.

IOM (Institute of Medicine). 1994. Fluid Replacement and Heat Stress, 3d ed., B.M. Marriott, ed. A report of the Committee on Military Nutrition Research, Food and Nutrition Board. Washington, D.C.: National Academy Press.

IOM (Institute of Medicine). 1995a. Not Eating Enough, Overcoming Underconsumption of Military Operational Rations, B.M. Marriott, ed. A report of the Committee on Military Nutrition Research, Food and Nutrition Board. Washington, D.C.: National Academy Press.

IOM (Institute of Medicine). 1997. Emerging Technologies for Nutrition Research, Potential for Assessing Military Performance Capability, S.J. Carson-Newberry and R.B. Costello, eds. A report of the Committee on Military Nutrition Research, Food and Nutrition Board. Washington, D.C.: National Academy Press.

II

Stage Setting:
The Military Situation

THE PAPERS PRESENTED AT THE WORKSHOP comprise parts II through VI. These chapters have undergone limited editorial change, have not been reviewed by an outside group, and represent the views of the individual authors. Selected questions and the speakers' responses are included to provide the flavor of the workshop discussion.

Part II provides an introduction to the workshop. Chapter 4 presents an overview and background of the basis for the Army's interest in nutrition and immune function. A detailed presentation of results of nutrition interventions on immune responses in soldiers participating in U.S. Ranger Training and Special Forces Assessment Schools is presented in Chapter 5, and Chapter 6 presents results of nutrition intervention studies during the Ranger Training Course at the Norwegian Military Academy.

Nutrition and Immune Function, 1999
Pp. 139–161. Washington, D.C.
National Academy Press

4

Why Is the Army Interested in Nutrition and Immune Function?

LTC Karl E. Friedl[1]

INTRODUCTION

The primary goal of the Army Operational Medicine Research Program is to develop physiological strategies to protect and sustain deployed soldiers. This research is valuable to the Army if it leads to a decisive improvement in the ability to accomplish the mission (i.e., enhanced readiness). One aspect of readiness is resistance to disease, and this may be compromised in soldiers when immune function is suppressed by operational stressors and other battlefield hazards. Combined stressors may reduce the normal ability of soldiers to resist pathogens, increase susceptibility to biological threat agents employed against them, and reduce effectiveness of vaccines intended to protect them.

Some immunological impairments may be prevented by ensuring adequate nutrition (e.g., preventing substantial energy or protein deficits) and by providing specific nutritional supplements to restore deficiencies (e.g., retinol). However, this report is focused primarily on approaches to enhance disease resistance in young men and women with an adequate baseline nutritional status. The main question to consider is "Do intakes of specific nutrients or vitamins,

[1] Karl E. Friedl, Army Operational Medicine Research Program, U.S. Army Medical Research and Materiel Command, Fort Detrick, MD 21702-5012

above normal levels, counter immunological impairments caused by operational stressors?"

BACKGROUND

The infectious disease threats facing soldiers vary with geography, but disease has usually accounted for more noneffective days than has combat or even nonbattle injury. In World War II, Rommel and his troops were seriously hampered by diarrheal disease (shigella) in North Africa, and the elite Merrill's Marauders and other units in the China-Burma theater were rendered ineffective by malaria (Reister, 1975). Malaria and diarrheal diseases remain high-priority research targets because of the consequences to the military mission and their widespread occurrence. Emerging infectious diseases and unexpected disease threats have occurred in recent conflicts (Heppner et al., 1993), presenting new challenges for which there may be no specific protection. This may also be true in the defense against some biological threat agents (Liu et al., 1996), for which physiological enhancements of immune protection may present one of the few options for protection. Enhancements of physiological defenses and the responsiveness to vaccines may center on nutritional strategies.

Even in military training, infectious diseases are a threat. For example, in 1990, half of the high attrition from Ranger school was attributed to medical problems, with one class decimated by pneumonia (Riedo et al,. 1991), and cellulitis continues to be a problem of Ranger students (Martinez-Lopez et al., 1993). The infectious disease problem in Ranger students appears largely to have been corrected through a nutritional intervention. Immune function deficits were attenuated with increased feeding, and dramatic reductions in infection (25% prevalence reduced to 2%) paralleled the changes in immune function tests (Kramer et al., 1997).

The interaction of nutrition and infection has been investigated extensively by military researchers in previous work. Most of this research centered on the consequences of infection to nutrition. COL William Beisel defined an entire field of research in the 1970s at the U.S. Army Medical Research Institute of Infectious Diseases with his work on cytokine-induced malnutrition (Beisel, 1995). His early work also described the physiological effects of lymphocytic endogenous mediator, properties of the cytokine now identified as interleukin-1 (IL-1). Beisel. demonstrated that a variety of diseases produced hypermetabolism, loss of protein and vitamins, and wasting of the muscle mass. These effects were mediated through cytokines. More recently, cytokines have been implicated in responses to inflammation as well as immunological responses to a wide variety of stressors (Roubenoff, 1993). These responses are largely responsible for modified immune function and, in some settings, suboptimal resistance to disease, which is a consequence of the accumulated stressors. With this common cytokine pathway, the effect on immune status may represent a generalized stress response to a diversity of stressors. These generalized cytokine responses to stress may be modified by specific nutrients. The focus of the Army's current research program is in this direction, examining the effect of nutrition on sustainment or enhancement of immune status in healthy individuals.

IMMUNE SUPPRESSION AND INFLAMMATORY RESPONSES TO OPERATIONAL STRESSORS

A current objective of Army operational medicine research is to identify the effect of operational stressors and other battlefield hazards on soldiers' immunological and/or inflammatory host defenses. Problems must be defined in relevant models of operational stress and in terms of actual disease susceptibility (Kusnecov and Rabin, 1994); research to develop nutritional countermeasures is appropriate after problems have been clearly identified. Stressors that are being investigated in military studies include chronic anxiety (referred to in the remainder of this chapter as "psychological stress"), inadequate restorative sleep, physical exertion, inadequate energy intake, industrial toxicological hazards, and mechanical/physical stresses (e.g., blast and laser injuries).

Psychological stressors are the best documented in terms of stress effects on immunological impairment, and an entire interdisciplinary field of psychoneuroimmunology is founded on studies linking the immune and central nervous systems (Ader and Cohen, 1993). The Department of Medical Neurosciences at the Walter Reed Army Institute of Research (WRAIR) has investigated acute and chronic rodent stress models actively (e.g., footshock in mice, learned helplessness in defeat-conditioned hamsters[2]), helping to define mechanisms of stress effects on the brain (Huhman et al., 1991, 1992). Footshock as well as chronic anxiety stress reliably suppresses T-cell proliferation and lymphocyte IL-2 production in rodents (Hardy et al., 1990). While adrenocorticoids suppress potentially maladaptive overresponses of immune function (Kapcala et al., 1995), LTC Ned Bernton has demonstrated that their effect is counterbalanced by other factors, such as dehydroepiandrosterone (DHEA) and some of the lactogens, that may reverse corticotropin-releasing factor-mediated decrements in immune function (Bernton et al., 1988, 1992; Rassnick et al., 1994). Studies of combat veterans with posttraumatic stress disorder suggest that, even with adrenal adaptation, anxiety may increase glucocorticoid receptors on lymphocytes (Yehuda et al., 1990, 1991); thus, circulating levels of cortisol may be low and still significantly affect immunogenic tissues (Dhabhar et al., 1995). These basic studies help to explain and verify observed links between psychological stress and illness (Cohen et al., 1991; Lee et al., 1995; Rubin et al., 1970, 1971),

---

[2] A model of stress in which the male hamster, accustomed to attacking unfamiliar hamsters introduced into his cage, is repeatedly defeated by larger, more aggressive intruders until his normal territorial aggression is replaced by defensive behavior and flight.

wound healing (Faist et al., 1996; Kiecolt-Glaser et al., 1995), and responses to vaccines (Kiecolt-Glaser et al., 1996; Moynihan et al., 1990).

Deployed soldiers suffer a wide variety of psychological stressors, including mission-related factors (e.g., ambiguity of the return date), family separation issues, and unit level issues (e.g., lack of time off); this was documented by Human Dimensions Teams (HDT) from the Army's research program in the Gulf War, Somalia, Haiti, and most recently Bosnia (Bliese and Wright, 1995; Gifford et al., 1996; Halvorsen et al., 1995; Rosen et al., 1993). Sixteen percent of soldiers in Bosnia indicated that they were coping poorly with stress in their life. This research is primarily centered on rapid identification of significant stress issues so that military leaders can pursue immediate interventions. Future HDT studies will include more comprehensive assessment of somatic complaints, including infections, as capabilities improve for quick turnaround of data acquisition and interpretation. This will also provide new information on the actual consequences of psychological stress in deployed forces.

At least part of the reason for high distress scores in soldiers in Bosnia is related to self-reported inadequate sleep (Gifford et al., 1996), and this has an impact on immune function that may be distinctly different from anxiety stress effects. Acute sleep restriction produces a reduction in natural immune responses (e.g., natural killer [NK] activity) and T-cell cytokine production (Irwin et al., 1996), but after more prolonged sleep deprivation, leukocytosis (an increase in the number of leukocytes) is observed and NK activity increases (Dinges et al., 1994). The immunosupportive function of sleep has been suggested on the basis of interactions between sleep and immunological challenges, mediated through cytokines such as IL-1 (Krueger et al., 1994; Pollmacher et al., 1995). For example, low-dose challenges with endotoxin suppress rapid eye movement (REM) sleep (Pollmacher et al., 1995). Sleep deprivation does not appear to affect mitogen-stimulated proliferative responses (Dinges et al., 1994), indicating a different effect on immune function than observed with energy deficit (Christadoss et al., 1984) or with an overlay of a substantial energy deficit even with a large sleep deficit (Kramer et al., 1997). In both of these latter examples, lymphocyte proliferation is suppressed. Immune function indices reflect a complex interrelationship among immune function, psychological stress, and sleep disruption (Kant et al., 1995), which is further complicated by physical work and energy deficit stressors. For example in rats, treadmill running can reduce some of the immune suppression produced by footshock stress (Dishman et al., 1995).

Physical exertion produces inflammatory changes as well as transient immunological responses. Moderate exercise is associated with enhanced immune function, but prolonged exercise, or exercise of very high intensity, causes at least transient suppression of immune function indices (Gray et al., 1992; Nieman et al., 1992; Shephard et al., 1994; Tvede et al., 1993). Thus, in female recruits participating in Army basic training involving a modest 2,800 kcal/d energy expenditure, T-cell proliferative responses to phytohemagglutinin (PHA, a mitogen) were increased (Westphal et al., 1995a). In a study of prolonged exhaustive exercise at the Defense and Civil Institute of Environmental Medicine, lymphocytosis (an increase in the number of lymphocytes) was produced, with reductions in the number of T-cells to 60 percent of pre-exercise levels by 2 hours post-exercise and marked suppression of NK cell counts even 7 days after the exercise challenge (Shek et al., 1995). These results are consistent with the field studies conducted at the Norwegian Defense Research Establishment (Bøyum et al., 1996), in a multistressor paradigm that includes strenuous exercise, followed by dramatic changes in immunological indices (see Wiik, Chapter 6). However, this stressful training does not result in a significant increase in infection rates (Bøyum et al., 1996). Thus, theorized connections between physical stress and disease susceptibility in athletes engaged in prolonged intensive training (Pedersen and Bruunsgaard, 1995) remain to be evaluated. It also remains to be established if it is always desirable to block some of the observed changes. For example, there may be adaptive value in obtaining some inflammatory responses if these are linked to muscle and bone remodeling responses to a change in habitual activity.

Deployed soldiers face higher health and performance risks from toxicological hazards than ever before. The modern battlefield includes unquantified but widespread agricultural and industrial toxins in developing and former Eastern bloc countries. Among the likely environmental pollutants are immunomodulators such as polychlorinated biphenyls, chlorinated dibenzo-*p*-dioxins, pesticides, and heavy metals. Although some immunotoxins may cause immune depression, the better known consequence of many of these is immunoenhancement, with potential health risks for autoimmune or allergic reactions (Krzystyniak et al., 1995). If the primary risk from these xenobiotics is via the disruption of brain and immune function interactions instead of through a direct effect on immunocompetent tissues (Fuchs and Sanders, 1994), conventional assays are unlikely to detect the hazard. Assessment of these deployment hazards may be difficult by conventional *in vitro* methods for other reasons as well: techniques have not been developed for identification of many toxins; even after a chemical is identified, health risks may be unstudied; and the effects of specific mixtures of chemicals will almost certainly be undefined. For these reasons, biosentinel species[3] and nonmammalian bioassays for the identification of environmental toxin risks are being actively investigated in the Center for Environmental Health Research (CEHR) at Fort Detrick, Maryland. Fish have been explored as biosentinels of immunotoxicity (Wester et al., 1994) and are part of the current program in the CEHR.

---

[3] Species of organisms used to detect and warn for presence of a toxin because of their sensitivity to the substance (e.g., canaries in coal mines) and/or because of their chronic contact with the environment.

Conceivably, a variety of stressors cause tissue damage and decrease healing capacity through oxidative stress, which could be countered with antioxidant feeding. For example, wound healing is accelerated with vitamin E treatment (Simon et al., 1994). Hypobaric hypoxia stress in the Operation Everest II experiment produced alterations in the indices of immune function (Meehan et al., 1988), and it was suggested in a previous CMNR workshop that increased antioxidant intakes could be beneficial to soldiers operating at altitude (Simon-Schnass, 1996). However, the issue must not be oversimplified. Blast overpressure from big weapons systems produces mechanical trauma to human airways, the gastrointestinal tract, and the musculoskeletal system. Basic research in the Department of Respiratory Research at WRAIR has demonstrated an interesting paradox, wherein antioxidants may increase oxidative stress following tissue damage due to blast overpressure through redox cycling of heme proteins and nonheme iron (Elsayed et al., 1996). *In vitro* studies also indicate that nitric oxide reactions may play an important role in the protection of tissues from oxidative damage (Gorbunov et al., 1996). These data highlight the importance of clarifying the basic mechanisms and problems associated with operational stressors before attempting to field solutions.

MILITARY MODELS TO STUDY OPERATIONAL STRESSORS

The models of operational stress that are appropriate to the military's research on immune function present some special challenges. Ideally, these should model actual deployments or realistic training scenarios in order to include stressors typical of military operations. Psychological stress and inadequate rest are probably the most important of these stressors to include because of their consistent appearance in current deployments. Significant rates of infectious disease problems should also be a key feature of the model. Ethical concerns limit the design of experimental models with these features; thus, much of the military's stress research involves opportunistic field studies where the investigators do not impose the stressors but are able to study the consequences. It is also likely that investigators will provide recommendations that will fix the problem, which, if incorporated, will reduce the future utility of the model. Thus, some of the best models are moving targets.

Some limited opportunities have existed for research during actual combat service. For example, during the Vietnam War, John Mason and his colleagues examined endocrine stress responses of helicopter air ambulance crews and Special Forces A-teams under attack (Bourne et al., 1967; Rose et al., 1969); also a Navy aeromedical research team studied stress responses of carrier pilots in combat (Lewis et al., 1967). Unfortunately, these studies preceded the recent advances in immune function testing and current understanding of the associations between stress and disease susceptibility. More recently, the Ranger course provided the Army with a very stressful training model, perhaps even exceeding the combined stress effects observed in actual combat but lacking the psychological components expected in a real deployment (Johnson et al., 1976; Moore et al., 1992; Pleban et al., 1990). Unfortunately for researchers, the participants in this test model are competitively evaluated against each other, making placebo-controlled studies difficult within a single course (i.e., no advantage can be ethically withheld from a portion of the participants).

Administering an infectious challenge is necessary to evaluate the efficacy of prospective interventions. For example, a study conducted in Panama demonstrated the efficacy of doxocycline prophylaxis in protection against leptospirosis infection (Takafuji et al., 1984). This placebo-controlled study took advantage of a known significant infectious hazard to which soldiers were exposed as a matter of course in jungle training and probably even in previous military nutrition studies (e.g., Consolazio et al., 1979). However, such studies tend to be one-time opportunities; if effective in demonstrating a solution to the problem, the model is no longer available for other intervention studies. In the absence of such opportunities, a safer infectious challenge may have to be considered such as respiratory tract viruses employed in the stress dose-response study of Cohen et al. (1991). Development of immunity in response to vaccines (e.g., hepatitis A vaccine) could also be evaluated in naive subjects in operationally relevant stress models. Bernton tried unsuccessfully to include such a trial in the 1992 Ranger studies; this would be invaluable in defining the practical consequences of the observed immune suppression and would offer information vital to the questions being posed in this report.[4]

One problem with studies of relatively short duration is that some of the changes noted may reflect acute-phase responses that could be triggered by a variety of novel stressors rather than identifying specific immune axis lesions. The Ranger training studies afforded a unique opportunity because of the duration of the course. In fact, by the end of the first study, immune function indices were returning to normal levels despite continued exposure to the course stressors (Kramer et al., 1997). This finding may indicate a recovery from acute-phase responses, an adaptation to the stressors, or a reduced energy deficit in the final phase of the course as behavioral and metabolic efficiencies decreased requirements to match intakes more accurately (Friedl et al., 1995a).

The many shorter-term models of operational stress range in length from 1 to 3 weeks, most typically about 1 week, as summarized elsewhere (Friedl, 1997). The Norwegian Ranger course is the best-defined model and is easily characterized for nutrition intakes because of the nearly total restriction on intakes (Opstad, 1995). Navy SEAL training "hell week" has also been characterized in nutrition studies (Singh et al. 1991; Smoak et al. 1988). A primary recommendation, which came out of the North Atlantic Treaty Organization workshop on "The Effect of Prolonged Exhaustive Military

---

[4] Since this workshop, a study involving hepatitis A vaccine administered to Ranger students has been designed and started (October 1997) by MAJ Jeffrey Kennedy (USARIEM, Natick, Mass.).

Activities on Man" (NATO, 1995), was to establish a multinational competition modeled along the lines of the 72-h Best Ranger competition to study efficacy of various interventions for enhancement of health and performance of elite soldiers. Buddy teams could be paired with both intervention and placebo members and the benefits of dietary supplements could be tested effectively in an acute operational stress scenario in motivated top performers.

MECHANISMS OF INCREASED INFECTION SUSCEPTIBILITY: ARMY-USDA COOPERATIVE RESEARCH DATA

In 1990, 14 Ranger students were hospitalized with pneumonia at Dugway Proving Ground, Utah; this unusual outbreak was investigated by a team from the Centers for Disease Control and Prevention (Riedo et al., 1991). The high level of stress and/or severity of disease was marked by negligible concentrations of testosterone in serum samples from nearly every student (Unpublished data, K. E. Friedl and L. J. Marchitelli, USARIEM, Natick, Mass., 1991). This outbreak prompted the commander of the Ranger Training Brigade to request help in determining if more sleep and changes in nutrition were necessary to ensure the health and safety of his trainees. This led to two Ranger studies in 1991 (Bernton et al., 1995; Moore et al., 1992) reviewed in a previous Committee on Military Nutrition Research workshop (IOM, 1992), which rekindled interest in the relationship between nutritional status and resistance to disease.

Measurement of immune function indices were included in these studies to provide sensitive markers of nutritional status (Sauberlich, 1984) and to address the primary concern of increased susceptibility to infection. A cooperative agreement with the U.S. Department of Agriculture (USDA) enabled Tim R. Kramer to contribute experience he gained from field immunology studies in China and Thailand (Kramer et al., 1993; Zhang et al., 1995). This exchange was an opportunity to address questions of importance to both agencies under a longstanding agreement (DoD, 1983; Kramer, 1992).

Since the first Ranger study, a series of studies between Kramer and U.S. Army Research Institute of Environmental Medicine investigators has led to an improved understanding of the role of energy deficit in immune function. The combined data from four separate studies involving methodology controlled by the same laboratory investigators in a consistent manner are summarized in Table 4-1. The methodology, including a whole blood method of lymphocyte proliferation measurement, and the challenges to carefully control field sample collection and handling are reviewed later in this report by Kramer (see Chapter 10). These data suggest that the degree of immune function suppression, as indicated by stimulated lymphocyte proliferative response, is proportional to the degree of energy deficit.

Although reliable energy expenditure data are available only for the two Ranger studies, body weight loss is a reasonable indicator of the scale of energy

TABLE 4-1 Energy Deficit and Its Relation to Stress Indices and PHA-Stimulated T-lymphocyte Proliferation

Study	N	Wks	% BW	% FFM	% IL-6	% PHA-T	% T
RGR-I	49	4	−9.2	—	−17	−52	−69
		8	−15.9	−6.9	−63	−21	−74
RGR-II	41	4	−7.0	—	+15	−32	−60
		8	−12.8	−6.1	−84	−5	−83
SFAS	37	3	−4.0	−1.0	−46	−20	−15
BCT	48	4	—	—	−37	+165	—
		8	−1.4	+5.0	+220	+144	—

NOTE: Values represent percent change from baseline measurements. BW, body weight; FFM, fat-free mass; IL-6, interleukin-6; PHA-T, phytohemagglutinin-stimulated T-cell proliferation; T, Testosterone.

SOURCE: Adapted from RGR-I, Ranger course, 1991 (Kramer et al., 1997); RGR-II, Ranger course, 1992 (Kramer et al., 1997); SFAS, Special Forces and Assessment course, 1993 (Unpublished data, B. Fairbrother and T. R. Kramer, USARIEM, Natick, Mass., 1993); BCT, Army Basic Combat Training, 1993 (Westphal et al., 1995a).

requirement supplied from body energy stores. The Special Forces Assessment and Selection (SFAS) course was only 3 weeks long, compared with 8 weeks for Ranger training and for Army basic training, and energy density of weight loss is likely to vary over time within a protracted energy deficit. Thus, the 4 percent weight loss figure in SFAS should be compared with 9 and 7 percent in the two Ranger classes at 4 weeks, confirming a substantially larger gap between intakes and requirements for Ranger students (Kramer et al., 1995).

IL-6 was used in all of these studies as a stress marker integrally related to activation of the hypothalamo-pituitary-adrenal axis as well as being produced by cells of immune origin (Zhou et al., 1993). After initial stress responses, the IL-6 response moves in the opposite direction. The lowest levels of IL-6 were found in soldiers with the highest stress conditions, including the very lowest level of IL-6 (along with the highest level of cortisol) in the individual soldier with the greatest relative weight loss (−23% of initial body weight). Because of the hypermetabolic effects of IL-6 (Stouthard et al., 1995), a decline in the levels of this cytokine is clearly adaptive during a continued energy deficit. This decline in IL-6 may also be important to stimulation of IL-1 and other cytokines involved in immune regulation (Zhou et al., 1996).

The gonadal steroids were also used as stress markers, but these steroids tend to reflect more specifically the energy deficit stressor as mediated through the hypothalamic control of the pituitary-gonadal axis. For women, progesterone was used as the female analog of the testosterone response. Mean levels of progesterone remained unchanged through the basic training studies, indicating not only the continuation of eumenorrheic cycles but also the absence of stress-induced deficient luteal phases (Friedl et al., 1995b).

Other indices of immune function measured in all of these studies, such as changes in IL-2 receptor, need further investigation. Changes in IL-2 receptor may reflect an increased activation of T-lymphocytes, causing increased release of receptor into circulation. Whether this increase indicates that the immune system is functioning better than the *in vitro* tests indicate, or that some immunopathological process is occurring, is unknown (Kramer et al., 1995).

Comprehensive vitamin and mineral analyses were performed in each of these four studies by the clinical laboratory at the Pennington Biomedical Research Center. No specific vitamin or mineral deficiencies could be identified, except for a small mid-study decline in serum retinol in the first Ranger study, probably related to a significant decline in measured retinol binding protein (Moore et al., 1992).

Delayed-type hypersensitivity (DTH) test results did not correspond to suppressed lymphocyte responsiveness *in vitro*. *In vivo* tests of immunocompetence using the Merieux multitine tests were applied at the beginning, at 6 weeks, and at the end (8 weeks) of the first Ranger study (after blood samples had been drawn for *in vitro* tests). There was no change in 72-h response rates across the course, except for a significant increase in the tuberculin responses (based on indurations ≥ 2 mm) (Martinez-Lopez et al., 1993). Thus, DTH testing was not performed in subsequent studies involving lower stress levels than in the first Ranger study.

A modest increase in caloric intake and a 20 percent reduction in energy deficit across the course may have been responsible for the marked reduction in infection rates noted between the first and the second Ranger study (Table 4-2). It is also possible that the attenuation of the immune function deficits observed in the *in vitro* tests offers a mechanism for the reduction in infection rates (Kramer et al., 1997). Infectious disease was negligible in the SFAS and basic training studies. These very tentative relationships suggest directions for more controlled laboratory studies.

SPECIFIC NUTRITIONAL FIXES AND THE PROMISE OF IMMUNE SUSTAINMENT AND POTENTIAL SUPERIMMUNITY

Specific nutrients or dietary supplements may improve host immune response in trauma or malnourished patients (Gallagher and Daly, 1993; Morgan, 1966); however, there are still few data to substantiate a role for dietary supplements (e.g., arginine, glutamine, antioxidant mixtures) in the enhancement of immune function in healthy individuals. This may be due to (1) the use of inadequate study models where infection is not an important problem or the effects of the stressors were not as profound as anticipated, and (2) the location of studies in difficult-to-control field settings that do not permit definitive conclusions.

TABLE 4-2 Infection Rates in Ranger Studies

Study	Phase 2 Wk 2–4	Phase 3 Wk 4–6	Phase 4 Wk 6–8
RGR-I (1991)	9/109 (8%)	19/75 (25%)	14/58 (24%)
RGR-II (1992)	14/121 (12%)	7/85 (8%)	1/58 (2%)

NOTE: These rates were determined by review of all recorded sick call visits by and medical treatments to students in the Ranger course. Cellulitis was the most common type of infection classified in both courses. The common diagnosis of "cellulitis of the knee" was not definitively distinguished from the noninfectious injury (bursitis) produced by frequently dropping to one knee during stops in patrolling operations; greater awareness of the need for knee protection in Ranger II (Caravalho, 1992; Kragh, 1993) may have contributed to the apparent differences in "infection" rates. RGR, Ranger training course.

SOURCE: Adapted from IOM (1993).

One study at the SFAS course tested a dose of oral glutamine (15 g/d) compared with an isonitrogenous dose of glycine and found no differences between treatments on any tests of immune function (Shippee et al., 1995). In LTC Barry Fairbrother's original SFAS study (Fairbrother et al., 1993), there was a suppression of immune function indices, although smaller than in the Ranger studies (Table 4-1). The *in vitro* lymphocyte responses cannot be compared directly between the glutamine study and the original study because of the timing of a DTH test at the end of the glutamine study; however, similar results were obtained for both treatment and control groups in the glutamine study. No statistically significant difference was obtained between the groups for the DTH test even when results were classified as positive for indurations greater than 5 mm diameter only (Shippee et al., 1995). Since infection is not a medical problem in the SFAS course, the most useful end point of modified infection rates is not testable in this setting. Eric Newsholme and others have suggested on theoretical grounds that glutamine may be an important link between immune function and exhaustive exercise because of the shared requirement for glutamine by both immune cells and skeletal muscle (Newsholme, 1994); however, a benefit from glutamine supplementation in these circumstances remains to be demonstrated.

Another study considered the effect of a carbohydrate beverage as a means of improving hydration status and energy balance. No differences in immune function outcomes were observed in this 3-d exercise by Ranger instructors, but there was also no change in any *in vitro* tests in the control group. The aspartame sweetener used in the control group beverage may have had an unexpected effect on immune indices (Montain et al., 1995).

New data from antioxidant studies in the field involving a mixture of vitamins and minerals (vitamin A, E, and selenium), will be presented later in this report by LTC Ronald Shippee (see Chapter 5). Another intervention study performed in the laboratory tested antioxidant vitamins and minerals to sustain immune function. In this study, funded under the Defense Women's Health Research Program (DWHRP94), Anita Singh tested zinc and vitamin E supplements to prevent exercise-induced changes in immune function parameters. Using a robust crossover placebo-controlled design, fit young women were tested with exercise to exhaustion on a treadmill. This exercise model was shown previously to produce suppression of immune function indices in men (Singh et al., 1994). The intervention study with women produced no differences in stress responses (e.g., serum levels of IL-6, cortisol, and adrenocorticotropic hormone) or indices of immune function (e.g., lymphocyte subsets and respiratory burst activity) (Singh, 1996).

An ambitious study conceived by LTC Kathleen Westphal and also funded under the DWHRP94 (Westphal et al., 1994) follows up on her finding of a significant prevalence of borderline iron deficiency and anemia in female Army recruits (Westphal et al., 1995a). This study examines iron status for a very large sample of Army women and includes a plan to compare immune function of soldiers in relation to iron status. These data are being analyzed by Shippee and CPT Tony Pusateri.

Perhaps the most promising line of investigation into nutritional interventions involves the effects of whole foods on immune function; such studies are being conducted by Kramer. A pilot study indicated that a modest daily supplement of kale, sweet potato, and tomato juice, providing beta-carotene, lutein, and lycopene for 3 weeks, produced a markedly enhanced response in mitogen-stimulated lymphocyte proliferation in unstressed individuals. The elevated response continued for several weeks after the feeding intervention (Unpublished data, T. R. Kramer, USDA Beltsville Human Nutrition Research Center, Beltsville, Md., 1996). A new study receiving partial support from the Army expands on these findings with a carefully controlled dose-response feeding study although initial analysis of the data with this study suggests confounding interactions from altered eating patterns and energy balance that will require experimental control (Kramer, 1996; Unpublished data, T. R. Kramer, USDA Beltsville Human Nutrition Research Center, Beltsville, Md., 1997).

DIETARY SUPPLEMENTS:
ARMY RESEARCHERS AS THE HONEST BROKERS

Many soldiers are using dietary supplements in an attempt to optimize their health and performance. Supplement use is reported to be widespread, especially among soldiers in elite units. Soldiers make the general assumption that if supplements can be sold, they must be effective for the purposes implied and they must be safe to use. The generalization goes further with the assumption that dietary supplements sold in the post exchanges and commissaries are endorsed by the Army leadership for use by soldiers. Fitness magazines sold in the same shops suggest the use of these products for a variety of health and performance benefits, quoting well-known athletes who have tried or tested the products, displaying scientific-looking graphs and tables, and carrying impressive lists of scientific citations. Associations with research performed by the USDA and other government agencies are also invoked as product endorsements, regardless of the actual research results. Such marketing gimmicks have been reviewed in detail elsewhere (Barrett and Herbert, 1994).

The following are some of the claims culled from four such magazines purchased in the local post exchange:

It's simple to boost your host resistance. You don't need fancy drugs nor exotic supplements. Plain old L-arginine or ornithine-alpha-ketoglutarate (OKG) will do it nicely. Multiple studies show increased T-lymphocyte counts, enhanced wound healing, increased strength of immune responses to mitogens, and other immune enhancements. Ten grams a day may keep you forever out of the dangerous hands of medicine.

Melatonin strengthens all cellular immunity in the body by its action on T-helper cells...Without them, your immune system cannot communicate with its troops and is almost powerless [suggests a dose of 20 mg/d].

We have found that the benefits to well-being, physique, and resistance to disease continued [through 4 years of DHEA use].

[Glutamine] *is the most depleted amino acid (and last to be replenished) during intense workouts. Many researchers believe it may be the single most important variable in determining optimum protein synthesis* [recommends 1.5 g/d of L-glutamine].

Whey peptides boost immune function better than any known protein. Medium and high molecular weight whey peptides with B vitamins raise cellular L-glutathione levels.

[Product] *is enriched with extra branched-chain amino acids and added L-glutamine—all anti-catabolic amino acids that can help minimize muscle protein breakdown caused by high intensity training (reductions in glutamine concentration in the blood following overtraining may also explain the immune deficiency reported in many athletes after strenuous exercise).*

Dietary supplements may carry some risk and can potentially impair rather than enhance military readiness. Even if marketed supplements are effective, there may be a tradeoff in problems associated with hyperresponsiveness of the immune system; thus, the strategy must be carefully evaluated. For example, Victor Herbert reported the case of an Air Force sergeant who used a well-known body building product; the young man was in good health until he died from what appears to have been an induced autoimmune disease (Herbert and Kasdan, 1994). Herbert suggests a similarity with other reports of serious consequences from enhanced immune activity associated with L-canavanine (found in alfalfa sprouts) and excessive vitamin E use and makes the recommendation that such immunomodulatory supplements should have warning labels (Herbert and Kasdan, 1994). Certainly, this points to the need for a new review of upper safe limits of nutrients and vitamins, including antioxidants.

Because the military is a performance-oriented subject population that is especially likely to be lured into use of dietary supplements, it becomes important for the military to counter misinformation with substantiated nutrition facts and guidance. There is currently no reliable information clearinghouse to which a soldier, dietitian, or physician can turn to identify bogus claims. Examples of how information might be better disseminated include Carol J. Baker-Fulco's "Performance Nutrition"/"Eat to Win" videotape instructional series, and general nutrition education centered on balanced and healthful diets (e.g., menu modification research efforts in collaboration with the Pennington Biomedical Research Center to develop good meals that will appeal to young soldiers). It is also important to publicize research findings on new supplements, including what does, and particularly what does not, appear to provide a benefit to soldiers.

AUTHOR'S CONCLUSIONS

Military operational medicine research is necessarily problem oriented. This does not preclude the need for basic research or the use of the best state-of-the-art science to overcome technological barriers and develop solutions that will make a difference to the deployed warfighter. Key technological barriers in nutritional immunology include an understanding of the relationship between immune function indices and disease susceptibility, a better understanding of the central role of cytokines in stress-induced suppression of immunological function, and a more complete understanding of the biological effects and modulation of oxidative stress. Practical limitations include diminishing resources and limited available expertise in the multiple disciplines required to accomplish this research. This further increases the need for efficient interlaboratory and interagency collaborations.

An Army nutritional immunology research program should include the following target objectives: (1) define the importance of nutritional status to effectiveness of immunizations and natural disease resistance in deployed soldiers, (2) identify a dietary supplement or feeding strategy that substantially reduces susceptibility of soldiers to infection in stressful operational settings, and (3) assess hazards to military readiness associated with dietary supplements commonly used by soldiers.

REFERENCES

Ader, R., and N. Cohen. 1993. Psychoneuroimmunology: Conditioning and stress. Annu. Rev. Psychol. 44:53–85.

Barrett S., and V. Herbert. 1994. The Vitamin Pushers. How the "Health Food" Industry is Selling America a Bill of Goods. Amherst, N.Y.: Prometheus Books.

Beisel, W.R. 1995. Herman Award Lecture, 1995: Infection-induced malnutrition—from cholera to cytokines. Am. J. Clin. Nutr. 62:813–819.

Bernton, E., H. Bryant, J. Holaday, and J. Dave. 1992. Prolactin and prolactin secretagogues reverse immunosuppression in mice treated with cysteamine, glucocorticoid, or cyclosporin-A. Brain Behav. Immunol. 6:394–408.

Bernton, E., D. Hoover, R. Galloway, and K. Popp. 1995. Adaptation to chronic stress in military trainees. Adrenal androgens, testosterone, glucocorticoids, IGF-I, and immune function. Ann. N.Y. Acad. Sci. 774:217–231.

Bernton, E., M.S. Meltzer, and J.W. Holaday. 1988. Suppression of macrophage activation and T-lymphocyte function in hypoprolactinemic mice. Science 239:401–404.

Bliese, P., and K. Wright. 1995. Stress in Today's Army: Human Dimension Research Team Findings. Information Briefing to Secretary of the Army. May 22, 1995. Washington, D.C.

Bourne, P.G., R.M. Rose, and J.W. Mason. 1967. Urinary 17-OHCS levels. Data on seven helicopter ambulance medics in combat. Arch. Gen. Psychiatry 17:104–110.

Bøyum, A., P. Wiik, E. Gustavsson, O.P. Veiby, J. Reseland, A.H. Haugen, and P.K. Opstad. 1996. The effect of strenuous exercise, calorie deficiency and sleep deprivation on white blood cells, plasma immunoglobulins and cytokines. Scand. J. Immunol. 43:228–235.

Caravalho Jr., J. 1992. Knee protection during Ranger school. Mil. Med. 157:A3.

Christadoss, P., N. Talal, J. Lindstrom, and G. Fernandes. 1984. Suppression of cellular and humoral immunity to T-dependent antigens by calorie restriction. Cell Immunol. 88:1–8.

Cohen, S, A.J. Tyrrell, and A.P. Smith. 1991. Psychological stress and susceptibility to the common cold. N. Engl. J. Med. 325:606–612.

Consolazio C.F., H.L. Johnson, R.A. Nelson, R. Dowdy, H.J. Krzywicki, T.A. Daws, L.K. Lowry, P.P. Warling, W.K. Calhoun, B.W. Schwenneker, and J.E. Canham. 1979. The relationship of diet to the performance of the combat soldier. Minimal calorie intake during combat patrols in a hot humid environment (Panama). Technical Report No. 76. Presidio of San Francisco, Calif.: Letterman Army Institute of Research.

DoD (Department of Defense). 1983. DoD Coordination on Food, Agriculture, Forestry, Nutrition, and Other Designated Research with the U.S. Department of Agriculture. Directive 3210.4. July 5, 1983. Washington, D.C.

Dhabhar, F.S., A.H. Miller, D.S. McEwen, and R.L. Spencer. 1995. Effects of stress on immune cell distribution. Dynamics and hormonal mechanisms. J. Immunol. 154:5511–5527.

Dinges, D.F., S.D. Douglas, L. Zaugg, D.E. Campbell, J.M. McMann, W.G. Whitehouse, E.C. Orne, S.C. Kapoor, E. Icaza, and M.T. Orne. 1994. Leukocytosis and natural killer cell function parallel neurobehavioral fatigue induced by 64 hours of sleep deprivation. J. Clin. Invest. 93:1930–1939.

Dishman, R.K., J.M. Warren, S.D. Youngstedt, H. Yoo, B.N. Bunnell, E.H. Mougey, J.L. Meyerhoff, L. Jaso-Friedmann, and D.L. Evans. 1995. Activity-wheel running attenuates suppression of natural killer cell activity after footshock. J. Appl. Physiol. 78:1547–1554.

Elsayed, N.M., Y.Y. Tyurina, V.A. Tyurin, E.V. Menshikova, E.R. Kisin, and V.E. Kagan. 1996. Antioxidant depletion, lipid peroxidation, and impairment of calcium transport induced by air-blast overpressure in rat lungs. Exp. Lung Res. 22:179–200.

Fairbrother, B., E.W. Askew, M.Z. Mays, R. Shippee, K.E. Friedl, R.W. Hoyt, M. Kramer, T.R. Kramer, and K. Popp. 1993. Nutritional assessment of soldiers during the special forces assessment and selection course. USARIEM Study Protocol, May 1993. Natick, Mass.: U.S. Army Research Institute of Environmental Medicine.

Faist, E., C. Shinkel, and S. Zimmer. 1996. Update on the mechanisms of immune suppression of injury and immune modulation. World J. Surg. 20:454–459.

Friedl, K.E. 1997. Variability of fat and lean tissue loss during physical exertion with energy deficit. Pp. 431–450 in Physiology, Stress, and Malnutrition: Functional Correlates, Nutritional Intervention, J. Kinney and H. Tucker, eds. New York: Lippincott-Raven.

Friedl, K.E, M.Z Mays, and T.R Kramer. 1995a. Acute recovery of physiological and cognitive function in U.S. Army Ranger students in a multistressor field environment. Workshop on the Effect of Prolonged Exhaustive Military Activities on Man—Physiological and Psychological Changes—Possible Means of Rapid Recuperation. NATO AC/243 Panel VIII. April 3–5. Holmenkollen, Oslo, Norway.

Friedl, K.E., K.A. Westphal, and L.J. Marchitelli. 1995b. Reproductive status and menstrual cyclicity of premenopausal women in Army basic combat training (BCT). FASEB J. 9:A292.

Fuchs, B.A., and V.M. Sanders. 1994. The role of brain-immune interactions in immunotoxicology. Crit. Rev. Toxicol. 24:151–176.

Gallagher, H.J., and J.M. Daly. 1993. Malnutrition, injury, and the host immune response: Nutrient substitution. Curr. Opin. Gen. Surg. 1993:92–104.

Gifford, R., R. Halverson, D. Ritzer, J. Valentine, and L. Newkirk. 1996. Operation Joint Endeavor: Psychological status of the deployed force—June 1996. Summary brief/report, July 1996. Washington, D.C.: Division of Neuropsychiatry, Walter Reed Army Institute of Research.

Gorbunov, N.V., A.N. Osipov, M.A. Sweetland, B.W. Day, N.M. Elsayed, and V.E. Kagan. 1996. NO-redox paradox: Direct oxidation of alpha-tocopherol and alpha-tocopherol-mediated oxidation of ascorbate. Biochem. Biophys. Res. Commun. 27:835–841.

Gray, A.B., Y.C. Smart, R.D. Telford, M.J. Weidemann, and T.K. Roberts. 1992. Anaerobic exercise causes transient changes in leukocyte subsets and IL-2R expression. Med. Sci. Sports Exerc. 24:1332–1338.

Halvorsen, R.R., P.D. Bliese, R.E. Moore, and C.A. Castro. 1995. Psychological well-being and physical health symptoms of soldiers deployed for Operation Uphold Democracy. A summary of Human Dimensions research in Haiti. Washington, D.C.: Division of Neuropsychiatry, Walter Reed Army Institute of Research.

Hardy, C.A., J. Quay, S. Livast, and R. Ader. 1990. Altered T-lymphocyte response following aggressive encounters in mice. Physiol. Behav. 47:245–251.

Heppner, D.G., A.J. Magill, R.A. Gasser, and C.N. Oster. 1993. The threat of infectious diseases in Somalia. N. Engl. J. Med. 328:1061–1068.

Herbert, V., and T.S. Kasdan. 1994. Alfalfa, vitamin E, and autoimmune disorders. Am. J. Clin. Nutr. 60:639–640.

Huhman, K.L., M.A. Hebert, J.L. Meyerhoff, and B.N. Bunnell. 1991. Plasma cyclic AMP increases in hamsters following exposure to a graded footshock stressor. Psychoneuroendocrinology 16:559–563.

Huhman, K.L., T.O. Moore, E.H. Mougey, and J.L. Meyerhoff. 1992. Hormonal responses to fighting in hamsters: Separation of physical and psychological causes. Physiol. Behav. 51:1083–1086.

IOM (Institute of Medicine). 1992. Nutritional Assessment of U.S. Army Ranger Training Class 11/91. A brief report of the Committee on Military Nutrition Research, Food and Nutrition Board, March 23. Washington, D.C.

IOM (Institute of Medicine). 1993b. Review of the Results of Nutritional Intervention, U.S. Army Ranger Training Class 11/92 (Ranger II), B.M. Marriott, ed. Report of the Committee on Military Nutrition Research, Food and Nutrition Board. Washington, D.C.: National Academy Press

Irwin, M., J. McClintick, C. Costlow, M. Fortner, J. White, and J.C. Gillin. 1996. Partial night sleep deprivation reduces natural killer and cellular immune responses in humans. FASEB J. 10:643–653.

Johnson, H.L., H.J. Krzywicki, J.E. Canham, J.H. Skala, T.A. Daws, R.A. Nelson, C.F. Consolazio, and P.P. Waring. 1976. Evaluation of calorie requirements for Ranger training at Fort Benning, Georgia. Technical Report No. 34. Presidio of San Francisco, Calif.: Letterman Army Institute of Research.

Kant, G.J., R.H. Pastel, R.A. Bauman, G.R. Meininger, K.R. Maughan, T.N. Robinson III, W.L. Wright, and P.S. Covington. 1995. Effects of chronic stress on sleep in rats. Physiol. Behav. 57:359–365.

Kapcala, L.P., T. Chautard, and R.L. Eskay. 1995. The protective role of the hypothalamic-pituitary-adrenal axis against lethality produced by immune, infectious, and inflammatory stress. Ann. N.Y. Acad. Sci. 771:419–437.

Kiecolt-Glaser, J.K., R. Glaser, S. Gravenstein, W.B. Malarkey, and J. Sheridan. 1996. Chronic stress alters the immune response to influenza virus vaccine in older adults. Proc. Natl. Acad. Sci. USA 93:3042–3047.

Kiecolt-Glaser, J.K., P.T. Marucha, W.B. Malarkey, A.M. Mercado, and R. Glaser. 1995. Slowing of wound healing by psychological stress. Lancet 346:1194–1196.

Kragh Jr., J.F. 1993. Use of knee and elbow pads during Ranger training. Mil Med. 158:A4.

Kramer, T.R. 1992. Support between USAMRDC and USDA for cooperative research under the Ration Sustainment Testing Program. Final report 1 July 1991–30 September 1991. Washington, D.C.: U.S. Department of Agriculture.

Kramer, T.R. 1996. Effects of various doses of vegetables on immune response and other health parameters in humans. USAMRMC Interagency Agreement C20M6770; ARS Agreement 60-3K47-6-060. Fredrick, Md.: U.S. Army Medical Research and Materiel Command.

Kramer, T.R., K.E. Friedl, and R.L. Shippee. 1995. Effects of caloric restriction in high-energy demanding U.S. Army training on T-lymphocyte functions in soldiers. Presentation to the 2nd International Society of Exercise and Immunology Convention, Brussels, Belgium, November 17–18.

Kramer, T.R., R.J. Moore, R.J. Shippee, K.E. Friedl, L. Martinez-Lopez, M.M. Chan, and E.W. Askew. 1997. Effects of food restriction in military training on T-lymphocyte responses. Int. J. Sports Med. 18:S84–S90.

Krueger, J.M., L.A. Toth, R. Floyd, J. Fang, L. Kapas, S. Bredow, and F. Obal Jr. 1994. Sleep, microbes and cytokines. Neuroimmunomodulation 1:100–109.

Kramer, T.R., E. Udomkesmalee, S. Dhanamitta, S. Sirisinha, S. Charoenkiatkul, S. Tuntipopipat, O. Banjong, N. Rojroongwasinkul, and J.C. Smith Jr. 1993. Lymphocyte responsiveness of children supplemented with vitamin A and zinc. Am. J. Clin. Nutr. 58:566–570.

Krzystyniak, K., H. Tryphonas, and M. Fournier. 1995. Approaches to the evaluation of chemical-induced immunotoxicity. Environ. Health Perspect. 103(suppl. 9):17–22.

Kusnecov, A.W., and B.S. Rabin. 1994. Stressor-induced alterations of immune function: Mechanisms and issues. Int. Arch. Allergy Immunol. 105:107–121.

Lee, D.J., R.T. Meehan, C. Robinson, M.L. Smith, and T.R. Mabry. 1995. Psychosocial correlates of immune responsiveness and illness episodes in U.S. Air Force Academy cadets undergoing basic cadet training. J. Psychosom. Res. 39:445–457.

Lewis, C.E., W.L. Jones, F. Austin, and J. Roman. 1967. Flight research program: IX. Medical monitoring of carrier pilots in combat-II. Aerospace Med. 38:581–592.

Liu, C.T., T.M. Kijek, C.A. Rossi, T.K. Bushe, C.B. Carpenter, S.D. Goodwin, A. Hail, D.A. Creasia, D.M. Walters, R.E. Dinterman, and K.A. Mereish. 1996. Staphylococcal enterotoxin B (SEB) kinetics after intratracheal instillation in Dutch rabbits. FASEB J. 10:A175.

Martinez-Lopez, L.E., K.E. Friedl, R.J. Moore, and T.R. Kramer. 1993A. Prospective epidemiological study of infection rates and injuries of Ranger students. Milit. Med. 158:433–437.

Meehan, R.U., U. Duncan, L. Neale, G. Taylor, H. Muchmore, N. Scott, K. Ramsey, E. Smith, P. Rock, R. Goldblum, and C. Houston. 1988. Operation Everest II: Alterations in the immune system at high altitudes. J. Clin. Immunol. 8:397–406.

Montain, S.J., R.L. Shippee, W.J. Tharion, and T.R. Kramer. 1995. Carbohydrate-electrolyte solution during military training: Effects of physical performance, mood state and immune function. Technical Report No. T95-13, AD-A297 258. Natick, Mass.: U.S. Army Research Institute of Environmental Medicine.

Moore, R.J., K.E. Friedl, T.R. Kramer, L.E. Martinez-Lopez, R.W. Hoyt, R.E. Tulley, J.P. DeLany, E.W. Askew, and J.A. Vogel 1992. Changes in soldier nutritional status and immune function during the Ranger training course. Technical Report No. T13-92, AD-A257 437. Natick, Mass.: U.S. Army Research Institute of Environmental Medicine.

Morgan, A.P., 1966. Energy Metabolism and Body Fuel Utilization, with Particular Reference to Starvation and Injury. Proceedings of the Committee on Metabolism in Trauma of the U.S. Army Research and Development Command. Cambridge, Mass.: Harvard University Printing Office.

Moynihan, J.A., R. Ader, L.J. Grota, T.R. Schachtman, and N. Cohen. 1990. The effects of stress on the development of immunological memory following low-dose antigen priming in mice. Brain Behav. Immun. 4:1–12.

NATO (North Atlantic Treaty Organization). 1995. Worskhop on the Effect of Prolonged Exhaustive Military Activities on Man—Physiological and Psychological Changes—Possible Means of Rapid Recuperation. NATO AC/243 Panel VIII. April 3–5. Holmenkollen, Oslo, Norway.

Newsholme, E.A. 1994. Biochemical mechanisms to explain immunosuppression in well-trained and overtrained athletes. Int. J. Sports Med. 15(suppl. 3):S142–S147.

Nieman, D.C., D.A. Henson, R. Johnson, L. Lebeck, J.M. Davis, and S.L. Nehlsen-Cannarella. 1992. Effects of brief, heavy exertion on circulating lymphocyte subpopulations and proliferative response. Med. Sci. Sports Exerc. 24:1339–1345.

Opstad, P.K. 1995. Medical consequences in young men of prolonged physical stress with sleep and energy deficiency. NDRE Publication 95/05586. Kjeller, Norway: Forsvarets Forskningsinstituttt, Norwegian Defence Research Establishment.

Pedersen, B.K., and H. Bruunsgaard. 1995. How physical exercise influences the establishment of infections. Sports Med. 19:393–400.

Pleban, R.J., P.J. Valentine, D.M. Penetar, D.P. Redmond, and G.L. Belenky. 1990. Characterization of sleep and body composition changes during Ranger training. Milit. Psychol. 2:145–156.

Pollmacher, T., J. Mullington, C. Korth, and D. Hinze-Selch. 1995. Influence of host defense activation on sleep in humans. Adv. Neuroimmunol. 5:155–169.

Rassnick, S., A.F. Sved, and B.S. Rabin. 1994. Locus coeruleus stimulation by corticotropin-releasing hormone suppresses *in vitro* cellular immune responses. J. Neurosci. 14:6033–6040.

Reister, F.A. 1975. Medical Statistics in World War II. Washington, D.C.: U.S. Government Printing Office.

Riedo, F.X., B. Schwartz, S. Glono, J. Hierholzer, S. Ostroff, J. Groover, D. Musher, L. Martinez-Lopez, R. Brelman, and the Pneumococcal Pneumonia Study Group. 1991. Pneumococcal pneumonia outbreak in a Ranger Training Battalion. Program and Abstracts of the Interscience Conference on Antimicrobial Agents and Chemotherapy. Abstract 48. Chicago, Ill.: American Society of Microbiology.

Rose, R.M., P.G. Bourne, R.O. Poe, E.H. Mougey, D.R. Collins, and J.W. Mason. 1969. Androgen responses to stress. II. Excretion of testosterone, epitestosterone, androsterone and etiocholanolone during basic combat training and under threat of attack. Psychosom. Med. 31:418–436.

Rosen, L.N., J.M. Teitelbaum, and D.J. Westhuis. 1993. Stressors, stress mediators, and emotional well-being among spouses of soldiers deployed to the Persian Gulf during Operation Desert Shield/Storm. J. Appl. Soc. Psychol. 23:1587–1593.

Roubenoff, R. 1993. Hormones, cytokines and body composition: Can lessons from illness be applied to aging? J. Nutr. 123:469–473.

Rubin, R.T., E.K. Gunderson, and R.J. Arthur. 1971. Life stress and illness patterns in the U.S. Navy: V. Prior life change and illness onset in a battleship's crew. Psychosom. Med. 15:89–94.

Rubin, R.T., R.G. Miller, R.J. Arthur, and B.R. Clark. 1970. Differential adrenocortical stress responses in naval aviators during aircraft carrier landing practice. Psychol. Rep. 26:71–74.

Sauberlich, H.E. 1984. Implications of nutritional status on human biochemistry, physiology and health. Clin. Biochem. 17:132–142.

Shek, P.N., B.H. Sabiston, A. Buguet, and M.W. Radomski. 1995. Strenuous exercise and immunological changes: A multiple-time-point analysis of leukocyte subsets, CD4/CD8 ratio, immunoglobulin production and NK cell response. Int. J. Sports Med. 16:466–474.

Shephard, R.J., S. Rhind, and P.N. Shek. 1994. Exercise and training: Influences on cytotoxicity, interleukin-1, interleukin-2 and receptor structures. Int. J. Sports Med. 15(suppl. 3):S154–S166.

Shippee, R., S. Wood, P. Anderson, T. Kramer, M. Nieta, and K. Wolcott. 1995. Effects of glutamine supplementation on immunological responses of soldiers during the Special Forces Assessment and Selection Course. FASEB J. 9:A731.

Simon, G.A., P. Schmid, W.G. Reifenrath, T. van Ravenswaay, and B.E Stuck. 1994. Wound healing after laser injury to skin. The effect of occlusion and vitamin E. Eur. J. Pharm. Sci. 83:1101–1106.

Simon-Schnass, I. 1996. Oxidative stress at high altitude and effects of vitamin E. Pp. 393–418 in Nutritional Needs in Cold and in High-Altitude Environments, Applications for Military Personnel in Field Operations, B.M. Marriott and S.J. Carlson, eds. Committee on Military Nutrition Research, Food and Nutrition Board, Institute of Medicine. Washington, D.C.: National Academy Press.

Singh, A. 1996. Micronutrient/antioxidant supplementation and immune function in women: Effects of physiological stress. Final report. Bethesda, Md.: Uniformed Services University of the Health Sciences.

Singh, A., M.L. Failla, and P.A. Deuster. 1994. Exercise-induced changes in immune function: Effects of zinc supplementation. J. Appl. Physiol. 76:2298–2303.

Singh, A., B.L. Smoak, K.Y. Patterson, L.G. LeMay, C. Veillon, and P.A. Deuster. 1991. Biochemical indices of selected trace minerals in men: Effect of stress. Am. J. Clin. Nutr. 53:126–131.

Smoak, B.L., A. Singh, B.A. Day, J.P. Norton, S.B. Kyle, S.J. Pepper, and P.A. Deuster. 1988. Changes in nutrient intakes of conditioned men during a 5-day period of increased physical activity and other stresses. Eur. J. Appl. Physiol. 58:245–251.

Stouthard, J.M.L, J.A. Romijn, T. van der Poll, E. Endert, S. Klein, P.J. Bakker, C.H. Veenhof, and H.P. Saverwein. 1995. Endocrinologic and metabolic effects of interleukin-6 in humans. Am. J. Physiol. 268(no. 5 pt. 1):E813–E819.

Takafuji, E.T., J.W. Kirkpatrick, R.N. Miller, J.J. Karwacki, P.W. Kelley, M.R. Gray, K.M. McNeill, H.L. Timboe, R.E. Kane, and J.L. Sanchez. 1984. An efficacy trial of doxycycline chemoprophylaxis against leptospirosis. N. Engl. J. Med. 310:497–500.

Tvede, N., M. Kappel, J. Halkjaer-Kristensen, H. Galbo, and B.K. Pedersen. 1993. The effect of light, moderate and severe bicycle exercise on lymphocyte subsets, natural and lymphokine activated killer cells, lymphocyte proliferative response and interleukin-2 production. Int. J. Sports Med. 14:275–282.

Wester, P.W., A.D. Vethaak, and W.B. van Muiswinkel. 1994. Fish as biomarkers in immunotoxicology. Toxicology 86:213–232.

Westphal, K.A., K.E. Friedl, M.A. Sharp, N. King, T.R. Kramer, K.L. Reynolds, and L.J. Marchitelli. 1995a. Health, performance, and nutritional status of U.S. Army women during basic combat training. Technical Report No. T96-2, AD-A32042. Natick, Mass.: U.S. Army Research Institute of Environmental Medicine.

Westphal K.A., A.E. Pusateri, and T.R. Kramer. 1994. Prevalence of negative iron nutriture and relationship with folate nutriture, immunocompetence, and fitness level in U.S. Army servicewomen. USARIEM Approved Protocol OPD94002-AP024-H016. Defense Women's Health Research Program 1994, Log No. W4168016. Natick, Mass.: U.S. Army Research Institute of Environmental Medicine.

Yehuda, R., M.T. Lowy, S.M. Southwick, D. Shaffer, and E.L. Giller Jr. 1991. Lymphocyte glucocorticoid receptor number in posttraumatic stress disorder. Am. J. Psychiatry 148:499–504.

Yehuda, R, S.M. Southwick, G. Nussbaum, V.S. Wahby, E.L. Giller Jr., and J.W. Mason. 1990. Low urinary cortisol excretion in patients with posttraumatic stress disorder. J. Nerv. Mental Dis. 178:366–369.

Zhang, Y.H., T.R. Kramer, P.R. Taylor, J.Y. Li, W.J. Blot, C.C. Brown, W. Guo, S.M. Dawsey, and B. Li. 1995. Possible immunologic involvement of antioxidants in cancer prevention. Am. J. Clin. Nutr. 62(suppl.):S1477–S1482.

Zhou, D., A.W. Kusnecov, M.R. Shurin, M. DePaoli, and B.S. Rabin. 1993. Exposure to physical and psychological stressors elevates plasma interleukin 6: Relationship to the activation of hypothalamic-pituitary-adrenal axis. Endocrinology 133:2523–2530.

Zhou, D., N. Shanks, S.E. Riechman, R. Liang, A.W. Kusnecov, and B.S. Rabin. 1996. Interleukin-6 modulates interleukin-1 and stress-induced activation of the hypothalamic-pituitary-adrenal axis in male rats. Neuroendocrinology 63:227–236.

DISCUSSION

DOUGLAS WILMORE: I am concerned with the field trials, and I am concerned with the dropouts in the field trials. If a hospitalized patient had a PHA level similar to the ones you report, we would not consider that abnormal.

KARL FRIEDL: That is not remarkable?

DOUGLAS WILMORE: Yes. Some of my learned colleagues can comment more about that. But we clearly see levels much, much lower, and we set ranges for normal that are broader than that. What I am concerned about, however, are figures that look at dropout rates with 121 entrants, 85 subjects looked at in the next go-round, and 58 subjects looked at in the last analyses. What may be of more interest would be what happened to the people who are not being measured.

KARL FRIEDL: We certainly tried to capture that. We captured it in those infection rates. When we looked at why people dropped out, the dropouts were not people who were having problems with infections. For the most part, the dropouts were the ones who were failing on peer reviews, that is, the subjective evaluation of their leadership capabilities and how well they could lead.

DOUGLAS WILMORE: It is not physical performance, as a general rule?

KARL FRIEDL: By and large, it is because they received a poor score in their leadership capabilities. Now, what goes into that though? Physical capabilities certainly do. These guys were fatigued and simply stopped performing because they couldn't think clearly anymore. I think that is the main reason they are dropping out. We looked very carefully for that because we were concerned about dropouts as well.

RONALD SHIPPEE: Karl and I have talked about this a lot. You have got to be extremely careful interpreting the attrition rates from these studies. I will give you an example. We do a lot of work with SFAS. SFAS is unique because we have complete access to the students. If a guy drops out academically, he gets out and we thank him for being in the course. If you go down to the building where the dropouts are waiting to be taken back to the post, there is a lot of hacking and coughing going on in there. So I know in my heart, when I look at these guys, a lot of the attrition that occurs when a guy says he failed to perform is probably due to illness. I was going to bring this up in my presentation.

We do all of these little immunological tests , and they are fine, and they give us some direction; but the true proof is going to be observing high infection rates at these schools. I will show you one approach to get at that. So, you are right. Be very careful when you look at attrition rates in these courses. They do not tell the whole story. I am sure that Karl will agree with that.

DOUGLAS WILMORE: I do not want to monopolize this at all; but just for the committee to realize, I have talked to some of the people who are getting ready to go on the Ranger courses. If you talk to them about the supplements that they are taking, the pictures that Karl showed do not do them justice. When I talked to them about doses, I found that they are really dosing. And the issue is, as I understand it, that they are withdrawing themselves from the supplements as they go out on the Ranger course. There is a classic example of withdrawal from high-dose vitamin C down to normal RDA [Recommended Dietary Allowance] vitamin C intake levels, and the functional effects of vitamin C deficiency are observed. That is an issue that I think really we have to come to grips with and address.

ROBERT NESHEIM: Any other questions? Yes.

JOSEPH CANNON: I have a question and comment. The question relates to the infection rates in the women who were undergoing basic training. Was that similar to the infection rates in the men?

KARL FRIEDL: No. I do not think we had any infection in the women. There was no significant problem with infection ratio. In fact, most of the sick call visits were for musculoskeletal injury.

JOSEPH CANNON: Just a comment. I would like to follow up on what Doug Wilmore was saying about PHA. In 1992, when we looked at U.S. Air Force cadets, they showed a similar falloff in PHA-induced lymphocyte proliferation. When we looked at the cadets who became ill, and compared them with those who remained perfectly healthy, there was no difference in those two groups in terms of their PHA response. So that certainly may not in itself tell the whole story.

KARL FRIEDL: But, in addition, you have got to consider what they are exposed to. They still have to come in contact with some kind of pathogen, unless there is some endogenous problem that will take over.

In the case of the Ranger students, in the last phase or towards the end of the course, when they are in this sort of suppressed stage, they are immersed in the Yellow River, and they spend a lot of time in water immersion in this fairly polluted river. At that point, they have a lot of knee abrasions. Every time they stop they drop down to one knee. So commonly we get these soft-tissue infections of the knee, cellulitis. It is because of exposure. I think that we have to have that piece of it. We have to have exposure on top of susceptibility.

ROBERT NESHEIM: Last comment?

ARTHUR ANDERSON: You mentioned that, with the first Ranger group study, you had an increase in positivity for T.B. [as demonstrated by the tine test] at the end of the study compared with the beginning of the study, but not in the second Ranger study, where individuals were knocked out early in the trial because of medical problems.

KARL FRIEDL: No. In the second study we did not do the tine study.

ARTHUR ANDERSON: Oh, you did not do the test?

KARL FRIEDL: No. We just saw that it did not show us much in the first study, so we did not repeat it.

ROBERT NESHEIM: Good. Well, thank you very much. I think that sets a real stage for the rest of this workshop.

Nutrition and Immune Function, 1999
Pp. 163–184. Washington, D.C.
National Academy Press

5

Physiological and Immunological Impact of U.S. Army Special Operations Training

A Model for the Assessment of Nutritional Intervention Effects on Temporary Immunosuppression

LTC Ronald L. Shippee[1]

INTRODUCTION

Historically, nutritional adequacy of operational (field) rations for soldiers has been defined by the ability of the rations to sustain blood levels of a particular nutrient or metabolite of the nutrient. Adequacy of certain vitamins and minerals has further been defined by the functional assessment of blood cell activity of selected enzymes. Based on these accepted criteria, the current military operational ration (Meal, Ready-to-Eat, MRE) has met the assessment for nutritional adequacy in a number of varied field settings over the past 10 years. Even when consumed at a rate of one MRE per day for periods of up to 10 days, the MRE appeared to supply adequate micronutrient nutrition in U.S. Army Ranger students (Moore et al., 1992).

[1] Ronald L. Shippee, U.S. Army Forensic Toxicology Drug Testing Laboratory, Fort Meade, MD 20755. *Formerly of* Military Nutrition Division, U.S. Army Research Institute of Environmental Medicine, Natick, MA 01760.

Many reports in the scientific literature are causing nutritional scientists to question the traditional assessments of nutritional adequacy. The current U.S. Recommended Dietary Allowances are in the process of being revised and updated; the Dietary Reference Intakes, as they will be known, will present recommended adequate levels of the nutrients for selected populations. The publicity concerning the recent research on the effect of perinatal folic acid supplementation on the incidence of congenital neural tube defects is a good example of a research finding that challenges the traditional view of nutrient adequacy.

One area of active research of particular concern to this readership involves assessment of nutritional adequacy based on immune responses. This is of particular importance to military operations during periods of extreme physical and psychological stress. Considerable interest in the exercise physiology and nutrition literature during the past 5 years focuses on the interaction of nutrition and susceptibility to infection in athletes training for competition. Although close analogies can be drawn between training for an athletic event and military combat training, some important differences need to be addressed. While an athlete is usually well rested and fed a diet specific to his or her sport and nutritional needs, individuals involved in combat training are often sleep deprived and fed "one-size-fits-all" military operational rations. Another important difference is that soldiers often suffer abrasions and cuts, which increases the chance for opportunistic infection.

Special Operations training offers the unique opportunity to determine the extent of immunological perturbations during military training. Furthermore, the structured nature of the training schools provides the opportunity to conduct controlled research studies designed to screen nutritional strategies that may be effective in sustaining immune responses during the stress of combat training. During the past 4 years, a number of field studies related to this issue have been conducted in collaboration with the Ranger Training Brigade (RTB), Fort Benning, Georgia, and the Special Warfare Training Center, Fort Bragg, North Carolina.

RESEARCH OBJECTIVES

The research conducted in these locations has been guided by two primary research objectives:

1. Combat training by its nature often involves risk of injury. The leadership must always balance training objectives with many safety issues. The primary goal of this research has been to provide physiological data that the commanders can use to develop guidelines for such issues as sleep deprivation, food restriction, and exposure to temperature extremes during strenuous physical training.

2. Access to young, healthy soldiers who are experiencing temporary alterations in immune responses has important implications for both military and civilian applications. The military relevance of this issue is obvious, considering that during all the major military conflicts in which the U.S. Armed Forces have been involved in modern history, nonbattle injury and infection account for far more casualties than those inflicted by enemy action (Palinkas, 1988; Seay, 1995). Most of the information concerning the interaction between nutrition and immune responses has been developed from research with individuals recovering from severe trauma injuries. Results from nutritional interventions during periods of combat training stress have the potential for contributing important scientific data to the field of nutritional immunology. This line of research will ultimately lead to the development of nutritional strategies designed to sustain host defense mechanisms during periods of extreme physiological and physical stress.

RESULTS

U.S. Army Ranger training and the Special Forces Assessment and Selection (SFAS) course are physically and psychologically demanding programs used by the U.S. Army to screen male officers and enlisted soldiers for entry into U.S. Army Special Operations units. Since the summer of 1992, a number of studies have been conducted with these Special Operations schools through collaborative research among the U.S. Army Medical Research and Materiel Command (USAMRMC), the Soldier System Command, U.S. Department of Agriculture, and Ross Products Division, Abbott Laboratories (ROSS).

Studies Involving Ranger Training

The RTB, Fort Benning, Georgia, conducts Ranger training continuously during the year, with classes starting approximately every 30 days. Until recently, Ranger training involved four, 2-wk phases conducted at geographically diverse training sites: Phase 1, Fort Benning, Georgia; Phase 2 (desert phase), Fort Bliss, Texas; Phase 3 (mountain phase), Dahlonega, Georgia; Phase 4, Eglin Air Force Base, Florida. Recently, the desert phase was eliminated, leaving three phases consisting of approximately 21 days each. At the end of each phase, soldiers are involved in 7- to 10-d field training exercises (FTX). Usually the soldiers conduct continuous operations during the FTX portions of the training and are not allowed to return to the barracks areas of the camps.

The severity of the Ranger training and episodic increases in accidents and infection resulted in two medical research studies during the mid-1960s and 1970s (Consolazio et al., 1966; Johnson et al., 1976). During the 1990–1991 training year, an unusually high number of *Streptococcal pneumonia* infections prompted a request from the RTB to the USAMRMC. This request resulted in two independent research studies conducted in 1991 by research teams from the Walter Reed Army Institute of Research and the U.S. Army Research Institute of Environmental Medicine (USARIEM). Based on the findings of these two studies, an additional study by USARIEM was conducted in the summer of 1992.

The salient results of the USARIEM study (Ranger I, RGR-I) are shown in Figures 5-1 through 5-10. The result of the energy expenditure (Figure 5-1) and intake (Figure 5-2) assessment was an average daily negative energy balance of −1,203 kcal (Figure 5-3). The feeding plan during the summer months in which the 1991 studies were conducted supplied one MRE during the FTX portions of the training. The impact of this negative energy balance was a 14 percent decrease in body weight (Figure 5-4) and a decrease in the average body fat from 16 percent to 5 percent (Figure 5-5). The impact of the severity of the training on physiological response is further reflected in changes in endocrine profiles. Figures 5-6 and 5-7 show the changes in circulating levels of testosterone and triiodothyronine (T3). Testosterone levels were suppressed below castration levels during the last three phases of the training.

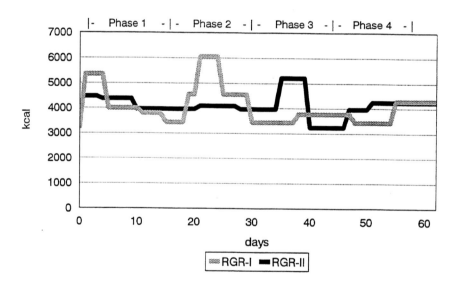

FIGURE 5-1 Energy expenditure during the Ranger I and Ranger II studies as measured by the doubly labeled water method.

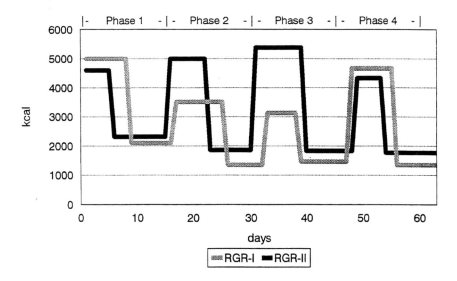

FIGURE 5-2 Caloric intake during the Ranger I and Ranger II studies.

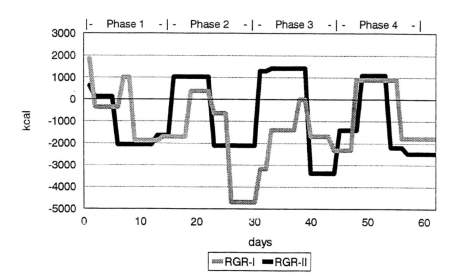

FIGURE 5-3 Energy balance during the Ranger I and Ranger II studies.

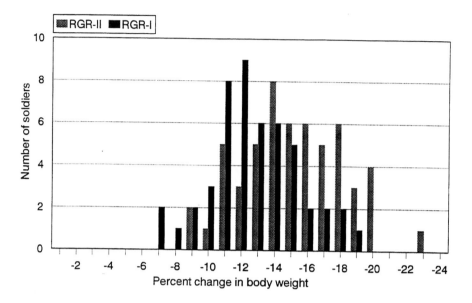

FIGURE 5-4 Percent body weight change during the Ranger I and Ranger II studies.

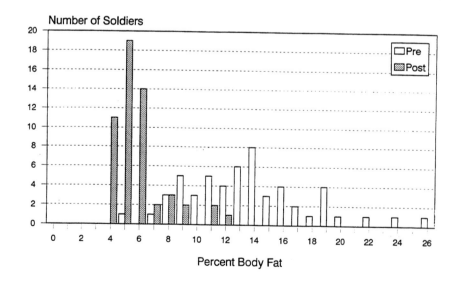

FIGURE 5-5 Percent body fat change during the Ranger I study.

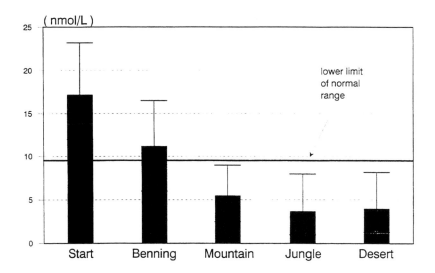

FIGURE 5-6 Serum testosterone concentration changes during the Ranger I study.

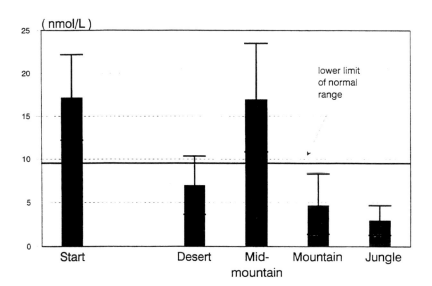

FIGURE 5-7 Serum triiodothyronine concentration changes during the Ranger I study.

Assessment of the impact of the training on immune responses was primarily determined using an *in vitro* proliferation assay. Details of the methodology used to perform the proliferation assay are outlined in Moore et al. (1992). Blood drawn at the various phases of training was transported from the training camps to the laboratory. In a sterile cell culture hood, the vacuum tube was uncapped, and a small portion of the blood was removed and diluted with cell culture medium. The diluted blood was pipetted into cell culture wells, followed by a volume of medium containing various compounds (mitogen) that are commonly used to stimulate white blood cells (lymphocytes) to proliferate in culture conditions. After 2 days, the culture cells were pulsed with a radioactively labeled nucleic acid. Over the next 24 hours, cells that were replicating took up the radioactive label and incorporated the nucleic acid into their DNA. After a total of 72 hours in culture, the cells were harvested with equipment that lyses the cells and traps both the labeled and unlabeled DNA on a small paper disk. This disk was then placed in a vial for subsequent determination of the amount of radiation it contained. The higher the radioactivity, the greater the cells' capacity to proliferate.

Data from the cells stimulated by the T-lymphocyte-stimulating mitogen (phytohemagglutinin) for RGR-I are shown in Figure 5-8. The immune response was significantly suppressed at the end of both the mountain and swamp phases of the training when compared with the other time points. The biological

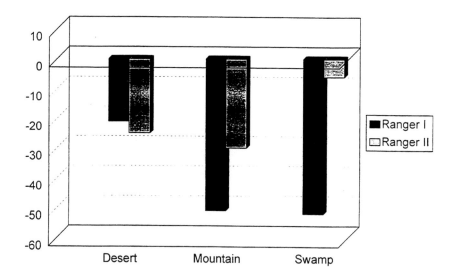

FIGURE 5-8 Percent change in peripheral blood lymphocyte proliferation during the Ranger I and Ranger II studies.

actions of T-lymphocytes are diverse and range from direct killing of invading pathogens to controlling the response of other lymphocyte cell types such as antibody production by B-lymphocytes. The fact that the T-lymphocyte proliferation response, or *cellular response*, was so adversely affected by the training was a very important finding of the RGR-I study.

Results from the study showing low body fat, altered endocrine patterns, perturbations in immune function, and undernutrition raised serious concern with a number of reviewers of the data. The National Academy of Sciences' Committee on Military Nutrition Research (CMNR) was particularly concerned with the impact of these altered physiological responses on thermogenic regulation of soldiers in response to cold exposure.

The final recommendation made to the RTB by the CMNR was to increase Rangers' ration intake during the FTX portions of the training such that no more than 10 percent of body weight was lost. This translated into an increase of 15 percent in food intake during Ranger training. The RTB agreed with this recommendation, and a second (follow-up) study, Ranger II (RGR-II), was conducted during the summer of 1992. To achieve the 15 percent increase in caloric intake, the Long Life Ration Packet (LLRP) was used instead of the MRE.

The salient findings from this study are summarized in Figures 5-1 through 5-10. The increased caloric intake of Rangers in training (in RGR-II) decreased the average daily negative energy balance of −1,203 kcal during RGR-I to −847 kcal (Figure 5-3). This resulted in an average 12 percent body weight loss and a final average percent body fat of 8 percent (Figures 5-4 and 5-9). The physiological impact of the increased caloric intake was also reflected in blood testosterone and T3 concentrations (Figures 5-10 and 5-11).

The infection rates during RGR-I for the desert, mountain, and swamp phases of training were 8, 25, and 24 percent, respectively, while the infection rates for the same phases during the caloric intervention study (RGR-II) were 12, 8, and 2 percent, respectively. This decrease in infection is supported by the proliferation data (Figure 5-8). However, although the cellular response was less suppressed during RGR-II when compared with RGR-I, the suppression during RGR-II was still considered clinically significant.

The research resulted in two significant changes to Ranger training. First, the RTB changed the MRE distribution to three meals per (every) 2 days, with additional supplementation during the winter classes. Second, the data were used by the RTB to support the request for additional medical support. This resulted in the permanent assignment of a physician's assistant at each of the three training camps.

It is impossible to determine by comparing data from RGR-I with that from RGR-II if the apparent benefit of the intervention with respect to immune responses was due to increased energy or specific nutrient(s) contained in the increased intake. The USARIEM research team attempted to answer this

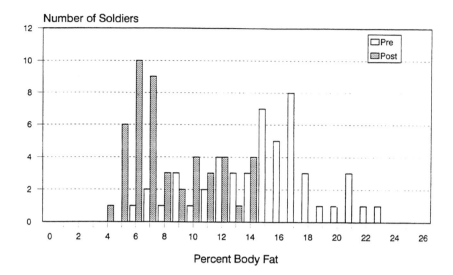

FIGURE 5-9 Percent body fat change during the Ranger II study.

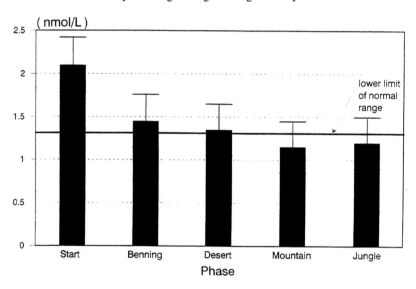

FIGURE 5-10 Serum testosterone concentration changes during the Ranger II Study.

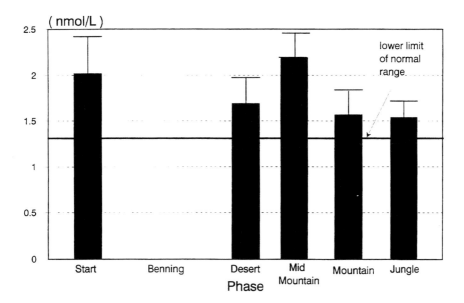

FIGURE 5-11 Serum triiodothyronine concentration changes during the Ranger II study.

question in a study conducted with volunteers from the Ranger training cadre stationed at Camp Merrill, Dahlonega, Georgia (Montain et al., 1995). The study's main purpose was to determine the effect of carbohydrate-electrolyte beverage on physical performance during 3 days of intense activity performing military-relevant tasks. Concurrently, the effect of energy intake on lymphocyte proliferation was tested. The total energy intake for the 3 days was 7,846 ± 1,460 and 5,312 ± 1,228 for the beverage test group and water control group, respectively. Energy intake from field rations was similar for each group. However, no significant difference in lymphocyte proliferation was measured between the two groups.

  Given these findings and some favorable results from specific nutrient intervention studies conducted with the SFAS as described below, USARIEM approached the RTB in February 1996 concerning possible nutrient intervention studies of Rangers in training. Encouraged by the data, the RTB recommended that a research protocol be developed. Shortly after this meeting four Ranger students died of hypothermia during the swamp phase of Ranger training.

  In a March 1996 meeting of the RTB and USARIEM, it was decided that a comprehensive research study would be conducted to reevaluate the physiological impact of Ranger training. The course had been reduced to three phases and the training events changed in response to the February tragedy.

The study was conducted in two parts (Young and Shippee, 1995). During November 1995, the effect of cold exposure was determined in 15 volunteers immediately after they had completed the swamp phase of Ranger training. The second part involved monitoring energy balance, body composition, nutritional status, and immune responses during each phase of the training. This part of the study was completed on April 7, 1996, and the data are being analyzed. From data on body composition and body weight changes of the 39 volunteers that remained in the study, some preliminary conclusions can be drawn. Percentage body fat decreased from a baseline of 15.3 percent down to 10.0 percent at the end of the 62 days of training. A net change in body weight of –7 lbs (3 kg) provides an estimate of energy balance of approximately –415 kcal/d. This is considerably less than the energy deficit shown for RGR-I and RGR-II and reflects the changes instituted by the RTB since February 1995.

Studies Involving Special Forces Assessment and Selection Training

Shortly after completing the RGR-II study, USARIEM received a request from the First Special Warfare Training Group to determine the physiological impact of SFAS training. The SFAS is a 21-d, physically and psychologically demanding course. Although food deprivation is not used as an overt training stressor, self-reported weight losses of between 10 and 15 lbs (4.5 and 6.8 kg) raised concern among the cadre.

The first study of SFAS (SFAS-I) was conducted in the summer of 1993 using a research design and methodology similar to that used in the RGR studies. The data are summarized in Figures 5-12 through 5-15. Although the volunteers were provided a mix of A rations and MREs 3 times per day, there was an average negative energy balance of 1,379 kcal/d (Figure 5-12). This level of negative energy balance resulted in an average weight loss of 7 lbs (3 kg) (Figure 5-13) and a change in percent body fat from 15.5 percent at baseline to 11.9 percent at the end of the training (Figure 5-14). Although infection did not contribute significantly to the medical attrition of the volunteers, there was a 23 percent reduction in lymphocyte proliferation (Figure 5-15).

Since this initial study, two additional studies have been conducted involving nutritional intervention. These studies were conducted under a Cooperative Research and Development Agreement (CRDA) with ROSS. The first intervention study used a sports drink-type beverage containing the amino acid glutamine.[2] The second intervention used a proprietary-based beverage containing increased levels of selected antioxidants nutrients.

---

[2] Daily intake from beverage: 35 g sucrose, 15.4 g glutamine, and 0.3 g fruit punch flavor.

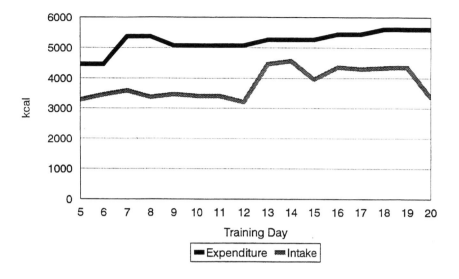

FIGURE 5-12 Energy expenditure and intake during the Special Forces Assessment and Selection Course.

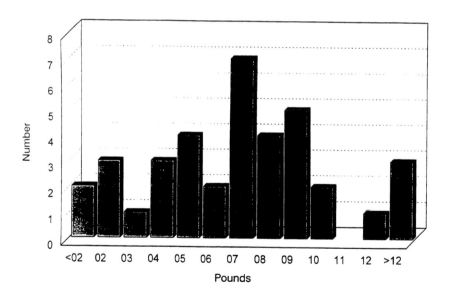

FIGURE 5-13 Body weight loss during the Special Forces Assessment and Selection Course.

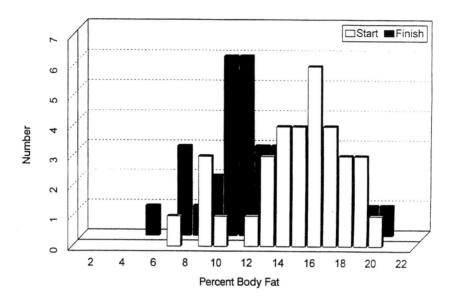

FIGURE 5-14 Percent body fat change during the Special Forces Assessment and Selection Course.

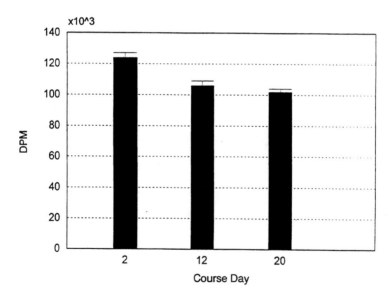

FIGURE 5-15 Peripheral blood lymphocyte proliferation during the Special Forces Assessment and Selection Course.

Although glutamine is not normally considered a dietary essential amino acid, evidence in the clinical, scientific literature indicates that dietary supplementation of glutamine is needed to sustain proper gut function and immune responses during recovery from severe trauma (Souba, 1992). Given the results of the work completed thus far with volunteers from Army Special Operations schools, a strong research hypothesis can be developed to support glutamine supplementation under severe training conditions.

Glutamine was given at a rate of 15 g/d for 18 days of the SFAS during the summer months of 1995 (SFAS-II). The lymphocyte proliferation suppression was equal to the level shown in the SFAS-I study; however, there was no significant effect of glutamine supplementation when compared to the glycine content group (Figure 5-16). To expand the assessment of the immune system, a skin test was included (Multi-Test CMI, Connaught Laboratories, Inc., Swiftwater, Pa.) during SFAS-II. The CMI test kit contains a glycerin negative control and seven antigens of culture filtrate from the following microorganisms: tetanus toxoid, diphtheria toxoid, *streptococcus*, tuberculin, and protease. The test was applied to the vertical forearm of each subject. After 48 hours, the response to each antigen was determined by measuring the diameters of the induration response at each of the eight tine administered sites. The test was administered at the end of the training, and the induration was

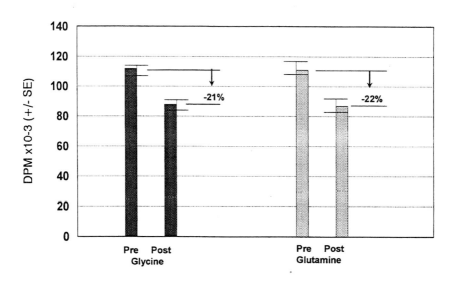

FIGURE 5-16 Peripheral blood lymphocyte proliferation during glutamine supplementation study with the Special Forces Assessment and Selection Course.

measured 24 hours later. Almost twice as many glutamine-supplemented volunteers responded with greater than 10 mm induration to tetanus toxoid when compared with the control group (Table 5-1). This result suggested a beneficial effect of the glutamine treatment. The discrepancies between the results of the two tests of the immune system are difficult to explain on the basis of one study.

During early 1996, an additional intervention study was performed with the SFAS (SFAS-III). This intervention involved a beverage containing four nutrients known to have biological antioxidant properties: vitamin A, vitamin E, vitamin C, and selenium. The beverage was given once a day during the SFAS. Results for the proliferation response and the skin test response to tetanus toxoid are shown in Figures 5-17 and 5-18. The group that received the antioxidant beverage had significantly less suppression of *in vitro* proliferation than the control group when suppression was expressed as a percentage change from baseline values. While more of the group that received antioxidant beverage gave a positive response to tetanus toxoid, the difference from the control group was not as dramatic as the responses shown in the glutamine study.

AUTHOR'S CONCLUSIONS AND RECOMMENDATIONS

During the past 4 years, a close working relationship has developed between USARIEM and the U.S. Army Special Operations groups. The value of this relationship was significantly demonstrated in the past year.

Because of the past experience with the RTB and close contact maintained during the months leading up to the February 1995 incident, the Military Nutrition Division (MND, currently the Military Nutrition and Biochemistry Division) in collaboration with the USARIEM Thermal Physiology Division provided immediate consultation to the RTB. This consultation was quickly followed up with field research studies. The primary objective of these studies

TABLE 5-1 Delayed-Type Hypersensitivity Response to Tetanus Toxoid and Diphtheria Antigens at the End of Special Forces Assessment and Selection Course

		Results			
		Tetanus		Diphtheria	
	Total Recorded	> 5 mm	> 10 mm	> 5 mm	> 10 mm
Glutamine	30	17	15	7	5
Control	27	18	8	5	3

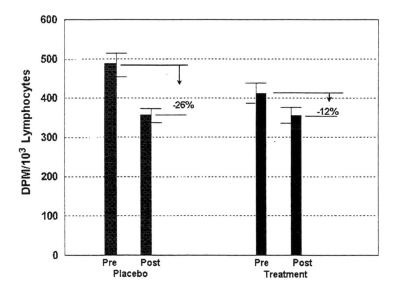

FIGURE 5-17 Peripheral blood lymphocyte proliferation during the antioxidant supplementation study with the Special Forces Assessment and Selection Course.

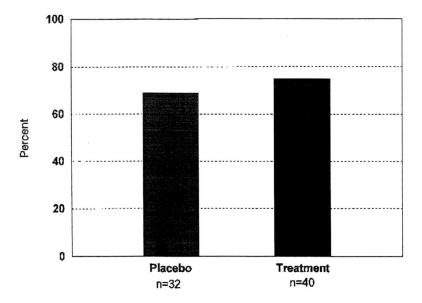

FIGURE 5-18 Delayed-type hypersensitivity response to tetanus toxoid during antioxidant supplementation study with the Special Forces Assessment and Selection Course.

was to provide the RTB with data to support the changes that had been made in the training protocol to ensure training safety. The secondary objective was to provide the necessary physiological and immunological background for future intervention studies.

Recently, a Memorandum of Agreement (MOA) has been developed that formalizes the working relationship between the SFAS and the MND. The salient features of this MOA include ready access to research volunteers and facilities support at Camp Mackall, North Carolina. Because of the MOA, planning and conducting field research is now accomplished at the company level. Building space and facilities support have been provided allowing for prepositioning laboratory equipment and supplies at the field site. These developments allow research to be conducted at significant monetary savings and with quick turnaround for planning and conducting the research and data analysis.

With this foundation of administrative support, the techniques can be refined to assess immunological responses at the cellular, molecular, and genetic levels. Techniques necessary to support this effort are currently being developed through the CRDA with ROSS and collaboration with academia.

In addition to collaboration with U.S. Army Special Operations units, areas for collaboration with Special Operations units in other countries should be explored. Lewis et al. (1991) have reported on changes in physiological and immunological parameters in Royal Marines. A review of this report shows both similarities and differences when compared with work from this laboratory over the past 4 years.

This research has a high degree of military relevance. While infection and disease susceptibility have always been a major concern to military activities, it is especially important now, considering the high rate of deployment of Army soldiers over the past 8 years. Prophylactic measures such as proper personal hygiene, vaccines, and antibiotics continue to play important roles. However, these measures alone may not always be enough. Antibiotic-resistant strains of bacteria are becoming more and more prevalent.

Although the immediate application of the findings from these studies is with Special Operations units, the implications of the research go far beyond this select army population. Nutritional strategies that will sustain host defense mechanisms during the stress of Special Operations training have important applications to sustaining the total force. Furthermore, this unique model may provide important insights into the cellular and molecular mechanisms involved in the complex interaction between nutrition and immune responses.

REFERENCES

Consolazio, C.F., L.O. Matoush, R.A. Nelson, R.S. Harding, and J.E. Canham. 1966. Nutritional survey: Ranger Department, Fort Benning, Georgia. Laboratory Report

No. 291. Denver, Colo.: U.S. Army Medical Research and Nutrition Laboratory, Fitzimons General Hospital.

Johnson, H.L., H.J. Krzywicki, J.E. Canham, J.H. Skala, T.A. Daws, R.A. Nelson, C.F. Consolazio, and P.P. Waring. 1976. Evaluation of calorie requirements for Ranger training at Fort Benning, Georgia. Technical Report No. 34. Presidio of San Francisco, Calif.: Letterman Army Institute of Research.

Lewis, D., M. Simmons, R. Pethybridge et al. 1991. The effect of training stress on the immune system in Royal Marine recruits. Alverstoke, GOSPORT, Hampshire: Institute of Naval Medicine.

Montain, S.J., R.L. Shippee, W.J. Tharion, and T.R. Kramer. 1995. Carbohydrate-electrolyte solution during military training: Effects of physical performance, mood state and immune function. Technical Report No. T95-13, AD-A297 258. Natick, Mass.: U.S. Army Research Institute of Environmental Medicine.

Moore, R.J., K.E. Friedl, T.R. Kramer, L.E. Martinez-Lopez, R.W. Hoyt, R.E. Tulley, J.P. DeLany, E.W. Askew, and J.A. Vogel. 1992. Changes in soldier nutritional status and immune function during the Ranger training course. Technical Report No. T13-92, AD-A257 437. Natick, Mass.: U.S. Army Research Institute of Environmental Medicine.

Palinkas, L.A. 1988. Disease and non-battle injuries among U.S. Marines in Vietnam. Milit. Med. 153:150–155.

Seay, W.J. 1995. Deployment medicine: Emporiatrics military style. Army Med. Dept. J. July/August:2–9.

Souba, W.W. 1992. Glutamine, Physiology, Biochemistry, and Nutrition in Critical Illness. Austin, Tx.: R.G. Landers Company.

Young, A., and R.L. Shippee. 1995. The impact of Ranger training on physiological responses and responses to thermoregulatory tolerance to cold. Human Research Protocol No. MND95009-AP027-H028, November 7. Natick, Mass.: U.S. Army Research Institute of Environmental Medicine.

DISCUSSION

ROBERT NESHEIM: Thank you, LTC Shippee. That was interesting to see what has progressed since the last time the Committee had a chance to review the Ranger studies.

GAIL BUTTERFIELD: In the study in which you fed [supplemental] carbohydrates, did you actually test for antigens?

RONALD SHIPPEE: If I could go back, I would do a lot of things knowing what I know now. But I wish. . . . That opportunity is open. The experiment was done in Dahlonega, Georgia, which is the mountain phase of Ranger. That is a very interesting training site, and that opportunity is open. The Ranger Academy is very open to using their cadre as a test model. I think it has been an underutilized model.

GAIL BUTTERFIELD: I have one other question. Is the rate of weight loss that was seen in the Special Forces over 3 weeks about the same as you find in your early work on your Rangers?

RONALD SHIPPEE: Yes.

GAIL BUTTERFIELD: But what is troubling to me is that it looks like the Special Forces [Assessment School trainees] are not doing as well as the Rangers are doing now, and that disturbs me.

RONALD SHIPPEE: It disturbs me, too.

ROBERT NESHEIM: A question over here.

RONALD SHIPPEE: I would like to comment first. Medical attention is much better [for SFAS trainees] because they don't spend as much time away from the base camp. Another significant observation for the Rangers, based on our data, too, is that even before the incident in February, is medical personnel have managed to travel out in the woods with these soldiers. So, there is more medical attention.

SUSANNA CUNNINGHAM-RUNDLES: I have a comment with respect to what you said about B-cells responding to PHA [phytohemagglutinin] activation. Up to 15 percent of peripheral blood mononuclear cells, which are B-cells, will respond to the change. Where you have stress with the T-cells, I think it is not surprising, but it is interesting. I also wonder what was your incubation period, 4 hours?

RONALD SHIPPEE: Yes, 4 hours. We were hoping, as Becton Dickinson has said, that this would be a replacement for PHA 3-d culture, but that is not quite working out right.

SUSANNA CUNNINGHAM-RUNDLES: I know. It is not so easy.

RONALD SHIPPEE: Yes, I thought I had found a good alternative for the 3-d culture method.

SUSANNA CUNNINGHAM-RUNDLES: I don't think they have done the number of studies that you have.

RONALD SHIPPEE: No. We attended the users' meeting in New England and discussed this with representatives from Becton Dickenson.

SUSANNA CUNNINGHAM-RUNDLES: Right.

DARSHAN KELLEY: In your Ranger and SFAS experience, there is calorie deficit, and there is physical exertion. We have done studies with overweight women with none of these things except calorie deprivation as a factor. Twelve to 15 weeks of 50 percent calorie restriction would cause a 25 to 40 percent increase in MPH the number of NK cells, the PHA-Con-A stimulation. There are, also, decreases in the serum and in the blood.

RONALD SHIPPEE: I am not denying that caloric deprivation isn't a component, but again I think this is where we must discuss the military relevance of what we are doing, there is going to be some caloric deprivation in a combat situation.

So, the question is, can single nutrients and nutritional strategies enhance or keep the immune response up? There is something else you need to consider in a military environment, and I learned this working at the Burn Center.

If you look at predictors of recovery from burns, it is age and weight, when they come into the burn unit, and another one is nutritional status.

So, in military soldiers you have got to think about whether we can give them a good immune system prior to getting wounded, and will that help the surgeon and speed recovery?

So, I am not denying that calories are a major component, but in our situation it may be practical for us to see if we can sustain immune responses with a single nutrient or multinutrient under a caloric restricted situation.

ROBERT NESHEIM: I think we will have to take just one more question and move on because we will have some time this afternoon for further discussion.

SIMIN NIKBIN MEYDANI: You saw a 10 percent response with the skin test. Was there a difference in the soldiers' prior exposure to tetanus, as far as isolation, when they were vaccinated?

RONALD SHIPPEE: I don't have access to that information. You would suspect in that age military population, they have probably had a booster shot within the last 4 or 5 years.

Now, I am interested in the way you present your data, and it has come up here before. You take the delayed-hypersensitivity skin test, and you will probably talk about this, and you present a cumulative value, right? I have not done that because I don't see much reaction to the other antigens, and I am starting to wonder whether maybe that in itself is significant. So, I always show the diphtheria and tetanus because I don't have any other reactions, and maybe that is the overall anergy that we are seeing.

ROBERT NESHEIM: Thank you very much. I think we have to move on. The committee will be dealing with this, and we will have some opportunities for further discussion later this afternoon.

Nutrition and Immune Function, 1999
Pp. 185–202. Washington, D.C.
National Academy Press

6

Immune Function Studies During the Ranger Training Course of the Norwegian Military Academy

Pål Wiik[1]

INTRODUCTION

Several reports have noted increased frequency of infectious disease especially in the respiratory system in athletes during high-intensity training (Fitzgerald, 1988; Hoffman-Goetz and Pedersen, 1994; Sharp and Koutedakis, 1992) and also during sustained military operations (Bernton et al., 1994; Kramer, 1994). From the substantial number of reports addressing this topic, the general view seems to be that light to moderate physical activities for up to a few hours stimulate immunity, while high-intensity acute exercise and chronic high-intensity training may suppress immune functions.

However, most of the published data on physical exercise consider duration of exercise of only up to a few hours. Because the strenuous physical exercise during military operations may last for weeks, sometimes with very little sleep and energy intake, the civilian data are inappropriate for purposes of

[1] Pål Wiik, Norwegian Defence Research Establishment, N-2007 Kjeller, Norway

comparison, and studies conducted under military conditions are necessary. In this chapter, findings from this laboratory documenting specific and nonspecific immune changes during 7 days of continuous Norwegian Ranger training will be summarized. Results of studies involving neuroendocrine modulators of immune functions will also be given.

The Ranger Training Course of the Norwegian Military Academy

The cadets of the Norwegian Military Academy take part in a Ranger training course lasting for 7 days as a part of their training program. During this course, cadets engage in continuous, physical, military activities of moderate intensity, day and night, such as marching with a rucksack, digging, and climbing. In a typical training course, activities have been found to correspond to an average of 32 percent of maximum oxygen uptake ($\dot{V}O_2$max) around the clock or about 8,500 kcal/24 h. This estimate is derived from continuous heart rate recordings, data on maximum heart rate and $\dot{V}O_2$max, and workload calculations and assumes a linear relationship between mean heart rate and the workload. However, increased heart rate due to dehydration or psychological stress, for example, may lead to an overestimation of the workload.

The energy supplied to each cadet during the actual training course was 0 kcal on days 1 and 2; about 700 and 950 kcal on days 3 and 4, respectively; 0 kcal on day 5; about 1,300 kcal on day 6; and 0 kcal on day 7. In one course, one group was given an extra 1,200 kcal per day per cadet in order to study the influence of reducing the calorie deficiency from about 95 to about 80 percent. No drugs, minerals, or vitamins were allowed.

Cadets were allowed no formal sleep time during the training course but got short periods of sleep between activities. On the basis of continuous heart rate recordings of individuals in a similar training course, total sleep time for Norwegian Ranger cadets was estimated to be less than 3 hours.

IMMUNE CHANGES DURING NORWEGIAN RANGER TRAINING

Changes in Parameters of Immune Function

Leukocyte Numbers

The total number of blood leukocytes in cadets increased during the Norwegian Ranger training course. Maximum numbers were observed in the first blood test administered to cadets, after 12 to 18 hours of activities, and submaximal numbers were observed on the following days (Bøyum et al., 1996). Of the various blood cells, granulocytes increased about two- to threefold, with maximum numbers reached after 1 to 2 days. Monocytes increased more gradually up to twofold, with maximum numbers reached after 4 to 5 days. In contrast, a reduction of 30 to 40 percent was observed in the number of the T-lymphocytes studied such as the natural killer (NK) cells, helper and suppressor cells, as well as B-lymphocytes, and a maximum reduction of these was observed already after 12 to 18 hours of activities. The same pattern was observed for eosinophils in peripheral blood, which were strongly reduced by 80 to 90 percent (Bøyum et al., 1996; Wiik et al., 1996).

Plasma Levels of Immunoglobulins

Serum concentrations of immunoglobulins in cadets decreased significantly throughout the course. IgG was reduced by 10 to 15 percent, IgA by 10 to 20 percent, and IgM by 20 to 35 percent (Bøyum et al., 1996).

Interleukins

No change in plasma levels of interleukin (IL)-1, IL-12, and IL-4 was found in cadets, but a 10 to 20 percent decrease of IL-6 (minimum after 5–7 days) and an approximately fourfold increase in granulocyte macrophage-colony stimulating factor (GM-CSF) has been demonstrated with maximum levels measured in cadets after 1 to 2 days (Bøyum et al., 1996).

Lymphocyte Mitogenic Response

For the lymphocyte mitogenic response, quite variable results were observed in cadets during the Norwegian Ranger training (Bøyum et al., 1996). In one course, a stimulation was observed, while in another course a suppression was observed.

Changes in Phagocyte Function

Granulocyte Functions

An accentuated chemiluminescence[2] response of the granulocytes (priming) to serum opsonized zymosan (SOZ)[3] was observed during the first few days of the course with a maximum increase in cadets on days 1 to 3 (+12 to +35%) (Wiik et al., 1996). Thereafter, a reduced response to SOZ below control values (−21 to −28%) was found during the final few days of the course. Extra supplementation of cadets with 1,200 kcal/24 h resulted in a more pronounced

---

[2] Chemiluminescence is used to measure the production of reactive oxygen molecules.

[3] SOZ is produced by incubating zymosan, a particulate extract from yeast, with human plasma. SOZ is commonly used as a stimulator of phagocyte function *in vitro*; it stimulates phagocytosis and production of reactive oxygen molecules.

priming (+57% vs. +21% of control response) during the first few days. The chemotactic response to the formylated bacterial tripeptide (*fMLP*) was also primed during the early days of the course, while a reduction toward control values was observed toward the end of the course (Bøyum et al., 1996). These data indicate that moderate, continuous, predominantly aerobic physical activity of individuals for 1 to 3 days, continuously, primes the production of reactive oxygen species in granulocytes, while longer, continuous military activities may also suppress granulocyte functions.

Monocytes

For the activated monocyte chemiluminescence production, a different pattern was observed from that of the granulocytes. A reduction was observed after 12 to 18 hours, followed by increasing values during the rest of the course, with the highest levels at the end (Wiik et al., 1989). Although no change in plasma levels of IL-1 and tumor necrosis factor was observed in cadets, increased secretion was observed *in vitro* after stimulation with endotoxin A (Personal communication, A. Bøyum, Norwegian Defence Research Establishment, Kjeller, Norway, 1996). These data support a long-lasting monocyte activation that is often associated with suppression of other immune functions (Tilz et al., 1993).

Effect of Reducing the Calorie Deficiency

Extra supplementing cadets with 1,200 kcal/24 h reduced the calorie deficiency from about 95 to 80 percent during the 7-d Norwegian Ranger training course, a rather small effect. A more significant priming was, however, observed in cadets' granulocytes, while a lower chemotactic response was observed. No significant difference was observed in leukocyte numbers (or lymphocyte subgroups), immunoglobulins, or interleukins (Bøyum et al., 1996; Wiik et al., 1996).

Neuropeptide Effect during Norwegian Ranger Training

Vasoactive Intestinal Peptide

The effect on leukocytes of the neuropeptide vasoactive intestinal peptide (VIP), which is released from autonomic nerve terminals in peripheral organs, including spleen, lymph nodes, and Peyer's patches in the gut, has been studied in this laboratory (Ottaway, 1991). VIP inhibits lymphocyte mitogenic response and monocyte production of oxygen radicals by stimulating adenylate cyclase in lymphocytes and monocytes, respectively (Ottaway, 1991; Wiik, 1989; Wiik et al., 1985). Increased plasma concentrations of VIP were observed during the

Ranger training course, which suggests an increased secretion or reduced degradation of the peptide (Øktedalen et al., 1984). It was also observed that the number of VIP receptors on leukocytes was upregulated (Wiik et al., 1988) and that a stronger inhibitory effect of VIP on monocytes occurred during the Norwegian Ranger training course (Wiik et al., 1989). *In vitro* studies have indicated that cortisol upregulates the VIP receptor (Wiik, 1991), which suggests that some of the inhibitory effects of glucocorticoids on phagocytes may be mediated by upregulation of receptors for inhibitory signal molecules like VIP (Wiik et al., 1988).

Furthermore, the effects of β-endorphins, enkephalins, and substance P on lymphocyte mitogenic response have been studied. The usual stimulatory effect of these peptides on the lymphocyte mitogenic response was inhibited during the Ranger training course (Unpublished data, P. Wiik, Norwegian Defence Research Establishment, Kjeller, Norway, 1995).

Catecholamines

Catecholamines may inhibit leukocyte function (Gibson-Berry et al., 1993), and catecholamine B$_2$ receptors and cyclic AMP response also were studied in leukocytes during the Norwegian Ranger training course. Receptor downregulation (Opstad et al., 1994a) reduced cyclic AMP response (Opstad et al., 1994b), and an impaired effect of catecholamines *ex vivo* were found (Unpublished data, P. Wiik, Norwegian Defence Research Establishment, Kjeller, Norway, 1995).

Adrenoglucocorticoid Regulation of Phagocyte Function in Animal Studies

It has generally been assumed that cortisol inhibits lymphocyte function and that it affects phagocyte function to a lesser extent. However, a strong correlation was observed between cortisol and a granulocyte respiratory burst in cadets during the Norwegian Ranger training course (Wiik et al., 1996). In contrast, further *in vitro* incubation of rat phagocytes with pharmacological concentrations of glucocorticoids for up to 24 hours induced no significant effect, while incubation for up to 5 days strongly inhibited a monocyte respiratory burst (Hauger and Wiik, 1997).

Exposing rats to corticosterone or fasting them for 48 hours reduced phagocyte production of reactive oxygen metabolites measured in peritoneal phagocyte preparations by luminol-amplified chemiluminescence after activation by SOZ (Wiik et al., 1995). Administration of corticosterone in the drinking water led to an increase in plasma corticosterone from 31 (control level) to 46 ng/ml, reducing chemiluminescence (per cell) by 31 percent. Fasting, which did not change plasma corticosterone or plasma ACTH concentrations, also had an inhibitory effect on chemiluminescence (–25%). Corticosterone administration and fasting when imposed concurrently strongly inhibited the chemiluminescence (–89%), which indicates that plasma corticosterone and fasting reduces chemiluminescence in a synergistic way (Wiik et al., 1995). Similar effects were observed on total leukocyte number; corticosterone administration, fasting, and the combined intervention reduced macrophage numbers –13, –19.7, and –55 percent respectively. Adrenalectomy induced no significant change in peritoneal leukocyte number or composition, while cells from adrenalectomized animals had significantly higher chemiluminescence reactions than cells from sham-operated (control) animals. Administration of corticosterone to adrenalectomized animals reduced chemiluminescence by 30 percent, while sham-operated animals had 49 percent lower chemiluminescence than adrenalectomized rats. The data from adrenalectomized rats also suggest that endogenous levels of corticosterone are inhibitory for chemiluminescence. These results are inconclusive for evaluating the effects of very low doses of corticosterone, since mechanisms other than the elimination of corticosterone could prime the chemiluminescence reaction after surgical adrenalectomy.

Further studies with synthetic glucocorticoids given to rats *in vivo* have confirmed and substantiated a strong negative effect on monocyte-macrophage function in nanomolar concentrations (Røshol et al., 1995). Studies of experimental inflammation in rats indicate that glucocorticoids *in vivo* strongly inhibit the chemotaxis of monocytes to the peritoneum but not the chemotaxis of granulocytes (Unpublished results, T. Haugedal, Norwegian Defence Research Establishment, Kjeller, Norway, 1995). However, the chemiluminescence responses of granulocytes as well as monocytes *ex vivo* were strongly inhibited by glucocorticoid administration.

AUTHOR'S SUMMARY AND RECOMMENDATIONS

During and after the Ranger training course of the Norwegian Military Academy, cadets had no significant increase in infectious disease (Bøyum et al., 1996). However, during a U.S. Army Ranger training course lasting for 62 days, a high rate of infections was observed in trainees including upper-respiratory infections, cellulitis, and even an epidemic of pneumococcal pneumonia (Bernton et al., 1994; Kramer, 1994). These results are supported by studies of infections in athletes during intense training (Fitzgerald, 1988; Hoffman-Goetz and Pedersen, 1994; Sharp and Koutedakis, 1992).

During the 7-d Norwegian Ranger training, cadets had increased numbers of granulocytes and monocytes in peripheral blood and a strong reduction of eosinophils and B- and T-lymphocytes, including helper, suppressor, and NK cells. A reduction in serum concentrations of immunoglobulins was also reported. However, no conclusion can be drawn from these data regarding lymphocyte mitogenic response since variable results were found. For granulocytes, a biphasic response pattern was observed, characterized by primed chemotactic and chemiluminescence responses at the beginning of the course and a normalization (chemotactic response) or a reduction to below control values (chemiluminescence) at the end of the 7-d course. Monocytes, however, remained activated during the entire course, with the highest chemiluminescence response toward the end. Other studies have reported that sustained monocyte activation is associated with suppression of other immune functions (Tilz et al., 1993).

Observed immune changes in Norwegian and U.S. Ranger training courses are largely in agreement. However, in contrast to the variable changes observed in lymphocyte mitogenic response during the Norwegian Ranger training, a significant reduction in lymphocyte mitogenic response was reported during the U.S. Army Ranger training (Kramer, 1994). This discrepancy may be due to the more acute stress observed in the Norwegian Ranger training. Moreover, methodological differences may have influenced the results; studies during Norwegian Ranger training were done in cell-adjusted preparations of mononuclear leukocytes, while whole-blood preparations were used in the U.S. Army studies (Kramer, 1994).

Data from the U.S. Army and Norwegian Ranger training courses comprise a complex picture of immune changes. Nonspecific granulocyte functions seem to be stimulated at the beginning of the course, followed by a period of suppression wherein the number of lymphocytes and several specific immune functions seem to be suppressed. Because these various immune parameters affect host defense against various infections differently, theoretically, these observed changes may affect the pathogenicity of different types of microorganisms differently. The priming of the phagocytic response at the beginning of Ranger training could indicate an increased resistance in soldiers' important "first line" of defense against invading microorganisms, and this may be one reason why no significant increase in infections during or after the 7-d Norwegian course was observed. However, it is also theoretically possible that this priming may contribute to inflammation associated with exercise-induced muscle fiber injury, ischemia-reperfusion injury of joints during exercise, and tendinitis (Armstrong et al., 1991).

Reduced caloric intake for several weeks seems to be of importance for impaired immunity, and with only a small increase in caloric intake during the U.S. Army Ranger training, infections were reduced and immune function improved (Shippee et al., 1994). However, during the Norwegian training, acute energy deprivation (by up to 95 percent of energy expenditure) during 7 days seems to have only moderately affected immunity, and by supplementing 1,200 kcal/24 h to reduce the caloric deficiency to 80 percent, only minor effects in cadets were observed. Furthermore, in a battlefield environment where the level of psychological stress is also high, such stress is known to cause immune suppression (Khansari et al., 1990; Kiecolt-Glaser and Glaser, 1991). It is difficult to determine the significance of each of these factors when combined, but the results from animal studies in this laboratory suggest that simultaneous fasting and high levels of glucocorticoids may synergistically inhibit immunity (Wiik et al., 1995).

No single test appears to predict immune competence, and since the immune changes observed in the Ranger studies are not indicative of a consistent change in immune function, the pathogenicity of different types of infectious agents may be differently affected by the changes in immune function. Leukocyte counts, which can be readily performed in the field, may give a simple although rough indication of the impact of the experienced stresses on immune status. In the laboratory, nonspecific phagocyte functions as well as lymphocyte subgrouping and different types of lymphocyte functions need to be studied. To evaluate immune competence, more complex immune functional studies, like skin reactions to antigens and vaccine responses, should be performed.

Understanding infectious disease and immune competence are of utmost importance for promoting peak military performance on the battlefield. Results from the Norwegian and U.S. Army Ranger training studies indicate that an association exists among the duration and intensity of physical activity, lack of nutrition, and immune competence. Even extreme military activities for up to 1 week with almost no sleep or food seem to be of little consequence to well-trained military personnel, while problems with immune competence seem to be of significance with deprivation of longer duration. It appears that a research program addressing the complex changes in immune system function during military challenges, including frequency of infections, and a systematic study of the influence of altering nutrient intakes and requirements of vitamins and minerals would be of utmost importance to military medicine.

REFERENCES

Armstrong, R.B., G.L. Warren, and J.A. Warren. 1991. Mechanisms of exercise-induced muscle fibre injury. Sports Med. 12:184–207.

Bernton, E., R. Galloway, and D. Hoover. 1994. Immune function II: Monocyte and granulocyte function. Chapter 10 in Nutritional and Immunological Assessment of Ranger Students with Increased Caloric Intake. Technical Report T95-5. Natick, Mass.: U.S. Army Research Institute of Environmental Medicine.

Bøyum, A., P. Wiik, E. Gustavsson, O.P. Veiby, J. Reseland, A.H. Haugen, and P.K. Opstad. 1996. The effect of strenuous exercise, calorie deficiency and sleep deprivation on white cells, plasma immunoglobulins and cytokines. Scand. J. Immunol. 43:228–235.

Fitzgerald, L. 1988. Exercise and the immune system. Immunol. Today 9:337–339.

Gibson-Berry, K.L., J.C. Whitin, and H.J. Cohen. 1993. Modulation of the respiratory burst in human neutrophils by isoproterenol and dibutyryl cyclic AMP. J. Neuroimmunol. 43:59–68.

Hauger, S.E., and P. Wiik. 1997. Glucocorticoid and ACTH regulation of rat peritoneal phagocyte chemiluminescence and nitric oxide production in culture. Acta Physiol. Scand. 161:93–101.

Hoffman-Goetz, L., and B.K. Pedersen. 1994. Exercise and the immune system: A model of the stress response? Immunol. Today 8:382–387.

Khansari, D.N., A.J. Murgo, and R.E. Faith. 1990. Effects of stress on the immune system. Immunol. Today 11:170–175.

Kiecolt-Glaser, J.K., and R. Glaser. 1991. Stress and immune function in humans. Pp. 849–864 in Psychoneuroimmunology, R. Ader, D.L. Felten, and N. Cohen, eds. Boston: Academic Press.

Kramer, T.R. 1994. Immune function I: Lymphocyte proliferation and subset analysis; Interleukin production. Chapter 9 in Nutritional and Immunological Assessment of Ranger Students with Increased Caloric Intake. Technical Report T95-5. Natick, Mass.: U.S. Army Research Institute of Environmental Medicine.

Øktedalen, O., P.K. Opstad, J. Fahrenkrug, and F. Fonnum. 1984. Plasma concentration of vasoactive intestinal peptide during prolonged physical exercise, calorie supply deficiency and sleep deprivation. Scand. J. Gastroenterol. 19:59–64.

Opstad, P.K., M. Bårtveit, P. Wiik, and A. Bøyum. 1994a. The dynamic response of β_2- and α_2-adrenoceptors in human blood cells to prolonged exhausting exercise, sleep and energy deficiency. Biogenic Amines 10:329–344.

Opstad, P.K., P. Wiik, A.H. Haugen, and K.K. Skrede. 1994b. Adrenaline stimulated cyclic adenosine monophosphate response in leucocytes is reduced after prolonged physical activity combined with sleep and energy deprivation. Eur. J. Appl. Physiol. 69:371–375.

Ottaway, C.A. 1991. Vasoactive intestinal peptide and immune function. Pp. 225–262 in Psychoneuroimmunology, R. Ader, D.L. Felten, and N. Cohen, eds. Boston: Academic Press.

Røshol, H., K.K. Skrede, C.E. Ærø, and P. Wiik. 1995. Dexamethasone and methylprednisolone effect on peritoneal phagocyte chemiluminescence after administration in vivo. Eur. J. Pharmacol. 286:9–17.

Sharp, N.C., and Y. Koutedakis. 1992. Sport and the overtraining syndrome: Immunological aspects. Br. Med. Bull. 48:518–533.

Shippee, R., K. Friedl, T. Kramer, M. Mays, K. Popp, E.W. Askew, B. Fairbrother, R. Hoyt, J. Vogel, L. Marchitelli, P. Frykman, L. Martinez-Lopez, E. Bernton, M. Kramer, R. Tulley, J. Rood, J. DeLany, D. Jezior, and J. Arsenault. 1994. Nutritional and immunological assessment of Ranger students with increased caloric intake. Report No. T95-5. Natick, Mass.: U.S. Army Research Institute of Environmental Medicine.

Tilz, G.P., W. Domej, A. Diez-Ruiz, G. Weiss, R. Brezinschek, H. P. Brezinschek, E. Hüttl, H. Pristautz, H. Wachter, and D. Fuchs. 1993. Increased immune activation during and after physical exercise. Immunobiology 188:194–202.

Wiik, P. 1989. Vasoactive intestinal peptide (VIP) inhibits the respiratory burst in monocytes by a cyclic AMP mediated mechanism. Regul. Pept. 25:187–97.

Wiik, P. 1991. Glucocorticoids upregulate the high affinity receptor for VIP on human mononuclear leucocytes in vitro. Regul. Pept. 35:19–30.

Wiik, P., P.K. Opstad, and A. Bøyum. 1985. Binding of vasoactive intestinal polypeptide (VIP) by human blood monocytes: Demonstration of specific binding sites. Regul. Pept. 12:145–163.

Wiik, P., P.K. Opstad, and A. Bøyum. 1996. Granulocyte chemiluminescence response to serum opsonized particles ex vivo during long-term strenuous exercise, energy, and sleep deprivation in humans. Eur. J. Appl. Physiol. 73:251–258.

Wiik, P., A.H. Haugen, D. Lovhaug, A. Bøyum, and P.K. Opstad. 1989. Effect of VIP on the respiratory burst in human monocytes *ex vivo* during prolonged strain and energy deficiency. Peptides 10:819–823.

Wiik, P., P.K. Opstad, S. Knardahl, and A. Bøyum. 1988. Receptors for vasoactive intestinal peptide (VIP) on human mononuclear luecocytes are upregulated during prolonged strain and energy deficiency. Peptides 9(1):181–186.

Wiik, P., K.K. Skrede, S. Knardahl, A.H. Haugen, C.E. Ærø, P.K. Opstad, and A. Bøyum. 1995. Effect of in vivo corticosterone and acute food deprivation on rat resident peritoneal cell chemiluminescence after activation ex vivo. Acta. Physiol. Scand. 154:407–416.

DISCUSSION

DONNA RYAN: You did not say much about how these Rangers did clinically.

PÅL WIIK: No, I did not. I just mentioned the infections.

DONNA RYAN: Is it a secret?

PÅL WIIK: No, it is not a secret. Of course, when they have not slept for 7 days, they hallucinate. They do not know where they are and what they are doing. They have problems with their balance, they have ataxia, and they have problems focusing. They are really in a bad state at the end of the course.

DONNA RYAN: Were there any problems with infection?

PÅL WIIK: No. As I mentioned, there was a small increase in the frequency of upper-respiratory infections during the weeks of the course, but it was not significant.

RONALD SHIPPEE: One of the reasons we are asked to study Ranger training was that the commander was very concerned about any lasting effects. They want to stress the soldiers, but not hurt them permanently. One aspect of the study was follow-up. The soldiers cannot control their body weight or their fat afterward. Soldiers continue to come up to me after they participate in the studies and complain that they cannot control their body weight. I was wondering whether you see any lasting effects with just this short 7-d stress?

PÅL WIIK: No, I do not think we have found that really. During the month after the training, some of them have hallucinatory flashbacks. They may have them while they are driving their cars so that they have to pull over and wait for the hallucinations to end. It is like an LSD flashback. But there is not, as far as I know, any documented permanent damage to the participants.

RONALD SHIPPEE: With the work I have done, one of the long-term effects that is observed is that because the Ranger trainees are allowed to use tobacco products to help them stay awake, most of the U.S. Rangers keep that habit. It is a big problem; in fact, the Regimental Command has asked us to take a look at it. Do you allow your folks to use tobacco products?

PÅL WIIK: In principle, they should not use tobacco, but some of them do. I must admit that we have a big problem with performing studies of the recovery period. We would love to explore that much more thoroughly than we have had a chance to do. When the soldiers are free, they go home to their families. They do not want to have any restrictions of their lives and their diets, including alcohol. It is very difficult for us to be able to look at this recovery phase both in the short and the long term because trainees are not motivated for it. As I told you, they are volunteers for the scientific part. During the course, it is easy to because they have half an hour of rest before a blood test. After the course, their motivation is gone.

GAIL BUTTERFIELD: I have asked this question of the Americans, and I will ask it of you. What is the justification for Ranger training in terms of real military experience? Are there real circumstances into which the troops are placed that warrant this type of training?

PÅL WIIK: I think that the important thing is that you hope that trainees can learn something from it. When the trainees have been put through this, you want them to remember what happens when they go too far, and you hope that as leaders, they won't take their men that far. You hope that they will permit the men food and sleep, plan their missions well, and not be "Rambos." Sometimes, if you do not remind the trainees how badly they did, their endorphins make them forget it, everything is rosy, they feel that they performed very well, and they feel that everybody should perform as well as they did themselves. So, in a way, they become supermen if you do not show them videos, talk to them afterwards, and have their comrades tell them how badly they behaved. I think that is a very important thing. Because, if you do not do that, there is absolutely no advantage going through a course like this.

GAIL BUTTERFIELD: Do the Ranger training commanders in the United States do that?

KARL FRIEDL: The debriefing?

GAIL BUTTERFIELD: Making the video?

KARL FRIEDL: Not to the extent the Norwegians do. I do not think we have ever tried doing anything like that. It sounds very interesting. They do this intense briefing in which the commanders show the trainees the videos.

GAIL BUTTERFIELD: It sounds like a good idea.

SCOTT MONTAIN: How many people participate in the course at any one time? Can you fail? If you can fail or get tossed out of the course, how many are failing because they cannot follow the rules of the game, in the sense of performing without sleep?

PÅL WIIK: About 60 every year in the military participate in this training course lasting 7 days. We take 10 or 15 or 20 for our studies. They are very well trained and selected before the course. It is in the second year of their education, so fewer than 10 percent fail.

SCOTT MONTAIN: So, if you are one of these people who is hallucinating quite badly, does your buddy just drag you along even though you are totally incoherent so you can pass? Do they slow down to the pace of the weakest man? What do they do?

PÅL WIIK: Well, if you have made the hallucinating person the leader, then you remove him from the leadership position. [Laughter.]
    If you are the leader, then you have a responsibility that is stimulatory to performance. As to your question, the trainees get some individual treatment in order to pass the course and still explore their individual limits.

SCOTT MONTAIN: With the sleep deprivation, if you give them monotonous tasks to do, they cannot do them, but if you give them tasks that are mentally stimulating, they can. So, if you put them into a leadership role, that is stimulating them.

PÅL WIIK: But if you see that an individual has a really bad tolerance for sleep deprivation, he will be told this, but he does not fail. You have to decide what these men will do after the military academy. A soldier with poor tolerance for sleep deprivation will not be able to choose positions where you have to have a decent tolerance for sleep deprivation. This is one of the experiences, or advantages, to derive from the course. You can tell people what they are suited for.

TIM KRAMER: I think, if I recall right from looking at your lymphocyte counts, that you had a U-shaped curve. You had your normal level at the beginning. It decreased. And then, if I am not mistaken, it began going back to baseline at day 7 or so.

PÅL WIIK: Yes, the lymphocyte number was found to be almost normalized on the last day. And in most of our functional studies, we find that on the last day or two there is a pattern of normalization. I always wonder why. After the soldiers have been able to keep up their high intensity training for all this time, they know that this is the last day, and perhaps this will give them a little relief. I had that same thought when you showed your data. I think that this relief can be a reason for this normalization pattern during the last days of training.

TIM KRAMER: That was the reason I brought that up. It is basically taking, I think, what you see in the Ranger I and Ranger II studies where you see a similar pattern but over a much longer period . . .

PÅL WIIK: . . . but it is always in the end.

TIM KRAMER: Yes, that is right. That is why I am wondering if really you are getting into a psychological effect, resulting in this slight increase.
  I guess the other question I have is, if I was reading your numbers right on the number of lymphocytes you had per what I reduced it to, which was microliters, you made the comment that the whole-blood assay system would not work on that. Is that because you do have a decrease? Or do you have an insufficient number of cells to observe any kind of a response?

PÅL WIIK: I think that with this kind of lymphopenia there is an obvious need for correction of the number of cells.

TIM KRAMER: You could do that, but I guess that does not mean you cannot do the assay, but you may want to express the results both ways. Your activity per volume, which would be circulating through your body, but also your activity per cell. Because, from the numbers that I was seeing there, you should get a very, very good level of activity, unless a functional capacity was impaired.

PÅL WIIK: I do not completely agree with you. Doing it both the traditional way and your way would be the best. But, if you do these whole-blood cultures, I would see it as an advantage also to have the ability to correct for lymphocyte numbers. Of course, you get very interesting information from the blood cultures that reflects the hormones, the interleukins, and the functional capacity of the cells in the blood, which we do not do with our method. We get the functional capacity of the cells in a culture medium with fetal bovine serum (in the culture).

TIM KRAMER: So you are really talking about a natural milieu versus an unnatural milieu?

PÅL WIIK: That is right. It is a natural milieu versus a standardized milieu.

JEFF KENNEDY: It brings me back to Gerald Keusch's comment earlier in the day. Your lymphocyte counts went down 80 percent. So 80 percent of your circulating lymphocytes disappeared from the blood. That means you are left with 20 percent of the original lymphocyte level. Now the question I have is, do those lymphocytes that are remaining show a decreased proliferative response; is that indicative of the lymphocyte pool in your body? Are you measuring the 20 percent that are remaining that nobody cares about or is not going to be needed or has not been honed? Or is nonproliferative, which is somehow selected against being very proliferative?

PÅL WIIK: That is a very important question when you are trying to evaluate the immune competence. When we work on peripheral blood cells, and you do not know anything about the rest of the body, and the blood is actually only a transport route for these cells. It is easily accessible so everybody uses it, but of course, we should have all of the other compartments also. Of course, it would be very interesting, for instance, to do some prominent labeling of cells, injecting them and see—trying to estimate how the total pool of these cells are behaving. I have the same feeling as you that for lymphocytes there is a significant reduction. But I do not think the reduction is as big as you estimated, since the sum of CD3, CD4, CD19, and CD16 cells was approximately 120 percent in the beginning and 77 percent towards the end of the course. Because some cells in the beginning appear to have more than one of these determinants and lose these at the end of the course.

DAVID NIEMAN: I have just a quick question on the timing of your samples relative to the last exertion of the trainees. Many of the changes that you were showing on day one are very similar to what we see during the one and a half to 3-h time period immediately following heavy exertion. When did you take those samples?

PÅL WIIK: Blood samples are taken at 8:00 in the morning every day.

DAVID NIEMAN: On day one after they have been exercising at 5:00 a.m. or 6:00 a.m.?

PÅL WIIK: They started in the afternoon the day before. So this first blood sample during the course is taken 12 hours after they started. In that time period, they have been exercising continuously at low impact, approximately 30 percent of maximum work capacity.

DAVID NIEMAN: So when they came at 8:00, what had they been doing for the couple of hours before?

PÅL WIIK: They had been running.

DAVID NIEMAN: What this looks like to me is an acute immune response to heavy exertion.

PÅL WIIK: It looks much like that. But it keeps up for most of the week.

DAVID NIEMAN: That is because they are exercising all of the time.

PÅL WIIK: At low impact, but for a long time.

ARTHUR ANDERSON: I have a question related to the answer to your first question. Would you say that vasoactive peptide intestinal receptors and liposomes were elevated during this stressful time?

PÅL WIIK: Yes, vasoactive intestinal peptide receptors are elevated.

ARTHUR ANDERSON: One of the vasoactive intestinal peptides does attract lymphocytes into the lymphatic tissue. It is not that common or customary attracting of lymphocytes during normal recirculation. The total circulating lymphocyte pool turns over 10 to 48 times in a 24-h period of time. An advanced mass of lymphatic pools is in lymphatic tissue. If you upregulated one of the signals for entering into lymphatic tissue because of this effect of stress, then you would change the rate of entry into lymphatic tissue without perhaps changing the rate of exit from the lymphatic tissue. So this is just a kinetic problem of turnover and not necessarily destruction or marginalization or, in any way, injury to the human body.

PÅL WIIK: I agree with you. But we do not know exactly what is going on.

DAVID NIEMAN: They are still there.

PARTICIPANT: How would you look at that?

PÅL WIIK: Actually, this is a very difficult problem to address, since no good antagonist exists to VIP. However, I personally think that catecholamines and cortisol are much more important.

JOHN FERNSTROM: Am I to suppose that these guys would have an increased susceptibility to disease because of these changes? If so, given all you have done with the guys, why not expose them to a standard cold, if you will, and get the question answered as to whether there is some increased susceptibility to infection, whether it is an upper-respiratory tract infection or some other thing. Because, to me, everybody is talking about this measurement and that measurement, but they are not really trying to make any connection that I can see to the physiology. The changes are dramatic, but I do not see the connection to reality. Maybe a functional-type test would be that additional step.

PÅL WIIK: It sounds logical that perhaps we should expose them to something like that. We have tried to evaluate the frequency of infections during the course. But doing a functional type test would, of course, be an ethical problem.

STEVE GAFFIN: Related to the reduction in IgM and IgA, do you see this as a general turning off of the production of antibodies, and that this is the expected disappearance of IgG, given its half-life? If so, I notice the IgM was still very high, at 60 percent of so. Yet IgM half-life is only a couple of days. So it looks like the body, on the face of it, appears still to be making IgM but maybe has turned off IgA production. Is that what you see? Do you have a different explanation?

PÅL WIIK: I really do not know. But Dr. Nieman told us today that IgA depletes very rapidly.

STEVE GAFFIN: From the nasal lavage.

PÅL WIIK: Yes. You observe a decrease very rapidly for IgM and more rapidly than the half-life.

STEVE GAFFIN: No, it is less rapidly. The half-life, as I recall, is a couple of days. Yet, after a week, you still have very high levels, 60 percent.

PÅL WIIK: But after 12 hours, a reduction of 20 or 30 percent was observed in IgM. If you shut off all of the new production, the primary response to antigens should be at a very low level.

DAVID NIEMAN: This has been found in the blood compartment after ultramarathons and marathons as well, almost the same percentage as you found.

RANJIT CHANDRA: I think that this is probably a reflection of leakage, for example, a huge stress like that and total energy deprivation within 24 hours could cause a leakage of proteins. I think it is a reflection of the size of the immunoglobulins. Those which are relatively smaller would show more leakage.

PÅL WIIK: But it is the opposite.

RANJIT CHANDRA: The IgM is higher.

PÅL WIIK: The IgM was reduced in our data more rapidly than IgG.

LEONARD KAPCALA: I just had a comment on your animal studies where your conclusions with the results of the adrenalectomy were kind of confusing. I would just comment on a couple of variables that may be contributing to that confusing picture, and that is that some cytokine systems may be differentially upregulated, playing a role that you do not know, and also adrenalectomized animals would have very high ACTH levels. ACTH is an immune modulator independent of glucocorticoids. β-endorphin would be high, and that is also an immune modulator. So you have several little variables that you do not know about, and those could then be partially responsible for some of the confusion of the results you are seeing with the adrenalectomy.

BRUCE BISTRIAN: There is a wide range of physiological function between what our daily lives are and what extreme stresses are. Are we really looking at normal variabilities? Unless there is some serious consequence, unless there is some serious [change in] infection rate, or some serious change in the quality of life, or unless there is some serious problem with this, is there any problem? Are we just investigating what is a normal variant when you put a human organism to another range?

PÅL WIIK: It is certain that what we are observing is a physiological response to exercise with no sleep and almost no food for 7 days. And we really have no problem during this period of time. However, if you are trying to make them go through this for a long period of time, you would have problems with immunity and consequently infections are demonstrated for the U.S. Ranger studies.

III

Introduction to Immune Function

Part III presents an overview of the current state of knowledge of immune function and the interaction of nutrition with immune response. Chapter 7 reviews the wealth of recent research that has led to exciting advances in the understanding of interactions among nutrition, immunity, and infection. It is now established that undernutrition is associated with consistent changes in immune responses that include number of T-cells, lymphocyte response to mitogens and antigens, phagocyte function, secretory IgA antibody response, complement activity, and NK cell activity. The nature of cytokines, the so-called hormones of the immune system, is explored in Chapter 8. Their biochemistry and classification, mode of action, and measurement are discussed as well as the potential of cytokines as an additional tool for assessing effects of nutrition and stress interactions.

Nutrition and Immune Function, 1999
Pp. 205–220. Washington, D.C.
National Academy Press

7

Nutrition and Immune Responses: What Do We Know?

Ranjit Kumar Chandra[1]

INTRODUCTION

Twenty-five years ago, the question "What do we know about nutrition and immunity?" could have been answered in a few minutes and written up on a few pages. The mutually aggravating interaction of malnutrition and infection has been known for centuries, but the concept of impaired immune responses mediating this interaction is relatively recent.

Three separate forces have driven the study of the immune system in nutritional deficiencies (Anonymous, 1987; Scrimshaw et al., 1968): (1) epidemiologic data showing an interaction, usually synergistic but sometimes antagonistic, between malnutrition and infection, (2) emerging new concepts and techniques in immunology, and (3) dramatic human interest cases. In the early 1970s, the results of the first systematic comprehensive studies were published (Chandra, 1972; Smythe et al., 1971). In young children with protein-calorie malnutrition, that is, both marasmus and kwashiorkor, alterations in a number of immune responses were shown. These alterations include

---

[1] Ranjit Kumar Chandra, Memorial University of Newfoundland, Janeway Child Health Centre, St. John's, Newfoundland A1A 1R8 Canada

histomorphology of lymphoid tissues, delayed hypersensitivity skin reactions, lymphocyte antibody production, and complement activity. Subsequently, these observations have been extended by experimentation in laboratory animals and in work on human subjects. It is now recognized that nutritional deficiencies are associated with impaired cell-mediated immunity; reduced number of circulating T-lymphocytes, particularly CD4+ helper T-cells and CD3+ CD25+ T-cells that bear the interleukin (IL)-2 receptor; decreased lymphocyte stimulation response to mitogens and antigens; altered production of cytokines; lower secretory IgA antibody response on mucosal surfaces; decreased antibody affinity; and phagocyte dysfunction. Similar alterations in immune responses have been reported with deficiencies of individual nutrients, such as protein, essential fatty acids, vitamin A, vitamin E, pyridoxine, folic acid, zinc, iron, copper, and selenium (Chandra, 1991, 1992a; Meydani and Hayek, 1992).

Today, nutritional immunology forms the basis of semester-long graduate courses, week-long symposia, and expansive monographs. Thus, to provide a complete answer to the question "What do we know about nutrition and immune responses?" is not easy or simple. Instead, a selective review and some recent observations are provided below.

GENERAL CONCEPTS

Several general principles and conclusions on nutrition and immunity can be stated:

• Protein-calorie malnutrition and deficiencies of individual nutrients, even subclinical deficits, are associated with impaired immune responses and altered risk of infection.

• Excessive intake of some nutrients may result in reduced immune responses.

• Dose-response curves should form the basis of recommendations for optimal nutrient intake.

• Immune responses are sensitive and functional indices of nutritional status and can aid in assessing prognosis in medical and surgical patients.

• Several factors other than nutrition can modulate immunocompetence.

• Basic knowledge of nutrition and immune interactions can be utilized to formulate nutritional recommendations and interventions that may reduce illness and improve chances of survival.

IMMUNE RESPONSES IN ALTERED NUTRITIONAL STATUS

Nutrient Deficiencies

Several review articles and monographs have analyzed data on nutrition and immunity (Alexander, 1995; Beisel, 1982, 1992; Bendich and Chandra, 1991; Chandra, 1991, 1992b, 1996; Chandra and Newberne, 1977; Chowdhury and Chandra, 1987; Gershwin et al., 1985; Good and Lorenz, 1992; Keusch et al., 1983; Santos, 1995; Suskind, 1977; Watson, 1984). Malnutrition penetrates many host defense mechanisms (Figure 7-1). For example, the proportion and absolute number of T-cells is reduced, particularly CD4+ helper cells (Figure 7-2), and the CD4+/CD8+ (helper/suppressor T-cell) ratio is decreased. There is reduced production of IL-1 and IL-2, interferon-γ, and tumor necrosis factor. Several antigen-nonspecific defenses also are altered, such as the microbicidal activity of phagocytes, levels of hemolytic complement and components C3 and Factor B, production of mucin, ciliary movement, and lysozyme.

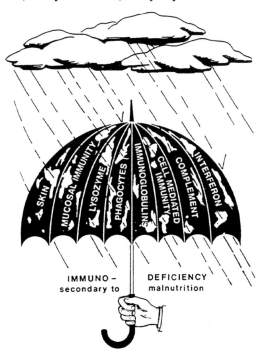

FIGURE 7-1 Immunity in malnutrition. A single view of host defenses as a protective umbrella, consisting of physical barriers (skin, mucous membranes), nonspecific mechanisms (complement, lysozyme, phagocytes), and antigen-specific processes (antibodies, cell-mediated immunity). In protein-energy malnutrition and in deficiencies of various nutrients, many of the host defenses are breached, allowing microbes to invade and produce clinical infection that is more severe and prolonged. SOURCE: Chandra, 1992b. Copyright ARTS Biomedical Publishers, reproduced with permission.

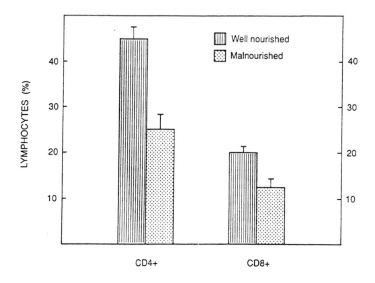

FIGURE 7-2 Proportion of T-lymphocyte subsets in malnourished and well-nourished subjects. There is a marked reduction in CD4+ cells.

Profound changes in immune responses have been observed in micronutrient deficiencies. For example, zinc deficiency results in lymphoid atrophy, impaired delayed cutaneous hypersensitivity, reduced lymphocyte response to mitogens, lower helper/suppressor T-cell ratio, decreased IL-2 production, and most importantly, reduced serum thymulin activity. Copper deficiency reduces the antibody response to T-cell-dependent antigens and impairs phagocyte function (Failla and Bala, 1992). Altered immune responses are readily reversed within weeks or months when nutritional counseling and appropriate supplements are provided; the one exception is the case of intrauterine growth retardation that is associated with prolonged reduction in cell-mediated immunity. In animal models of nutritional deficiency produced before and/or during gestation, the adverse effects on immune responses are observed in the first- and second-generation offspring (Chandra, 1975).

Serum thymulin activity is the prime example of a nutrient-specific immunologic function test that correlates significantly with zinc intake and therefore can serve as a specific functional measure *par excellence* of zinc deficiency. Other immunologic tests that may be used singly or in combination as indicators of nutrition are listed in Table 7-1. The choice will depend upon the clinical and population setting where the study is done (Sarchielli and Chandra, 1991).

TABLE 7-1 Immunologic Tests as Indicators of Nutritional Status

Lymphocyte number (CD3, CD4)
Terminal deoxynucleotidyl transferase activity
Lymphocyte response to mitogens and antigens
Complement C3 and Factor B concentration
Interleukin-2 production
Delayed cutaneous hypersensitivity
Serum Thymulin activity

Nutrient Excesses

If reduced intake of an essential nutrient impairs immunity, this does not imply that large amounts will be beneficial. In fact, there may be a negative impact on immune responses and even infectious morbidity as has been shown for zinc and vitamin A (Chandra, 1984, 1991; Semba et al., 1995). Dose-response curves (Figure 7-3) should be constructed to assess the amount of nutrient intake associated with optimal high immune response.

There is much recent work on lipid modulation of immune responses, and this is reviewed by other authors in this volume (see Kelley, Chapter 14). Briefly, dietary intake of large quantities of fats impairs immune responses. The results of studies are conflicting on the effects of individual dietary fatty acids on various immune responses, such as lymphocyte stimulation in the presence of mitogen. The confounding variables include the amount and degree of unsaturation of fatty acid, age of subjects, species and genetic background of animals, source of mononuclear cells tested, nature and dose of infectious or tumor challenge, and the time and duration of observation (Erickson et al., 1992). Modest amounts of omega-3 fatty acids contained in marine oils reduce inflammatory responses (Endres et al., 1993) and may decrease the severity of autoimmune arthritis, improve survival following endotoxin challenge, and slow the growth of cancer (Fernandes et al., 1992; Venkatraman and Fernandes, 1992). In one study, feeding of flax seed oil rich in α-linolenic acid (18:3n-3) to healthy young adults suppressed the lymphocyte proliferation response to phytohemagglutinin (PHA) and concanavalin A and decreased the delayed hypersensitivity response to seven recall antigens. However, serum concentrations of immunoglobulins, complement C3, C4, salivary IgA, the number of T- and B-cells, and their subsets were not affected (Kelley et al., 1991).

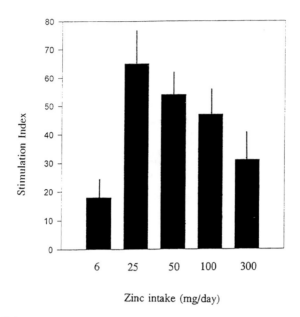

Zinc intake (mg/day)

FIGURE 7-3 Lymphocyte stimulation response to optimal dose of phytohemagglutinin (PHA) in adult men with a range of zinc intakes from dietary and supplemental sources. Results are shown as stimulation index calculated as counts per minute in PHA-stimulated culture divided by counts per minute in unstimulated cultures. Bars represent mean ± standard deviation. There were 6 to 10 subjects in each group.

OTHER FACTORS INFLUENCING IMMUNE RESPONSES

The evaluation of the effects of nutrition on immunity demands an awareness of other confounding variables that also influence immune responses. The prominent factors are listed in Table 7-2. Physical and thermal trauma alters a variety of immune responses; most are decreased, and this change may be beneficial to the host since clones of immunocompetent cells that react against the host are suppressed transiently. Both extreme cold and hot environmental temperatures, which in turn would change the body temperature, impair some immune responses, such as phagocyte function, and can contribute to the increased risk of infections seen at extremes of temperature. Infection itself can suppress immune responses and worsen malnutrition. The prime examples of this are measles and acquired immunodeficiency syndrome. Measles is associated with impaired cell-mediated immunity for 12-16 weeks. Emotional stress, such as bereavement on the part of the elderly (Table 7-3) and fear of scholastic examinations on the part of medical school students, is associated with reductions

TABLE 7-2 Confounding Nonnutritional Factors Influencing Immune Responses

Genetics
Trauma: physical, thermal
Environmental and body temperature
Infection
Emotional stress
Physical activity

in immune responses such as natural killer (NK) cell activity, lymphocyte stimulation response to mitogens, and IL-2 production. Physical activity has an interesting correlation with immune response (Gleeson et al., 1995) and susceptibility to infection. Moderate, graded exercise is associated with enhanced immune responses and decreased incidence of infection, particularly among those groups such as the elderly who show compromised immunity and experience frequent infections (Table 7-4). In contrast, strenuous exercise—both severe and prolonged exercise—reduces immunity and increases the incidence of infection in the short term. Thus, a reverse J-shaped curve best describes the relationship between physical activity and immunocompetence (Figure 7-4).

TABLE 7-3 Immunologic Responses in 11 Elderly Subjects

Immunologic Response	Prebereavement	Postbereavement	P
Lymphocyte stimulation response to PHA*	47 ± 9	23 ± 12	< 0.05
Interleukin-2 production, U/ml	10 ± 2	7 ± 2	< 0.05
Natural killer cell activity, %	43 ± 4	28 ± 7	< 0.01

NOTE: P was calculated by paired Student's t-test. Prebereavement tests were done 1 to 3 months prior to loss of spouse as part of a longitudinal study. Postbereavement assessment was conducted 1 to 2 weeks after loss of spouse. U, units. The data respesent means $\pm$ SD.

* PHA, phytohemagglutinin. Results were expressed as counts per minute in PHA-stimulated culture/counts in unstimulated cultures.

TABLE 7-4 Immunologic Responses in 14 Elderly Subjects Enrolled in an Exercise Program

Immunologic Response	Pre-exercise Period	Post-exercise Period	P
Lymphocyte stimulation response to PHA*	39 ± 8	63 ± 13	< 0.05
Interleukin-2 production, U/ml	7 ± 3	16 ± 2	< 0.01
Natural killer cell activity, %	32 ± 6	49 ± 8	< 0.01

NOTE: P was calculated by paired Student's t-test. After base-line assessment, the subjects were enrolled in a graded program of gentle exercise, consisting of walking and low-impact aerobic activity, ~40 minutes, 4 times a week for a total of 6 months. Blood was withdrawn on a nonexercise day. U, units. The data respesent means ± SD.

* PHA, Phytohemagglutinin. Results were expressed as counts per minute in PHA-stimulated culture/counts in unstimulated cultures.

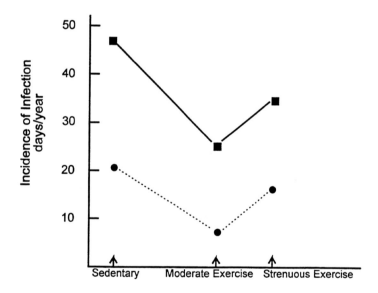

FIGURE 7-4 Schematic relationship among intensity of exercise, immune responses, and incidence of respiratory infection. Strenuous and/or prolonged physical activity lowers immunity, and regular moderate exercise for short periods enhances immunity. ●, young subjects (n=8–12 in each group); ■, elderly subjects (n=8–11 in each group).

NUTRITIONAL SUPPLEMENTS FOR BOOSTING IMMUNITY

In population groups with a high prevalence of nutritional deficiencies, supplementation to prevent or treat specific nutrient deficiency may be expected to decrease morbidity and improve survival. This has been documented for vitamin A, iron, and zinc (Sazawal et al., 1996; Sommer et al., 1986; Vyas and Chandra, 1984), although a few studies have failed to show beneficial results (Arthur et al., 1992; Rahmathullah et al., 1991), and in others, the effect on diarrheal disease was negated by an increase in respiratory illness. The potential significance of the negative effect of massive dosing of single nutrients should be borne in mind. Nevertheless, population-wide efforts to eradicate highly prevalent nutritional deficiencies can have a major impact on immunity and risk of illness and death. A significant correlation between serum retinol levels and long-term morbidity has been observed in infants with respiratory syncytial virus bronchiolitis[2] (Figure 7-5). It should be noted that none of the serum retinol levels were below 20 µg/dl, a threshold commonly accepted to demarcate clinically significant deficiency of vitamin A. Thus, even within the "normal"

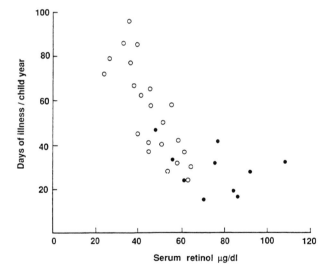

FIGURE 7-5 Relationship between serum retinol concentration and respiratory morbidity in 32 infants with acute bronchiolitis caused by respiratory syncytial virus. Blood was drawn approximately 7 to 10 days after recovery from the acute illness, and the infants were followed monthly for 1 year. Morbidity data were recorded on a questionnaire, completed daily at home and reviewed by the study team every month. Retinol was estimated by high performance liquid chromatography. ●, infants (n=10) receiving multivitamin supplements at home; ○, infants (n=22) who had not been given any multivitamin supplement ($r = 0.87$).

---

[2] Respiratory syncytial virus is the most common cause of lower-respiratory tract infections in infants and children throughout the world and can cause bronchiolitis (inflammation of the bronchioles) or pneumonia.

TABLE 7-5 Immunostimulant Nutrients

Vitamins: vitamin A, β-carotene, vitamin E
Minerals: zinc, selenium
Amino acids: glutamine, arginine

range of retinol values, there was a correlation between nutrient levels and the burden of illness. A limited trial with physiologic amounts of vitamin A—5,600 retinol equivalents once a week for 1 year—was associated with reduced respiratory morbidity (Unpublished data, R. K. Chandra, Memorial University of Newfoundland, Janeway child Health Centre, St. John's, 1994).

Whereas deficiencies of most nutrients impair immune responses, a modest increase in the intake of some micronutrients may be associated with an enhancement of selected immune responses. The principal nutrients for which such evidence exists are listed in Table 7-5. Thus, a feeding regimen that includes an extra amount of some or all of these micronutrients can enhance immunity particularly in individuals with a compromised immune system. This concept has been used successfully to devise feeding formulas with purported immunostimulant properties, for example, IMPACT® (Sandoz) and IMMUN-AID® (McGaw). Both these products contain additional amounts of arguinine, glutamine, omega-3 fatty acids and micro-nutrients. Indeed, rodents fed on these special formulas have higher immune responses and improved survival after challenge with *Listeria monocytogenes* (Chandra et al., 1991, 1992). Limited clinical data such as incidence of wound infections, other postoperative complications, and length of hospital stay support these observations (Bower, 1995). The era of designer feeding cocktails has just dawned.

Another population group in whom nutrient deficiencies are common is the elderly (Chandra, 1991, 1992a; Herbeth et al., 1992; Lesourd et al., 1992; Meydani et al., 1995). As many as 40 percent of elderly have reduced dietary intake and/or low blood levels of one or more nutrients. This is associated with impaired immune responses and a high incidence of infections. In a randomized, double-blind, placebo-controlled study of noninstitutionalized elderly, supplementation with all micronutrients in physiological amounts or modest excess was associated with enhanced cell-mediated immune responses, higher antibody level after immunization with influenza virus vaccine, higher NK cell activity, and increased IL-2 production (Chandra, 1992a). Most importantly, those receiving the micronutrient supplement experienced fewer respiratory infections and therefore were prescribed fewer antibiotics.

CONCLUDING REMARKS

Several exciting advances have contributed to an understanding of interactions among nutrition, immunity, and infection. A new facet of host-parasite interaction includes the possibility of viral mutation with altered virulence brought about by nutrient deficiency. It is now established that undernutrition is associated with consistent changes in immune responses such as the number of T-cells, lymphocyte response to mitogens and antigens, phagocyte function, secretory IgA antibody response, complement activity, NK cell activity, and production of cytokines. Immunocompetence is a sensitive and functional index of nutrition. Nutrient-specific immunological tests, such as thymulin for zinc status, hold promise for estimating optimum intake. The prevention and correction of nutrient deficiencies, even subclinical ones, can reduce the burden of illness and decrease mortality.

REFERENCES

Alexander, J.W. 1995. Specific nutrients and the immune response. Nutrition 11(suppl. 2):229–232.

Anonymous. 1987. This week's Citation Classic. Current Contents 30:15.

Arthur, P., B. Kirkwood, D. Ross, J. Gyapong, A. Tomkins, and A. Hutton. 1992. Impact of vitamin A supplementation on childhood morbidity in northern Ghana. Lancet 339:361–362.

Beisel, W.R. 1982. Single nutrients and immunity. Am. J. Clin. Nutr. 35:417–468.

Beisel, W.R. 1992. History of nutritional immunology. J. Nutr. 122:591–596.

Bendich, A., and R.K. Chandra. 1990. Micronutrients and Immune Functions. New York: New York Academy of Sciences.

Bower, R.H., F.B. Cerra, B. Bershadksy, J.J. Licari, D.B. Hoyt, G.L. Jensen, C.T. Van Buren, M.M. Rothkopf, J.M. Daly and B.R. Adelsberg. 1995. Early enteral administration of a formula (Impact) supplemented with arginine, nucleotides, and fish oil in intensive care unit patients: results of a multicenter, prospective, randomized, clinical trial. Crit. Care Med. 23(3):436–449.

Chandra, R.K. 1972. Immunocompetence in undernutrition. J. Pediatr. 81:1194–1200.

Chandra, R.K. 1975. Antibody formation in the first and second generation offspring of nutritionally deprived rats. Science 19:289–290.

Chandra, R.K. 1984. Excessive intake of zinc impairs immune responses. J. Am. Med. Assoc. 252:1443–1446.

Chandra, R.K. 1991. 1990 McCollum Award lecture. Nutrition and immunity: lessons from the past and new insights into the future. 53(5):1087–101.

Chandra, R.K. 1992a. Effect of vitamin and trace-element supplementation on immune responses and infection in elderly subjects. Lancet 340:1124–1127.

Chandra, R.K. 1992b. Experience of an old traveller and recent observations. Pp. 9–43 in The First INIG Award Lecture: Nutrition and Immunology. St. John's, Newfoundland: ARTS Biomedical Publishers and Distributors.

Chandra, R.K. 1996. Nutrition, immunity and infection: From basic knowledge of dietary manipulation of immune responses to practical application of ameliorating suffering and improving survival. Proc. Natl. Acad. Sci. USA 93:14304–14307.

Chandra, R.K., and P.M. Newberne. 1977. Nutrition, Immunity, and Infection: Mechanisms of Interactions. New York: Plenum.

216   RANJIT KUMAR CHANDRA

Chandra, R.K., M. Baker, S. Whang, and B. Au. 1991. Effect of two feeding formulas on immune responses and mortality in mice challenged with *Listeria monocytogenes*. Immunol. Lett. 27:45–48.

Chandra, R.K., S. Whang, and B. Au. 1992. Enriched feeding formula and immune responses and outcome after *Listeria monocytogenes* challenge in mice. Nutrition 8:426–429.

Chowdhury, B.A., and R.K. Chandra. 1987. Biological and health implications of toxic heavy metal and essential trace element interactions. Prog. Food Nutr. Sci. 11:55–113.

Endres, S., S.N. Meydani, R. Ghorbani, R. Schindler, and C.A. Dinarello. 1993. Dietary supplementation with n-3 fatty acids suppresses interleukin-2 production and mononuclear cell proliferation. J. Leukoc. Biol. 54:599–603.

Erickson, K.L., N.E. Hubbard, and S.D. Sommers. 1992. Dietary fat and immune function. Pp. 81–104 in Nutrition and Immunology, R.K. Chandra, ed. St. John's, Newfoundland: ARTS Biomedical Publishers.

Failla, M., and S. Bala. 1992. Cellular and biochemical functions of copper in immunity. Pp. 129–142 in Nutrition and Immunology, R.K. Chandra, ed. St. John's, Newfoundland: ARTS Biomedical Publishers.

Fernandes, G., J.T. Venkatraman, and N. Mohan. 1992. Effect of omega-3 lipids in delaying the growth of human breast cancer cells in nude mice. Pp. 283–296 in Nutrition and Immunology, R.K. Chandra, ed. St. John's, Newfoundland: ARTS Biomedical Publishers.

Gershwin, M.E., R.S. Beach, and L.S. Hurley. 1985. Nutrition and Immunity. New York: Academic Press.

Gleeson, M., W.A. McDonald, A.W. Cripps, D.B. Pyne, R.L. Clancy, and P.A. Fricker. 1995. The effect on immunity of long-term intensive training in elite swimmers. Clin. Exp. Immunol. 102:210–216.

Good, R.A., and E. Lorenz. 1992. Nutrition and cellular immunity. Int. J. Immunopharmacol. 14:361–366.

Herbeth, B., A. Lemoine, B.P. Zhu, and M. Chavance. 1992. Vitamin status, immunity and infections in the elderly. Pp. 225–237 in Nutrition and Immunology, R.K. Chandra, ed. St. John's, Newfoundland: ARTS Biomedical Publishers.

Kelley, D.S., L.B. Branch, J.E. Love, P.C. Taylor, Y.M. Rivera, and J.M. Iacono. 1991. Dietary α-linolenic acid and immunocompetence in humans. Am. J. Clin. Nutr. 53:40–46.

Keusch, G.T., C.S. Wilson, and S.D. Waksall. 1983. Nutrition, host defenses and the lymphoid system. Arch. Host Def. Mech. 2:275–359.

Lesourd, B.M., R. Moulias, M. Favre-Beffone, and C.H. Rapin. 1992. Nutritional influences on immune responses in the elderly. Pp. 211–224 in Nutrition and Immunology, R.K. Chandra, ed. St. John's, Newfoundland: ARTS Biomedical Publishers.

Meydani, S.N., and M. Hayek. 1992. Vitamin E and the immune response. Pp. 105–128 in Nutrition and Immunology, R.K. Chandra, ed. St. John's, Newfoundland: ARTS Biomedical Publishers.

Meydani, S.N., D. Wu, M.S. Santos, and M.G. Hayek. 1995. Antioxidants and immune response in aged persons. Overview of present evidence. Am. J. Clin. Nutr. 62(suppl.):1462S–1476S.

Rahmathullah, L., B.A. Underwood, R.D. Thulasiraj, and R.C. Milton. 1991. Diarrhoea, respiratory infections and growth are not affected by a weekly low dose vitamin A supplement: A masked controlled field trial in children in Southern India. Am. J. Clin. Nutr. 54:568–577.

Santos, J.I.. 1995. Nutrition, infection, and immunocompetence. Infect. Dis. Clinics North Am. 8:243–267.

Sarchielli, P., and R.K. Chandra. 1991. Immunocompetence methodology. Pp. 425–545 in Nutrition Status Assessment, F. Fidanza, ed. London: Chapman and Hall.

Sazawal, S., R.E. Black, M.K. Bhan, S. Jalla, N. Bhandari, A. Sinha, and S. Majumdar. 1996. Zinc supplementation reduces the incidence of persistent diarrhea and dysentery among low socioeconomic children in India. J. Nutr. 126(2):443–450.

Scrimshaw, N.S., C.E. Taylor, and J.E. Gordon. 1968. Interactions of nutrition and infection. Monograph. Geneva: World Health Organization.

Smythe, P.M., M. Schonland, G.G. Brereton-Stiles, H.M. Coovadia, H.J. Grace, W.E.K. Loening, A. Mafoyne, M.A. Parent, and G.H. Vos. 1971. Thymolymphatic deficiency and depression of cell-mediated immunity in protein-calorie malnutrition. Lancet 2(7731):939–943.

Sommer, A., I. Tarwotjo, E. Djunaedi, K.P. West Jr., A.A. Loeden, R. Tilden, L. Mele. 1986. Impact of vitamin A supplementation on childhood mortality. A randomised controlled community trial. 1(8491):1169–1173.

Suskind, R.M., ed. 1977 Malnutrition and the Immune System. New York: Raven Press.

Venkatraman, J.T., and G. Fernandes. 1992. Mechanisms of delayed autoimmune disease in B/W mice by omega-3 lipids and food restriction. Pp. 309–323 in Nutrition and Immunology, R.K. Chandra, ed. St. John's, Newfoundland: ARTS Biomedical Publishers.

Vyas, D. and R.K. Chandra. 1984. Functional implications of iron deficiency. In Iron Nutrition in Infancy and Childhood, A. Stekel, ed. New York: Raven Press.

Watson, R.R., ed. 1984. Nutrition, Disease Resistance and Immune Functions. New York: Marcel Dekker.

DISCUSSION

RONALD SHIPPEE: That was great, Dr. Chandra. In our human model in the field, we can only look at one compartment or lymphoid system as well as peripheral blood. I often wonder if we are trying to fix something that is not broken. We have already had some comments questioning the Army's interpretation of the PHA stimulation data for peripheral blood lymphocytes. Maybe we are just looking at the effect of margination of blood vascular leukocytes in these soldiers, and maybe it is a protective mechanism, and maybe we should not be in there trying to change it.

RANJIT CHANDRA: I think that Dr. Wilmore certainly addressed this as well: that in the surgical patient or in some of the acute stress patients, sometimes for a short period it is beneficial for the host to turn down immune responses. I think there may be some stressful situations where it is useful to let immune response stay depressed for a period of time. But there are other aspects of immunity which I think need to be brought up to normal. So, once again, I cannot overemphasize that your end point has to be what the biological outcome will be, even if you are looking at low lymphocyte responses to mitogens. If you are seeing no change in infection, then what does it mean?

RONALD SHIPPEE: I worked for 8 years at the Burn Center in San Antonio. Studies employing a burned rat model have demonstrated that if you have a 30 percent scald burn on a rat, the circulating blood [lymphocytes] show a decrease in ConA [concanavalin A]-stimulated proliferation, but proliferation in the draining lymph node and the spleen is actually decreased.

HARRIS LIEBERMAN: Thank you for a wonderful presentation. My question is, you had noted at the beginning of your talk that there appeared to be some association between the progression of AIDS and nutritional status. Can you indicate how strong that association typically has been found to be, and what sort of populations have been studied with that issue in mind, that is, in developed world or third-world kinds of populations?

RANJIT CHANDRA: There are three groups [that are studying the relationship of the progression of AIDS and nutritional status] in three areas of the world that I am aware of. The first group of studies are those originating in the United States—one from the Baltimore area, led by Neil Graham and his group in epidemiology. I have been associated with a couple of those studies. Secondly, there is also a group from Johns Hopkins working in Uganda, working mostly on maternal and maternal-child transmission. I know that Dr. Semba has worked on vitamin A status on maternal child transmission. Then there are studies coming from Florida. Dr. Beach, among others, has shown that the micronutrient levels in the blood correlate with some progression indices. Now, these studies are in an early phase. As you might expect, different studies are coming up with different nutrients that correlate best. Also, I think one earlier study from the Hopkins group suggested some B vitamins as being very important, and lastly, another study from Africa showing that a higher B_{12} level is, in fact, more ominous than a low B_{12} level. So I think we are in an early phase. But there seems to be some indication that there may be a relationship between the progression of AIDS and nutritional status that we need to look at carefully.

MELVIN MATHIAS: I have been very interested in following this literature and making the transition from the deficiency model to a supplemental model. I am not sure that the biochemical mechanism is continuous. You have done a lot of work with zinc in immunity. Is there a transposition from deficiency—that is, is there a change in the biochemical mechanism in the deficient state to the supplemental state?

RANJIT CHANDRA: I think there is. I really appreciate this question because we know very little. For example, we know that zinc deficiency affects several enzymes that are key for protein synthesis and for cellular proliferation, and certain aspects of immune responses. But when you go beyond deficiency to large amounts, other mechanisms come into play. I am thinking of the membrane transport of nutrients. Even calcium transport across the lymphocyte cell membrane is affected by large amounts of zinc. I am looking at stability of lymphocyte membranes. I am looking at the composition of lymphocyte membrane in terms of fatty acid composition, which is affected by zinc intake.

We know, from earlier studies, that even serum levels of fatty acids are affected, which, in turn, might impair or influence immune responses. So you are perfectly correct to say that the mechanisms whereby a zinc deficiency impairs immune responses are probably quite different from mechanisms where very large amounts of zinc may also impair immune response.

DOUGLAS WILMORE: The committee is faced with different types of questions, and I wonder whether you would reflect on them. My view really jives very much with the English church records, that is, malnutrition results in immunological impairment and infection. But what we are faced with are several sorts of objectives. One is to keep the military personnel well nourished before they go into a stress situation. We are asked, can we take those people shortly before they go into a stress situation and give them something, possibly a supplement, to make them superimmune or superresponsive, or superresistant? Then I guess the last thing that we are asked is when soldiers are in the field and in these other stress situations and probably suboptimally nourished, is there some way we can alter nutrient intake in that situation to enhance immunologic response?

We have a fourth concern, and that is, once they are injured or infected how to return them to function, but let's stay away from that for right now. Give us your sense about where we can realistically accomplish some of these goals, sort of along these various pathways.

RANJIT CHANDRA: To my mind, the answers to these questions are yes, yes, and yes. That is, there are things that one can do to optimize nutritional status and, therefore, immunity prior to anybody going into a stressful situation, even with the best optimal military diet. First, I am sure that, if you assess the nutritional status of these individuals going into the Ranger training, not all of them will be at an optimum level in all nutrients. If, for a period of time, be it 2 weeks, or 4 weeks, or 4 months, you can not only assess but optimize their status, it will prepare them for a period of stress, maybe increased utilization and need for nutrients, and, therefore, minimize the decline that will occur, not only in nutritional status but also in functional consequences like immunity.

Secondly, certainly during a stressful period, there could be elements that we can look at which are more important than others in sustaining immune response.

To your last question, there is no doubt, as we have seen in many other scenarios, that once you are depleted, there are certain ways in which you can not only replete nutrient status more rapidly but also replete immune responses. So I think what we need is to fine-tune these "yeses" to identify the nutrients, the amounts, and the period over which such repletion has to take place.

DOUGLAS WILMORE: Those may all be different in different situations.

RANJIT CHANDRA: Certainly.

ROBERT NESHEIM: I think we need to take our coffee break. Actually, I think that those questions you pose are ones that the committee is going to have to deal with in the next couple of days, and hopefully, from an analysis of all of the information we have, we can make some recommendations. That certainly spells out our task.

Nutrition and Immune Function, 1999
Pp. 221–232. Washington, D.C.
National Academy Press

8

Cytokines and Nutritional Status: Possible Correlations and Investigations

Jeffrey L. Rossio[1]

INTRODUCTION

What Are the Cytokines?

The cytokines are a relatively diverse group of low molecular weight (8,000–30,000 daltons) proteins that act to transmit information among the cells involved in immunological responses. On one level, they can be thought of as the "hormones" of the immune system. However, as will be explained shortly, the cytokines can have many important roles including cell activation, effector function (for example, killing of virus-infected cells), immune suppression, and induction of cell differentiation. The main function of the cytokines is to promote, sustain, and terminate an immunological response that is appropriate for the pathogen or other antigen toward which the response is directed. This chapter will give an overview of the cytokine system and the variables to be

---

[1] Jeffrey L. Rossio, AIDS Vaccine Program, National Cancer Institute-Frederick, Cancer Research and Development Center, Frederick, MD 21702

considered when studying the relationships that may exist between the cytokines and nutritional status.

The Nature of the Cytokines

Biochemistry

Almost all cytokines are glycoproteins secreted from a variety of cell types (Casciari et al., 1996). Recombinant cytokines have been expressed in bacterial systems where glycosylation does not occur and seem to have equivalent biological activity, at least vitro. However, the state of glycosylation may have some effect on the stability of cytokines in the circulation, and perhaps on biological half-life. Most cytokines work as monomers, although some exist as homodimers (for example, interleukin [IL]-10), heterodimers (for example, IL-12), and trimers (for example, tumor necrosis factor-alpha [TNF-α]).

Mode of Action

The cytokines act by binding specifically to receptors on the surface of target cells. Most cytokine receptors have been well characterized, and many have been isolated, sequenced, and cloned. Some receptors belong to the immunoglobulin superfamily, that is, they consist of glycoproteins with characteristic intra- and interchain disulfide bonds forming looped structures. Other cytokines use receptors in the 7-transmembrane family, which is known to work through the activation of intracellular G-proteins. Receptor structures vary from single chains to multimers of two or three chains. Also, some receptor peptide chains are shared among receptors for more than one cytokine. In some cases the receptors may be present (at low levels) on resting target cells; when these cells are activated during immune responses, the receptors increase in number. In other cases, receptors appear *de novo* following activation. This is an important characteristic of cytokine regulation.

Principles of Cytokine Action

Janis Kuby, in her textbook, *Immunology* (1994), notes three basic principles that must be taken into account when studying cytokines. First, the cytokine molecules tend to be very pleiotropic. That is, each one has numerous biological functions. At first, the cytokines were described in terms of their functional activities, for example "T-cell growth factor" (now, IL-2). However, when the cytokines were isolated and their amino acid sequences were determined, it was found that many molecules with diverse biological activities were, in fact, the same. So for instance, the molecule called interleukin-1 or IL-1 has at least 50 unique, separate names related to unique, separate biological activities. The "interleukin" nomenclature was, in part, developed to unify all the various names for the cytokines into a coherent system.

A second important principle regarding cytokines is that they are redundant. That is, several unique cytokine molecules have the same biological function. One example is the ability of some cytokines to act as an endogenous pyrogen, to induce fevers. This was a property originally ascribed to IL-1, but later, at least two other cytokines, IL-6 and TNF-α, were shown to have similar activity. This feature makes sense in terms of natural processes, since redundancy ensures that if a problem develops in the production of a single cytokine, the entire immunological process will not become ineffective. However, the redundant nature of cytokines often poses problems in measurement of single cytokines using biological assays. It is important to realize that a single biological effect might be due to several different cytokines.

A third characteristic of cytokine biology is that the cytokines are often synergistic. A single cytokine molecule may not have a strong biological effect, but when it is combined with other cytokines, the effect emerges. It is now known that the cytokines often work in cascading pathways, with one cytokine inducing the production of one or more cytokines so that the effect becomes amplified.

Cytokine Experimentation

Quite a bit is known about the cytokines and how they control immunological reactions. The cytokine system is quite similar in all vertebrates, and models developed in mice and other laboratory animals have been used extensively to dissect the roles of the various regulatory factors. In recent years, the techniques of molecular biology and genetics have allowed the development of transgenic mice that overproduce individual cytokines, as well as gene knockout animals that are unable to produce specific cytokines.

The study of cytokine biology is complicated somewhat by the regulation imposed on *in vivo* cytokine activity. Cytokines are induced during the course of immunological responses, and their measured levels can correlate with the extent and nature of these responses. However, as discussed earlier, the cytokines work by binding to cell surface receptors, and these also are regulated during immunological responses. So, it is necessary to measure not only cytokine production but also the ability of an individual to respond in a given circumstance as a result of appropriate receptor display. Other authors in this volume have noted that during periods of high stress, such as those that occur during Ranger training, a substantial proportion of cells from the trainees had lost many surface markers. If the cytokine receptors are among these markers that are lost, this could explain the lack of proper cytokine regulation of an immune response and increased disease susceptibility in this population. This possibility has not been studied and would be a fruitful area of investigation.

Classification of the Cytokines

Since cytokine biology is so complicated, it is a good idea to try to compartmentalize the various cytokines by function. Joost Oppenheim of the National Cancer Institute's Frederick Cancer Research and Development Center, who is a codiscoverer of two of the cytokines (IL-1 and IL-8), and this author have suggested such a classification scheme, which may make it easier for a nonexpert to understand what to look at when studying cytokine actions (Oppenheim et al., 1993). An outline of the scheme is presented in Table 8-1.

Inflammatory Cytokines

The first group, and one of the most important, includes cytokines that are important in the development of inflammatory responses. There have been many studies of these activities because of the desire to control inflammation. Among the cytokines that fall in this category are IL-1, TNF-α, interferon-gamma (INF-γ), IL-8, and IL-17.

T- and B-Lymphocyte Growth Factors

This group is large and includes many cytokines that control the growth and differentiation of T- and B-lymphocytes, the cells that recognize foreign materials, initiate immunological responses, regulate those responses, and conduct many of the immunological effector activities (cell killing, antibody production, etc.). Cytokines in this group are the T-cell growth enhancers IL-1α, IL-1β, IL-2, IL-4, IL-7, IL-9, and IL-15 and the B-cell growth factors IL-4, IL-6, and IL-14. Note that some cytokines appear in more than one category, which emphasizes the pleiotropic nature of these molecules.

TABLE 8-1 Classification of the Cytokines

Inflammatory cytokines

T- and B-lymphocyte growth factors

Hematopoietic growth and differentiation factors

Chemotactic agents

Inhibitory/regulatory factors

Cytotoxic/cytostatic inducers and effectors

Other factors

A distinction is sometimes made, which has been mentioned by other authors, between cytokines in this group that primarily enhance cell-mediated immune responses (Th1 responses) versus those that promote antibody or B-cell responses (Th2 responses). In mice, it appears that two different populations of helper T-cells produce different profiles of cytokines, but the situation is less clear in humans. At any rate, the Th1 group of cytokines includes IL-2 and IFN-γ, while the Th2 group includes IL-4, IL-5, IL-6, IL-9, IL-10, and IL-13.

Hematopoietic Growth and Differentiation Factors

The first cytokines licensed for clinical use fall in the category of hematopoietic growth and differentiation. These molecules encourage the production of new white blood cells (WBC) from precursor cells in the bone marrow. Whenever WBC are consumed or killed (inflammatory reactions, blood loss, AIDS, chemotherapeutic insult, radiation exposure, etc.), these cytokines can be administered to hasten the recovery of normal cell numbers. Factors to enhance recovery include GM-CSF (granulocyte-macrophage colony-stimulating factor), G-CSF (granulocyte colony-stimulating factor), M-CSF (macrophage/monocyte colony-stimulating factor), SCF (stem cell [activating] factor), IL-3, IL-5, and IL-11.

Chemotactic Agents

A growing family of cytokines acts to attract various types of cells to the site of nascent or ongoing immune or inflammatory responses. These "chemokines" are the newest group of cytokines and include IL-8, RANTES[2], MIP (macrophage inflammatory protein)-1α, and MIP-1β.

Inhibitory/Regulatory Factors

Several cytokines are important in the control of immune responses by limiting the extent of response, for example, by terminating a reaction when the inducing substance has been removed. These include IL-10; IL-13; IFN-α, -β, and -γ; and transforming growth factor (TGF)-β.

Cytotoxic/Cytostatic Inducers and Effectors

Some cytokines have direct or indirect effects resulting in the killing of cells bearing foreign antigens, such as viral-infected cells, cells infected with intracellular parasites, or cancer cells. These include IL-12, TNF-α, and TNF-β.

---

[2] RANTES: Regulated on Activation, Normal T-Cell-Expressed and -Secreted; a chemoattractant and activating factor for T-lymphocytes (mononuclear leukocytes).

Other Growth Factors

The above list is not exhaustive; many other cytokines have been described. Also, the list keeps growing as new factors are described, isolated, and characterized (Aggarwal and Puri, 1995; Callard and Gearing, 1994).

Measurement of Cytokines

Fortunately, the measurement of cytokines is becoming routine in the research laboratory, thanks to the development of sensitive and specific enzyme-linked immunosorbent assays (ELISAs) (Kopp and Holmlund, 1996; Whiteside, 1994). In the past, reliance on assays for the biological activity of cytokines made measurement much more difficult, partly due to the inherent variability of biological systems and partly due to the pleiotropic and redundant activities of the cytokines themselves (Coligan et al., 1994). Several manufacturers offer ELISA capture assay[3] kits with all the required reagents and standards necessary to evaluate cytokines in serum or plasma. In addition, several sources sell matched antibody pairs in bulk, including a capture antibody and a biotinylated secondary antibody. With these reagents, laboratories that are capable of performing internal quality control and standardization functions can save a considerable amount of money when evaluating cytokines.

Sample Types and Preparation

Cytokines are present in trace amounts in serum and plasma under normal circumstances. Fortunately, the current ELISA tests are sensitive to about 5 to 50 picograms of cytokine per ml, which is a useful range. Cytokine can be quantitated equally well in either serum or plasma. Levels of cytokines measured by ELISA are the same in both fluids. The test format (capture assay) eliminates most competitive substances present in these fluids. One important consideration is that the cytokines are not very stable and have short half-lives. Therefore, samples must be collected and tested fresh, or rapidly deep frozen for later evaluation. Freeze-thaw cycles tend to break down the cytokines and must be avoided. Most cytokine activity is stable for up to 8 hours in serum or plasma in a refrigerator. Isolated or purified cytokines (e.g., standards) are far less stable.

---

[3] A capture assay is an immunoassay in which a microtiter plate is first coated with a "capture antibody" (usually polyclonal) to the antigen to be measured; the antigen-containing test solution is then applied, and antigen is captured by (bound to) the capture antibody. The captured antigen is then detected using a secondary antibody (often monoclonal) that is covalently bound to a substance that can be converted to a detectable species (for example, a biotinylated secondary antibody becomes detectable when reacted with enzyme-labelled streptavidin and appropriate substrate.)

Clinical Use of Cytokines

A large number of cytokine clinical trials (Phase I, Phase II and Phase III) are underway in the United States and throughout the world. The indications for such trials are wide-ranging, spanning the spectrum of diseases from cancer, to autoimmune conditions, inflammatory conditions, and infectious diseases due to bacteria, parasites and viruses (cf, Oppenheim et. al., 1993). Since cytokines have such broad regulatory influences on immunological responses, they could theoretically be applied in almost any case where host defenses need to be boosted or suppressed. Unfortunately, our understanding of the full scope of activities of individual cytokines, and of the interactions among the cytokines, is not sufficiently sophisticated to allow trials of mixtures of cytokines; the first trials involve careful observations following the administration of individual cytokines to patients who generally have failed all conventional modes of therapy.

Several general observations may be made concerning these studies. First, as expected, cytokines administered parenterally in large amounts can result in numerous undesirable side effects, since the cytokine concentrations reached in body fluids during these trials far exceed levels normally observed. Major side effects have included fevers, loss of vascular integrity (capillary leakage) with accompanying hemodynamic problems, and flu-like syndromes. Since there are so many cytokines, and their properties and actions differ so greatly, it is difficult to generalize regarding side effects. The clinical approach to cytokine use is still basically an empirical one, and testing of new cytokines must be undertaken only with great caution.

Even so, the use of some cytokines, such as the hematopoietic growth factors, is already routine for some uses (e.g., enhanced recovery of white blood cells following chemotherapy for cancer). Other approved indications will be added in the near future.

Cytokines and Nutrition:
Author's Observations and Recommendations

The inclusion of an independent presentation on the topic of cytokine biology as related to nutritional status represents a major new direction of investigation in both immunology and nutrition. Although some information on cytokine responses to stresses such as exercise or infection is available (and, in fact, is liberally represented in data offered in this volume), there are as yet relatively few published studies (Gallagher and Daly, 1993; Grimble, 1995; Harbige, 1996). It is logical to assume that the cytokines, acting as the hormones of the immune system, would be affected generally by nutritional status in the same way that other physiological systems would be affected. For example, chronic nutritional deficiencies adversely affect the immune response, including reductions in the production and activity of cytokines. However, little information is available concerning whether cytokine deficits would occur gradually as nutritional adequacy becomes limiting, or whether there would be a threshold effect, where cytokines would suddenly cease to be produced at a certain level of nutritional deficit.

Another way to look at the current data is to think about what can be done now, versus what can be done later, after more knowledge is acquired. Mechanisms are important and will need to be understood to get a full picture of the cytokine-nutrition interrelationship. However, considering the current status of knowledge in this area, more data probably need to be collected. "Phenomenology," often used as a pejorative in science, meaning that one is looking for descriptions and not for theory, may be the order of the day; theory will come later.

It is not unlikely that the measurement of cytokines in an acute stress situation will offer some picture of the way the body is responding, especially if the stressors have been shown to impair general health. To date, the cytokines most closely examined have been those in the "inflammatory cytokine" group, since physical stress is well known to result in generalized and specific inflammation in the tissues. Exercise, for example, induces changes in cytokines such as IL-1 (see Nieman, Chapter 17 in this volume).

As monitors of the body's attempts to achieve homeostasis, the cytokines may be good "leading indicators" of future health status. It would be straightforward to design a study to investigate this point, along the lines of existing studies on military trainees reported at this meeting. Malnutrition and problems related to subnormal caloric intake may be evident quite early by using cytokine levels as surrogate markers of health status. Since so little has been done to investigate this possibility, there is strong rationale for measuring many cytokines in a controlled study and then checking to see if a single cytokine or (more likely) a "profile" of cytokine activity is predictive of disease susceptibility and outcome.

Another fruitful line of investigation would be to examine the *in vitro* ability of blood cells from various individuals (for example, military trainees) to respond to stimulators such as antigens (tetanus, influenza, etc.) or mitogens (phytohemagglutinin, concanavalin A) with appropriate cytokine responses. These data could be correlated with the ability of these individuals to cope with stresses such as malnutrition and strenuous physical activity. Perhaps cytokine responsivity can predict which individuals could withstand better the rigors of training, with less chance of infection and disease. This knowledge would be of value in choosing appropriate personnel for specific missions. No data currently exist that address this topic.

In summary, the new area of cytokine biology, in which the so-called hormones of the immune system are monitored in order to assess disease resistance and general health, may be a fruitful area of study. The fact that the cytokines are short-lived, and that their production represents an accurate "snapshot" of current immune status, may prove valuable in assessing both the effects of experimental modification of diet and nutritional factors and interactions between diet and stresses such as exercise or fatigue in terms of impact on health and resistance. However, the field is so new that considerable groundwork needs to be done to assess the feasibility and applicability of cytokine measurement as an adjunct to other tools used to monitor nutrition and health.

REFERENCES

Aggarwal, B.B., and R.K. Puri, eds. 1995. Human Cytokines: Their Role in Disease and Therapy. Cambridge, Mass.: Blackwell Scientific.
Callard, R., and A.J.H. Gearing. 1994. The Cytokine Facts Book. London: Academic Press.
Casciari, J.J., H. Sato, S.K. Durum, J. Fiege, and J.N. Weinstein. 1996. Reference databases of cytokine structure and function. Cancer Chemother. Biol. Response Modif. 16:315–346.
Coligan, J.E., A.M. Kruisbeek, D.H. Margulies, E.M. Shevach, and W. Strober, eds. 1994. Current Protocols in Immunology. New York: John Wiley & Sons.
Gallagher, H.J., and J.M. Daly. 1993. Malnutrition, injury and the host immune response: Nutrient substitution. Curr. Opin. Gen. Surg. 93:92–104.
Grimble, R.F. 1995. Interactions between nutrients and the immune system. Nutr. Health 10:191–200.
Harbige, L.S. 1996. Nutrition and immunity with emphasis on infection and autoimmune disease. Nutr. Health 10:285–312.
Kopp, W.C., and J.T. Holmlund. 1996. Cytokines and immunological monitoring. Cancer Chemother. Biol. Response Modif. 16:189–238.
Kuby, J. 1994. Immunology. New York: W.H. Freeman and Company.
Oppenheim, J.J., J.L. Rossio, and A.J.H. Gearing, eds. 1993. Clinical Applications of Cytokines: Role in Pathogenesis, Diagnosis and Therapy. New York: Oxford University Press.
Whiteside, T.L. 1994. Cytokines and cytokine measurements in a clinical laboratory. Clin. Diagn. Lab. Immunol. 1:257–260.

DISCUSSION

RONALD SHIPPEE: In our field studies, we typically draw blood quite a bit. Could you give us some guidance on handling those samples, how fast we have to get it out of the glass, suggested temperature, and surely regarding shipping samples.

JEFFREY ROSSIO: Cytokines are small proteins, and they are relatively susceptible to proteolysis. They have relatively short half lives.

In order to store cytokines themselves for shipment, if you are specifically looking for plasma cytokines, I think that the samples would have to be frozen fairly quickly. They are stable once frozen.

RONALD SHIPPEE: In getting the cells separated from the plasma, are there guidelines?

JEFFREY ROSSIO: In terms of what things to measure, there are two things we can look at. We can look at the capability of the cells to produce cytokines or we can look at a snapshot of what cytokines are already there.

If you want to deal with the cells the way Tim Kramer is dealing with the cells, then I think it is fairly important to keep the cells in the milieu where they are happy (which is not too cold because cold inhibits the ability of the cells to recover their cytokine production) and to get them to the laboratory as quickly as possible.

We have a lot of experience with shipping samples across the country, and if they are shipped across the country in the winter, even in those insulated Styrofoam Federal Express mailers, the cells lose almost all the biological activity when they get cold.

ARTHUR ANDERSON: We actually have been able to measure two of the signal cytokines like IFN-γ or TNF. The IFN-γ and TNF activity was measured in serum that was shipped from Korea during the Korean War, and after all these years after the Korean War and being stored in a $-70°$ walk-in freezer, we are still able to measure the INF-γ and TNF.

JEFFREY ROSSIO: Had it been stored at $-70°$ since its collection?

ARTHUR ANDERSON: It had been stored at $-70°$ but was shipped in wet ice.

ROBERT NESHEIM: Any other questions or comments?

STEVE GAFFIN: Is it known whether the cytokines pass through the gut wall?

JEFFREY ROSSIO: I don't know. It is known that the gut makes, or the enterocyte makes, IL-4.

STEVE GAFFIN: What about the permeability of the gut wall?

JEFFREY ROSSIO: We don't think they are present in the lumen, but there is little data to address this point.

ARTHUR ANDERSON: We fed cytokines to mice as an adjuvant for an oral vaccine study, and found that fed cytokines will increase immune response in a cytokine-appropriate way. So, you can have both. You can have enterocytes making cytokines and also cytokine absorption present.

JEFFREY ROSSIO: One of the things in my manuscript that I didn't have time to talk about involves the intervention with cytokines; you have to remember that the cytokines are designed to be intercellular messengers.

Most of the cytokines work at very short distances and for very short times. When cytokines are administered in large amounts in an adjuvant-type setting, the side effects of those cytokines are often very severe.

We have a lot of experience with using cytokine therapy in cancer patients, and there are very major problems with administering nonphysiological or large amounts of cytokines, and that is something that will have to be overcome. The delivery problem is something that needs much more study.

GERALD KEUSCH: I am thinking about the complexity of the issue of cytokines in the gut. In model systems using cultured human intestinal epithelial cells in regions where the membrane forms very nice tight junctions, they will make IL-8, but it is almost all at the basal side. IL-8 appears to have a very important physiological effect as a chemokine to attract neutrophils. The neutrophil response actually goes through the monolayer of epithelial cells and will facilitate the transfer of bacteria from the apical side to the luminal side.

In shigellosis, the cytokine cascade including IL-8 and IL-1 in particular, is part of the pathogenesis of the disease. The inflammatory response of those cytokines is essential for creating the disease.

So, we have heard about double-edged swords. Clearly at the level of the gut in intestinal disease, that is one of the critical infectious diseases in the military for fighting capacity. We have got to be very careful about understanding what happens when you put cytokines on the surface or just below the gut surface.

JEFFREY ROSSIO: And depending on cytokine status, the balance of cytokines, especially the Th1-Th2 balance, may affect the outcome of the disease process depending on the pathogen.

There is a lot of study in parasitology looking at leishmaniasis and other types of parasites where the Th1-Th2 cytokine balance, determines the outcome of the disease.

DAVID NIEMAN: In regard to the use, let us say you are measuring total inflammatory cytokines in response to exertion. The lab that we have been working with is trying to get us to send them serum instead of plasma, but it is easier for us to use plasma. Do you have an opinion on which is better?

JEFFREY ROSSIO: We have done a lot of measurements both ways. Plasma is usually easier to get and more available. We haven't had a lot of trouble in measuring cytokines in plasma. So, probably you have to talk to the laboratory and see if they have a problem with standardizing their assays one way, and they don't want to go to the trouble of standardizing them again or not. We haven't found interfering substances.

Now, in some of our studies in cancer patients, we have gone to the extent of doing a double molecular filtration to remove everything with a molecular weight of over 50,000 and everything under a molecular weight of 15,000 or 10,000 with centrifugal filters to see if there were inhibitors around that were affecting our results. The conclusion of that study was that it was not worthwhile to go to the trouble of performing a double molecular filtration.

DAVID NIEMAN: One follow up question. Immediately after heavy exertion when we take a sample and separate the plasma and try to freeze it within 30 minutes, on doing that we find that IL-6 goes up about sixfold. Is there anything you can recommend like deliverance timing for freezing, or is 30 minutes okay?

JEFFREY ROSSIO: I don't know. We usually just recommend as fast as possible. I think 30 minutes is probably okay. When cytokines are present in low concentrations, like any protein in low concentration, they have a tendency to adhere to glass, to adhere to polystyrene. So, we are usually trying to do it as quickly as possible and get it frozen as quickly as possible.

IV

Assessment

Measurement of "immunity" has often focused on measurement of humoral immunity to determine the presence of protective antibodies. Cellular immune function is fundamentally more complex and difficult to measure. Chapter 9 emphasizes the importance of the rationale for undertaking immune assessment to selecting the appropriate assessment method. It also provides a brief description of a variety of *in vivo*, and *in vitro* assessment methodologies. The use of whole-blood cultures for evaluation of functional activity of lymphoid cells *in vitro* is explored in Chapter 10 with an emphasis on the feasibility of their use for field studies.

Nutrition and Immune Function, 1999
Pp. 235–248. Washington, D.C.
National Academy Press

9

Methodological Issues in Assessment of Human Immune Function

Susanna Cunningham-Rundles[1]

INTRODUCTION

Assessment of immune function in the context of studies presented in this volume is based on the underlying premise that *in vitro* or *ex vivo*[2] measurements of immune response during the stress of training reflect the innate status of the immune system and, furthermore, may be interpreted to predict future response. However, the fundamental relationships that are valid in other well-studied settings may be different for two main reasons. First, stress associated with military training conditions does not have an exact parallel with conditions associated with military deployment. Second, a greater or more

---

[1] Susanna Cunningham-Rundles, Immunology Research Laboratory and Department of Pediatrics, The New York Hospital-Cornell University Medical College, New York, NY 10021
[2] *Ex vivo* measurements are those made on cells or tissues that have been sampled (taken) from an experimental subject and placed (in a test tube) under short-term culture conditions.

severe stress reaction does not necessarily predict poorer recovery, and recovery may be the critical parameter for assessing potential response to future stress and long-term health of the immune system.

Factors influencing immune response of the individual to potential environmental pathogens at any single point in time include such interacting host factors as genetic predisposition, general fitness or state of health, previous history of exposure, and nutrient status. Although immunization can be protective against known pathogens (that is, where exposure can be predicted), nutrients may support general improvement of immune function or act as specific cofactors, which suggests that repletion or supplementation could ultimately provide an approach for optimizing immune response.

Evidence is increasing that nutrients are involved specifically with the development of an immune response (Cunningham-Rundles, 1993). Further, current studies suggest that key elements in the diet, for example some trace elements, have a profound influence on immune response even within a period of days (Prasad et al., 1988). Conversely, nutrient deprivation may have long-term consequences, especially when these deprivations are unrecognized and uncorrected (Ohshima et al., 1991).

Development of a rational experimental design for the measurement of general immune function and how this may relate to future immunity is important if the operation of these nutrition-immune function interactions is to be clarified in essentially healthy persons under stress. Quantitative measures of response to a test stimulus may indicate but may not predict response to an unforeseen pathogen. In contrast, the relationship among immunization, subsequent development of serum antibody titer, and protection against encounter with the immunizing pathogen can be more easily quantified and predicted.

The subsequent discussion presents some key elements in the evaluation of immune response. Some of the key questions that must be considered are:

- How is immune function defined?
- What is the setting?
- How is immune function measured?
- Is there change over time?
- Do measures of immune response *in vitro* or *ex vivo* correlate with immune response *in vivo*?
- Can measures of immune response predict future response?

RATIONALE FOR IMMUNE ASSESSMENT

The rationale for undertaking immune assessment is an important consideration in selecting the tests. Immune tests have been developed from several areas of primary research, including susceptibility to and recovery from specific infections, development of vaccines, study of congenitally impaired host defense, investigations into the basis of graft rejection, and the science of blood transfusion (Paxton et al., 1995).

Although the impact of chronic protein calorie deprivation on susceptibility to infection has been well documented, less is known about the impact of acute deprivation. The fundamental premise that nutritional status has a major impact on immune function is soundly based on a wide range of studies indicating that nutritional deprivation, especially chronic deprivation, produces a measurable impairment of immune response that reflects both duration and degree of nutrient deficit (Cunningham-Rundles and Cervia, 1996; Shronts, 1993). For most human studies, the circumstances of nutritional status impairment have been either in the context of (1) pathological disease states associated with altered nutrient intake, altered absorption, or changes in utilization, or (2) increased and unmet special nutrient requirements such as those that occur during childhood development, during aging, or under conditions of inadequate nutrient intake and food scarcity. Although it is generally thought to be relatively rare in this country, malnutrition is frequently associated with immune deficiency and causes significant vulnerability to infections (Chandra, 1993). Taken together, these studies indicate that nutrients are critical cofactors for immune response and suggest that (1) there is a potential benefit from repletion where deficits are found and (2) better long-term nutrient status is associated with better immune response, lowered incidence of infections, and possibly cancer prevention.

The critical questions about immune status in Special Forces troops, however, are how acute nutrient deprivation of the fundamentally healthy person undergoing highly stressful training in preparation for possible defense activities may influence long-term host defense and whether temporary nutritional deficits incurred during training or in combat conditions may produce long-term vulnerability. The studies of nutrient immune interaction in the settings noted above do not provide an adequate blueprint for answering these questions.

The central question of how the stress of military training influences immune response must be posed in the context of relevance to recovery. The immune system responds to challenge via a vast array of interrelated processes, and the healthy person may be made essentially stronger by these encounters if recovery can be supported properly.

The generalized lack of response to immune signals, called *anergy*, may indicate failure of immune response, as is commonly encountered in primary immune deficiency, granulomatous diseases, acute infection, trauma, and cancer. However, simple malnutrition, for example that associated with aging or other conditions where nutrient intake is inadequate, can produce anergy, as measured by loss of the secondary response to recall (memory) antigens in the delayed-type hypersensitivity skin test *in vivo* and *in vitro* (Blot et al., 1993; Peretz et al., 1991; Smythe et al., 1971). Thus, conditions resulting in acquired anergy may be improved with appropriate intervention.

THE IMMUNE SYSTEM

The immune system is an organ system consisting of primary tissues (bone marrow, fetal liver, and thymus) and secondary lymphoid tissues (spleen and lymph nodes). The work of two main immune cell types (Haynes et al., 1990; Paul, 1993) is often used to define immune activity. T-lymphocytes (T-cells) are defined by expression of (1) the T-cell receptor that binds to antigen, and (2) CD3, a surface determinant associated with the T-cell receptor that is essential for activation. T-cells have an array of clonally variable receptors for a large range of antigens, require thymic maturation for normal function, and mediate cellular immunity. B-lymphocytes (B-cells) are identified by surface immunoglobulin (detected by monoclonal antibodies such as CD19, CD20) and, upon appropriate activation, develop into plasma cells secreting specific antibody and thus mediate humoral immunity.

The normal functions of these cells have been defined in situations of pathological absence or loss. Loss of the normal thymus has been found to compromise T-cell function and affect T-dependent B-cell activation. Failure at the bone marrow level has been observed to affect both T-cell and B-cell immune response.

The distinction between specific and nonspecific immune response is an intrinsic feature of immunity that permits differentiation between self and nonself at the cellular level. In general, this is accomplished by the integration of the molecular complex called the major histocompatibility complex (MHC) "self"-antigen system into the antigen recognition phase. Antigen must be processed and presented in the context of self-MHC to be recognized and to lead to the development of immune response. T-cell activation is a highly controlled event. Antigens are recognized by T-cells only after the antigen has been processed and presented on the surface of an antigen-presenting cell, APC, which may be a monocyte, dendritic cell, or B-cell. The antigen is presented as a MHC/peptide combination. The antigen-processing function is carried out by antigen-presenting cells, the best studied of which is the monocyte. This response triggers lymphocyte activation and proliferation and leads to the production of effector cells (natural killer cells, phagocytes, or cytotoxic T-cells) and triggering of B-cells to produce antibody. This kind of immunity, often termed *adaptive immunity*, is retained as "memory" and is typically elicited following immunization or natural infection (Owen and Jenkinson, 1993).

A second fundamental type of immunity can be described as *innate immunity*, as it is not stored as a memory function and is not improved by repeated contact. This immunity is mediated by phagocytic cells, some of which, like the monocyte, can also process and present antigen. Innate immunity is mediated by certain cytokines such as interferons (Cohen, 1994; Germain and Margulies, 1993), which confer nonspecific protection. Natural killer (NK) cells are an integral component of the nonadaptive, innate immune system. Unlike phagocytic cells, NK cells are not functionally developed at birth (Cunningham-Rundles et al., 1993), probably because the key cytokine, interferon-gamma (INF-γ), which is needed for development and maturation of this system, is also downregulated at birth.

This third arm, represented by the NK cell, can be defined as neither B-cell nor exactly T-cell-like, in having neither surface immunoglobulin nor a rearranged T-cell receptor. This cell, once called the "K" cell, "null" cell, or "third population," has eluded conventional classification by cell lineage analysis. Currently, CD56 is considered the most definitive marker of the NK cell (Trinchieri, 1992). However, NK cells are best known as cells that can kill nonspecifically (naturally) viral-infected cells and bacteria and prevent tumor cell metastasis. If activated by a key cytokine, interleukin (IL)-2, NK cells will differentiate into lymphokine-activated killer (LAK) cells (Ortaldo and Longo, 1988). These cells can kill many tumor cell types. The NK cell system is constitutively active and does not have to be primed by antigen to kill. When armed with specific antibody, however, these cells can kill specifically. Functional evaluation of this cell population can be readily achieved using a short-term chromium release assay (known as NK cell cytotoxicity assay and using NK cell-sensitive tumor cell lines as targets) and is a valuable tool in assessing immune response.

Although assessment of all aspects of immunity is not required to implement immune testing, examination of the range of possible changes in a pilot study is advisable so that possible critical interactions are not overlooked.

SELECTION AND DEVELOPMENT OF THE TEST SYSTEM

Measurement of "immunity" has often focused on measurement of humoral immunity to detect the presence of potentially protective antibodies to an infectious agent introduced by natural infection or by immunization. Cellular immune function is fundamentally more complex and less easy to measure. Basic humoral immune tests are usually carried out to measure the specific antibody product of a response formed in the past *in vivo* to a specific virus or microbe. An outline of tests for humoral immunity appears in Figure 9-1.

In contrast, cellular immune assays measure current response *in vitro*, and sometimes *in vivo*, by elicitation of a functional response at the time of the test. An outline of cellular immune tests appears in Figure 9-2.

Human studies have been based on observation of peripheral blood immune cells because the peripheral compartment is most accessible and readily measured, but this approach may not reflect regional events (Cunningham-Rundles, 1994). Knowledge of the differences between systemic and mucosal immune response may ultimately explain many current paradoxes arising when immune response measured *in vitro* or *ex vivo* is compared with host defense *in vivo*.

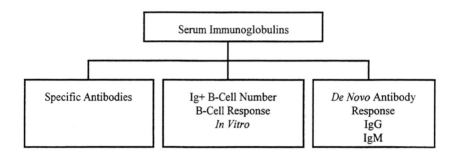

FIGURE 9-1 Evaluation of humoral immune response includes assessment of the general level of serum immunoglobulins and specific antibodies. This reflects previous immunization and serves to assess intrinsic integrity of the B-cell system. In addition, studies may include examination of B-cell response *in vitro* and response to *de novo* immunization that may show differences associated with current, perhaps transient, immune impairment.

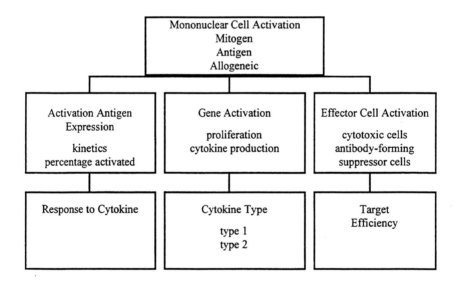

FIGURE 9-2 Evaluation of cellular immune response is characteristically conducted as a three-step process. First, the level of activation is studied using the three basic types of activators: mitogen, antigen, and allogeneic activation. Then the activation pathway is examined for integrity of the process in general terms. Finally, the effector phase is examined for specificity of cytokine production, and response capacity towards key intermediates, the cytokines, and strength of the effector process. All aspects of this process may reflect current immune deficits since response is elicited *in vitro*.

Systemic cellular immune function appears to be regulated through functionally distinct T-helper-type cytokine patterns, such that when T-helper type 1 (Th1) cytokines, IL-2, and INF-γ are produced, cellular immune host defense is favored, and when T-helper type 2 (Th2) cytokines IL-4, IL-5, IL-6, and IL-10 are produced, B-cell response is induced (Barnes et al., 1993; Yamamura et al., 1991).

In contrast to systemic immunity, the primary activity of mucosal immune response is to protect the mucosa by blocking microbial, toxin, and antigen entry; this protection is mediated by secretion and transport of IgA to the lumen of the gut, a process mediated by a special type of memory T-cells with reduced proliferative capacity and capability to promote B-cell activation (Kagnoff, 1993; Marsh and Cummins, 1993).

Recent studies suggest that normal mucosa may downregulate mucosal T-cell reactivity (Qiao et al., 1993). Triggering of these cells, however, can produce an inflammatory response. Although there are few noninvasive methods to evaluate the gastrointestinal immune response, events in this compartment of the immune system may be crucial during response to stress.

In Vivo Assessment of Immune Response

In vivo skin testing and examination of humoral immune response to previously encountered vaccines can be useful in establishing both a baseline response and a response due to the impact of military training.

An issue that frequently must be confronted in immune studies is how to evaluate the potential significance of impaired immune response detected *in vitro* as a reliable reflection of susceptibility to future infection *in vivo*. Studies of even relatively well-defined disorders have shown that there may be very significant differences in the clinical impact of immune deficiency. One way to test this is to undertake a planned immunization, which can be accomplished, for example, by assessing response to a flu vaccine. If proliferative response is measured *in vitro* to the immunizing antigen, both T- and B-cell response can be assessed.

The use of a skin test panel can be an important way to measure delayed-type hypersensitivity *in vivo* (Kniker et al., 1979). Experience with the delayed-type hypersensitivity skin test during previous decades has shown good overall correlation between lack of reactivity, or anergy, and immune deficiency in a variety of settings. The skin test is not very quantifiable. The use of the purified protein derivative (PPD) skin test to assess possible presence of *Mycobacterium tuberculosis* is an exception, although anergic individuals do not respond. In addition, there are false positives with persons who have been vaccinated with BCG (Bacillus Calmette-Guerin[3]).

---

[3] A vaccine used as an adjuvant (immunomodulator) for cancer treatment, as well as for tuberculosis immunization.

Some studies have been based on a *de novo* immunization skin test using dinitrofluorobenzene (DNFB). Although this approach was once used rather extensively, it is no longer considered useful because of ambiguities in the underlying mechanism of reaction, which produces some contact sensitivity, and because of lingering alteration in skin. The introduction of the "skin window"[4] (Black et al., 1988) test may ultimately provide a more quantitative and informative measure of *in vivo* immune response because the reaction can be used to test autologous response, and the types of cells entering the region can be studied.

Despite some reservations (including issues with variable level of response with this test and difficulties in interpretation of negative results), the importance of the skin test as a convincing demonstration that immune defects noted *in vitro* may have prognostic significance *in vivo* should not be underestimated (Kniker et al., 1979). The use of test systems that provide a broad range of test antigens as well as positive and negative controls are particularly recommended.

In Vitro Assessment of Immune Response

Functional studies need to be carried out on fresh anticoagulated blood whenever possible (or blood stored at room temperature in the dark for under 24 hours) before mononuclear cells are isolated. When blood is being sent by air or transported to a distant lab, it is advisable to include a control specimen drawn in parallel from control persons (those not subjected to the military training conditions) to serve as an internal standard for the shipping process.

The question of when the blood should be drawn is important. In general, most data have been obtained with blood drawn in the morning as there are circadian effects that may influence results. When this schedule cannot be followed, it is helpful to continue to maintain a uniformity of drawing time for individual subjects.

Proliferative Response

Since peripheral blood lymphocytes are resting cells (not cycling), the cellular immune reaction must be generated *de novo* in the test system with the introduction of the stimulant; this stimulant must be potentially capable of triggering the response. In addition, the culture system must be capable of supporting the reaction by providing all needed elements, and there must be a measurable end point.

---

[4] The skin window test involves removal of the surface epithelial layer of skin, often from a blister, followed by topical application of an antigen of interest, and subsequent enclosure of the incision within an air-tight space (cell or window).

All of these tests require experience and are best used in the context of defined questions. The establishment of laboratory normal ranges and maintenance of reagent quality control, especially for certain variable elements such as serum, is essential for accuracy and sensitivity of these tests.

The use of whole blood to assess immune response is a valuable approach because it approximates *in vivo* conditions and, further, is often more practical in field conditions. However, use of this system to pinpoint critical interactions appears to require further development.

The choice of stimulant is very important. If the stimulant is "nonspecific" (for example, mitogens that directly trigger response or allogeneic cells that express MHC class II antigens recognized as "foreign"), a relatively large fraction of isolated mononuclear cells from all healthy persons will be capable of reacting in an appropriately designed system. If the test signal is an antigen previously encountered *in vivo*, then a smaller proportion of the cells from the donor will react. This latter type of reaction, the classic delayed-type hypersensitivity type IV reaction (Kirkpatrick, 1988), is a secondary response comparable to a humoral immune response to a "booster" immunization.

Development of Effector Cell Response

The development of an effector response (appearance or activity of effector cells such as NK cells or cytotoxic cells) may be affected or altered by the kinetics of the proliferative response. This may occur because of delayed secondary recruitment during the amplification phase of the response or because of changes in cytokine production. Cytokine patterns are critical for the development of effector activity. Effector functions may be missing or impaired during a stress response. Evaluation of this may require a detailed approach, however, since alterations in subpopulations and kinetics must be considered. Attempts to restore response by cytokine addition may be useful as a means of identifying the lesion.

When suppressor cell mechanisms (actions of specific cell types or cytokines that serve to inhibit the immune response) are suspected, removal of cells by magnetic or flow cytometric approaches may be useful. Monitoring population characteristics in these cases is also critical. Studying the response of subpopulations will also require careful evaluation of normal cells in parallel since, to a large degree, immune response is under negative control.

Assessment of Cell Types by Flow Cytometry

The development of monoclonal antibodies directed against human immune cell surface determinants has provided a more accurate and ultimately quantifiable way to define lymphocyte subpopulations (Lanier et al., 1986; Reinherz and Schlossman, 1980).

Flow cytometry also has the potential to become a major approach to the study of immune function. Certain key cellular events occurring along the T-cell activation-proliferation pathway can be measured directly in a flow cytometer.

As shown in Figure 9-3, several different approaches can be combined in the development of test systems. Although early events, such as the rapid increase in intracellular free calcium that leads to change in pH and in membrane potential, can be measured cytometrically, lack of standardization is a limitation at present. However, increased expression of cell surface molecules, which occurs following lymphocyte activation, is relatively easily measured. For example, after T-cell activation, the first measurable surface marker induced is CD69, which is not expressed on resting T-cells. The kinetics of appearance and decline have been well defined (Lopez-Cabrera et al., 1993). Other cell surface markers appearing on activated T-cells following activation include CD25 (the alpha chain of the IL-2 receptor), CD71, and HLA-DR.[5] Use of these markers as a means of probing critical events in lymphocyte activation provides a new approach to the development of methods that can measure subtle but clinically significant events (Cunningham-Rundles et al., 1990).

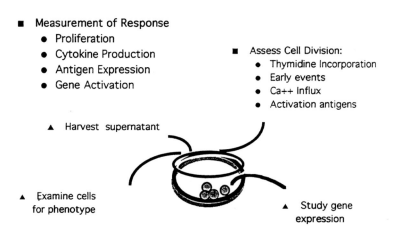

- ■ Measurement of Response
  - Proliferation
  - Cytokine Production
  - Antigen Expression
  - Gene Activation

- ■ Assess Cell Division:
  - Thymidine Incorporation
  - Early events
  - Ca++ Influx
  - Activation antigens

▲ Harvest supernatant

▲ Examine cells for phenotype

▲ Study gene expression

FIGURE 9-3 Measurement of immune response can be performed in microtiter tissue culture plates, typically in triplicate. The figure depicts how parallel studies may be performed under the same culture conditions using the same activator, shown here at the level of the single well, and then be used to follow the consequences of activation through the ensuing stages: (1) early events such as gene activation, (2) activated antigen expression, (3) cytokine production, (4) proliferation (cell division), and (5) effector cell activity.

---

[5] Human leukocyte antigen (comparable to MHC)-DR is one family of class II human histocompatibility gene products. Presence or absence of certain alleles in this genetic region have been associated with altered risk for several chronic diseases.

AUTHOR'S CONCLUSIONS

The central question of how the stress of military training influences immune response must be posed in the context of significance for recovery. The immune system provides response to challenge at several levels. The fundamentally healthy person may become essentially stronger by these encounters if recovery can be supported properly.

The key question involving the immune status of Special Forces troops is how acute nutrient deprivation during training may influence long-term host defense and whether temporary nutritional and immune deficits incurred during training might produce long-term vulnerability. Studies of nutrient-immune interaction in most previous settings are not necessarily relevant to this question. Undertaking a properly organized and implemented study for the purpose of establishing the exact range and nature of changes in immune response that occur during the stress of training is an important first step. As discussed here, it is critical to standardize and quantify an approach that includes several levels of immune response.

Further research is needed to determine how specific immune deficits emerging during emotional and physical stress are influenced by other imposed stressors such as caloric and micronutrient deprivation. Knowledge is also needed about how these stressors may affect the kinetics and the degree of recovery of immune response leading to the support of host defense.

REFERENCES

Barnes, P.F., L. Shuzhuang, J.S. Abrams, E. Wang, M. Yamamura, and R.L. Modlin. 1993. Cytokine production at the site of disease in human tuberculosis. Infect. Immun. 61(8):3482–3489.

Black, M.M., R.E. Zachrau, and R.H. Ashikari. 1988. Skin window reactivity to autologous breast cancer: An index of prognostically significant cell-mediated immunity. Cancer 62:72–83.

Blot,W.J., J.Y. Li, P.R. Taylor, W. Guo, S. Dawsey, G.Q. Wang, C.S. Yang, S.F. Zheng, M. Gail, G.Y. Li, Y. Yu, B. Liu, J. Tangrea, Y. Sun, F. Liu, J.F. Fraumeni Jr., Y.H. Zhang, and B. Li. 1993. Nutrition intervention trials in Linxian, China: Supplementation with specific vitamin/mineral combinations, cancer incidence, and disease specific mortality in the general population. J. Natl. Cancer Inst. 85(18):1483–1491.

Chandra, R.K. 1993. Nutrition and the immune system. Proc. Nutr. Soc. (England) 52(1):77–84.

Cohen, J.J. 1994. Cells involved in host defense: The new immunology. J. Nutr. Immunol. 2(4):73–86.

Cunningham-Rundles, S., ed. 1993. Nutrient Modulation of Immune Response. New York: Marcel Dekker.

Cunningham-Rundles, S. 1994. Malnutrition and gut immune function. Curr. Opin. Gastroenterol. 10: 664–670.

Cunningham-Rundles, S., and J.S. Cervia. 1996. "Malnutrition and host defense" in nutrition. Pp. 295–307 in Pediatrics: Basic Science and Clinical Application, 2d ed., W.A. Walker and J.B. Watkins, eds. Basel, Switzerland: Marcel Dekker.

Cunningham-Rundles, C., C. Chen, J.B. Bussel, C. Blankenship, M.B. Veber, D. Sanders-Laufer, T. Hinds, J.S. Cervia, and P. Edelson. 1993. Human immune development: Implications for congenital HIV infections. Ann. N.Y. Acad. Sci. 693:20–34.

Cunningham-Rundles, S., R.R. Yeger-Arbitman, R. Nachman, S.A. Kaul, and M. Fotino. 1990b. New variant of MHC class II deficiency with interleukin-2 abnormality. Clin. Immunol. Immunopathol. 56:116–123.

Germain, R.N., and D.H. Margulies. 1993. The biochemistry and cell biology of antigen processing and presentation. Ann. Rev. Immunol. 11:403–450.

Haynes, B.F., S.M. Denning, P.T. Le, and K.H. Singer. 1990. Human intrathymic T-cell differentiation. Semin. Immunol. 2:67–77.

Kagnoff, M.F. 1993. Immunology of the intestinal tract. Gastroenterology 105(5):1275–1280.

Kirkpatrick, C.H. 1988. Delayed hypersensitivity. Pp. 261–277 in Immunological Diseases, M. Sampter, D.W. Talmage, M.M. Frank, K.F. Austem, and H.N. Claman, eds. Boston and Toronto: Little, Brown.

Kniker, W.T., C.T. Anderson, and M. Roumiantzeff. 1979. The MULTITESTR system: A standardized approach to evaluation of delayed-type hypersensitivity and cell-mediated immunity. Ann. Allergy 43:73–79.

Lanier, L., J.H. Phillips, J. Hackett Jr., M. Tutt, and V. Kumar. 1986. Natural killer cells: Definition of a cell type rather than a function. J. Immunol. 137: 2735–2739.

Lopez-Cabrera, M., A.G. Santis, E. Fernandez-Ruis, R. Blacher, F. Esch, P. Sanchez-Mateos, and F. Sanchez-Madrid. 1993. Molecular cloning, expression, and chromosomal localization of the human earliest lymphocyte activation antigen AIM/CD69, a new member of the C-type animal lectin superfamily of signal transmitting receptors. J. Exp. Med. 178:537–547.

Marsh, M.N., and A.G. Cummins. 1993. The interactive role of mucosal T-lymphocytes in intestinal growth, development, and enteropathy. J. Gastroenterol. Hepatol. 8:270–278.

Ohshima, T., T. Nakaya, K. Saito, H. Maeda, and T. Nagano. 1991. Child neglect followed by marked thymic involution and fatal systemic pseudomonas infection. Int. J. Legal Med. 104(3):167–171.

Ortaldo, J.R., and D.L. Longo. 1988. Human natural lymphocyte effector cells: Definition, analysis of activity, and clinical effectiveness. J. Natl. Cancer Inst. 80:999–1010.

Owen, M.J., and E. Jenkinson. 1993. Ontogeny of the immune response. Pp. 3–12 in Clinical Aspects of Immunology, P.J. Lachman, D.K. Peters, F.S. Rosen, and M.J. Walport, eds. London: Blackwell Scientific.

Paul, W.E. 1993. Fundamental Immunology, 3d ed. New York: Bauer Press.

Paxton, H., S. Cunningham-Rundles, and M.R.G. O'Gorman. 1995. Laboratory evaluation of the cellular immune system. Pp. 887–912 in Clinical diagnosis and Management by Laboratory Methods, J.B. Henry, ed. Philadelphia: W.B. Saunders and Company.

Peretz, A., J. Neve, J. Duchateau, V. Siderova, K. Huygen, J.P. Famaey, and Y.A. Carpentier. 1991. Effects of selenium supplementation on immune parameters in gut failure patients on home parenteral nutrition. Nutrition 7(3):215–221.

Prasad, A.S., S. Meftah, J. Adballah, J. Kaplan, G.J. Brewer, J.F. Bach, and M. Dardenne. 1988. Serum thymulin in human zinc deficiency. J. Clin. Invest. 82:1202–1210.

Qiao, L., G. Schurmann, F. Autschbach, R. Wallich, and S.C. Meuer. 1993. Human intestinal mucosa alters T-cell reactivities. Gastroenterology 105:814–819.

Reinherz, E.L., and S.F. Schlossman. 1980. The differentiation and function of human T-lymphocytes. Cell 19:821–827.

Shronts, E.P. 1993. Basic concepts of immunology and its application to clinical nutrition. Nutr. Clin. Pract. 8(4):177–183.

Smythe, P.M., M. Schonland, G.G. Brereton-Stiles, H.M. Coovadia, H.J. Grace, W.E.K. Loening, A. Mafoyne, M.A. Parent, and G.H. Vos. 1971. Thymolymphatic deficiency and depression of cell-mediated immunity in protein-calorie malnutrition. Lancet 2:939–943.

Trinchieri, G. 1992. The hematopoietic system and hematopoiesis. Pp. 1–25 in Neoplastic Hematopathology, D.M. Knowles, eds. Baltimore: Williams and Wilkins.

Yamamura, M.K., R.J. Uyemura, K. Deans, T.H. Weinberg, B. Rea, B. Bloom, and R.L. Modlin. 1991. Defining protective responses to pathogens: Cytokine profiles in leprosy lesions. Science 254: 277–279.

DISCUSSION

JOHANNA DWYER: I was wondering, in the slides you presented of the dietary fat and PGE_2 response, what specific fatty acids were in the fat?

SUSANNA CUNNINGHAM-RUNDLES: We do not have that information yet. It has all been done by food recall. But basically what we are going to do in the future in that particular study is provide people with a standardized diet. This was actually done with free-living people. The results were helped by taking out all of the noncompliant people.

JOHANNA DWYER: This must have reduced your sample size.

SUSANNA CUNNINGHAM-RUNDLES: With human subjects, it does not always work out.

ARTHUR ANDERSON: Regarding giving several oxygenase inhibitors to mimic the effect of high-stress training, would that have an effect similar to the dietary change?

SUSANNA CUNNINGHAM-RUNDLES: I think it well might. It would be very interesting to know that. Prostaglandin secretion is not normally activated. Prostaglandin level would be undetected unless we stimulated cells *in vitro*. Clearly, this was a person who probably did have a genuine risk for tumor development. The level of prostaglandin that was documented was very interesting. You do not see that commonly. But, in terms of responsiveness to PHA and the development of prostaglandin, yes, in that setting [of a high-stress training environment] you probably would see a suppression of that. I think it would be interesting to do the study and find out what the effects would be.

STEVE GAFFIN: While the subject is mainly the problem of malnutrition and immunosuppression, among those tests that you have just described, are there any populations of humans in whom overstimulation of the immune system is observed, in whom there is immuno-activation, and through whom we could then search for dietary components to that, apart from genetic factors?

SUSANNA CUNNINGHAM-RUNDLES: This is not easy to do, but I would suggest using a model of chronic viral infections. We do have chronic activation of the immune system in those settings, in the development of cytokines that then eventually produce the loss of lean body mass. There are some good studies. I would very much approve of what Dr. Chandra said, for example, about parallels between HIV-associated malnutrition and protein calorie malnutrition. The problem is that HIV is such a hellish infection that you hesitate to extrapolate from that. But you could look at other chronic viral infections with that kind of evidence. You could look at autoimmune disease. But I personally think that autoimmune disease is a very unusual setting, and you would be on very shaky ground when you tried to apply it because you would have deregulation of the immune mechanisms. I am not sure that that would really apply to a healthy person under stress.

STEVE GAFFIN: I meant healthy people in different populations around the world. Are any of them relatively more resistant to certain infections, which might relate to that?

SUSANNA CUNNINGHAM-RUNDLES: That is true. Generally, however, those things appear to be somewhat more related to genetics. This actually is quite an interesting area to talk about. It is not easily addressed. But different MHC genes do affect response to particular stimulants, basically, most of the stimulants that we encounter. Personally, as a microbiologist, I believe it is all microbes. So I think that our response to microbes is extraordinarily fundamental. I do not know of anything that would exactly fit what you are looking for, though.

MELINDA BECK: We know that a lot of response to infection occurs locally and in the blood. What is your feeling about looking at, say, nasal lavage to study a respiratory infection?

SUSANNA CUNNINGHAM-RUNDLES: I really think that is very excellent and very much on target.

Nutrition and Immune Function, 1999
Pp. 249–262. Washington, D.C.
National Academy Press

10

Application of Whole-Blood Cultures to Field Study Measurements of Cellular Immune Function *In Vitro*

Tim R. Kramer[1]

This chapter describes the use of whole-blood cultures in evaluating the functional activity of blood lymphoid cells *in vitro*, with emphasis on the feasibility of their use in field studies. Results are presented from experiments to establish optimal mitogenic lymphocyte proliferation, interleukin production, and release of interleukin receptors in whole-blood cultures.

BACKGROUND

In vitro measurements of mitogen- and antigen-induced blood lymphocyte proliferation, interleukin production, and release of soluble interleukin receptors are commonly used to determine the functional activity of T-lymphocytes. Such measurements are routine when the volume of blood is abundant, the number of samples is small, and the blood can be processed by an experienced worker in a well-equipped laboratory. They are not routine when a large number of blood samples must be processed on a given day, when blood volume is limited, or

---

[1] Tim R. Kramer, U.S. Department of Agriculture-Agricultural Research Service, Beltsville Human Nutrition Research Center, Phytonutrients Laboratory, Beltsville, MD 20705-2350

when facilities and expertise are limited. Each of these scenarios independently can prohibit the traditional use of density gradient-separated (Bøyum, 1977) peripheral blood mononuclear cells (PBMC) for measurement of T-lymphocyte functions *in vitro*. Preparation of a PBMC suspension requires an abundance of blood and well-trained laboratory workers, and it is time consuming. In an effort to demonstrate various effects on the cellular immune system of humans, several investigators have established the use of whole-blood cultures for measurement *in vitro* of lymphocyte proliferation (Bloemena et al., 1989; Bocchieri et al., 1995; Fletcher et al., 1992; Fritze and Dystant, 1984; Kramer and Burri, 1997; Kramer et al., 1997, in press; Leroux et al., 1985; Zhang et al., 1995) and interleukin production (DeForge and Remick, 1991; DeGroote et al., 1992; Desch et al., 1989; Ellaurie et al., 1991; Elsässer-Beile et al., 1993; Kirchner et al., 1982; Lyte, 1987; Nerad et al., 1992; Oliver et al., 1993). The use of whole-blood cultures offers four advantages: (1) only small amounts of blood are required; (2) many samples can be processed at once; (3) samples contain their own natural milieu of blood components, both cellular and humoral (fluid components of blood); and (4) whole-blood cultures are more cost effective than are cultures containing PBMC.

Using whole-blood cultures has helped to establish associations between suppressed mitogenic proliferative responsiveness of T-lymphocytes *in vitro* and each of the following: marathon running (Eskola et al., 1978), intense treadmill exercise (Nieman et al., 1994), intense military training with reduced caloric intake (Kramer et al., 1997b), certain types of cancer (Fritze and Dystant, 1984), infection with human immunodeficiency virus (Bocchieri et al., 1995; Kramer and Chan, 1994), marginal zinc status (Kramer et al., 1990), and a diet low in carotene (Kramer and Burri, 1997). Whole-blood cultures have also been used to demonstrate the suppressive effects of treatment with oral corticosteroids on production of interferon-gamma (INF-γ) in response to dust mite antigen *in vitro* (Ellaurie et al., 1991), and to monitor the effects of biologic response modifiers on interleukin production by immune cells (Elsässer-Beile et al., 1993).

METHODS AND RESULTS

Blood Donors

Healthy adults donated blood for this series of experiments. Study of the donors was approved by the Institutional Review Board of Johns Hopkins University and by the U.S. Department of Agriculture Human Studies Review Committee. The project was conducted in accord with the Helsinki Declaration of 1975 as revised in 1983.

Blood Collection

Tests of leukocyte function, lymphocyte proliferation, interleukin production, and receptor release were conducted on 12-h fasting blood samples collected in sterile 3-ml VACUTAINER® tubes containing 45 USP units of sodium heparin (Becton Dickinson Co., Rutherford, N.J.). The blood was held at room temperature (20–22°C) until processed. Processing of blood for *in vitro* lymphocyte responses was started within 3 hours after collection.

Lymphocyte Proliferation in Whole-Blood Cultures

Through a series of experiments, the procedure described in Table 10-1 was established as optimal for this laboratory for maximum mitogenic proliferative responsiveness of blood lymphocytes in whole-blood cultures to phytohemagglutinin (PHA).

Amount of Blood per Culture

Maximum mitogenic proliferative responsiveness of lymphocytes to optimal-dose PHA in whole-blood cultures has been reported to occur in round-bottom microculture wells containing 12.5 µl of heparinized blood in a total volume of 200 µl of combined blood plus RPMI-1640 tissue culture medium (Kramer et al., in press). Table 10-2 lists results of a representative experiment to determine the optimal blood volume needed for maximum mitogenic proliferative responsiveness of blood lymphocytes to PHA in whole-blood cultures. As observed previously, cultures containing 12.5 µl of heparinized blood showed the highest mean level of maximum mitogenic proliferative responsiveness of lymphocytes to optimal-dose PHA *in vitro*. This amount of blood per microculture was obtained by the addition of 50 µl of 1:4 diluted blood into each culture well (Steps 1 and 2, Table 10-1). Cultures containing 8.3 and 6.25 µl of blood (blood-to-RPMI-1640 dilutions of 1:24 and 1:32, respectively) showed lower lymphocyte proliferation than did those with 12.5 µl of blood (a 1:16 dilution). Microcultures containing 25 µl of blood were too concentrated (1:8 final dilution) with erythrocytes for proper harvester collection of the whole-blood cultures (data not presented). Microcultures containing 6.25 and 12.5 µl of whole blood showed similar and lower intersubject ($N = 11$) coefficients of variation (CV) in lymphocyte proliferation than did cultures containing 8.3 µl of blood. Building on these results, the following experiments on lymphocyte proliferation were conducted with cultures containing 12.5 µl of heparinized blood.

TABLE 10-1 Mitogenic Proliferative Responsiveness of Lymphocytes in Whole-Blood Cultures[*]

Step	Procedure
1	Place 400 mL heparinized blood into 1200 TL RPMI-1640.[†]
2	Add 50 mL 1:4 diluted blood to each culture well.[‡]
3	Add 50 mL PHA at 1.25-80 μg/ml to each well.[§]
4	Add 100 mL RPMI-1640 to each culture well.[∥]
5	Incubate in 5% CO2, 95% humidified air at 37°C for 96 hours.
6	Add 1 μCi 3H-thymidine to each culture.[#]
7	Harvest cultures onto fiberglass filters.[**]
8	Count 3H-thymidine incorporation by blood lymphocytes.[††]
9	Tabulation of lymphocyte proliferative responsiveness.[‡‡]

[*] According to the method of Kramer et al. (in press).

[†] Dilution prepared in 4.0 ml polystyrene tubes (FALCON®, Becton Dickinson Co., Rutherford, N.J.). The RPMI-1640 contains GlutaMAX-I (GibcoBRL, Grand Island, N.Y.) at 2.0 mmol/liter and penicillin streptomycin at 100,000 U/liter and 100 mg/liter, respectively; referred to herein as RPMI-1640.

[‡] Typically, wells 1 to 12 of two consecutive rows of round-bottom, 96-well tissue culture plates (Corning Glass Works, Corning, N.Y.) prepared per diluted blood sample.

[§] PHA (Sigma Chemical Co., St. Louis, Mo.) added at twofold concentrations to each set of triplicate cultures starting at 1.25 μg/ml. RPMI-1640 alone added to first set of triplicate for unstimulated responsiveness.

[∥] Each culture contains a final volume of 200 μl, with the final blood dilution at 1:16.

[#] At 18 hours before termination of culture incubation.

[**] With a multicell harvester (Skatron Inc., Sterling, Va.).

[††] In a beta liquid scintillation counter (Beckman LS 3801) using a single-label disintegrations per minute (dpm) program with the activity reported in dpm per culture.

[‡‡] The median value of each set of triplicate cultures is chosen as the activity for a given concentration of stimulant. Final presentation of the data is in becquerels (Bq, disintegrations per second) per culture or per lymphocyte, when lymphocyte numbers are available. Depending on the distribution of lymphocyte proliferation data among subjects, values may be transformed (log or square root) to conform with normality assumptions.

TABLE 10-2 Volume of Blood Needed per Culture for Maximum Mitogenic Proliferative Responsiveness of Lymphocytes to PHA

	Blood Quantity (μl)		
	6.25	8.3	12.5
Mean*	3,653	4,302	4,806
SD†	907	1,319	˙1,164
CV‡	25	31	24

* $N = 11$. Maximum lymphocyte proliferative responsiveness (Bq) to PHA at twofold concentrations (starting with the lowest concentration), 1.25–80 μg/ml, 96-h CO_2 incubation, 24-h label with ^{3}H-thymidine.

† Standard deviation.
‡ Intersubject coefficient of variation.

Duration of Incubation of Whole-Blood Cultures

Seventy-two hours of incubation is the standard for evaluating the mitogenic proliferative responsiveness of PBMC to PHA *in vitro*. PBMC cultures for lymphocyte proliferation are free of erythrocytes and isologous (syngeneic) plasma. Because whole-blood cultures contain both of these blood components, a series of experiments was conducted to determine the optimal duration of incubation for maximum mitogenic proliferative responsiveness of

TABLE 10-3 Duration of Incubation for Mitogenic Proliferative Responsiveness of Lymphocytes to PHA in Whole-Blood Cultures

	Duration (hours)				
	72	96	120	144	168
Mean*	1,954	4,501	6,087	4,217	2,120
SD†	510	1,157	1,283	1,272	1,254
CV‡	26	26	21	30	59

* $N = 8$. Lymphocyte proliferative responsiveness (Bq) to PHA at twofold concentrations (starting with the lowest concentration), 2.5–10 μg/ml, 24-h label with ^{3}H-thymidine.
† Standard deviation.
‡ Intersubject coefficient of variation.

lymphocytes to PHA in whole-blood microcultures containing 12.5 μl of heparinized blood. Table 10-3 presents the results of a representative experiment, which indicated that the optimal duration of incubation was 120 hours.

Duration of ^{3}H-Thymidine Label of Whole-Blood Cultures

Estimates of DNA synthesis by mitogen-stimulated lymphocytes are frequently accomplished in microcultures containing 5×10^4 to 2×10^5 PBMC in a 200 μl volume labeled with 0.5 to 1.0 μCi of ^{3}H-thymidine during the final 3 to 24 hours of incubation. Table 10-4 presents the results from a representative study to determine the optimal duration of labeling PHA-stimulated whole-blood cultures with 1.0 μCi (37 KBq)^2 of ^{3}H-thymidine ([methyl-^{3}H], specific activity of 248 GBq [6.7 Ci]/mmol; Dupont NEN Products, Boston, Mass.) for maximum mitogenic proliferative responsiveness of blood lymphocytes cultured for a total of 120 hours *ex vivo*. PHA-stimulated whole-blood cultures labeled with ^{3}H-thymidine during the final 18 hours of the 120-h incubation showed a higher mean ^{3}H-thymidine incorporation than did those labeled for 3, 6, 12, and 24 hours. These cultures and those labeled with ^{3}H-thymidine for only 3 hours showed the lowest intersubject CV.

TABLE 10-4 Duration of ^{3}H-Thymidine Label for Mitogenic Proliferative Responsiveness of Lymphocytes to PHA in Whole-Blood Cultures

	Duration (hours)				
	3	6	12	18	24
Mean*	2,782	4,416	5,504	5,580	5,165
SD†	470	923	1,179	975	1,046
CV‡	17	21	21	17	20

* $N = 8$. Lymphocyte proliferative responsiveness (Bq) to PHA at twofold concentrations (starting with the lowest concentration), 2.5–10 μg/ml, 120-h incubation.
† Standard deviation.
‡ Intersubject coefficient of variation.

---

^{2} One Becquerel (Bq) is equal to 0.027×10^{-9} Curies (Ci) or 1 disintegration per second (dps); thus, 1 Ci equals 3.7×10^{10} dps and 2.2×10^{12} dpm.

Finalized Durations of Cell Culture and ^{3}H-Thymidine Labeling

The results in Table 10-3 showed that 120-h incubation was optimal for maximum lymphocyte proliferation in response to PHA in whole-blood cultures. This differs from the current recommendation of 96 hours (Table 10-1; Kramer et al., in press). Because of the results presented in Tables 10-3 and 10-4, a follow-up experiment was conducted to determine whether maximum mitogenic proliferative responsiveness of lymphocytes to PHA in whole-blood cultures occurs in cultures incubated for 96 or 120 hours and labeled with ^{3}H-thymidine during the final 18 or 24 hours. The results presented in Table 10-5 show that PHA-stimulated whole-blood cultures labeled with ^{3}H-thymidine during the final 18 hours of a 96-h incubation had higher lymphocyte proliferation with lower intersubject CV than did those labeled for 24 hours and those cultured for 120 hours and labeled with ^{3}H-thymidine for 18 and 24 hours.

Data Presentation of Lymphocyte Proliferation in Whole-Blood Cultures

Traditionally, *in vitro* lymphocyte proliferation data are presented as activity for a constant number of PBMCs per culture. Lymphocyte proliferation in whole-blood cultures is most frequently presented as becquerels of ^{3}H-thymidine incorporated per culture, thus, per volume of blood. However, when the number of absolute lymphocytes is known by automated cell count, the proliferative responsiveness also can be presented as activity per

TABLE 10-5 Optimized Duration of Cell Culture Incubation and ^{3}H-Thymidine Labeling for Maximum Proliferative Responsiveness of Lymphocytes to PHA in Whole-Blood Cultures

Hours of ^{3}H-thymidine[*]	Incubation[†]	Mean[‡]	CV[§]
18	96	5,961	13
24	96	5,050	16
18	120	4,815	19
24	120	4,672	23

[*] 1.0 µCi ^{3}H-thymidine.
[†] In 5% CO_2 at 37°C. [‡] $N = 8$. Maximum proliferative responsiveness (Bq) to doses of PHA at twofold concentrations (starting with the lowest concentration), 1.25–80 µg/ml.
§ Intersubject coefficient of variation.

TABLE 10-6 Lymphocyte Proliferative Responsiveness
per Blood Volume and per Cell

Unit	Mean[*]	SD[†]	CV[‡]
Volume	4,368	786	18
Lymphocyte	0.204	0.045	22

[*] $N = 15$. Maximum proliferative responsiveness (Bq).
[†] Standard deviation.
[‡] Intersubject coefficient of variation.

lymphocyte. As illustrated in Table 10-6, higher intersubject variation is routinely found when the proliferative activity is presented as the amount of ^{3}H-thymidine incorporated per blood lymphocyte compared with blood volume. Whenever conditions and facilities permit, hematologic data are collected that allow the results to be presented in both forms: per blood volume and per lymphocyte.

Effects of Holding and Shipping Blood on Whole-Blood Lymphocyte Proliferation

The traditional practice of setting up cell cultures for lymphocyte proliferation within a few hours after blood collection has limited the use of this *in vitro* test in many studies. In efforts to expand the use of *in vitro* lymphocyte proliferation tests in field studies, this laboratory has studied the effects of 24-h holding and shipping of blood on PHA-induced lymphocyte proliferation in whole-blood cultures. In general, holding blood for 24 hours has presented mixed effects. Results presented in Table 10-7 show that holding blood at room

TABLE 10-7 Effects of Holding Blood on Maximum Proliferative Responsiveness of Lymphocytes to PHA in Whole-Blood Cultures

Holding time (hours)	Mean[*]	SD[†]	CV[‡]
~4	4,112	560	14
~29	4,270	802	19

[*] $N = 14$. Maximum proliferative responsiveness (Bq).
[†] Standard deviation.
[‡] Intersubject coefficient of variation.

temperature (22–25°C) for approximately 29 hours after blood collection did not cause a change in mean ($N = 14$) maximum proliferative responsiveness of blood lymphocytes to PHA in whole-blood cultures. There was, however, suppressed activity in cultures from the blood that had been held for 24 hours and stimulated with suboptimal concentrations of PHA for maximum lymphocyte proliferation *in vitro* (data not presented). As presented in Table 10-7, and routinely observed in other unpublished results, holding blood for 24 hours before setup in culture causes an increase in intersubject variation. This laboratory found that heparinized blood held up to 30 hours (total length of time from collection to setup in incubation) after collection at temperatures of 11 to 25°C (including time/temperature during air shipment) shows 0 to ±10 percent change in mean ($N = 15$) maximum proliferative responsiveness (unpublished data).

Cytokine Production and Receptor Release *In Vitro*

Table 10-8 shows the procedure currently used to measure release of tumor necrosis factor-alpha (TNF-α), INF-γ, interleukin-10 (IL-10), and the release of soluble receptor for IL-2 (sIL-2R) in response to PHA in whole-blood cultures. The procedure is based on the results presented in Table 10–9, using PHA as the

TABLE 10-8 Cytokine Production and Release of sIL-2R

Step	Procedure
1	Place 200 mL heparinized blood into 2 sterile tubes.[*]
2	Add 200 mL RPMI-1640 to the control-culture.[†]
3	Add 200 mL RPMI-1640 with PHA to test-culture.[†‡]
4	Incubate in 5% CO_2 at 37°C for designated time.[§]
5	Centrifuge culture tubes.[∥]
6	Collect supernatants and store at –70°C until analyzed.[#]

[*] 4.0 ml polystyrene tubes (FALCON®, Becton Dickinson Co.). One tube serves as the unstimulated control; the other is the stimulated-test culture.

[†] Total volume, 400 mL; final blood dilution, 1:2.

[‡] PHA at appropriate concentration for designated cytokine test culture; suggested concentrations presented in Table 10-9.

[§] Suggested times presented in Table 10-9.

[∥] 10 min at $1,000 \times g$ in 10°C.

[#] Measured according to directions of ELISA kit for each cytokine or receptor.

stimulant. The use of other stimulants, especially specific antigens, will require changes in incubation time for production of the various cytokines and for the release of sIL-2R. Using the procedure outlined in Table 10-8, from 2.5 ml of heparinized whole-blood, cultures are prepared for the measurement of TNF-α, INF-γ, and IL-10 and the release of sIL-2R. This is in addition to preparation of 48 microcultures for lymphocyte proliferation *in vitro*, as described in Table 10-1.

Concentration of Stimulant per Culture

Based on results of preliminary experiments (data not presented), the durations of incubation and concentrations of PHA listed in Table 10-9 are chosen to determine the amounts of PHA stimulant needed per whole-blood culture, according to the procedure presented in Table 10-8, for optimal production of TNF-α, INF-γ, and IL-10 and for release of sIL-2R. The mean concentration of TNF-α was high in whole-blood cultures stimulated with 48 μg of PHA per culture for 24 hours (Table 10-9). The mean concentrations of INF-γ, IL-10, and sIL-2R were higher in whole-blood cultures stimulated with 16 μg than in those stimulated with 32 μg of PHA per culture. It is encouraging

TABLE 10-9 Dose-Response Cytokine Production and Release of Soluble Interleukin Receptor

Cytokine/Receptor	Hours	μg PHA[*]	Mean[†]	SD[‡]	CV[§]
TNF-α[I] (pg/ml)	24	48	7,019	1,364	19
INF-γ[#] (pg/ml)	48	16	14,195	7,959	56
	48	32	11,496	5,996	52
IL-10[**] (pg/ml)	96	16	8,967	3,607	40
	96	32	7,061	2,423	34
sIL-2R[††] (U/ml)	96	16	4,774	1,032	22
	96	32	4,206	833	20

[*] Concentration per culture (value × 2.5 = μg/ml).
[†] $N = 13$.
[‡] Standard deviation.
[§] Intersubject coefficient of variation.
[I] Tumor necrosis factor-α (Medgenix Diagnostics, Belgium).
[#] Interferon-γ (Endogen, Inc., Cambridge, Mass.).
[**] Interleukin-10 (Endogen, Inc., Cambridge, Mass.).
[††] Soluble interleukin-2 receptor (T-Cell Diagnostics/Endogen, Inc., Cambridge, Mass.).

that the intersubject CV for TNF-α and sIL-2R was similar to that for PHA-stimulated lymphocyte proliferation per blood volume placed in culture within 6 hours after collection (Tables 10-6 and 10-8). However, it is of concern that intersubject variation is so high for supernatants evaluated for INF-γ and IL-10 content. Studies are currently under way to determine whether the variation can be reduced, even as cytokine production is maintained.

AUTHOR'S CONCLUSION

As an alternative to the traditional use of PBMCs to determine the functional activity of blood lymphocytes *in vitro*, the use of whole-blood cultures presents several advantages: they require less blood, less laboratory work time, and less worker expertise, and thus they are more cost effective than are cultures of PBMCs. The use of whole-blood cultures is well established for measurement of lymphocyte proliferation. Less established is their use in the study of interleukins. This area, however, is currently receiving increased attention. The feasibility of conducting cost-effective cellular immunity tests *in vitro* is greatly increased by the use of whole-blood cultures in conjunction with overnight shipment of fresh blood to central laboratories for delayed processing or for study in remote field laboratories in partnership with a central laboratory.

REFERENCES

Bloemena, E., M.T.L. Roos, J.L.A.M. Van Heijst, J.M.J.J. Vossen, and P.T.A. Schellekens. 1989. Whole-blood lymphocyte cultures. J. Immunol. Meth. 122:161–167.

Bocchieri, M.H., M.A. Talle, L.M. Maltese, I.R. Ragucci, C.C. Hwang, and G. Goldstein. 1995. Whole blood culture for measuring mitogen induced T-cell proliferation provides superior correlations with disease state and T-cell phenotype in asymptomatic HIV-infected subjects. J. Immunol. Meth. 181:233–243.

Bøyum, A. 1977. Separation of lymphocytes, lymphocyte subgroups and monocytes: A review. Lymphology 10:71–76.

DeForge, L.E., and D.G. Remick. 1991. Kinetics of TNF, IL-6, and IL-8 gene expression in LPS-stimulated human whole blood. Biochem. Biophys. Res. Commun. 174:18–24.

De Groote, D., P.F. Zangerle, Y. Gevaert, M.F. Fassotte, Y. Beguin, F. Noizat-Pirenne, I. Pirenne, R. Gathy, M. Lopez, I. Dehart, D. Igot, M. Baudrihaye, D. Delacroix, and P. Franchimont. 1992. Direct stimulation of cytokines (IL-1J, TNF-I, IL-6, IL-2, IFN-K and GM-CSF) in whole blood. I. Comparison with isolated PBMC stimulation. Cytokine 4:239–248.

Desch, C.E., N.L. Kovach, W. Present, C. Broyles, and J.M. Harlan. 1989. Production of human tumor necrosis factor from whole blood ex vivo. Lymphokine Res. 8:141–146.

Ellaurie, M., S.L. Yost, and D.L. Rosenstreich. 1991. A simplified human whole blood assay for measurement of dust mite-specific gamma interferon production in vitro. Ann. Allergy 66:143–147.

Elsässer-Beile, U., S. von Kleist, A. Lindenthal, R. Birken, H. Gallati, and J.S. Mönting. 1993. Cytokine production in whole blood cell cultures of patients undergoing therapy with biological response modifiers or 5-fluorouracil. Cancer Immunol. Immunother. 37:169–174.

Eskola, J., O. Ruuskanen, E. Soppi, M.K. Viljanen, M. Järvinen, H. Toivonen, and K. Kouvalmnen. 1978. Effect of sport stress on lymphocyte transformation and antibody formation. Clin. Exp. Immunol. 32:339–345.

Fletcher, M.A., N. Klimas, R. Morgan, and G. Gjerset. 1992. Lymphocyte proliferation. Pp. 213–219 in Manual of Clinical Laboratory Immunology, 4th ed., N.R. Rose, E. Conway DeMacario, J.L. Fahey, H. Friedman, and G.M. Penn, eds. Washington, D.C.: American Society for Microbiology.

Fritze, D., and P. Dystant. 1984. Detection of impaired mitogen responses in autologous whole blood of cancer patients using an optimized method of lymphocyte stimulation. Immunol. Lett. 8:243–247.

Kirchner, H., C. Kleinicke, and W. Digel. 1982. A whole-blood technique for testing production of human interferon by leukocytes. J. Immunol. Meth. 48:213–219.

Kramer, T.R., and B.J. Burri. 1997. Modulated mitogenic proliferative responsiveness of lymphocytes in whole-blood cultures by low carotene diet and mixed-carotenoid supplementation of women. Am. J. Clin. Nutr. 65:871–875.

Kramer, T.R., and M.M. Chan. 1994. Use of whole-blood cultures to monitor mitogenic responsiveness (MR) of lymphocytes in HIV+ children. FASEB J. 8:A494.

Kramer, T.R., R.J. Moore, R.L. Shippee, K.E. Friedl, L. Martinez-Lopez, M.M. Chan, and E.W. Askew. 1997. Effects of food restriction in military training on T-lymphocyte responses. Int. J. Sports Med. 18 (suppl. 1):S84–S90.

Kramer, T.R., K. Praputpittaya, Y. Yuttabootr, R. Singkamani, and M. Trakultivakorn. 1990. The relationship between plasma zinc and cellular immunity to *Candida albicans* in young females of northern Thailand. Ann. N.Y. Acad. Sci. 587:300–302.

Kramer, T.R., M.P. Howard, and J. Chittams. In Press. Mitogen-induced T-lymphocyte proliferation in whole-blood cultures: Optimization based on activity and variation. J. Nutr. Immunol.

Leroux, M., L. Schindler, R. Braun, H.W. Doerr, H.P. Geisen, and H. Kirchner. 1985. A whole-blood lymphoproliferative assay for measuring cellular immunity against herpes viruses. J. Immunol. Meth. 79:251–262.

Lyte, M. 1987. Generation and measurement of interleukin-1, interleukin-2, and mitogen levels in small volumes of whole blood. J. Clin. Lab. Anal. 1:83–88.

Nerad, J.L., J.K. Griffiths, J.W.M. Van der Meer, S. Endres, D.D. Poutsiaka, G.T. Keusch, M. Bennish, M.A. Salam, C.A. Dinarello, and J.G. Cannon. 1992. Interleukin 1J (IL-1J), IL-1 receptor antagonist, and TNF-α production in whole blood. J. Leukoc. Biol. 52:687–692.

Nieman, D.C., A.R. Miller, D.A. Henson, B.J. Warren, G. Gusewitch, R.L. Johnson, J.M. Davis, D.E. Butterworth, J.L. Herring, and S.L. Nehlsen-Cannarella. 1994. Effect of high- versus moderate-intensity exercise on lymphocyte subpopulations and proliferative response. Int. J. Sports Med. 15:199–206.

Oliver J.C., L.A. Bland, C.W. Oettinger, M.J. Arduino, S. K. McAllister, S.M. Aguero, and M.S. Favero. 1993. Cytokine kinetics in an *in vitro* whole blood model following an endotoxin challenge. Lymphokine Cytokine Res. 12:115–120.

Zhang, Y.H., T.R. Kramer, P.R. Taylor, J.Y. Li, W.J. Blot, C.C. Brown, W. Guo, S.M. Dawsey, and B. Li. 1995. Possible immunologic involvement of antioxidants in cancer prevention. Am. J. Clin. Nutr. 62(suppl.):1477S–1482S.

DISCUSSION

RONALD SHIPPEE: Do you supplement the whole-blood cultures with fetal bovine serum?

TIM KRAMER: No. We had found that the addition of fetal bovine serum to whole-blood cultures decreased the mitogenic responsiveness of lymphocytes to phytohemagglutinin.

SYDNE CARLSON-NEWBERRY: What is the number of peripheral blood lymphocytes needed to reliably measure the proliferative responsiveness of lymphocytes in whole-blood cultures?

TIM KRAMER: We have not done a definitive study to determine the minimal absolute lymphocyte number needed for reliable lymphocyte proliferation results in whole-blood cultures. However, in collaboration with Dr. Maria M. Chan of Children's National Hospital in Washington, D.C., children being treated for bone marrow transplantation failed to show functional lymphocyte proliferation.

JEFFREY ROSSIO: I think the issue of logistics in shipping blood overnight is very important. We have found that shipping blood when the temperature is very cold can be suppressive on the functional capacity of the blood.

TIM KRAMER: I agree. We have found suppressed lymphocyte proliferation when the blood had been held overnight at near freezing or at 39°C.

SEYMOUR REICHLIN: There are many places where immune function can be regulated in stress. You could have marginations so that part of the cell population of interest does not even appear in the blood anymore, and is stuck to the walls of the endothelium. That is a catecholamine-mediated function. You can have changes in the population of cells being synthesized in the thymus and spleen. You can have transient changes in glucocorticoids, growth hormone, and prolactin, all of which can change the activity of the cells at the time that they are exposed to this level of hormone when one takes a sample from a stressed individual; so, that was really my question. You are diluting the blood so that the steroid levels have been reduced. You are diluting the blood so that the growth hormone and prolactin levels have been reduced. You are only measuring the functions of the cells that appear in the blood, not the ones that are stuck in the tissues somewhere. I think that is the question. That is especially true in acute stress situations. If you look at the literature on short-term stress, for example, one-day stresses, [academic] examinations, as with the work of the Glasers at Ohio State, all of that is very short-term stuff and might not even be reflected in these kinds of studies.

TIM KRAMER: I can totally relate to your concern about that. Except for probably the skin test response, the whole- blood culture system is probably the closest that we can get to what is going on in the body. This is one of the reasons that we have been interested in it, because it keeps the milieu constant.

V

Nutrition

A variety of nutrients have been identified as having direct effects on both humoral and cellular immune responses. Chapters 11 through 16 each present recent information on the role of specific individual nutrients in the immunity response.

Glutamine, the subject of Chapter 11, is a nonessential amino acid that comprises approximately 60 percent of the free amino acid pool in skeletal muscle. It is thought that major illnesses such as injury, burns, and/or other disease states associated with significant inflammatory response initiate an increased glutamine requirement. Studies in bone marrow transplant patients and postoperative patients support the concept that glutamine is a specific growth factor for lymphocytes.

In Chapter 12, the author provides a brief review of vitamin A deficiency as a nutritionally acquired immunodeficiency disorder that primarily affects infants, preschool children, and pregnant and lactating women. Healthy adult men and women are at low risk of deficiency except under conditions of chronic infection or prolonged dietary deprivation.

Recent advances on the immune function response to interventions with vitamins E and/or C are described in Chapter 13. By virtue of their role as antioxidants, these two nutrients have increasingly been applied to clinical situations including aging, cancer, AIDS, asthma, and exercise. Most studies show that vitamin E can improve the immune response during aging, but results have been variable in other situations.

In Chapter 14, the author provides a detailed review of research on the effects of intake of total fat and individual fatty acids on immune response. There are complex interactions between total fat intake, fat composition, ratios of individual fatty acids, duration of feeding, antioxidant nutrient status, and age and health status of the subjects which make it difficult to determine the net effect of fats on immune response. Different indices of immune response respond differently to changes in fat intake. Current recommendations of the American Heart Association of only 30 percent of energy from fat, with 10 percent of energy each from saturated, monounsaturated and polyunsaturated fatty acids will improve immune response in most individuals.

The controversy that has developed in recent years over the relationship between iron nutritional status and susceptibility to infection, mediated by the effects of iron on the host and the pathogen is explored in Chapter 15. The evidence reviewed suggests that iron deficiency provides little nonspecific protection against infections and that iron overload stimulates growth of a very limited number of pathogens, but results in real damage of the immune system. The author believes there are no convincing data that show oral iron supplements for repletion of stores and treatment of iron-deficiency anemia have any adverse impact on response to infectious disease.

A number of studies that have examined the effects of trace elements on immune function are reviewed in Chapter 16. Most of these are important as they demonstrate which immune parameters are sensitive to specific nutrients. However, they are limited in that most do not correlate immune dysfunction with an actual increase in illness. The author's own research with selenium indicates that host nutrition not only affects the host immune response, but also affects the pathogen. Host nutrient deficiency may cause the pathogen to mutate to a more virulent form.

Nutrition and Immune Function, 1999
Pp. 265–278. Washington, D.C.
National Academy Press

11

Glutamine

Douglas W. Wilmore[1]

INTRODUCTION

In humans, glutamine has traditionally been thought of as a nonessential amino acid probably because of its abundance within the body's various amino acid pools. Almost all human cells contain the enzyme glutamine synthetase, which can, under appropriate conditions, produce glutamine. However, it recently has been postulated that during catabolism, the tissue demands for glutamine exceed the endogenous production of this amino acid, resulting in a state of glutamine deficiency (Lacey and Wilmore, 1990). It is thought that major illness such as injury, burns (Gore and Jahoor, 1994; Parry-Billings et al., 1990), infection (Shabert and Wilmore, 1996), and/or other disease states associated with a significant inflammatory response initiate this increased glutamine requirement. Exogenous glutamine may be helpful during these conditions to restore an adequate supply of this important nutrient.

Glutamine provides a ready source of energy through its conversion to citric acid cycle intermediates and the generation of ATP. It serves as a major substrate involved in the intraorgan transport of nitrogen and is highly efficient

---

[1] Douglas W. Wilmore, Department of Surgery, Brigham and Women's Hospital, Boston, MA 02115

because it contains two nitrogen moieties. It is important in the generation of purines and pyrimidines necessary for DNA biosynthesis (Martin, 1985) and serves as a precursor in some tissues for metabolically generated bases (Welbourne, 1995) (that is, endogenously synthesized purines and pyrmedines; those not from dietary sources) and glycoproteins. Glutamine is also a regulator (or co-regulator) of cell proliferation (Kandil et al., 1995), the generation of heat-shock proteins[2] (Ehrenfried et al., 1995), and the expression of certain cell surface receptors (Spittler et al., 1995). It is not known if some of these specific activities involve direct or indirect genetic regulatory mechanisms.

Glutamine may also be rate limiting for the synthesis of glutathione, one of the most important intracellular antioxidants. Studies show that in the presence of cysteine, the provision of glutamine will enhance glutathione stores and reduce oxidant damage (Hong et al., 1992).

This chapter reviews the pertinent clinical studies that suggest an association between glutamine and the immune defenses of the body.

PHYSIOLOGIC BIOCHEMISTRY

Although almost all tissues contain the enzymes for glutamine synthesis, most glutamine is synthesized in skeletal muscle and brain, and these are the major organs that export glutamine. Liver, however, has the capacity to both consume and produce glutamine, depending on a variety of controlling factors. Because of the large mass of skeletal muscle, most glutamine comes from this tissue and is exported via the bloodstream to visceral organs (Souba et al., 1985). Under normal conditions, glutamine is maintained in high concentrations within the skeletal muscle free amino acid pool. Excluding taurine, glutamine represents about 60 percent of the free amino acids in skeletal muscle and maintains an intracellular concentration of about 20 mmol/Liter intracellular water. With normal plasma concentrations ranging from 600 to 650 μmol/Liter, this large concentration gradient (about 30:1) favors rapid transfer of a large quantity of glutamine from this intracellular store into the bloodstream (Muhlbacher et al., 1984). Because skeletal muscle intracellular glutamine concentrations fall with starvation and the stress of illness, muscle biopsy followed by analysis of intracellular glutamine concentration has been used as a marker of nutritional status in depleted patients and may even be predictive of a fatal outcome (Roth et al., 1982). Other studies have demonstrated that the skeletal muscle intracellular concentration of glutamine is related to the rate of protein synthesis in skeletal muscle (Jepson et al., 1988; MacLennan et al., 1987). Finally, the exogenous administration (supplementation) of glutamine (by addition to total parenteral nutrition [TPN]) attenuates the usual fall in

---

[2] Heat-shock proteins are a class of proteins whose synthesis is stimulated by thermal temperatures (greater than normal growth temperatures) and other stressors. These proteins are believed to play an essential role in adaptation and protection of cells from damage.

skeletal muscle intracellular concentrations following stress (Hammarqvist et al., 1989) and improves net synthesis of skeletal muscle protein.

During catabolic states, elaboration (synthesis and secretion) of a variety of stress hormones, including glucocorticoids, occurs; this latter steroid has been shown to induce the expression of glutamine synthetase in skeletal muscle (Hickson et al., 1996) and thus initiate *de novo* glutamine synthesis and enhanced skeletal muscle glutamine production and release into the bloodstream. In normal humans in the postabsorptive state, approximately 40 percent of plasma glutamine is thought to be derived from other amino acids, and an additional 45 percent originates from its direct release from tissue protein (Perriello et al., 1995). The remainder of glutamine comes from the conversion of glucose and glutamate to glutamine. Studies have not yet been performed in stressed individuals to determine the relative contribution of various disease states to the accelerated rate of glutamine production during stress, but data from animal models (Muhlbacher et al., 1984) suggest that all pathways are accelerated to enhance glutamine production during catabolic states.

The glutamine produced by skeletal muscle is transported via the bloodstream and taken up by various visceral organs (Souba et al., 1985). The distribution of blood glutamine is concentration dependent but also relies on membrane transporters that are distributed throughout the various visceral tissues. These transporters are regulated by a variety of metabolic factors that modify the rate of glutamine transported into the cell (Fischer et al., 1995). During stress states, organs compete for glutamine, and a hierarchy of priorities is established among tissues to determine glutamine uptake and subsequent utilization. Organs or tissues such as liver, gastrointestinal mucosa, kidney, and immunological tissue are the major consumers of glutamine. As blood concentrations fall, cell transport along with blood flow to specific organs become the rate-limiting factors that determine cell uptake and subsequent utilization. These regulating events and the intraorgan competition for glutamine have major impact on cell protection, proliferation, and function.

Glutamine is consumed by the kidney to aid acid-base homeostasis; as the amide nitrogen is cleaved, it joins with a H+ (hydrogen ion/proton) to excrete NH4+ (ammonium) in the urine; simultaneously, a bicarbonate group (HCO_3-) is released into the bloodstream (Pitts et al., 1972). Tissues like the enterocytes (Windmueller, 1982), colonocytes (Ardawi and Newsholme, 1985), lymphocytes, and macrophages (Parry-Billings et al., 1990) utilize glutamine as a primary fuel, but glutamine also serves as a molecule that supports the proliferative response (Kandil et al., 1995). Finally, the liver utilizes this amino acid in a host of metabolic functions, depending on the requirements of the body. Glutamine plays an active role in gluconeogenesis, and recently it has been demonstrated (Perriello et al., 1995) that in postabsorptive individuals, glutamine, not alanine or lactate, is the predominant precursor for the transfer of new carbon to the glucose pool. Because glutamine is such an efficient molecule for the shuttling of nitrogen throughout the body, it serves as a major nitrogen donor for the hepatic synthesis of amino acids and/or hepatic proteins. Efficient pathways also exist for excess glutamine nitrogen to be converted to urea, which is then excreted from the body. Finally, glutamine is extracted by the liver from the bloodstream and used for the synthesis of glutathione (Welbourne et al., 1993).

GLUTAMINE AND IMMUNE FUNCTION

In the 1950s, it was realized that glutamine was an essential nutrient *in vitro* necessary for the growth of some bacteria and almost all cultured cells. Eagle and coworkers (1956) reported that both mouse fibroblasts and HeLa cells died in culture unless the media was supplemented with glutamine. When this amino acid was added to the culture media, cell proliferation occurred in a dose-responsive manner with increasing concentrations of glutamine. Ardawi and Newsholme (1983) studied lymphocytes harvested from rat mesenteric lymph nodes to determine the influence of glutamine on cell function. Glutamine addition caused a fourfold increase in [3H] thymidine incorporation, a marker of cell proliferation. This effect was not observed when glutamine was substituted by other amino acids or by ammonia.

Glutamine uptake in these and other experiments far exceeded the requirements for oxidative metabolism of the cells studied. In proliferative cells, glutamine yields such compounds as ammonia, glutamate, aspartate, and lactate, a process termed glutaminolysis (McKeehan, 1982; Newsholme et al., 1988a, b). This pathway makes available essential precursors—ammonia, glutamine, and aspartate—for purine and pyrimidine biosynthesis. Glutamine also provides the nitrogen for the formation of glucosamine, guanosine triphosphate (GTP) and nicotinamide adenine dinucleotide (NAD), all important substances necessary for normal cell function.

A variety of *in vitro* experiments have demonstrated the importance of glutamine in maintaining or improving immunological function. Parry-Billings et al. (1990) demonstrated that glutamine was necessary for the proliferative response of lymphocytes. In addition, a dose-response relationship was found between *in vitro* glutamine concentration and the rate of phagocytosis achieved by mouse macrophages.

Others have isolated neutrophils from burn patients and studied the ability of these cells to kill *Staphylococcus aureus* in the presence or absence of glutamine. Glutamine enhanced bactericidal function in normal neutrophils and generally restored this function to normal levels in neutrophils taken from burn patients (Ogle et al., 1994). Others have demonstrated that glutamine plays a supportive role in the generation of lymphokine-activated killer cells (LAK cells), which are also important for effective host defense (Juretic et al., 1994). Finally, *in vitro* studies demonstrated an important role for glutamine in the upregulation and/or maintenance of specific cell surface antigens of human monocytes, which may be important in the host response to infection (Roth et al., 1982).

Glutamine has also been administered to patient populations to evaluate the effect of this amino acid on clinical outcome, specifically the impact of supplementing this amino acid on infection. Ziegler et al. (1992) studied 45 adult patients receiving allogeneic bone marrow transplant for hematologic malignancies. After a week of intensive chemotherapy and total body radiation, parenteral nutrition was initiated the day after bone marrow transplantation. Patients were randomized to receive glutamine-supplemented (0.57 g/kg/d) or standard (glutamine-free) isonitrogenous, isocaloric, intravenous, nutritional formulas for the next 3 to 4 weeks, when oral intake was resumed.

MacBurney and coworkers (1994) found that hospital stays were shorter in the patients receiving glutamine supplementation (29 vs. 36 days, $p = 0.017$), and this was primarily due to the reduction in clinical infection (three compared with nine in the control group, $p = 0.041$). The incidence of bacterial contamination was also significantly reduced. This resulted in a cost savings to the hospital of about $10,700 per patient, plus the revenues gained from the increased bed availability.

Ziegler and coworkers (1994) also evaluated circulating white blood cells in the glutamine-treated and control bone marrow transplant patients. Lymphocytes were isolated and subjected to flow cytometry using monoclonal antibodies. The glutamine-treated subjects demonstrated a significant increase in total lymphocytes, CD3, CD4, and CD8 cells when compared with the patients receiving standard therapy. These data are consistent with a more rapid recovery in lymphocytes of the patients receiving glutamine.

Two other trials have been performed in similar populations. One demonstrated a decreased length of stay in the treatment group, but retrospective analysis did not identify a relationship between glutamine administration and reduced infection rate (Schloerb and Amare, 1993). The other trial was performed in Europe using a glutamine dipeptide (Van Zaanen et al., 1994). Patient selection and treatment protocols varied from the initial reported studies. These findings showed no difference between groups, although the glutamine administered was only about two-thirds the amount given in the other two studies.

A final study has evaluated the effect of glutamine-supplemented parenteral nutrition solutions on the immunological effects following an elective operation (O'Riordain et al., 1994). Patients were randomized to receive postoperative standard or glutamine-supplemented TPN. After 5 days of infusion, T-cell DNA synthesis was increased in the glutamine-supplemented group but did not change in the control group. Other outcome variables were not evaluated in this study.

These data, when taken together, suggest that the *in vitro* proliferative response mediated by glutamine can be translated to whole body experiments. Studies in bone marrow transplant patients and postoperative patients support the concept that glutamine is a specific growth factor for lymphocytes. Whether these effects can be universally translated to all critically ill individuals is not known; to date the populations studied are highly specific and results are dependent on the dose and duration of glutamine administered.

GLUTAMINE AND THE GASTROINTESTINAL TRACT

The gut is another important target organ for glutamine metabolism, and the maintenance of normal function of this organ may be invaluable to host defense against intestinal flora and/or their by-products. Animal studies demonstrate that a variety of stresses—starvation, infection, injury—result in the increased movement of bacteria from the bowel lumen to local and regional lymph nodes (Deitch et al., 1989). This process, termed *bacterial translocation*, is well characterized in animals, particularly rodents. It is not known if this process occurs in normal bowel in humans sustaining a similar stress. However, a second process also occurs in the intestinal tract of stressed animals, and this change has clearly been demonstrated in humans. This process involves changes in the permeability of the small bowel to small intraluminal molecules that enter the body during various diseases. Channels exist between the enterocytes, and the entrances to these pericellular pathways are highly regulated and energy dependent. During hypoperfusion, hypoxia, malnutrition, or injury, these pathways become more permeable to luminal molecules that would otherwise be excluded from the body. This enhanced intestinal permeability is well documented in patients with burns (Deitch, 1990), infection (Ziegler et al., 1988), and inflammatory bowel disease (Hollander et al., 1986) and raises the possibility that endotoxin, or other bacterial factors that are found in the intestinal lumen, may gain entrance to the body during these disease states. Thus, strategies that will maintain bowel mucosal vitality and barrier function also may contribute to the enhanced immune defenses of patients.

Glutamine is able to enhance mucosal growth and improve gut barrier function during certain situations. Windmueller (1982) demonstrated that glutamine provided a major portion of the energy required by the enterocytes, and Ardawi and Newsholme (1985) showed similar effects in colonocytes. Rhoads and colleagues demonstrated that glutamine activates a variety of early response genes, essential to the proliferative response of the enterocyte (Kandil et al., 1995). In addition, glutamine enhances the effect of growth factors on enterocyte DNA synthesis (Jacobs et al., 1988) and stimulates ornithine decarboxylase activity in a dose- and time-dependent manner. This latter enzyme regulates the rate-limiting step in polyamine biosynthesis, which is critical for intestinal cell generation and repair.

When glutamine was added to parenteral nutrition solutions and administered to animals as their sole nutrient source, the villus atrophy that is ordinarily associated with intravenous nutrition was greatly attenuated (O'Dwyer et al., 1989). Similar support of villus growth has been observed by van der Hulst and coworkers (1993) in humans. Patients requiring preoperative intravenous feedings were randomized into two groups, one receiving glutamine-supplemented and the other receiving standard (glutamine-free) parenteral nutrition. Intestinal biopsies were taken before and at the end of the parenteral infusions, and tests of intestinal permeability also were performed. After 2 weeks of parenteral glutamine, villus height was unaltered in the glutamine-supplemented group, and it decreased significantly in the group receiving standard parenteral feedings. In addition, the patients receiving glutamine had no changes in intestinal permeability, whereas permeability increased in the group receiving glutamine-free nutrition.

Other studies in humans have demonstrated improvement in bowel function with glutamine administration. For example, when oral glutamine was administered to a small group of patients with Crohn's disease, body weight increased and bowel permeability significantly improved (Zoli et al., 1995). Glutamine administration to premature infants enhanced their ability to take full enteral feeds, compared with a nonsupplemented control group (Lacey et al., 1996). Finally, glutamine administered to patients in an intensive care unit enhanced absorption from the gastrointestinal tract when compared to that of patients receiving glutamine-free intravenous solutions (Tremel et al., 1994).

Taken together, these studies demonstrate that glutamine enhances normal structure and function of the gastrointestinal tract in humans. Additional trials are under way to evaluate the effect of administering this amino acid to populations at risk for infectious diarrhea and those with known bowel disorders.

AUTHOR'S DISCUSSION AND CONCLUSIONS

Glutamine serves many important functions in the body that may be beneficial and support the host's immunologic defenses. For example, glutamine supports skeletal muscle protein synthesis and also enhances bicarbonate production, which may neutralize the acid load that is generated by moderate to severe exercise or catabolism (Welbourne, 1995). Glutamine also supports glutathione biosynthesis, and this antioxidant attenuates tissue damage associated with free-radical production. Over the past several years, glutamine has been studied in several groups of critically ill patients, for whom a specific effect may not be able to be identified, but the multiple effects of this amino acid may benefit the individual patient. For example, Griffiths et al. (1997) randomly divided 84 intensive care patients who were admitted to their unit into two groups: one group received glutamine supplementation (25 g) and the second received standard glutamine-free feedings. The groups were well matched in terms of their general characteristics and received similar quantities of calories and protein. Mortality was significantly greater at 6 months in the patients receiving standard therapy when compared with the glutamine group (67% vs. 43%). Although the pattern of early deaths was similar, length of stay and increased late mortality were observed in the group receiving standard therapy. It is not known how glutamine supplementation prevented these later deaths. Effects could occur via enhanced immunologic function, improved repair of bowel mucosa associated with augmented absorptive and barrier function, enhanced skeletal muscle function, augmented acid-base homeostasis, or improved antioxidant activity. Whatever the mechanism, glutamine appears to serve an essential function in selected patient groups.

Because of the favorable cost-benefit ratio of this amino acid, other populations are currently being evaluated in an effort to improve outcome and quality of life with glutamine supplementation. Over the next several years, data should be forthcoming to direct the use of this therapy to specific groups of highly responsive individuals.

REFERENCES

Ardawi, M.S.M., and E.A. Newsholme. 1983. Glutamine metabolism in lymphocytes of the rat. Biochem. J. 212:835–842.

Ardawi, M.S.M., and E.A. Newsholme. 1985. Fuel utilization in colonocytes of the rat. Biochem. J. 231:713–719.

Deitch, E.A. 1990. Intestinal permeability is increased in burn patients shortly after injury. Surgery 107:411–416.

Deitch, E.A., J. Wintertron, M.A. Li, and R. Berg. 1989. The gut is a portal of entry for bacteremia. Ann. Surg. 205:681–690.

Eagle, H., V.L. Oyama, M. Levy, C.L. Horton, and R. Fleischman. 1956. The growth response of mammalian cells in tissue culture to L-glutamine and L-glutamic acid. J. Biol. Chem. 218:607–616.

Ehrenfried, J.A., J. Chen, J. Li, and B.M. Evers. 1995. Glutamine-mediated regulation of heat shock protein expression in intestinal cells. Surgery 118:352–357.

Fischer, C.P., B.P. Bode, S.F. Abcouwer, G.C. Lukaszewicz, and W.W. Souba. 1995. Hepatic uptake of glutamine and other amino acids during infection and inflammation [editorial]. Shock 3:315–322.

Gore, D.C., and F. Jahoor. 1994. Glutamine kinetics in burn patients. Arch. Surg. 129:1318–1323.

Griffiths, R.D., C. Jones, and T.E. Palmer. 1997. Six month outcome of critically ill patients given glutamine-supplemental parenteral nutrition. Nutrition 13:295–302

Hammarqvist, F., J. Wernerman, R. Ali, A. von der Decken, and E. Vinnars. 1989. Addition of glutamine to total parenteral nutrition after elective abdominal surgery spares free glutamine in muscle, counteracts the fall in muscle protein synthesis, and improves nitrogen balance. Ann. Surg. 209:455–461.

Hickson, R.C., L.E. Wegrzyn, D.F. Osborne, and I.E. Karl. 1996. Glutamine interferes with glutamine-induced expression of glutamine synthetase in skeletal muscle. Am. J. Physiol. 270:E912–E917.

Hollander, D., C.M. Vadheim, E. Brettholz, G.M. Petterson, T. Delahunty, and J.I. Rotter. 1986. Increased intestinal permeability in patients with Crohn's disease and their relatives. Ann. Int. Med. 105:883–885.

Hong, R.W., J.D. Rounds, W.S. Helton, M.K. Robinson, and D.W. Wilmore. 1992. Glutamine preserves liver glutathione after lethal hepatic injury. Ann. Surg. 215:114–119.

Jacobs, D.O., D.A. Evans, K. Mealy, S.T. O'Dwyer, R.J. Smith, and D.W. Wilmore. 1988. Combined effects of glutamine and epidermal growth factor on the rat intestine. Surgery 104:358–364.

Jepson, M.M., P.C. Bates, P. Broadbent, J.M. Pell, and D.J. Millward. 1988. Relationship between glutamine concentration and protein synthesis in rat skeletal muscle. Am. J. Physiol. 255:E166–E172.

Juretic, A., G.C. Spagnoli, H. Hörig, R. Babst, K. von Bremen, F. Harder, and M. Heberer. 1994. Glutamine requirements in the generation of lymphokine-activated killer cells. Clin. Nutr. 13:42–49.

Kandil, H.M., R.A. Argenzio, W. Chen, H.M. Berschneider, A.D. Stiles, J.K. Westwick, R.A. Rippe, D.A. Brenner, and J.M. Rhoads. 1995. L-glutamine and L-asparagine stimulate ODC activity and proliferation in a porcine jejunal enterocyte line. Am. J. Physiol. 269:G591–G599.

Lacey, J.M., and D.W. Wilmore. 1990. Is glutamine a conditionally essential amino acid? Nutr. Rev. 48(8):297–309.

Lacey, J.M., J.B. Crouch, K. Benfell, S.A. Ringer, C.K. Wilmore, D. Maguire, and D.W. Wilmore. 1996. The effects of glutamine-supplemented parenteral nutrition in premature infants. JPEN J. Parenter. Enteral Nutr. 20:74–80.

MacBurney, M., L.S. Young, T.R. Ziegler, and D.W. Wilmore. 1994. A cost-evaluation of glutamine-supplemented parenteral nutrition in adult bone marrow transplant patients. J. Am. Diet. Assoc. 94:1263–1266.

MacLennan, P.A., R.A. Brown, and M.J. Rennie. 1987. A positive relationship between protein synthesis rate and intracellular glutamine concentration in perfused rat skeletal muscle. FEBS Lett. 215:187–191.

Martin, D.W.. 1985. Metabolism of purine and pyrimidine nucleotides. P. 357–375 in Harper's Review of Biochemistry, D.W. Martin, P.A. Mayes, V.W. Rodwell, and D.K. Granner, eds. Los Altos, Calif.: Lang Medical Publishers.

McKeehan, W.L. 1982. Glycolysis, glutaminolysis, and cell proliferation. Cell Biol. Int. Rep. 6:635–650.

Muhlbacher, F., C.R. Kapadia, M.F. Colpoys, R.J. Smith, and D.W. Wilmore. 1984. Effects of glucocorticoids on glutamine metabolism in skeletal muscle. Am. J. Physiol. 247:E75–E83.

Newsholme, E.A., P. Newsholme, and R. Curi. 1988a. The role of the citric acid cycle in cells of the immune system and its importance in sepsis, trauma, and burns. Biochem. Soc. Symp. 54:145–162.

Newsholme, E.A., P. Newsholme, R. Curi, E. Challoner, and M.S.M. Ardawi. 1988b. A role for muscle in the immune system and its importance in surgery, trauma, sepsis, and burns. Nutrition 4:261–268.

O'Dwyer, S.T., R.J. Smith, T.L. Hwang, and D.W. Wilmore. 1989. Maintenance of small bowel mucosa with glutamine enriched parenteral nutrition. JPEN J. Parenter. Enteral Nutr. 13:579–585.

Ogle, C.K., J.D. Ogle, J-X. Mao, J. Simon, J.G. Noel, B-G. Li, and J.W. Alexander. 1994. Effect of glutamine on phagocytosis and bacterial killing by normal and pediatric burn patient neutrophils. JPEN J. Parenter. Enteral Nutr. 18:128–133.

O'Riordain, M.G., K.C.H. Fearon, J.A. Ross, P. Rogers, J.S. Falconer, D.C. Bartolo, O.J. Gardern, and D.C. Carter. 1994. Glutamine-supplemented total parenteral nutrition enhances T-lymphocyte response in surgical patients undergoing colorectal resection. Ann. Surg. 220:212–221.

Parry-Billings, M., J. Evans, P.C. Calder, and E.A. Newsholme. 1990. Does glutamine contribute to immunosuppression after major burns? Lancet 336:523–525.

Perriello, G., R. Jorde, N. Nurjhan, M. Stumvoll, G. Dailey, T. Jenssen, D.M. Bier, and J.E. Gerich. 1995. Estimation of glucose-alanine-lactate-glutamine cycles in postabsorptive humans: Role of skeletal muscle. Am. J. Physiol. 269:E443–E450.

Pitts, R.F., L.A. Pilkington, M.B. MacLeod, and E. Leal-Pinto. 1972. Metabolism of glutamine by the intact functioning kidney of the dog. J. Clin. Invest. 51:557–565.

Roth, E., J. Funovics, F. Muhlbacher, P. Sporn, W. Mauritz, and A. Fritsch. 1982. Metabolic disorders in severe abdominal sepsis: Glutamine deficiency in skeletal muscle. Clin. Nutr. 1:25.

Schloerb, P.R., and M. Amare. 1993. Total parenteral nutrition with glutamine in bone marrow transplantation and other clinical applications (a randomized, double-blind study). JPEN J. Parenter. Enteral Nutr. 17:407–413.

Shabert, J.K., and D.W. Wilmore. 1996. Glutamine deficiency as a cause of human immunodeficiency virus wasting. Med. Hypotheses 46:252–256.

Souba, W.W., R.J. Smith, and D.W. Wilmore, 1985. Glutamine metabolism by the intestinal tract. JPEN 9:608–617.

Spittler, A., S. Winkler, P. Gotzinger, R. Oehler, M. Wilheim, C. Tempfer, G. Weigel, R. Fuggar, G. Boltz-Nitulescu, and E. Roth. 1995. Influence of glutamine on the phenotype and function of human monocytes. Blood 86:1564–1569.

Tremel, H., B. Kienle, L.S. Weilemann, P. Stehle, and P. Furst. 1994. Glutamine dipeptide-supplemented parenteral nutrition maintains intestinal function in the critically ill. Gastroenterology 107:1595–1601.

Van der Hulst, R.R., B.K. van Kreel, M.F. von Meyenfeldt, R.J. Brummer, J.W. Arends, N.E. Deutz, and P.B. Soeters. 1993. Glutamine and the preservation of gut integrity. Lancet 334:1363–1365.

Van Zaanen, H.C.T., H. van der Lelie, J.G. Timmer, P. Furst, and H.P. Sauerwein 1994. Parenteral glutamine dipeptide supplementation does not ameliorate chemotherapy-induced toxicity. Cancer 74:2879–2884.

Welbourne, T.C. 1995. Increased plasma bicarbonate and growth hormone after an oral glutamine load. Am. J. Clin. Nutr. 61:1058–1061.

Welbourne, T.C., A.B. King, and K. Horton. 1993. Enteral glutamine supports hepatic glutathione efflux during inflammation. J. Nutr. Biochem. 4:236–242.

Windmueller, H.G. 1982. Glutamine utilization and the small intestine. Adv. Enzymol. 53:202.

Ziegler, T.R., R.L. Bye, R.L. Persinger, L.S. Young, J.H. Antin, and D.W. Wilmore. 1994. Glutamine-enriched parenteral nutrition increases circulating lymphocytes after bone marrow transplantation. JPEN J. Parenter. Enteral Nutr. 18(suppl.):17S.

Ziegler, T.R., R.J. Smith, S.T. O'Dwyer, R.H. Demling, and D.W. Wilmore. 1988. Increased intestinal permeability associated with infection in burn patients. Arch. Surg. 123:1313–1319.

Ziegler, T.R., L.S. Young, K. Benfell, M. Scheltinga, K. Hortos, R. Bye, F.D. Morrow, D.O. Jacobs, R.J. Smith, J.H. Antin, and D.W. Wilmore. 1992. Clinical and metabolic efficacy of glutamine-supplemented parenteral nutrition following bone marrow transplantation: A double-blind, randomized, controlled trial. Ann. Intern. Med. 116:821–828.

Zoli, M., M. Carè, C. Falco, R. Spanò, G. Bernardi, and I. Gasbarrini. 1995. Effect of oral glutamine on intestinal permeability and nutritional status in Crohn's disease. Gastroenterology 108:A766.

DISCUSSION

GAIL BUTTERFIELD: Should weight lifters take glutamine supplements to increase their muscle mass?

DOUGLAS WILMORE: If they really want to increase their muscle mass, anabolic steroids and growth hormone are much better. They are also much more expensive, and you can walk down to the corner store and get [glutamine]. So, glutamine is a very inexpensive and really safe agent.

GAIL BUTTERFIELD: But are there data to suggest that in a normal healthy person, increase in glutamine intake is going to have an anabolic effect?

DOUGLAS WILMORE: There is only anecdotal data in normals. There are some randomized trials going on in AIDS patients following weight loss, for example, where there is an early increase in body weight, which in fact may be due to water because glutamine helps transport water across the gastrointestinal tract.

    Realize that with all the anabolic agents, protein synthesis is associated with water retention and cell swelling. So, you always have to see water going into a person or water uptake increasing, and this at least fits that criterion so far. However, I don't think the data are available to show that a normal individual will increase their muscle mass.

SIMIN NIKBIN MEYDANI: How much of the effect on the immune system is due to glutamine itself and how much is due to [glutathione]?

DOUGLAS WILMORE: I don't know. It is quite clear that if you deplete those immune cells of glutathione that you will really cause cellular dysfunction.

    The other thing I don't know is the role that glutamine plays as an acid-base buffer system within cells. Clearly this may be a major role that glutamine plays in the gastrointestinal tract because tight junctions are quite sensitive to acidosis of the enterocyte. So, I think we just don't know the answers to these issues, and really *in vitro* studies would have to provide this information.

LEONARD KAPCALA: Is it known if there are any central effects of supplemental glutamine that would be influencing the glutamic acid and MDA [methyldopanine] receptor activation in brain?

DOUGLAS WILMORE: There are central effects from glutamine, and these are known effects. There is an old body of data in the European psychiatric literature where glutamine was used both in animals and in people to reduce addiction, and it has been used in alcoholics to reduce alcohol ingestion. It has been used in rats to reduce drug ingestion and alcohol ingestion, so that there may be central effects that can be perceived somehow in that role.

Nobody has moved further with that. We were quite concerned with the administration of glutamine in the premature infants because of their immature brains and actually did very careful dose-response studies to be sure that we didn't see toxicities in those infants.

So, yes, there are known central effects. The brain makes glutamine and glutamic acid and exports them. Brain and lung and muscle are the big exporters.

JEFFERY ZACHWIEJA: This is a follow-up on Gail [Butterfield]'s question. When I was at Washington University, we infused normal healthy males with either an amino acid solution without glutamine or an amino acid solution supplemented with glutamine and looked at the effects on muscle protein synthesis by carbon-13 level and leucine incorporation in skeletal muscle and found no difference in those young healthy males.

So, at least in terms of what we did, it appears that unless the muscle glutamine pool has become rapidly depleted by some condition, the extra glutamine won't have an effect on the muscle.

DOUGLAS WILMORE: I think that that is the point that always has to be re-emphasized, particularly if you propose a hypothesis that this is a conditional essential amino acid. The point is that you have to have the condition, and the condition clearly isn't [present in] well-nourished people, because it is not an essential amino acid in well-nourished people, and in fact, even in the military troops that take a large amount of protein and amino acids in their diet, it may in fact not be conditional under those circumstances. Of course, we really need the skeletal muscle biopsy data and concentration data and things of that sort to prove that fact.

However, there may be some functional outcome data that enhance performance, and there are a number of Olympic teams that are now using glutamine during training. So, we can see how that works out.

NED BERN: Is the mechanism by which glutamine stimulates growth hormone release known?

DOUGLAS WILMORE: Not specifically, no. I suspect it is quite similar to the same mechanism by which leucine stimulates hormone release.

NED BERN: Have you any idea how long that stimulation lasts?

DOUGLAS WILMORE: It is very short. A glutamine concentration curve with oral ingestion, if you ingest enough, looks very much like a glucose tolerance curve. So, you will get your peak stimulation at a couple of hours, something like that.

RANJIT CHANDRA: The question is, do you have any idea about the threshold for both deficiency and where the effects of glutamine occur?

DOUGLAS WILMORE: The question is thresholds, and I guess that implies or asks about dose-response curves and at what levels can we achieve those kinds of responses? In the hospital, we are moderately aggressive with glutamine administration, and it is not unusual to give one-third of the amino acid load as glutamine. That comes from the fact that that is what your skeletal muscle is producing. If in fact, we mimic what skeletal muscle does under stressed states, it puts out one-third of glutamine, one-third of alanine, and the rest a variety of amino acids.

If we were to feed an adult patient under a stressed state 1½ g of protein per kilogram body weight, ½ g of that would be glutamate. So, a 70 kg person would receive about 30 g of glutamate.

Now with babies, we give 20 percent of their amino acid load as glutamine, and their total amino acid load is about 2½ to 3 g/kg.

BRUCE BISTRIAN: I was interested when you talked about what was essential. In most of the conditions you mentioned, potential essentiality is also characterized by increased acid production. Has anyone done anything to see what the effect of just providing an equivalent amount of base would be?

DOUGLAS WILMORE: When we first started the studies with uptake across the bowel, the control was actually to give bicarbonate. That is really the proper control under those conditions.

You don't achieve those same effects. There are much greater effects of glutamine than [would be achieved by] just giving an equivalent amount of bicarbonate, but you know, those were stable physiologic preparations that we used, and the question has come up in the audience from time to time about people exercising and diminishing splanchnic blood flow, and that clearly is a phenomenon that I think Loren B. Rowell looked at in the 1960s or early 1970s. He ran students from the University of Washington so hard, he could make their liver enzymes go up and had simultaneous splanchnic blood flow measurements, which demonstrated splanativic ischemia.

So, that is a phenomenon that occurs, and acidosis of the gastrointestinal epithelium is probably a real thing. It appears to be important in clinical practice because the tonometry data has suggested that the mucosa becomes acidotic. One of the effects of glutamine is to neutralize this intracellular acidosis.

BRUCE BISTRIAN: I was thinking, also, about the effect of the base on Philmidge. When used in acidosis conditions like renal failure, it has profound effects on muscle metabolism where the effect on the muscles may be its base effect.

DOUGLAS WILMORE: I don't think we know the answer to that. There are some Swedish data looking at that in postoperative patients that could possibly address that with intracellular pH probes, but I don't think anyone has done that study.

Nutrition and Immune Function, 1999
Pp. 279–288. Washington, D.C.
National Academy Press

12

Vitamin A and Immune Function

Richard D. Semba[1]

INTRODUCTION

Vitamin A is an essential micronutrient for immunity, cellular differentiation, growth, reproduction, maintenance of epithelial surfaces, and vision. Vitamin A is found as preformed vitamin A in foods such as liver, cod-liver oil, butter, eggs, and dairy products and as provitamin A carotenoids in foods such as spinach, carrots, and orange fruits and vegetables. Among the micronutrients, vitamin A plays a central role in normal immune function. In a comprehensive review of the literature, Scrimshaw et al. (1968) concluded "no nutritional deficiency is more consistently synergistic with infectious disease than that of vitamin A" (p. 94). Although conventionally it has been thought that the main clinical manifestations of vitamin A deficiency involve the eye (for example, night blindness and xerophthalmia), it is now well established that widespread immune alterations, anemia, and increased infectious disease morbidity and mortality occur during vitamin A deficiency. The use of vitamin A supplements to enhance immunity has been demonstrated in the recent series

---

[1] Richard D. Semba, The Johns Hopkins University, Department of Ophthalmology, Ocular Immunology Service, Baltimore, MD 21205

of clinical trials involving children in developing countries (Beaton et al., 1993). This chapter will review the potential importance of vitamin A to immune function in adult men and women.

CLINICAL MANIFESTATIONS OF VITAMIN A DEFICIENCY

The most commonly recognized clinical manifestations of vitamin A deficiency involve the eye, and a complete description of the clinical staging is described in Sommer (1982). The occurrence of ocular signs and symptoms of mild and advanced vitamin A deficiency have relevance to immune status as their presence signals a high risk of vitamin A-related immune abnormalities in the individual. Night blindness is one of the earliest symptoms of mild vitamin A deficiency. Typically the vision is normal during the day, but the ability to distinguish objects under less well-illuminated conditions—at dusk or during the night—is impaired. Vitamin A is involved in the generation of rhodopsin, the visual pigment in rod photoreceptors, which allows the retina to detect light in dark-adapted conditions. Other conditions besides vitamin A deficiency can cause night blindness, including advanced glaucoma, pupillary abnormalities involving a small pupil, retinitis pigmentosa, and certain rare retinal disorders involving rod function of the retina. Mild vitamin A deficiency is also characterized by keratinizing, squamous metaplasia of the conjunctiva. A well-defined, raised area of conjunctival metaplasia can sometimes be recognized, typically on the temporal and/or nasal bulbar conjunctiva, and this lesion, known as a Bitot's spot, is considered pathognomonic for vitamin A deficiency.

Advanced vitamin A deficiency is characterized by corneal xerosis, in which the clear, shiny corneal epithelium is replaced by areas of keratinized epithelium, giving the cornea a dull, grayish-white appearance. Cornea ulcers may occur in advanced vitamin A deficiency, and typically these ulcers are small, round or oval, full-thickness ulcers that may allow the aqueous humor to drain from the anterior chamber of the eye. The most advanced eye lesion of vitamin A deficiency is keratomalacia, a condition in which the cornea undergoes widespread ulceration and necrosis, with or without concomitant bacterial or fungal superinfection. Usually under these circumstances, the affected individual will become blind in the affected eye(s) and is at greatly increased risk of immunodeficiency and death.

EPIDEMIOLOGY OF VITAMIN A DEFICIENCY

Vitamin A deficiency is one of the most common micronutrient deficiencies in the world, affecting an estimated 125 million individuals (Sommer and West, 1996). The groups at highest risk for the development of vitamin A deficiency are infants, preschool children, pregnant women, and lactating women. Vitamin A deficiency is the most common in developing countries, affecting areas of the world such as Southeast and southern Asia, sub-Saharan Africa, areas of the South Pacific, and parts of South and Central America (Sommer and West, 1996). Vitamin A deficiency was once common in Europe and the United States prior to improvements in diet, fortification of foods with vitamin A, and general advances in public health. Pregnant women are at higher risk of developing vitamin A deficiency because of increased demands for vitamin A by the growing fetus. Breastfeeding provides the vitamin A for infants before weaning, and lactating women are at risk of vitamin A deficiency during this period.

Several factors may contribute to the development of vitamin A deficiency, including inadequate intake of vitamin A-containing foods, malabsorption due to infections in the gut, liver disease, the acute phase response and abnormal urinary losses of vitamin A, zinc deficiency, concomitant protein energy malnutrition, and increased utilization of vitamin A during infections. Diarrheal disease and intestinal parasites may interfere with the absorption of vitamin A. Liver disease, such as hepatitis, may impair the capacity of the liver to store and release vitamin A. Zinc deficiency has been shown to impede the release of retinol-binding protein and vitamin A from the liver (Smith, 1980). During infections, circulating vitamin A levels usually decrease because of the acute phase response, possible increased utilization of vitamin A by peripheral tissues, and abnormal urinary losses of vitamin A (Alvarez et al., 1995).

The Recommended Dietary Allowance (RDA [NRC, 1989]) of vitamin A for adult men and women in the United States is 800 μg RE (retinol equivalents)/d. For lactating women, the RDA is 1,200 to 1,300 μg RE/d. In general, healthy adult men and women who receive the RDA of vitamin A would be at low risk of developing vitamin A deficiency. This is primarily due to the fact that the liver, which stores about 90 percent of the body's vitamin A, has a capacity to store vitamin A for a prolonged period. In healthy children, the liver can store enough vitamin A to last for a few months, whereas in healthy adults, it seems that the adult liver can store enough vitamin A to last for several months to a year or more.

VITAMIN A DEFICIENCY IN ADULTS

Vitamin A deprivation experiments have been conducted among adults in order to determine the minimal requirements of vitamin A, and these experiments illustrate the capacity of the liver to store vitamin A. Impaired dark adaptation was noted in five subjects after various periods from 16 to 124 days of vitamin A and carotenoid deprivation (Booher et al., 1939). Wagner (1940) deprived 10 subjects of dietary vitamin A and carotenoids for 6 months and noted signs of vitamin A deficiency. Brenner and Roberts (1943) noted no signs of deficiency in three subjects who were deprived of vitamin A and carotenoids for over 7 months.

During World War II, a vitamin A deprivation experiment was conducted by the Medical Research Council on 20 men and 3 women, most of them between the ages of 20 and 30 years (Hume and Krebs, 1949). These individuals were conscientious objectors to military service who volunteered for human experimentation at a research institute in Sheffield, England. The plan was to give 16 adults a diet devoid of vitamin A and carotene until signs of deficiency appeared and then determine the dose of vitamin A or carotene that was necessary to return their levels to normal. The original experiment was expected to last 6 to 8 months; however, the experiment continued for over 18 months in several of the volunteers because no signs of deficiency developed. After 8 months, the plasma vitamin A levels began to decline in most subjects. Only 3 men became deficient, as evident by a gradual drop in plasma vitamin A levels that was accompanied by impaired dark adaptation. After 16 to 20 months of deprivation, 2 previously healthy volunteers developed tuberculosis.

Xerophthalmia and keratomalacia have been infrequently reported in adult men and women, usually under conditions of extreme dietary deprivation or in association with chronic infections and wasting. Night blindness and keratomalacia were reported among adults in a prison in Kampala, Uganda, where the diet was monotonous and contained little vitamin A (Mitchell, 1933; Owen, 1933). Vitamin A deficiency has been reported in concentration camps (Salus, 1957). Scattered case reports exist of keratomalacia in adults (Pillat, 1929), and these cases occurred mostly among adults with liver disease, malnutrition, or severe diarrheal disease. Alcoholic liver disease can increase the risk of vitamin A deficiency. Low vitamin A levels consistent with deficiency have been described in adults with HIV infection (Karter et al., 1995; Semba et al., 1993a, 1994). There is little evidence that noninfectious stress such as heat or cold will affect vitamin A status. It should be noted that vitamin A deficiency was once a major problem in the nineteenth century for American sailors involved in long voyages and was widely reported in both Union and Confederate armies during the Civil War.

Pregnancy and lactation represent a period of high risk in women for the development of vitamin A deficiency. Night blindness is not uncommon among pregnant women in developing countries, and a recent case control study from Nepal suggests that pregnant women with night blindness have increased infectious disease morbidity (Christian et al., 1996). In sub-Saharan Africa, HIV-infected pregnant women with vitamin A deficiency have higher risk of passing HIV infection to their infants, and their infants have lower birthweight and higher infant mortality (Semba et al., 1994, 1995). Vitamin A deficiency has been reported in pregnant women of lower socioeconomic class in the United States (Duitsman et al., 1995). The requirements for vitamin A may increase in pregnant women because of needs for vitamin A by the growing fetus. During lactation, the daily requirement for vitamin A is higher because of the transfer of circulating vitamin A into breastmilk.

VITAMIN A DEFICIENCY AS AN IMMUNODEFICIENCY DISORDER

Epidemiologic studies, clinical trials, and experimental studies in animal models have firmly established that vitamin A deficiency is a nutritionally acquired immunodeficiency disorder that is characterized by widespread immune alterations and increased infectious disease morbidity and mortality (Semba, 1994). In humans, most of the understanding of vitamin A-related immunodeficiency comes from studies involving children rather than adults. Autopsy studies in children have shown that vitamin A deficiency is associated with atrophy of the thymus, lymph nodes, and spleen (Blackfan and Wolbach, 1933; Sweet and K'ang, 1955). Vitamin A deficiency is often associated with protein-energy malnutrition (PEM), making it difficult to attribute these pathologic alterations in the immune system to vitamin A deficiency alone. However, under well-controlled conditions, animal models have shown a similar association between vitamin A deficiency and atrophy of the thymus, lymph nodes, and spleen (Ahmed et al., 1990; Krishnan et al., 1974).

Vitamin A deficiency is associated with widespread alterations in mucosal surfaces, including that of the eye (Natadisastra et al., 1987), oropharynx, respiratory tract, gastrointestinal tract, and genitourinary tract (Brown et al., 1979; Sweet and K'ang, 1955). Pathologic changes in the conjunctiva associated with night blindness include keratinizing metaplasia of the conjunctiva and loss of goblet cells and mucus (Natadisastra et al., 1987). In the respiratory tract, vitamin A deficiency is associated with loss of ciliated respiratory epithelium, goblet cells, and mucus (Goldblatt and Benischek 1927; Wolbach and Howe, 1925). Squamous metaplasia has been reported to occur in the tracheal epithelium of vitamin A-deficient animals (McDowell et al., 1984). Loss of microvilli from enterocytes and loss of goblet cells and mucus have also been observed in animals deficient in vitamin A (Rojanapo et al., 1980). These pathologic alterations in mucosal surfaces constitute a violation in the first line of defense of the immune system and may explain the more severe morbidity from respiratory and diarrheal disease in children with mild vitamin A deficiency.

T-cell subset alterations have been reported in vitamin A deficiency. In preschool children in rural Indonesia, clinical and subclinical vitamin A deficiency is associated with T cell subset alterations such as lower circulating percentage of CD4 cells and lower CD4/CD8 ratio (Semba et al., 1993b). A study involving HIV-seronegative injection drug users from inner city Baltimore showed that adults with vitamin A levels consistent with deficiency (serum vitamin A < 1.05 µmol/liter) had significantly lower CD4 counts than those without deficiency (Semba et al., 1993a). Studies in HIV-infected adults have shown a fairly consistent association between low vitamin A levels and low CD4 counts (Phuapradit et al., 1996; Semba et al., 1993a, b). Other T-cell subset alterations include lower circulating natural killer (NK) cells in vitamin A-deficient animals, and treatment with retinoic acid is associated with increases in circulating NK cells (Zhao and Ross, 1995). In children with AIDS, high-dose vitamin A supplementation increases circulating CD4 T-cells and NK cells (Hussey et al., 1996). Vitamin A appears to play a key role in lymphopoiesis, which may explain the increases in total lymphocyte counts, CD4 T-cells, and NK cells associated with vitamin A supplementation or improvement of vitamin A status.

A hallmark of vitamin A deficiency is depressed antibody responses to T-cell-dependent antigens, such as tetanus toxoid; viral and parasite antigens; and T-cell independent type 1 antigens; such as meningococcal polysaccharides (Ross, 1992; Semba, 1994). The mechanisms by which vitamin A deficiency impairs antibody responses include alterations in interleukin (IL)-4 and interferon-gamma production (Cantorna et al., 1996) and IL-2 receptor expression (Sidell et al., 1993). In addition, the growth and activation of T- and B-cells are dependent on vitamin A and its metabolites (Buck et al., 1990; Garbe et al., 1992; Wang et al., 1993). Vitamin A-deficient animals that are experimentally infected with different pathogens generally have impaired immune responses and increased morbidity and mortality. Children with clinical or subclinical vitamin A deficiency have depressed IgG responses to tetanus toxoid compared with children supplemented with vitamin A (Semba et al., 1992). There are few data regarding antibody responses in vitamin A-deficient adults, probably because deficiency is generally uncommon, except in those with chronic infections such as HIV infection.

CONSIDERATIONS FOR ADULT MEN AND WOMEN

In healthy adult men and women, it is reasonable to expect that a diet that meets or exceeds the RDA of vitamin A of 800 µg RE/d will be sufficient to avoid a deficiency state. Such requirements could be met through a diet that includes butter, cheese, egg yolks, whole milk, vitamin A-fortified skim milk, and liver. Foods such as carrots and spinach contain β-carotene and other provitamin A carotenoids that are converted to vitamin A. The absorption of provitamin A carotenoids is improved if accompanied by dietary fat, such as cooking oil. Recent data suggest that the bioavailability of carotenoids in vegetables and fruits for conversion to vitamin A is much lower than previously estimated (de Pee et al., 1995), and currently further studies are being undertaken to address this issue. Individuals with prolonged infections such as diarrhea or malaria may have reduced their hepatic reserves of vitamin A during the period of infection, and it would be reasonable to encourage increased consumption of vitamin A-containing foods during infection and convalescence. If periods of dietary deprivation are anticipated, it would be reasonable to expect that a daily supplement that contains 800 to 1,500 µg RE (2,666 to 5,000 IU) could minimize the risk of vitamin A deficiency and associated immunodeficiency. Because vitamin A is an immune enhancer, another issue is whether supplementation beyond the daily requirement for vitamin A will increase immunity. There are few data to suggest that megadoses of vitamin A will confer additional protection against infections, and supplementation above levels of 3,000 μg RE (10,000 IU)/d in healthy adults may increase the risk of vitamin A toxicity or of birth defects in women of childbearing age.

AUTHOR'S CONCLUSIONS

Vitamin A deficiency is a nutritionally acquired immunodeficiency disorder that primarily affects infants, preschool children, pregnant women, and lactating women. Healthy adult men and women of military age represent the lowest risk group for the development of vitamin A deficiency. However, under certain conditions such as chronic infection or prolonged dietary deprivation, the risk of vitamin A deficiency and associated immune abnormalities may be significant. Under such circumstances, daily supplementation with the RDA for vitamin A would be expected to minimize such risk. Individuals who meet the RDA of vitamin A per day would be likely to avoid the risk of vitamin A deficiency under normal circumstances. Because of the capacity of the adult liver to store several months or more of vitamin A, adults are generally buffered against developing vitamin A deficiency.

REFERENCES

Ahmed, F., D.B. Jones, and A.A. Jackson. 1990. The interaction of vitamin A deficiency and rotavirus infection in the mouse. Br. J. Nutr. 63:363–373.

Alvarez, J.O., E. Salazar-Lindo, J. Kohatsu, P. Miranda, and C.B. Stephensen. 1995. Urinary excretion of retinol in children with acute diarrhea. Am. J. Clin. Nutr. 61:1273–1276.

Beaton, G.H., R. Martorell, K.J. Aronson, B. Edmonston, G. McCabe, A.C. Ross, and B. Harvey. 1993. Effectiveness of vitamin A supplementation in the control of young child morbidity and mortality in developing countries. State-of-the-Art Series Nutrition Policy Discussion Paper No. 13. Geneva, Switzerland: Administrative Committee on Coordination/ Subcommittee on Nutrition of the United Nations.

Blackfan, K.D., and S.B. Wolbach. 1933. Vitamin A deficiency in infants. A clinical and pathological study. J. Pediatr. 3:679–706.

Booher, L.E., E.C. Callison, and E.M. Hewston. 1939. An experimental determination of the minimum vitamin A requirements of normal adults. J. Nutr. 17:317–331.

Brenner, S., and L.J. Roberts. 1943. Effects of vitamin A depletion in young adults. Arch. Intern. Med. 71:474–482.

Brown, K.H., A. Gaffar, and S.M. Alamgir. 1979. Xerophthalmia, protein-calorie malnutrition, and infections in children. J. Pediatr. 95:651–656.

Buck, J., G. Ritter, L. Dannecker, V. Katta, S.L. Cohen, B.T. Chait, and U. Hämmerling. 1990. Retinol is essential for growth of activated human B-cells. J. Exp. Med. 171:1613–1624.

Cantorna, M.T., F.E. Nashold, T.Y. Chun, and C.E. Hayes. 1996. Vitamin A downregulation of IGN-γ synthesis in cloned mouse Th1 lymphocytes depends upon the CD28 costimulatory pathway. J. Immunol. 156:2674–2679.

Christian, P., K.P. West Jr., S.K. Khatry, J. Katz, R.J. Stoltzfus, and R.P. Pokhrel. 1996. Epidemiology of night blindness during pregnant in rural Nepal. P. 8 in Abstracts of the XVII International Vitamin A Consultative Group Meeting, March 1996, Guatemala City, Guatemala.

de Pee, S., C.E. West, Muhilal, D. Karyadi, and J.G. Hautvast. 1995. Lack of improvement in vitamin A status with increased consumption of dark-green leafy vegetables. Lancet 346:75–81.

Dresser, D.W. 1968. Adjuvanticity of vitamin A. Nature 217:527–529.

Duitsman, P.K., L.R. Cook, S.A. Tanumihardjo, and J.A. Olson. 1995. Vitamin A inadequacy in socioeconomically disadvantaged pregnant Iowan women as assessed by the modified relative dose response (MRDR) test. Nutr. Res. 15:1263–1276.

Garbe, A., J. Buck, and U. Hämmerling. 1992. Retinoids are important cofactors in T-cell activation. J. Exp. Med. 176:109–117.

Goldblatt, H., and M. Benischek. 1927. Vitamin A deficiency and metaplasia. J. Exp. Med. 46:699–707.

Hume, E.M., and H.A. Krebs. 1949. Vitamin A requirements of human adults: An experimental study of vitamin A deprivation in man. Medical Research Council Special Report Series 264. London: Her Majesty's Stationery Office.

Hussey, G., J. Hughes, S. Potgieter, G. Kessow, J. Burgess, D. Beatty, M. Keraan, and E. Carelse. 1996. Vitamin A status and supplementation and its effects on immunity in children with AIDS. P. 6 Abstracts of the XVII International Vitamin A Consultative Group Meeting, March 1996, Guatemala City, Guatemala, March.

Karter, D.L., A.J. Karter, R. Yarrish, C. Patterson, P.H. Kass, J. Nord, and J.W. Kislak. 1995. Vitamin A deficiency in non-vitamin-supplemented patients with AIDS: A cross-sectional study. J. Acquir. Immune Defic. Syndr. Hum. Retrovirol. 8:199–203.

Krishnan, S., U.N. Bhuyan, G.P. Talwar, and V. Ramalingaswami. 1974. Effect of vitamin A and protein-calorie undernutrition on immune responses. Immunology 27:383–397.

McDowell, E.M., K.P. Keenan, and M. Huang. 1984. Effects of vitamin A-deprivation on hamster tracheal epithelium: A quantitative morphologic study. Virchows Arch. B 45:197–219.

Mitchell, J.P.. 1933. Observations on health in relation to diet in H.M. Central Prison, Uganda. I. Prison diets and morbidity. East Afr. Med. J. 10:38–53.

Natadisastra, G., J.R. Wittpenn, K.P. West Jr., Muhilal, and A. Sommer. 1987. Impression cytology for the detection of vitamin A deficiency. Arch. Ophthalmol. 105(9):1224–1228.

NRC (National Research Council). 1989. Recommended Dietary Allowances, 10th ed. Subcommittee on the Tenth Edition of the RDAs, Food and Nutrition Board, Commission of Life Sciences. Washington, D.C.: National Academy Press.

Owen, H.B. 1933. Observations on health in relation to diet in H.M. Central Prison, Uganda. II. The ocular manifestations of vitamin A deficiency. East Afr. Med. J. 10:53–58.

Phuapradit, W., K. Chaturachinda, S. Tannepanichskul, J. Sirivarasry, K. Khupulsup, and N. Lerdvuthisopon. 1996. Serum vitamin A and β-carotene levels in pregnant women infected with human immunodeficiency virus-1. Obstet. Gynecol. 87:564–567.

Pillat, A. 1929. Does keratomalacia exist in adults? Arch. Ophthalmol. 2:256–287, 399–415.

Rojanapo, W., A.J. Lamb, and J.A. Olson. 1980. The prevalence, metabolism and migration of goblet cells in rat intestine following the induction of rapid, synchronous vitamin A deficiency. J. Nutr. 110:178–188.

Ross, A.C. 1992. Vitamin A status: Relationship to immunity and the antibody response. Proc. Soc. Exp. Biol. Med. 200:303–320.

Salus, R. 1957. Ophthalmology in a concentration camp. Am. J. Ophthalmol. 44:12–17.

Scrimshaw, N.S., C.E. Taylor, and J.E. Gordon. 1968. Interactions of Nutrition and Infection. Geneva: World Health Organization.

Semba, R.D. 1994. Vitamin A, immunity, and infection. Clin. Infect. Dis. 19:489–499.

Semba, R.D., N.M.H. Graham, W.T. Caiaffa, J.B. Margolick, L. Clement, and D. Vlahov. 1993a. Increased mortality associated with vitamin A deficiency during human immunodeficiency virus type 1 infection. Arch. Intern. Med. 153:2149–2154.

Semba, R.D., P. Miotti, J.D. Chiphangwi, G. Liomba, L.P. Yang, A. Saah, G. Dallabetta, and D.R. Hoover. 1995. Infant mortality and maternal vitamin A deficiency during HIV infection. Clin. Infect. Dis. 21:966–972.

Semba, R.D., P. Miotti, J.D. Chiphangwi, A. Saah, J. Canner, G. Dallabetta, and D.R. Hoover. 1994. Maternal vitamin A deficiency and mother-to-child transmission of HIV-1. Lancet 343:1593–1597.

Semba, R.D., Muhilal, A.L. Scott, G. Natadisastra, S. Wirasasmita, L. Mele, E. Ridwan, K.P. West Jr., and A. Sommer. 1992. Depressed immune response to tetanus in children with vitamin A deficiency. J. Nutr. 122:101–107.

Semba R.D., Muhilal, B.J. Ward, A.L. Scott, G. Natadisastra, K.P. West Jr., and A. Sommer. 1993b. Abnormal T-cell subset proportions in vitamin A-deficient children. Lancet 341:5–8.

Sidell, N., B. Chang., and L. Bhatti. 1993. Upregulation by retinoic acid of interleukin-2 receptor mRNA in human T-lymphocytes. Cell. Immunol. 146:28–37.

Smith, J.C. 1980. The vitamin A-zinc connection: A review. Ann. N.Y. Acad. Sci. 355:62–74.

Sommer, A. 1982. A Field Guide to the Detection and Control of Xerophthalmia. Geneva: World Health Organization.

Sommer, A., and K.P. West Jr. 1996. Vitamin A Deficiency: Health, Survival, and Vision. New York: Oxford University Press.

Sweet, K.L., and H.J. K'ang. 1955. Clinical and anatomic study of avitaminosis A among the Chinese. Am. J. Dis. Child. 50:699–734.

Wagner, K.H. 1940. Die experimentelle Avitaminose A beim Menschen. Hoppe-Seyler's Zeitschr. f. physiol. Chemie 264:153–188.

Wang, W., J.L. Napoli, and M. Ballow. 1993. The effects of retinol on in vitro immunoglobulin synthesis by cord blood and adult peripheral blood mononuclear cells. Clin. Exp. Immunol. 92:164–168.

Wolbach, S.G., and P.R. Howe. 1925. Tissue changes following deprivation of fat-soluble A vitamin. J. Exp. Med. 42:753–777.

Zhao, Z., and A.C. Ross. 1995. Retinoic acid repletion restores the number of leukocytes and their subsets and stimulates natural cytotoxicity in vitamin A-deficient rats. J. Nutr. 125:2064–2073.

DISCUSSION

ROBERT NESHEIM: Are there questions or discussion of this paper? I guess you had a question, Dr. Chandra?

RANJIT CHANDRA: The first question is what was your perception of the two studies related to mortality? The second question or comment is that I think the nutrient that probably has not a very widespread effect or is not as clear as for instance, zinc—perhaps the discrimination would come from antibody responses to those agents which I think have a more flexible response.

RICHARD SEMBA: I don't think I understand your second question, quite as well, but of the eight clinical trials I showed, all showed reductions in mortality except one.

The one study in India showed a 6 percent reduction in mortality. I cannot explain that study, but I can explain the Sudan study. The Sudan study showed actually a negative effect, but it is quite puzzling because those investigators also showed that vitamin A supplementation had no impact on vitamin A deficiency. In other words, in children who had night blindness or xerophthalmia, it did not reduce that at all, which makes me a little bit concerned. I am quite puzzled over that.

So, one would expect that [a decrease in night blindness] at least as a minimum, and those investigators concluded that maybe they weren't giving enough vitamin A.

I think if I understand your second question, I don't think anybody has looked at effects of vitamin A supplementation in humans on antigens that are less immunogenic, such as Dresser (1968) did in mice with, I think, bovine serum albumin. That hasn't been done. It would be very interesting to see.

We are doing a study in adults with conjugated pneumococcal vaccine in Baltimore using vitamin A and zinc in a factorial design to see whether that will increase their immune responses.

RANJIT CHANDRA: Have you looked at the secretory immune system?

RICHARD SEMBA: No.

ROBERT NESHEIM: Thank you very much. We appreciate your comments on vitamin A, and I think it has been very helpful to us.

Nutrition and Immune Function, 1999
Pp. 289–303. Washington, D.C.
National Academy Press

13

Vitamin E, Vitamin C, and Immune Response: Recent Advances

Laura C. Rall and Simin Nikbin Meydani[1]

INTRODUCTION

Tocopherols (the major group of compounds with vitamin E biological activity) are known chemically as antioxidants; they prevent propagation of the oxidation of unsaturated fatty acids by trapping peroxyl free radicals (NRC, 1989). Vitamin E is found in cellular membranes of animal tissues, associated with polyunsaturated fatty acids in phospholipids. Here, vitamin E serves as the primary defense against potentially harmful oxidation reactions (NRC, 1989).

In addition to vitamin E, ascorbic acid (vitamin C) is one of the other essential nutrients, assisting in this antioxidant defense system by protecting against lipid peroxidation (Frei et al., 1988). In fact, vitamin C has been shown to function by sparing or reconstituting vitamin E, thus protecting lipid membranes (Packer et al., 1979). Although it is widely believed that the basic role of vitamin E is its function as an antioxidant (NRC, 1989), vitamin C has other important functions in numerous biological systems, including the synthesis of hormones, neurotransmitters, collagen and carnitine; the

---

[1] Simin Nikbin Meydani, Nutritional Immunology Laboratory, U.S. Department of Agriculture-Human Nutrition Research Center on Aging at Tufts, Boston, MA 02111

detoxification of exogenous compounds; and cytochrome P-450 activity (reviewed in NRC, 1989). However, recent evidence has also shown that vitamins E and C are needed for normal function of the immune system (Anderson et al., 1980) (reviewed in M. Meydani, 1995).

The present Recommended Dietary Allowance (RDA) for vitamin E is 10 mg of α-tocopherol equivalents (TE)/d for male adults and 8 mg/d for women; for vitamin C the RDA is 60 mg/d for adults regardless of gender (NRC, 1989). The recommendation for vitamin E is based on customary dietary intakes from U.S. food sources, while in the case of vitamin C, the RDA represents a balance between the amount necessary to prevent overt symptoms of deficiency and the amount beyond which the nutrient is not retained by the body (NRC, 1989). In both instances, the recommendation is admittedly somewhat arbitrary (NRC, 1989), and in neither case was the RDA designed with the aim of promoting optimal health benefits.

Although vitamins E and C have long been recognized for their antioxidant properties, increasing attention has been focused on their abilities, along with those of other antioxidants, to reduce the risk of chronic disease. The question of an optimal level of intake for health promotion and chronic disease prevention is beyond the scope of this chapter. Instead, this review will focus on the effects of vitamins E and C on immunity and the implications of vitamin status and supplementation for various populations and disease states. Specifically, the effects of these nutrients during aging, acquired immunodeficiency disease (AIDS), coronary heart disease (CHD), cancer, allergy, and exercise will be considered.

AGING

Most evidence indicates a progressive decline in immune response in both laboratory animals and human subjects with advancing age. Those parameters that seem to decrease with age include thymic tissue mass, antibody response, delayed-type hypersensitivity (DTH) response, T-cell proliferative response to mitogen stimulation, and the proportion of T-cell subsets with naive cell surface markers (Makinodan, 1995). However, other immune parameters frequently increase with age, including variability in immune responses among individuals, production of autoantibodies, production of monoclonal immunoglobulins, and the proportion of T-cell subsets with memory membrane markers (Makinodan, 1995). The net result of these changes is a dysregulated immune response accompanied by increased morbidity and mortality among the elderly (reviewed in Goodwin, 1995).

Research efforts are now directed at finding ways to alleviate this dysregulation of immunity and, ultimately, to reduce the age-associated increase in morbidity and mortality. Interestingly, most of the nutritional interventions that are successful in improving immunologic vigor in aging humans are antioxidant in nature (S.N. Meydani et al., 1995).

Vitamin E

A series of controlled clinical trials by S.N. Meydani et al. (1990, 1997a) and M. Meydani et al. (1994) have demonstrated that vitamin E supplementation of elderly persons may enhance the immune response. In the first study (S.N. Meydani et al., 1990), healthy elderly men ($\geq$ 60 years old) were supplemented with 800 mg 2-*ambo*-α–tocopherol or placebo/d for 30 days. Their diets provided adequate amounts of vitamin E and other nutrients. All subjects resided and consumed all of their food in the Metabolic Research Unit at the Jean Mayer U.S. Department of Agriculture-Human Nutrition Research Center on Aging at Tufts University.

Before and after supplementation, blood samples were collected for measurement of various biochemical and immunologic indexes, and DTH was measured as an *in vivo* indicator of cell-mediated immunity (CMI). Results showed that vitamin E supplementation was associated with increased plasma vitamin E, DTH score, mitogenic response to concanavalin A (Con-A), and interleukin (IL)-2 production. Vitamin E supplementation was also associated with decreased prostaglandin (PG)E$_2$ production by peripheral blood mononuclear cells (PBMCs) and decreased plasma lipid peroxide concentrations.

Although this study did demonstrate a beneficial effect of vitamin E on immune response, the study was of relatively short duration, using a high dosage of vitamin E. Therefore, to further investigate the effect of long-term supplementation and optimal concentration of vitamin E on the immune response of elderly individuals, a double-blind, placebo-controlled study with 80 free-living, healthy, elderly persons (> 65 years of age) was conducted (S.N. Meydani et al., 1997a). Subjects were randomly assigned to receive either placebo, 60, 200, or 800 mg vitamin E/d. Fasting blood samples were collected before and after 1 and 4.5 months of supplementation, and mitogenic response, cytokine production, lymphocyte subpopulations, and biochemical indexes were measured. In addition, DTH and antibody response to vaccination were also measured as *in vivo* indices of immune response. Subjects' health status, weight, dietary intake, and physical activity were monitored for the duration of the study. All three vitamin E-supplemented subject groups demonstrated a significant increase in plasma vitamin E levels and DTH response, while the placebo group showed no increase in plasma vitamin E levels, mitogenic response, or DTH.

An additional study was also performed to assess further the effect of long-term vitamin E supplementation on immune response of young versus elderly subjects (M. Meydani et al. 1994). Sixty healthy young and elderly men and women were supplemented with either 400 mg *RRR*-α–tocopherol or placebo for 6 months. Fasting blood samples were collected before and after 2, 4, and 6 months of supplementation. Levels of plasma α–tocopherol increased among subjects in both age groups after 2 months of supplementation and remained elevated for the duration of the study. Furthermore, vitamin E reduced levels of plasma lipid peroxides among subjects in all age groups after 2 months of supplementation, but by 6 months, this effect was only observed among the elderly subjects. Vitamin E supplementation also resulted in an increased DTH response in both age groups, although the effect was stronger in elderly compared with young individuals.

The findings of this series of clinical trials suggest that vitamin E supplementation of elderly individuals leads to enhancement of *in vivo* and *in vitro* measures of immune response. Furthermore, supplementation with large amounts of vitamin E (800 mg) has not been found to have adverse health effects among healthy elderly individuals (S.N. Meydani et al., 1997b). Additional research is currently being conducted to determine the mechanism of the immunoenhancing effect of vitamin E.

Vitamin C

Compared with vitamin E, there have been fewer studies specifically examining the effects of vitamin C on immune response, particularly among elderly individuals. One study utilized a combination of vitamin A, C, and E supplements among 30 elderly long-stay patients (Penn et al., 1991). Nutritional status and cell-mediated immune function were assessed before and after 28 days of supplementation. CMI was enhanced in the supplemented but not the placebo group, as indicated by an increase in the absolute number of T-cells, T4 subsets, the T4:T8 ratio, and the proliferation of lymphocytes in response to phytohemagglutinin (PHA). The findings of this study suggest that supplementation with antioxidant nutrients can improve cell-mediated immune parameters among elderly long-stay patients; however, the study design prevents the independent effects of each of the nutrients from being determined.

Studies that have looked exclusively at vitamin C in terms of its effect on immunocompetence have had inconsistent results. A depletion-repletion study designed to determine the dietary ascorbate requirement to optimize the functions of the vitamin other than prevention of scurvy was carried out in healthy, young-to-middle-aged men (25–43 years of age) (Jacob et al., 1991). Immune and oxidant defense parameters were measured while subjects consumed 5 to 250 mg/d of ascorbic acid over 92 days while residing in a metabolic unit. No changes in proliferation of PBMCs or erythrocyte antioxidant enzymes were observed during depletion or repletion. In contrast, DTH response did decrease during ascorbic acid deficiency; however, repletion for 21 days at 60 or 250 mg ascorbic acid/d did not restore the mean DTH score to predepletion levels. Therefore, there were no clear differences in the immune and oxidative damage parameters among healthy, young-to-middle-aged men during this depletion-repletion study.

Unlike these findings of Jacob et al. (1991), others have found that vitamin C may improve selected immune responses in elderly individuals. For example, vitamin C supplementation (500 mg daily, given intramuscularly, for 1 month) enhanced lymphocyte proliferative response *in vitro* and skin reactivity to tuberculin antigen *in vivo* among elderly individuals with low blood vitamin C levels (Kennes et al., 1983). In addition, increased vitamin C intake (1–3 g/d for 1 week) has been shown by others to stimulate lymphocyte proliferative response (Anderson et al., 1980). Inconsistent findings among studies may be explained by one or more of the following factors: the population studied (young versus elderly), the dosage of vitamin C (pharmacologic levels versus physiologic levels), and the duration of supplementation. Additional studies to examine the effects of vitamin C on immune response, taking into account these various factors, are required before any definitive conclusions can be drawn.

CANCER

Some experimental and epidemiologic studies have suggested that both vitamins E and C may reduce the risk of various types of cancer. However, the evidence remains controversial either because of the nutrient source (diet or supplement) or the cancer site studied. Both nutrients, via their antioxidant function, may eliminate free radicals and decrease DNA damage by reducing mutagenesis and cell transformation (Block, 1992; M. Meydani, 1995). In addition to its role as an antioxidant, vitamin E may also directly affect various cells of the immune system (i.e., natural killer [NK] and inflammatory cells), leading to an enhanced ability to inhibit tumor production (M. Meydani, 1995).

Byers and Guerrero (1995) have recently reviewed all epidemiologic studies on the topic of diet and cancer prevention in which intakes of vitamins E and C or fruit and vegetable consumption were estimated. Results showed that diets high in fruits and vegetables (≥ 5 servings/d) and, therefore, high in vitamin C are associated with lower risk of cancer of the oral cavity, esophagus, stomach, colon, and lung. The hormone-associated cancers of the breast and prostate appear to be less related to fruit and vegetable intake. Diets high in added vegetable oils, presumably high in vitamin E, have been less consistently associated with reduced cancer risk. However, when studies of vitamins E and C consumed as supplements are considered, there is little support for a protective role of either nutrient against cancer. Therefore, if vitamins E or C are protective against cancer, this effect may be due to their consumption in whole foods, where they are combined with other nutrients or bioactive compounds that together provide a protective effect against cancer. The most prudent approach seems to be one of increasing fruit and vegetable consumption in the diet, thus maximizing the potential benefits of antioxidant nutrients in terms of cancer prevention.

AIDS

Considerable evidence has accumulated that HIV-infected patients are under chronic oxidative stress as evidenced by increased levels of hydroperoxides and malondialdehyde (MDA) in serum (Pace and Leaf, 1995). This oxidative stress may contribute to various aspects of immune dysfunction in HIV disease pathogenesis, including viral replication, inflammation, decreased immune cell proliferation, loss of immune function, and apoptosis (Pace and Leaf, 1995). Furthermore, changes in levels of antioxidant nutrients have also been observed in various tissues of these patients (Pace and Leaf, 1995). Therefore, vitamins E, C, and other antioxidants may have immunoenhancing properties that could help normalize immune dysfunctions that lead to full-blown AIDS (Wang and Watson, 1993).

A number of studies by Watson and colleagues illustrate this point with regard to vitamin E (Wang et al., 1994a,b, 1995). These researchers have used C57BL/6 mice infected with LP-BM5 retrovirus to cause murine AIDS, which is functionally similar to human AIDS. Animals were supplemented with at least a 15-fold increase of vitamin E in a liquid diet (160 IU/liter). Vitamin E supplementation led to increased NK cell cytotoxicity, splenocyte proliferation, and IL-2 and interferon-γ levels, all of which are suppressed by retrovirus infection. Vitamin E also led to decreased IL-6, IL-10, and tumor necrosis factor [TNF]-α production, all of which had been increased by retrovirus infection. These findings suggest that high levels of vitamin E supplementation can modulate cytokine production and normalize immune dysfunctions during the development of murine AIDS. It is not clear, however, whether these immunological changes alter the clinical outcome of the disease.

Human studies have also suggested that vitamin E is involved in HIV pathogenesis, perhaps via its effect on IgE production (Shor-Posner et al., 1995). Elevated production of IgE has been demonstrated in persons infected with HIV-1 (Israel-Biet et al., 1992) and is associated with T-cell dysregulation, opportunistic infections, and an increase in allergic reactions (Carr et al., 1991; Gruchalla and Sullivan, 1991; Pedersen et al., 1991; Schwartzman et al., 1991; Wolf et al., 1991; Wright et al., 1990). Furthermore, IgE production has been shown to be affected by vitamin E status in an animal model (Inagaki et al., 1984). In a study of 100 asymptomatic HIV-1 seropositive and 42 HIV-1 seronegative homosexual men, Shor-Posner et al. (1995) found that the HIV-1 seropositive subjects with biochemical evidence of vitamin E deficiency had elevated IgE levels (independent of CD4 counts) compared with the seronegative controls and tended to have higher levels than the vitamin E-adequate seropositive subjects. In addition, subjects with low plasma vitamin E levels also had low dietary intakes of vitamin E compared with nondeficient HIV-seropositive subjects. Therefore, nutritional status seems to be an important factor in the IgE elevation observed during the early stages of HIV-1 disease, and supplementation may be warranted in HIV-1-infected individuals with vitamin E deficiency. Indeed, a study of HIV-infected patients has shown that, among HIV-seropositive individuals, the consumption of vitamins E and C in the form of supplements is in the megadose range (mean intake of 239 and 905 mg/d, respectively), driven in part by information received from health professionals and the media regarding the possible benefits of increased intakes of these nutrients (Martin et al., 1991).

In the Multicenter AIDS Cohort Study of 281 HIV-1 seropositive homosexual or bisexual men, it has been shown that individuals with the highest level of total intake of vitamin C from food and supplements had a significantly decreased rate of progression to AIDS (Tang et al., 1993). In a multinutrient statistical model, however, vitamin C remained only marginally significant, which suggests that when taken in combination with other nutrients, vitamin C may have less of an effect compared to the benefits of other nutrients.

Although AIDS is ultimately a fatal disease, improved means of treating infections can greatly prolong survival (Gorbach et al., 1993). Supplements of vitamins and minerals, including vitamins E and C, to combat increased oxidative stress are a recommended part of dietary interventions for AIDS patients (Gorbach et al., 1993). However, appropriate dosages have not yet been determined.

ASTHMA AND LUNG FUNCTION

It is possible that antioxidant defenses are of particular importance in the lung since a naturally high exposure to oxygen may be further increased by oxidative processes during inflammation and inhalation of oxidant air pollutants (Burney, 1995). Such damage could lead to permanent loss of lung function over time. It has, therefore, been hypothesized that vitamins E and C, acting either as antioxidants or through a direct effect on immune function, may reduce airway inflammation, thereby decreasing the severity of asthma or even preventing its occurrence in susceptible individuals (Hatch, 1995; Troisi et al., 1995).

Associations between several dietary factors assessed by a semiquantitative food frequency questionnaire and the incidence of asthma over a 10-y period were evaluated as part of the Nurses' Health Study of 77,866 women 34 to 68 years of age (Troisi et al., 1995). Women in the highest quintile of vitamin E intake from diet alone had a reduced risk of asthma (relative risk 0.53, $p = 0.0005$) compared with women in the lowest quintile of dietary intake. However, the use of vitamin C or E supplements was associated with a significant increase in the risk of asthma, although this seemed to be due to women at high risk of asthma initiating the use of vitamin supplements prior to diagnosis. These data suggest that although antioxidant supplementation is not an important determinant of adult-onset asthma, dietary intake of vitamin E may have a modest protective effect.

In another epidemiologic study, stronger evidence is provided that vitamin C and possibly vitamin E may influence lung function in middle and later life (Britton et al., 1995). In a cross-sectional survey of 2,633 subjects 18 to 70 years of age living in England, researchers found that higher dietary intakes of both vitamins C and E were associated with improved lung function (measured by spirometry). However, these two nutrients were significantly correlated, and after adjustment, there was no independent effect of vitamin E on lung function after allowing for the effect of vitamin C.

These findings are supported by results from NHANES I, which have also suggested that dietary vitamin C intake has a protective effect on pulmonary function (Schwartz and Weiss, 1994). Although these studies must be interpreted with caution, they do suggest that dietary intake of foods rich in vitamins C and E may be beneficial in decreasing the risk of asthma or reduced lung function, particularly among individuals at increased risk for these conditions (for example, smokers).

EXERCISE

Evidence exists that lipid peroxidation products suggestive of oxidative stress increase after exercise (Davies et al., 1982), although this has not been consistently observed, even after an acute bout of exercise (Cannon et al., 1990). Whether or not oxidative damage occurs during exercise seems to depend on a number of factors, including the intensity of exercise, the location of the sampling site, and the state of training of the subjects (Witt et al., 1992). Intense or exhaustive exercise in untrained individuals is more likely to result in oxidative damage, which is more likely to be detected in muscle samples than blood (Witt et al., 1992). Furthermore, if oxidative stress is great enough to overcome antioxidant defense systems in the body, then oxidative damage will inevitably occur (Witt et al., 1992). Therefore, a great deal of attention has recently been focused on whether antioxidant nutrients, in particular vitamins E and C, may help to reduce oxidative stress and damage during exercise.

Most studies do demonstrate a benefit of vitamins E and C in reducing measures of oxidative stress following exercise. Levels of breath pentane and serum MDA, indirect measures of free radical generation, have been shown to be lower at rest and after an acute bout of exercise among young healthy men consuming 1,000 mg vitamin C and 592 mg α-tocopherol equivalents per day compared with subjects receiving a placebo (Kanter et al., 1993).

In addition, both nutrients individually have also been shown to have beneficial effects in terms of reducing exercise-induced oxidative injury. M. Meydani et al. (1993) have demonstrated that vitamin E (800 IU dl-α-tocopherol) taken daily for 48 days by a group of young (22–29 years) and older (55–74 years) men led to lower urinary thiobarbituric acid excretion after a bout of eccentric exercise,[2] suggesting that vitamin E provides protection against exercise-induced oxidative injury. Furthermore, in a double-blind, placebo-controlled study, when 21 male subjects took vitamin E supplements (800 IU/d) for 48 days and then ran downhill on an inclined treadmill (Cannon et al., 1991), endotoxin-induced secretion of IL-1β was increased 154 percent in cells obtained from placebo subjects 24 hours postexercise; however, no significant exercise-related changes were observed in cells from vitamin E-supplemented subjects. This IL-1β response to vitamin E supplementation is consistent with a mechanism involving oxygen radicals. Specifically, exercise-induced oxygen radicals increased IL-1β secretion after an acute bout of eccentric exercise in cells from subjects taking a placebo but not from subjects taking vitamin E. In addition, urinary 3-methylhistidine, a measure of muscle proteolysis, was associated with IL-1β production. These findings suggest that vitamin E may be beneficial in reducing the oxygen radical-induced muscle damage of eccentric exercise.

In support of these findings, others have also shown that vitamin E supplementation reduces expired pentane and MDA levels in response to exercise (Dillard et al., 1978; Sumida et al., 1989). In addition, vitamin C supplementation (600 mg/d) has also been shown to reduce the incidence of upper respiratory tract infections in ultramarathon runners compared with subjects taking a placebo (Peters et al., 1993).

In summary, there is considerable evidence regarding the benefits of vitamin E and C supplementation in terms of reducing oxidative stress and/or damage during exercise. However, data remain incomplete, particularly in terms of the optimal amount of supplementation that should be recommended to achieve these benefits.

AUTHORS' CONCLUSIONS

By virtue of their role as antioxidant and immuno-enhancing nutrients, the benefits of vitamins E and C have been increasingly recognized and applied to various clinical situations including aging, cancer, AIDS, asthma, and exercise. The ultimate impact of these nutrients has been variable however, due to differences in whether dietary or supplemental sources of the vitamin are considered, and if supplements are utilized, the dosage and whether combinations of antioxidants are administered.

Most studies show that vitamin E can improve the immune response during aging and suggest that it can reduce the oxidative damage that may contribute to cancer, to the complications of AIDS, and to asthma as well as the damage that may occur during exercise. The strongest evidence seems to be associated with higher dietary intakes of vitamin E, as opposed to consumption of vitamin E in

---

[2] Eccentric exercise is when external resistance exceeds muscle force, the muscle lengthens and develops tension.

the form of supplements. The exceptions seem to be in the case of exercise and aging, for which supplementation with high levels of vitamin E have been utilized in order to achieve beneficial effects.

In terms of vitamin C, the evidence seems less conclusive for a benefit of this nutrient during aging, although as with vitamin E, a reduction in oxidative stress has been observed as a result of high dietary intake (or supplementation in the case of exercise) of vitamin C in cancer, AIDS, and asthma patients and with exercise. Additional research is necessary in order to further define the possible benefits of vitamins E and C in various disease states as well as their optimal dosages. Further investigation is also warranted to elucidate more fully the antioxidant and immuno-enhancing properties of these nutrients.

ACKNOWLEDGMENTS

This project has been funded at least in part with federal funds from the U.S. Department of Agriculture, Agricultural Research Service, under contract number 53-K06-01. The contents of this publication do not necessarily reflect the views or policies of the U.S. Department of Agriculture, nor does mention of trade names, commercial products, or organizations imply endorsement by the U.S. government.

The authors would like to thank Timothy S. McElreavy for preparation of this manuscript.

REFERENCES

Anderson, R., R. Oosthuizen, R. Maritz, A. Heron, and A. J. VanRensburg. 1980. The effects of increasing weekly doses of ascorbate on certain cellular and humoral immune function in volunteers. Am. J. Clin. Nutr. 33:71–76.
Block, G. 1992. Vitamin C status and cancer: Epidemiologic evidence of reduced risk. Ann. N.Y. Acad. Sci. 669:280–292.
Britton, J.R., I.D. Pavord, K.A. Richards, A.J. Knox, A.F. Wisniewski, S.A. Lewis, A.E. Tattersfield, and S.T. Weiss. 1995. Dietary antioxidant vitamin intake and lung function in the general population. Am. J. Respir. Crit. Care Med. 151:1383–1387.
Burney, P. 1995. The origins of obstructive airways disease: A role for diet? Am. J. Respir. Crit. Care Med. 151:1292–1293.
Byers, T., and N. Guerrero. 1995. Epidemiologic evidence for vitamin C and vitamin E in cancer prevention. Am. J. Clin. Nutr. 62:1385S–1392S.
Cannon, J.G., S.N. Meydani, R.A. Fielding, M.A. Fiatarone, M. Meydani, M. Farhangmehr, S.F. Orencole, J.B. Blumberg, and W.J. Evans. 1991. Acute phase response in exercise. II. Associations between vitamin E, cytokines, and muscle proteolysis. Am. J. Physiol. 260:R1235–R1240.
Cannon, J.G., S.F. Orencole, R.A. Fielding, M. Meydani, S.N. Meydani, M.A. Fiatarone, J.B. Blumberg, and W.J. Evans. 1990. Acute phase response in exercise: Interaction of age and vitamin E on neutrophils and muscle enzyme release. Am. J. Physiol. 259:R1214–R1219.

Carr, A., D.A. Cooper, and R. Penny. 1991. Allergic manifestations of human immunodeficiency (HIV) infection. J. Clin. Immunol. 11:55–64.

Davies, K.J.A., L. Packer, and G.A. Brooks. 1982. Free radicals and tissue damage produced by exercise. Biochem. Biophys. Res. Commun. 107:1198–1205.

Dillard, C.J., R.E. Litov, W.M. Savin, E.E. Dumelin, and A.L. Tappel. 1978. Effects of exercise, vitamin E, and ozone on pulmonary function and lipid peroxidation. J. Appl. Physiol. 45:927–932.

Frei, B., R. Stocker, and B.N. Ames. 1988. Antioxidant defenses and lipid peroxidation in human blood plasma. Proc. Natl. Acad. Sci. USA 85:9748–9752.

Goodwin, J.S. 1995. Decreased immunity and increased morbidity in the elderly. Nutr. Rev. 53:S41–S46.

Gorbach, S.L., T.A. Knox, and R. Roubenoff. 1993. Interactions between nutrition and infection with human immunodeficiency virus. Nutr. Rev. 51:226–234.

Gruchalla, R.S., and T.J. Sullivan. 1991. Detection of human IgE to sulfamethoxazole by skin testing with sulfamethoxazoyl-poly-l-tyrosine. J. Allergy Clin. Immunol. 88:784–792.

Hatch, G.E. 1995. Asthma, inhaled oxidant, and dietary antioxidants. Am. J. Clin. Nutr. 61:625S–630S.

Inagaki, N., H. Nagai, and A. Koda. 1984. Effect of vitamin E on IgE antibody formation in mice. J. Pharmacobiodynamics 7:70–74.

Israel-Biet, D., F. Labrousse, J.M. Tourani, H. Sors, J.M. Andrieu, and P. Even. 1992. Elevation of IgE in HIV-infected subjects: A marker of poor prognosis. J. Allergy Clin. Immunol. 89:68–75.

Jacob, R.A., D.S. Kelley, F.S. Pianalto, M.E. Swendseid, S.M. Henning, J.Z. Zhang, B.N. Ames, C.G. Fraga, and J.H. Peters. 1991. Immunocompetence and oxidant defense during ascorbate depletion of healthy men. Am. J. Clin. Nutr. 54:1302S–1309S.

Kanter, M.M., L.A. Nolte, and J.O. Holloszy. 1993. Effects of an antioxidant vitamin mixture on lipid peroxidation at rest and postexercise. J. Appl. Physiol. 74:965–969.

Kennes, B., I. Dumont, D. Brohee, C. Hubert, and P. Neve. 1983. Effect of vitamin C supplements on cell-mediated immunity in old people. Gerontology 29:305–310.

Makinodan, T. 1995. Patterns of age-related immunologic changes. Nutr. Rev. 53:S27–S34.

Martin, J.B., T. Easley-Shaw, and C. Collins. 1991. Use of selected vitamin and mineral supplements among individuals infected with human immunodeficiency virus. J. Am. Diet. Assoc. 91:476–478.

Meydani, M. 1995. Vitamin E. Lancet 345:170–175.

Meydani, M., W.J. Evans, G. Handelman, L. Biddle, R.A. Fielding, S.N. Meydani, J. Burrill, M.A. Fiatarone, J.B. Blumberg, and J.G. Cannon. 1993. Protective effect of vitamin E on exercise-induced oxidative damage in young and older adults. Am. J. Physiol. 264:R992–R998.

Meydani, M., S.N. Meydani, L. Leka, J. Gong, and J.B. Blumberg. 1994. Effect of long-term vitamin E supplementation on lipid peroxidation and immune responses of young and old subjects. FASEB J. 8:A415.Meydani, S.N. M. Meydani, J.B. Blumberg, L. Leka, M. Pedrosa, B.D. Stollar, and R. Diamond. 1997b. Safety assessment of long-term vitamin E supplementation in healthy elderly. FASEB J. 10:A448.

Meydani, S.N., M.P. Barklund, S. Liu, M. Meydani, R.A. Miller, J.G. Cannon, F.D. Morrow, R. Rocklin, and J.B. Blumberg. 1990. Vitamin E supplementation enhances cell-mediated immunity in healthy elderly subjects. Am. J. Clin. Nutr. 52:557–563.

Meydani, S.N., M. Meydani, J.B. Blumberg, L. Leka, M. Pedrosa, B.D. Stollar, and R. Diamond. 1997a. Safety assessment of long-term vitamin E supplementation in healthy elderly. FASEB J. 10:A448.

Meydani, S.N., M. Meydani, J.B. Blumberg, L.S. Leka, G. Siber, R. Loszewski, C. Thompson, M.C. Pedrosa, R.D. Diamond, and B.D. Stollar. 1997b. Vitamin E supplementation enhances *in vivo* immune response in healthy elderly: A dose-response study. J. Am. Med. Assoc. 277:1380–1386.

Meydani, S.N., D. Wu, M.S. Santos, and M.G. Hayek. 1995. Antioxidants and immune response in aged persons: Overview of present evidence. Am. J. Clin. Nutr. 62:1462S–1476S.

NRC (National Research Council). 1989. Recommended Dietary Allowances, 10th ed. Subcommittee on the Tenth Edition of the RDAs, Food and Nutrition Board, Commission of Life Sciences. Washington, D.C.: National Academy Press.

Pace, G.W., and C.D. Leaf. 1995. The role of oxidative stress in HIV disease. Free Radical. Biol. Med. 19:523–528.

Packer, J.E., T.F. Slater, and R.L. Willson. 1979. Direct observation of a free radical interaction between vitamin E and vitamin C. Nature 278:737–738.

Pedersen, M., C.M. Nielsen, and H. Permin. 1991. HIV-antigen-induced release of histamine from basophils from HIV infected patients: Mechanism and relation to disease progression and immunodeficiency. J. Allergy 46:206–212.

Penn, N.D., L. Purkins, J. Kelleher, R.V. Heatley, B.H. Mascie-Taylor, and P.W. Belfield. 1991. The effect of dietary supplementation with vitamins A, C and E on cell-mediated immune function in elderly long-stay patients: A randomized controlled trial. Age Ageing 20:169–174.

Peters, E.M., J.M. Goetzsch, B. Grobbelaar, and T.D. Noakes. 1993. Vitamin C supplementation reduces the incidence of postrace symptoms of upper-respiratory-tract infection in ultramarathon runners. Am. J. Clin. Nutr. 57:170–174.

Schwartz, J., and S.T. Weiss. 1994. Relationship between dietary vitamin C intake and pulmonary function in the First National Health and Nutrition Examination Survey (NHANES I). Am. J. Clin. Nutr. 59:110–114.

Schwartzman, W.A., M.W. Lambertus, C.A. Kennedy, and M.B. Goetz. 1991. Staphylococcal pyomyositis in patients infected by the human immunodeficiency virus. Am. J. Med. 90:595–600.

Shor-Posner, G., M.J. Miguez-Burbano, Y. Lu, D. Feaster, M. Fletcher, H. Sauberlich, and M.K. Baum. 1995. Elevated IgE level in relationship to nutritional status and immune parameters in early human immunodeficiency virus-1 disease. J. Allergy Clin. Immunol. 95:886–892.

Sumida, S., K. Tanaka, H. Kitao, and F. Nakadomo. 1989. Exercise-induced lipid peroxidation and leakage of enzymes before and after vitamin E supplementation. Int. J. Biochem. 21:835–838.

Tang, A.M., N.M. Graham, A.J. Kirby, L.D. McCall, W.C. Willett, and A.J. Saah. 1993. Dietary micronutrient intake and risk of progression to acquired immunodeficiency syndrome (AIDS) in human immunodeficiency virus type 1 (HIV-1)-infected homosexual men. Am. J. Epidemiol. 138:937–951.

Troisi, R.J., W.C. Willett, S.T. Weiss, D. Trichopoulos, B. Rosner, and F.E. Speizer. 1995. A prospective study of diet and adult-onset asthma. Am. J. Resp. Crit. Care Med. 151:1401–1408.

Wang, Y., and R.R. Watson. 1993. Is vitamin E supplementation a useful agent in AIDS therapy? Prog. Food Nutr. Sci. 17:351–375.

Wang, Y., D.S. Huang, C.D. Eskelson, and R.R. Watson. 1994a. Long-term dietary vitamin E retards development of retrovirus-induced disregulation in cytokine production. Clin. Immunol. Immunopathol. 72:70–75.

Wang, Y., D.S. Huang, B. Liang, and R.R. Watson. 1994b. Nutritional status and immune responses in mice with murine AIDS are normalized by vitamin E supplementation. J. Nutr. 124:2024–2032.

Wang, Y., D.S. Huang, S. Wood, and R.R. Watson. 1995. Modulation of immune function and cytokine production by various levels of vitamin E supplementation during murine AIDS. Immunopharmacology 29:225–233.

Witt, E.H., A.Z. Reznick, C.A. Viguie, P. Starke-Reed, and L. Packer. 1992. Exercise, oxidative damage, and effects of antioxidant manipulation. J. Nutr. 122:766–773.

Wolf, R., J. Oph, and I. Yust. 1991. Atopic dermatitis provoked by AL721 in a patient with acquired immunodeficiency syndrome. Ann. Allergy 66:421–422.

Wright, D.N., R.P. Nelson, D.K. Ledford, E. Fernandez-Caldas, W.L. Trudeau, and R.F. Lockey. 1990. Serum IgE and human immunodeficiency virus (HIV) infection. J. Allergy Clin. Immunol. 85:445–452.

DISCUSSION

HARRIS LIEBERMAN: I just wanted to say that I think not only are the methods that you have used in your work of direct relevance to the military population, but the population that you are working with actually has many similarities with regard to the kind of problems that we have.

We are talking about studying healthy people who have potentially subclinical deficits in function as opposed to more severe kinds of deficits in function associated with severe illness.

I did want to ask you a question, too. You had some sort of informal data on illness levels in the patients in your vitamin E-supplemented study. What was the shape of the dose-response function in those self-reports? Did it appear that the 200 mg was also optimal?

SIMIN NIKBIN MEYDANI: It looked like it, but that is just about it. You know, the numbers are very small, and I am even stretching it showing the combined data [all three vitamin E-supplement group vs. placebo], but it looks like that.

STEVE GAFFIN: Any possible additional benefits from omega-3 fatty acids?

SIMIN NIKBIN MEYDANI: We have done work with the elderly and omega-3 fatty acids. Actually, if you give it to the elderly, it causes a decrease in T-cell proliferation—also in DTH—and we think that is because when you give omega-3 fatty acids, you increase the requirement for vitamin E.

Now, if you combine vitamin E with omega-3 fatty acids, you might see a very different picture, but by itself, it actually decreases T-cell function, but it also decreases cytokines—the inflammatory cytokines like IL-1 and TNF, which could be useful.

BRUCE BISTRIAN: This comment really refers to both Dr. Shippee's talk and yours also. I was involved in the early assessment of CMI, the skin test, and I would like to mention to you because of the importance of this that whereas it looks like transformation data have, to my knowledge, never been collated with any clinical outcome, the anergy data have been extraordinarily well collated with many, many different populations, and in that regard if you recategorize, it is very important, the antigen should be very strictly defined, that being less than 2 mm to any of the antigens because if you have people like that, their risk if they were like that for a long period of time, we have known from the elderly, the risk of outcome is dramatically impaired. Most important for the military: if you have true anergy and those soldiers are wounded, they are often in the hospital and would probably be impaired by that. I would be very careful and concerned how much anergy is truly defined, how much you are producing. If you are already producing substantial amounts of anergy, then you have a very serious concern.

SIMIN NIKBIN MEYDANI: I think that is a very good point.

ERHARD HAUS: Basically that is what I think. First of all, you cannot comment that antioxidants cause decantenation, which in a military environment with sleep deprivation might try to convince them it is all right. Any thoughts about this?

SIMIN NIKBIN MEYDANI: I would be able to tell you probably in 3 or 5 months because we are doing a study with that currently. So, I will be able to tell you that.

ROBERT NESHEIM: Thank you very much. Because of the time schedule, with the commander coming at lunch, we have to move fast. But go ahead.

HARRIS LIEBERMAN: Is arachidonic acid released?

SIMIN NIKBIN MEYDANI: That, of course, could be a possibility. The reason we didn't concentrate on it was that as I said we don't see any difference in the level of arachidonic acid in the macrophages, and also if you noticed, there was only an increase in cyclooxygenase and 5-lipoxygenase products and not in the 12 and 15-lipoxygenase products. So, that indicates to me that perhaps it is not the release of arachidonic acid, because if it was release of arachidonic acid and a change in phospholipase activity, it would be likely that all the products of arachidonic acid would be affected. But I think that is a possibility.

DR. KENNEDY: This is a comment more than a question because I am about to go on study for a month, but what did you use to stimulate IL-2?

SIMIN NIKBIN MEYDANI: PHA and Con-A. We either used PHA or Con-A, and both of them work.

DR. KENNEDY: Ron didn't present all our work. We have some interesting data to suggest that part of the stress response in Special Forces may be due to a shift in the paradigm from Th2 [T-helper 2] to Th1, and also we are interested in some recent data that look at surgical stress. Have you looked at FOS[3] or AP1[4]?

SIMIN NIKBIN MEYDANI: Not yet, but as part of looking at the mechanism, that is something we will be looking at. I do want to mention that we have done flow cytometry, and so far we have not seen any effect of vitamin E on the percentage of T-cells or B-cells. It doesn't mean that Th1 and Th2 are not being affected, and in fact some of our cytokine data indicate that perhaps that will be affected, but the total number of cells, you know the CD3s and so forth, is not affected by vitamin E supplementation. Neither is the total immunoglobulin level.

So, the specific response to the vaccine is affected but not the total immunoglobulin level.

---

[3] FOS is a nuclear protooncogene protein, also characterized as an immediate early gene product because of the time of its expression in relation to the cell cycle. FOS transcription is stimulated by injury.

[4] AP1 is a transcription factor known to play a key role in the regulation of transcription of IL-2 and some other immune responses.

Nutrition and Immune Function, 1999
Pp. 305–316. Washington, D.C.
National Academy Press

14

Fatty Acids and Immune Functions

Darshan S. Kelley[1]

INTRODUCTION

Dietary lipids comprise mainly triglycerides and only small amounts of phospholipids, cholesterol, and other sterols. Chemically triglycerides are the triacylglycerols or glycerol molecules esterified with three fatty acids. Fatty acids without any double bond in their carbon chain are called saturated, and those with one or more double bonds are called unsaturated. Unsaturated fatty acids with more than one double bond are called polyunsaturated fatty acids (PUFAs). Based on the position of the first double bond from the methylene end, unsaturated fatty acids are classified into the n-3, n-6, and the n-9 series, which cannot be interconverted in animals. The first double bond for the n-3 series is between C3 and C4 from the methylene end, for the n-6 series it is between C6 and C7, and for the n-9 series it is between C9 and C10. Examples of the saturated fatty acids include palmitic acid, 16:0, and stearic acid, 18:0; for the n-9 type include palmitoleic acid, 16:1n-9, and oleic acid, 18:1n-9; for the n-6 type, linoleic acid, 18:2n-6 (LA), and arachidonic acid, 20:4n-6 (AA); for the n-3 type, α-linolenic acid, 18:3n-3 (ALA), eicosapentaenoic acid, 20:5n-3

---

[1] Darshan S. Kelley, U.S. Department of Agriculture-Agricultural Research Service, Western Human Nutrition Research Center, Presidio of San Francisco, CA 94129

(EPA), and docosahexaenoic acid, 22:6n-3 (DHA). Dietary sources of fatty acids include animal fats, coconut and palm oils for saturated fatty acids; olive and canola oils for oleic acid; sunflower, corn, and soybean oils for LA; organ meats and eggs for AA; flaxseed and pyrilla oils for ALA; marine oils for EPA and DHA. Humans cannot synthesize PUFA of the n-3 and n-6 series, which are termed essential fatty acids (EFAs); they can however, elongate LA to AA and convert ALA to EPA and DHA by a complex pathway. The same desaturases and elongases are involved in the elongation of the n-3 and n-6 PUFA, and these enzymes seem to have a preference for n-3 over the n-6 PUFA.

AA is the major PUFA in most cell membranes, and it is a precursor for a number of compounds termed *eicosanoids*. AA is converted into prostaglandins, prostacyclins, and thromboxanes through the cyclooxygenase pathway and to leukotrienes and lipoxins through the lipoxygenase pathway. Depending on their concentration and type, prostaglandins and leukotrienes stimulate or inhibit the activity of the immune cells. Other 20-C fatty acids, like dihomo-gamma linolenic acid (DGLA, 20:3n-6) and EPA compete with AA for the lipoxygenase and cyclooxygenase enzymes and reduce the products formed from AA, including eicosanoids of the 2-series and leukotriene B4, which are potent modulators of the immune cells.

Both the total fat intake and the ratios between fatty acids of different classes influence the activity of immune cells. Such information was initially obtained through epidemiological human studies and studies conducted with cultured cells and animal models. These studies showed that EFAs are required for the growth and maintenance of the immune cells, and FFAs (free fatty acids) are produced and secreted during the activation of these cells. A number of intervention studies regarding the effects of the amount and composition of dietary fat on human immune response have been conducted in the last decade, results from these human studies are discussed here.

AMOUNT OF FAT INTAKE AND HUMAN IMMUNE RESPONSE

Reduction in total fat intake has been found to enhance immune response (IR) in humans as noted in several studies. We noted that the proliferation of peripheral blood mononuclear cells (PBMCs) cultured with T- and B-cell-specific mitogens almost doubled when the level of fat in the diet of healthy men was reduced from 30 to 25 energy percent (en%) for 11 weeks (Kelley et al., 1989). Similar results were found in another study conducted in healthy women whose fat intake was reduced from 40 en% to 25 or 31 en% for 6 weeks (Kelley et al., 1992a). In these studies, the reduction in fat intake also resulted in an increase in the number of circulating T- and B-lymphocytes, while the ratio between the Th- (helper) and Ts- (suppressor) cells did not change. An increase in the proliferation of PBMCs in response to the T-cell mitogen concanavalin A (Con-A) and in the *in vitro* secretion of interleukin (IL)-1 and tumor necrosis factor (TNF) was also found in a group of elderly men and women when their fat intake was reduced from 36 to 27 en% for 6 months (Meydani et al., 1993). An increase in PBMC proliferation suggests a faster response in the event of pathogenic attack. Results from two other studies show an increase in the number (Rasmussen et al., 1994) and activity (Barone et al., 1989) of natural killer (NK) cells when the fat intake was reduced by about 10 en%. Other indices of IR tested in these studies, including delayed-type hypersensitivity (DTH) and the secretion of IL-6 were not altered, which suggests that not all indices of IR are equally affected by the reduction in fat intake. This is to be expected because different immune cells have different half lives and respond to different stimuli.

n-6 PUFA AND HUMAN IR

The intake of n-6 PUFA was also changed in the two studies dealing with total fat intake mentioned earlier (Kelley et al., 1989, 1992a). In one of the studies, the level of LA was changed from 5 en% to 3 en% for one-half of the subjects and to 13 en% for the remaining half of subjects for 11 weeks (Kelley et al., 1989). The other study was a cross-over type, wherein each subject was fed a diet with 3 and 10 en% LA for 6 weeks (Kelley et al., 1992a), and the stabilization diet contained 5 en% LA. In these two studies, changing the level of LA from 3 to 13 en% had no adverse effect on several indices of IR tested, when the total fat contents of the intervention diets were maintained constant. Inhibition of IR may have happened if the increase in n-6 PUFA was accompanied by an increase in total fat intake. When the increase in LA intake was accompanied with an increase in total fat (22 to 28 en%), it did inhibit NK cell activity in the healthy men (Barone et al., 1989). In this study, inhibition may have resulted from the additive inhibitory effects of total fat and of n-6 PUFA. In general, these studies indicate that moderate levels of LA consumption have no adverse effects on human IR. The plasma and adipose tissue levels of n-6 PUFA presumably reflect their dietary intake, and significant negative correlations were found between NK cell activity and the plasma levels of total PUFA, n-6 PUFA, and LA (Rasmussen et al., 1994) in a group of Danish men with mean age of 71 years. However, no correlation was found between the adipose tissue PUFA and NK cell activity or PBMC proliferation in American men with mean age of 47 years (Berry et al., 1987). The difference in the age of the subjects and the tissue being investigated may account for the difference in these two studies. Other factors that may explain inconsistencies between some of the results from various studies include differences in total fat intake, antioxidant nutrients, duration of feeding, and the index being examined.

In the above studies regarding n-6 PUFA, the level of LA and not that of AA in the diets was changed. LA is rapidly metabolized with only a limited conversion to AA. Studies conducted in animals indicate that dietary AA may be metabolized differently from the endogenously synthesized AA (Whelan et al., 1993), and preliminary human studies indicated harmful effects of dietary

AA (Seyberth et al., 1975). AA and its metabolites have been found to inhibit activity of immune cells *in vitro*. In a recent study, this author examined the effect of dietary AA on IR and several other health parameters of young men (Kelley et al., 1997). Ten healthy men were fed a basal diet containing 30 en% fat (10:10:10; saturated: monounsaturated: polyunsaturated) and 200 mg/d of AA for 15 days, after which the diet of six men was supplemented with 1.5 g of additional AA from ARASCO Oil (Martek Biosciences Corporation, Columbia, Md.) for 50 days, and the other four men remained on the basal diet. The diets of the two groups were crossed over for the next 50 days. AA supplementation had no adverse effect on a number of indices of IR tested, including DTH response, NK cell activity, lymphocyte proliferation in response to Con-A, phytohemagglutinin (PHA), and pokeweed mitogens, as well as *in vitro* secretion of IL-1, IL-2, and TNF. However, it significantly increased the number of circulating neutrophils and the secondary response to influenza vaccine. The feeding of the low-fat, nutritionally balanced diet was found in this study to enhance several indices of IR including PBMC proliferation and cytokine production, which was also found in the earlier studies from this laboratory (Kelley et al., 1989, 1992a). The results of this study show that moderate levels of AA fed as natural triglycerides have no adverse effects on human IR, even if AA is a precursor for the inflammatory eicosanoids. It is possible that higher amounts of AA may have adverse effects on human IR; however, for nutritional purposes, the amount of AA fed was adequate.

n-3 PUFA AND HUMAN IMMUNE RESPONSE

In the last few years, interest in examining the effect of n-3 PUFA on immune status has increased, because these fatty acids have been found (1) to be beneficial in the management of some human autoimmune diseases and (2) to reduce the incidence of certain types of cancer in animal models. Studies examining the effect of n-3 PUFA on human IR have used both plant sources (containing ALA) and marine oils (containing EPA and DHA). Most of these human studies indicate inhibition of human IR by n-3 PUFA. Adding flax seed oil to provide 6 en% ALA for 8 weeks to a basal diet containing 23 en% fat inhibited the PBMC proliferation and DTH response of male soldiers (Kelley et al., 1991). The design of this study does not permit one to distinguish if this inhibition by flaxseed oil was due to increased fat intake or increased ALA intake or both. The feeding of flax seed oil caused small but significant increases in the ALA and EPA levels of the PBMC (Kelley et al., 1993), making it difficult to distinguish if the inhibition was caused by ALA or EPA or both. Several other indices of IR, including serum and salivary immunoglobulin levels, serum levels of complement proteins C_3 and C_4, and the number of circulating lymphocytes bearing markers for T-, Th-, Ts-, and B-cells were not changed in the study with flax seed oil (Kelley et al., 1991). ALA supplementation has also been reported to inhibit PBMC proliferation in ALA-deficient patients (Bjerve et al., 1989) and the *in vitro* secretion of TNF-α and IL-1β in healthy men (Caughey et al., 1996). The latter study with healthy men provided 14 g of ALA for 4 weeks and included a control group that provided only 1.1 g ALA. The total fat contents of the ALA and control diets were comparable (29.4 en%), which indicates that the inhibition of cytokine production was specifically caused by ALA.

Fish oils have been found to inhibit several aspects of neutrophil, monocyte, and lymphocyte functions in several human studies (Endres et al., 1989, 1993; Kramer et al., 1991; Lee et al., 1985; Meydani et al., 1991; Molvig et al., 1991; Payan et al., 1986; Virella et al., 1989). Fish oil intake of 18 g/d, in addition to the fat content of the basal diet, inhibited neutrophil and monocyte functions within 6 weeks of its supplementation, while it failed to inhibit T-cell functions as determined from IL-2 production within this time of intake (Caughey et al., 1996; Endres et al., 1989). The production of IL-2 was, however, significantly inhibited 10 weeks after the discontinuation of fish oil intake. The inhibition of neutrophil functions by fish oils could be overcome within 10 weeks of discontinuation, while it took 20 weeks to overcome the inhibition of lymphocyte and monocyte functions. The differences in the time taken to cause or overcome inhibition are presumably due to different half-lives of various immune cells, as mentioned earlier for the total fat intake. In this study, inhibition of IR may have resulted from both the intake of n-3 PUFA and the added fat. The amount of fish oil has varied from 6 to 20 g/d, and the inhibition of immune parameters was observed within 6 or more weeks of fish oil intake in various studies (Endres et al., 1989, 1993; Kramer et al., 1991; Lee et al., 1985; Meydani et al., 1991; Molvig et al., 1991; Payan et al., 1986; Virella et al., 1989). Since 1 g of fish oils contains on an average 180 mg EPA and 120 mg DHA, the intake of EPA and DHA in these studies ranged from 2 to 6 g/d.

In addition to the above studies with fish oils, the effect of fish intake on human IR has also been examined in several studies (Kelley et al., 1992b; Meydani et al., 1993). Reducing total fat intake from 36 to 27 en%, with a concomitant increase in fish intake (EPA + DHA = 1.23 g/d or 0.54 en%) by men and women over the age of 40 years for 6 months significantly inhibited several indices of IR, including DTH, lymphocyte proliferation, and secretion of IL-1, IL-6, and TNF, when compared with the corresponding values when subjects were fed the high-fat diet (Meydani et al., 1993). However, the switch to low-fat and low-fish intake (EPA + DHA = 0.27 g/d or 0.13 en%) for the same period did not inhibit any of these indices. The lymphocyte proliferation and the secretion of TNF and IL-1 were actually enhanced by the low-fish diet, which was perhaps caused by the reduction in fat intake from 36 to 27 en%, rather than by the low n-3 PUFA intake. In a cross-over study young, healthy men (25–40 years) were fed salmon, 500 g/d (EPA + DHA = 2.1 en%) for 40 days. None of the indices of IR tested were inhibited by the consumption of this amount of salmon (Kelley et al., 1992b). However, the DTH response was significantly increased, which was perhaps due to the reduction in total fat intake from 29 to 23 en%. Thus, it is important not to view just the changes in n-3 PUFA intake but also in total fat and the ratios between n-6 and n-3 PUFA. The age and antioxidant nutritional status are other important factors that determine the impact of n-3 PUFA on human IR.

CLINICAL TRIALS WITH n-3 PUFA

The immuno-inhibitory effects of n-3 PUFA along with their beneficial effects for cardiovascular health prompted a number of studies with these fatty acids in the management of autoimmune and inflammatory diseases. The overall health of the patients was improved by fish oil supplementation in these studies, although the laboratory tests usually did not show corresponding improvements. The diets of rheumatoid arthritis patients when supplemented with fish oils led to a reduction in swollen and tender joints, morning stiffness, and pain index (Kremer et al., 1995). Fish oil supplementation has also been reported to decrease symptoms of lupus (Walton et al., 1991), psoriasis (Kojima et al., 1989), cystic fibrosis (Lawrence and Sorrell, 1993), ulcerative colitis (Stenson et al., 1992), and inflammatory bowel disease (O'Marn, 1987). Early restenosis after angioplasty decreased (Gapinski et al., 1993) and renal functions in patients maintained on cyclosporin after kidney or liver transplant improved (Badalamenti et al., 1995; Berthoux et al., 1992) with fish oil supplementation. The intake of fish oils in these studies ranged from 4 to 20 g/d for 6 weeks to 6 months. The circulating levels of several cytokines including IL-1, IL-2, IL-4, IL-6, TNF, and interferon-γ decreased with fish oil consumption in patients with advanced colorectal cancer compared with the corresponding values prior to fish oil consumption (Purasiri et al., 1994). It took from 2 to 6 months to lower the levels of various cytokines, which were restored to the original levels within 3 months of fish oil discontinuation. In healthy adults, the maximal increase in oral temperature following typhoid vaccination was attenuated by the prior consumption of fish oils (4.5 g/d) for 6 to 8 weeks (Cooper et al., 1993). Thus, evidence from both *in vitro* and *in vivo* studies shows the inhibition of IR by n-3 PUFA. In contrast to the results from these *in vivo* studies with several patient groups and results from *in vitro* studies conducted with the cells isolated from healthy subjects after the feeding of n-3 PUFA, where n-3 PUFA was found to inhibit IR, in patients with asthma (Payan et al., 1986) and ALA deficiency (Bjerve et al., 1989), n-3 PUFA supplementation was found to enhance PBMC proliferation and the number of circulating T-lymphocytes, respectively. Interaction with the drugs taken or the effects of EFA deficiency may have resulted in the stimulation of these indices of IR in these patients.

Although the results from clinical trials with fish oils seem encouraging, any benefit from their intake must outweigh the risk associated with the overall suppression of IR. The clinical relevance of such immune suppression is not now known and must be evaluated before the intake of fish oils can be recommended in the management of such disorders. Because most fish oils are rich in cholesterol, the risk of increased cholesterol intake should also be considered. Moreover, the increased need for antioxidant nutrients should be considered whenever the diet is supplemented with fish oils. The risk/benefit ratios may vary in different individuals and for the same individual under various set of conditions. Thus, fish oil supplementation should not be done without clinical supervision. The safe level of fish oil intake for subjects over 40 years is probably between 0.27 and 1.23 g/d of EPA + DHA, because 1.23 g/d inhibited several indices of IR, while 0.27 g/d did not. From a nutritional point of view, the consumption of fish 2 to 3 times a week or that of ALA up to 5 g/d by the general adult population should not have any adverse effect on IR. Further studies are needed to determine the requirements and the safe levels for EPA and DHA intake in various population groups. Because fish oils contain both EPA and DHA, it is also important to establish the role of these fatty acids individually. The author has just completed a metabolic unit study in which the effect of adding DHA to the diets of healthy men was examined. Results from this study should be available shortly.

MECHANISMS BY WHICH DIETARY FAT ALTERS IMMUNE RESPONSE

A number of substances and/or mechanisms listed below may be involved in mediating the effects of dietary fat on IR:

• *Serum lipoproteins*. Both the concentration and composition of dietary fat (fatty acids as well cholesterol) can alter serum lipoprotein profile, which influences the activity of the immune cells. *In vitro* studies have shown that low-density lipoproteins (LDL) inhibited lymphocyte and neutrophil functions, while high-density lipoproteins (HDL) enhanced neutrophil chemotaxis and phagocytosis. Other studies have indicated that lymphocyte proliferation *in vitro* was positively correlated with the number of HDL receptors and negatively correlated with the number of LDL receptors. One of the mechanisms by which LDL inhibits lymphocyte and monocyte functions is through apo proteins B and E (apo B and E). Other lipoproteins (very low density, intermediate density and chylomicrons) that are enriched in apo B and apo E also inhibit immune cells. Whether the serum lipoprotein changes caused by dietary fat are large enough to affect IR *in vivo* needs to be investigated.

• *Eicosanoid type and concentration*. Fatty acids of the n-3 and n-6 type yield different types of eicosanoids, which have different effects on immune cells. Changing the ratios between n-3 and n-6 PUFA intake alters the type and concentration of eicosanoids produced, since the same enzymes are involved in the metabolism of both types of PUFA. In general, eicosanoids derived from the n-3 PUFA are less potent mediators of inflammation than those derived from

AA. Furthermore, the effects of these eicosanoids are dose dependent, that is, small concentrations $(10^{-10} - 10^{-12} \, M)$ of prostaglandin-E$_2$ (PGE$_2$) and leukotriene-B$_4$ (LTB$_4$) stimulate some of the immune cells, while concentrations higher than $10^{-9} \, M$ inhibit the same cells.

• *Oxidative stress.* Increasing the PUFA intake increases oxidative stress, which if not counterbalanced by antioxidant nutrients, can damage cells and inhibit IR. The clearance of oxidized lipoproteins is through the scavenger receptors on the macrophages, and this receptor is not subject to the same feedback inhibition by the intracellular cholesterol as is the receptor for the native LDL. Thus, the antioxidant nutrient status can have profound effects on the IR, and it must be considered when evaluating the effects of dietary fat on IR.

• *Membrane fluidity.* Dietary fatty acids incorporated into membrane lipids can change membrane fluidity, which increases with an increased content of unsaturated membrane lipids. Changes in membrane fluidity can affect intercellular interaction, receptor expression, nutrient transport and signal transduction. All these factors can affect cell growth.

Any single dietary intervention may involve more than one of the above substances and/or mechanisms. It is also possible that some fatty acids directly affect the cells of the immune system.

AUTHOR'S CONCLUSIONS AND RECOMMENDATIONS

Interaction between several factors, including total fat, its composition, and the ratios between various classes of fatty acids; duration of feeding; antioxidant nutrient status; and age and health status of the subjects determines the net effect of dietary fat on IR. Because of this complex interaction, not all individuals respond equally to changes in fat intake. Furthermore, different indices of IR respond differently to changes in fat intake. In general, when other factors are maintained constant, reduction in total fat intake enhances several indices of human IR, and the converse is true when fat intake is increased. If total fat intake is not changed, a moderate increase in the consumption of n-6 PUFA (LA or AA) does not adversely affect several indices of IR tested. A number of studies indicate inhibition of several indices of human IR, with an increased consumption of n-3 PUFA (ALA, EPA, and DHA). Most of these studies lacked a concomitant control group, or the studies did not maintain a constant total fat intake. The inclusion of a control group is important in order to rule out the effects of seasonal changes or the inhibition in IR due to increased fat intake. There has been limited success in the management of autoimmune disorders by supplementing the diets of such patients with n-3 PUFA. However, such practice is not recommended without clinical supervision because of the risk of overall inhibition of IR. Current recommendations by the American Heart Association to reduce total fat intake to 30 en%, with 10 en% from each of the saturated, monounsaturated, and polyunsaturated fatty acids to improve cardiovascular health, will also improve IR in most individuals who consume diets containing more than 30 en% fat. There are currently no recommendations in the United States regarding the intake of n-3 PUFA. However, daily intakes of 200 to 400 mg of EPA+ DHA or up to 5 g of ALA should have no adverse effects on the IR of healthy adults.

These findings regarding the effects of total fat and n-3 PUFA have significant implications for developing nutritional guidelines for the military. The current fat content of the military rations is well above 30 en percent and reducing it to 30 en percent will improve not only the cardiovascular health but will also enhance several indices of IR. However, this improvement in IR must outweigh the reduction in energy density and palatability of military rations. Enhanced IR may improve general health under a variety of situations, but it can be deleterious under several other conditions like autoimmune disorders or organ transplant. We need to develop guidelines tailored to individual needs, however for the general public including the military, a reduction in total fat with some increase in the intake of n-3 PUFA should prove to be generally healthy. There may also be specific situations under which the incorporation of small amounts of n-3 PUFA into the diet of the military personnel will be useful in the management of autoimmune disorders.

REFERENCES

Badalamenti, S., F. Salerno, E. Lorenzano, G. Paone, G. Como, S. Finnazzi, A.C. Sacchetta, A. Rimola, G. Graziani, D. Galmarini, and C. Ponticelli. 1995. Renal effects of dietary fish oil supplementation with fish oil in cyclosporine-treated liver transplant recipients. Hepatology 22:1695–1701.

Barone, J., J.R. Hebert, and M.M. Reddy. 1989. Dietary fat and natural killer cell activity. Am. J. Clin. Nutr. 50:861–867.

Berry, E.M., J. Hirsch, J. Most, D.J. McNamara, and S. Cunningham-Rundles. 1987. Dietary fat, plasma lipoproteins, and immune functions in middle-aged American men. Nutr. Cancer 9:129–142.

Berthoux, F.C., C. Guerin, and G. Burgard. 1992. One-year randomized controlled trial with omega-3 fatty acid-fish oil in clinical renal transplant. Transplant. Proc. 24:2578–2582.

Bjerve, K.S., S. Fischer, F. Wammer, and T. England. 1989. α-linolenic acid and long-chain omega-3 fatty acid supplementation in three patients with omega-3 fatty acid deficiency. Am. J. Clin. Nutr. 49:290–300.

Caughey, G.E., E. Montzioris, R.A. Gibson, L.G. Cleland, and M.J. James. 1996. The effect on human tumor necrosis factor-α and interleukin-1β production of diets enriched in n-3 fatty acids from vegetable oil or from fish oil. Am. J. Clin. Nutr. 63:116–122.

Cooper, A.L., L. Gibbons, M.A., Horan, R.A. Little, and N.J. Rothwell. 1993. Effect of dietary fish oil supplementation on fever and cytokine production in human volunteers. Clin. Nutr. 12:321–328.

Endres, S., R. Ghorbani, V.E. Kelley, K. Georgilis, G. Lonnemann, J.W.M. van der Meer, J.G. Cannon, T.S. Rogers, M.S. Klempner, P.C. Weber, E.J. Schaefer, S.M. Wolff, and C.A. Dinarello. 1989. The effect of dietary supplementation with n-3 polyunsaturated fatty acids on the synthesis of interleukin-1 and tumor necrosis factor by mononuclear cells. N. Engl. J. Med. 320:265–271.

Endres, S., S.N. Meydani, R. Ghorbani, R. Schindler, and C.A. Dinarello. 1993. Dietary supplementation with n-3 fatty acids suppresses interleukin-2 production and mononuclear cell proliferation. J. Leukocyte Biol. 54:599–603.

Gapinski, J.P., J.V. VanRuiswyk, G.R. Henderbert, and G.S. Schectman. 1993. Preventing restenosis with fish oils following coronary angioplasty. Arch. Intern. Med. 153:1595–1601.

Kelley, D.S., L.B. Branch, and J.M. Iacono. 1989. Nutritional modulation of human status. Nutr. Res. 9:965–975.

Kelley, D.S., L.B. Branch, J.E. Love, P.C. Taylor, Y.M. Rivera, and J.M. Iacono. 1991. Dietary α-linolenic acid and immunocompetence in humans. Am. J. Clin. Nutr. 53:40–46.

Kelley, D.S., R.M. Dougherthy, L.B. Branch, P.C. Taylor, and J.M. Iacono. 1992a. Concentration of dietary n-6 polyunsaturated fatty acids and human immune status. Clin. Immunol. Immunopathol. 62:240–244.

Kelley, D.S., G.J. Nelson, L.B. Branch, P.C. Taylor, Y.M. Rivera, and P.C. Schmidt. 1992b. Salmon diet and human immune status. Eur. J. Clin. Nutr. 46:397–404.

Kelley, D.S., G.J. Nelson, J.E. Love, L.B. Branch, P.C. Taylor, P.C. Schmidt, B.E. Mackey, and J.M. Iacono. 1993. Dietary α-linolenic acid alters tissue fatty acid composition, but not blood lipids, lipoproteins or coagulation status in humans. Lipids 28:533–537.

Kelley, D.S., P.C. Taylor, G.J. Nelson, P.C. Schmidt, and B.E. Mackey. 1997. Effects of dietary arachidonic acid on human response. Lipids 32:449–456.

Kojima, T., T. Terano, E. Tanabe, S. Okamoto, Y. Tamura, and S. Yoshida. 1989. Effect of highly purified eicosapentaenoic acid on psoriasis. J. Am. Acad. Dermatol. 21:150–151.

Kramer, T.R., N. Schoene, L.W. Douglass, J.W. Judd, J.T. Ballard-Barbash, R. Taylor, P.R. Bhagavan, and P.P. Nair. 1991. Increased vitamin E intake restores fish oil-induced suppressed blastogenesis of mitogen-stimulated T-lymphocytes. Am. J. Clin. Nutr. 54:896–902.

Kremer, J.M., D.A. Lawrence, G.F. Petrillo, L.L. Litts, P.M. Mullaly, R.I. Rynes, R.P. Stocker, N. Parhami, N.S. Greenstein, B.R. Fuchs, A. Mathur, D.R. Robinson, R.I. Sperling, and J. Bigaouette. 1995. Effects of high-dose fish oil on rheumatoid arthritis after stopping nonsteroidal anti-inflammatory drugs. Arthritis Rheum. 38:1107–1114.

Lawrence, R., and T. Sorrell. 1993. Eicosapentaenoic acid in cystic fibrosis. Lancet 342:465–469.

Lee, T.H., R.L. Hoover, J.D. Williams, R.I. Sperling, J. Ravalese, B.W. Spur, D.R. Robinson, E.J. Corey, R.A. Lewis, and K.F. Austen. 1985. Effect of dietary enrichment with eicosapentaenoic acid and docosahexaenoic acids on *in vitro* neutrophil and monocyte leukotriene generation and neutrophil function. N. Engl. J. Med. 312:1217–1224.

Meydani, S.N., S. Endres, M.N. Woods, B.R. Goldin, C. Soo, A. Morrill-Labrode, C.A. Dinarello, and S.L. Gorbach. 1991. Oral n-3 fatty acid supplementation suppresses cytokine production and lymphocyte proliferation: Comparison between young and old women. J. Nutr. 121:547–555.

Meydani, S.N., A.H. Lichtenstein, S. Cornwall, M. Meydani, B.R. Goldin, H. Rasmussen, C.A. Dinarello, and E.J. Schaefer. 1993b. Immunologic effects of national cholesterol education panel step-2 diets with and without fish-derived n-3 fatty acid enrichment. J. Clin. Invest. 92:105–113.

Molvig, J., F. Pociot, H. Worssaae, L.D. Wogensen, L. Baek, P. Christensen, T. Mandrup-Poulsen, K. Anderson, P. Madsen, J. Dyerberg, and J. Nerup. 1991. Dietary supplementation with omega-3 polyunsaturated fatty acids decreases mononuclear cell proliferation and interleukin-1β content but not monokine secretion in healthy and insulin-dependent diabetic individuals. Scan. J. Immunol. 34:399–410.

O'Mam, C.A. 1987. Nutritional therapy in ambulatory patients. Digest. Dis. Sci. 32:95S–99S.

Payan, D.G., M.Y.S. Wong, T. Chernov-Rogan, F.H. Valone, W.C. Pickett, V.A. Blake, and W.M. Gold. 1986. Alteration in human leukocyte function induced by ingestion of eicosapentaenoic acid. J. Clin. Immunol. 6:402–410.

Purasiri, P., A. Murray, S. Richardson, D. Heys, D. Horrobin, and O. Eremin. 1994. Modulation of cytokine production *in vivo* by dietary essential fatty acids in patients with colorectal cancer. Clin. Sci. 87:711–717.

Rasmussen, L.B., B. Kiens, B.K. Pederson, and E.A. Richter. 1994. Effect of diet and plasma fatty acid composition on immune status in elderly men. Am. J. Clin. Nutr. 59:572–577.

Seyberth, H.W., O. Oelz, T. Kennedy, B.J. Sweetman, A. Danon, J.C. Frolich, M. Helmberg, and J.A. Oates. 1975. Increased arachidonic acid in lipids after administration to man: Effects on prostaglandin biosynthesis. Clin. Pharmacol. Ther. 18:521–529.

Stenson, W.F., D. Cort, J. Rogers, R. Burakoff, K. Deschyver-Kecskemeti, T.L. Gramlich, and W. Beeken. 1992. Dietary supplementation with fish oil in ulcerative colitis. Ann. Intern. Med. 116:609–614.

Virella, G., J.M. Kilpatrick, M.R. Rugeles, B. Hayman, and R. Russell. 1989. Depression of humoral responses and phagocytic functions *in vivo* and *in vitro* by fish oil and eicosapentaenoic acid. Clin. Immunol. Immunopathol. 52:257–270.

Walton, A.J.E., M.L. Snaith, M. Locniskar, A.G. Cumberland, W.J.W. Morrow, and D.A. Isenberg. 1991. Dietary fish oil and the severity of symptoms in patients with systemic erythematosus. Ann. Rheum. Dis. 50:463–466.

Whelan, J., M.E, Surette, I. Hardardottir, G. Lu, K.A. Golemboski, E. Larsen, and J.E. Kinsella. 1993. Dietary arachidonic acid enhances tissue arachidonate levels and eicosanoid production in Syrian hamsters. J. Nutr. 123:2174–2185.

DISCUSSION

MELVIN MATHIAS: The decrease in dietary fat seems to be very clear-cut and reproducible with many investigators, in many investigator's hands, but the mechanism of that response—you had a shopping list of possible interactions. From your reading of the literature is there any particular mechanism that might jump out?

All the other parameters could involve eicosanoids, but just a decrease in fat is so clear and profound that we don't have a good—I don't have a good—mechanism. Do you have one?

DARSHAN KELLEY: I have a slide on the various mechanisms; somehow it got buried somewhere. The decrease in fat intake is very difficult to attain without changing the ratios between fatty acids, and also other nutrients. Now, we can maintain the ratios, but in most of the studies when you change the fat, you are changing the ratios within fatty acids, and also some of the other nutrients.

Even if you are maintaining the ratios, if you decrease the total fat, you are decreasing the antioxidant load. You also would decrease the lipoproteins in the serum, particularly lipoprotein B and E are significantly inhibitory of the immune cells.

So, any of those two mechanisms could easily account for the increase in IR by the decrease in fat intake on the activity of the immune cells, in addition to eicosanoids that you mentioned.

STEVE GAFFIN: A number of studies show that fish oil omega-3 fatty acids are beneficial, effective against endotoxin shock or gram negative sepsis. Your studies show the opposite general effect, that it is actually immunosuppressive. Can you explain why it should be protective in one case and not beneficial in another?

DARSHAN KELLEY: I think probably fish oils have more than one kind of effect. One is that the inhibitory effect may be mediated through the eicosanoid production, decreasing the production of series-2 eicosanoids. But I think in the beneficial effects, we are talking about in sepsis, that could be the increased production of free radicals that could be harmful to the pathogens. Again, a double-edged sword.

Nutrition and Immune Function, 1999
Pp. 317–336. Washington, D.C.
National Academy Press

15

Iron Metabolism, Microbial Virulence, and Host Defenses

Gerald T. Keusch[1]

INTRODUCTION

The relationship between iron nutritional status and susceptibility to infection, mediated by the effects of iron on the host and the pathogen, has become a topic of controversy in recent years. This controversy has followed the clear demonstration that iron is removed from the circulation into metabolically inaccessible forms during acute infection and the understanding that iron is required by both host and pathogen for survival and cellular replication. This documented "iron withholding" by the host has been seen by proponents of the so-called nutritional immunity hypothesis as evidence to suggest that it is of utility to host defense, providing a means to control infectious agents by limiting pathogen multiplication. The extension of this hypothesis has been that giving iron may be clinically harmful, either during an acute infection or as a supplement to control nutritional anemia. There is another camp, however, which believes that iron deficiency impairs immune function and increases susceptibility to infection.

---

[1] Gerald T. Keusch, Division of Geographic Medicine and Infectious Diseases, Tupper Research Institute, New England Medical Center, Boston, MA 02111

This chapter addresses the physiology of iron metabolism by host and pathogen, discusses the immunological data, reviews the clinical studies in humans, and draws conclusions about the benefits and risks for military personnel, particularly premenopausal women, of giving iron supplements.

IRON METABOLISM

Iron is a highly reactive metal able to generate oxygen free radicals that are toxic to cells. However, the aerobic nature of the earth creates a problem, because oxygen is also needed for life. Because iron can shift between the ferrous and ferric states and can readily and reversibly bind with oxygen, while containing it in a nonreactive state, iron-containing proteins have been selected as the predominant carrier of oxygen. In the environment, the problem of reactive free oxygen has been solved by converting inorganic iron to oxyhydroxide polymers, which reduces the amount of uncomplexed ferric (Fe^{+++}) in solution at biological pH to tolerable levels $(< 10^{-18} M)$. In the mammalian host, iron is present predominantly as protein complexes, including transport, storage, enzyme, and oxygen transporter systems, primarily as heme, iron-sulfur proteins, and ferritin intracellularly, or bound to extracellular transport glycoproteins such as transferrin in serum or lactoferrin on mucosal surfaces. Mammals have overcome the environmental restrictions and biological imperatives of bound, insoluble iron by developing an effective iron acquisition system able to compete with hydroxyl ion for ferric iron. Iron absorption, transport to and into cells, and storage are closely regulated by systems that sense the amount of available free iron and rapidly respond to maintain iron homeostasis.

This mechanism has been essential, because iron is the most abundant transition metal in humans, amounting to approximately 4 g in adult males, with about 1 g in storage forms. In young adult women, the amount of storage iron is considerably reduced to around 300 mg because of continuing iron losses during menstruation. Iron balance is tightly controlled, amounting to only 1 to 2 mg lost per day in men, but more in menstruating females, which is why iron-deficiency anemia is common among adult women.

In addition to oxygen transport, iron is essential for many physiological processes, as iron metalloproteins are able to accept electrons from various donors, to shift oxidation state, and to participate in redox reactions and hence serve in the electron transport chain in the form of cytochromes and mitochondrial iron-sulphur proteins (Griffiths, 1987). Many iron metalloproteins are enzymes, including enzymes involved in oxygen metabolism itself (catalase, peroxidase, superoxide dismutase), as well as flavoproteins such as xanthine oxidase and dehydrogenase; NADH/NADPH dehydrogenases; amino acid hydroxylases; and a key enzyme for DNA synthesis, ribonucleotide reductase.

Thus, to limit iron-mediated catalysis of oxygen to produce extremely reactive oxygen radicals such as the hydroxyl radical, OH·, which is highly toxic to cell membranes and can totally degrade DNA, virtually all iron in mammalian hosts is tied up with proteins, and the "free iron" pool is maintained at exceedingly low levels. The plasma-iron binding protein, transferrin, and a related protein, lactoferrin, released from the secondary granules of polymorphonuclear neutrophils (PMNs) (and also present in milk), keep the circulating free iron concentration close to zero. A major function of iron-transferrin is to provide a continuous source of iron for the rapid enzyme turnover, such as demonstrated by DNA synthesis, because the rate limiting enzyme for the production of nucleotides, ribonucleotide reductase is required for DNA synthesis. Uptake of iron from transferrin to the cell follows the binding of iron-transferrin to the transferrin receptor (TfR), a transmembrane protein for receptor-mediated endocytosis of iron-transferrin (Pollack, 1992). Transport of the TfR-iron complex into an acidified endosome results in the release of iron, with recirculation of the apotransferrin-TfR complex to the cell surface where the apotransferrin is released (Harford et al., 1990). If iron is taken up in excess, it is rapidly complexed within the cell by ferritin, a large, hollow, spherical protein that can accumulate large amounts of iron (Theil, 1987) and modulate iron-mediated reactions under conditions of excess intracellular iron (Joshi and Zimmerman, 1988). Ferritin is present in small amounts in the circulation and mirrors iron nutrition, with low levels found in people with iron deficiency and high levels in people with normal amounts of iron. Thus, serum ferritin serves in the diagnosis of iron-deficiency anemia (Worwood, 1986), and every µg per liter is equivalent to 8 to 10 mg of storage iron (Bothwell, 1995).

Transport and storage of iron are finely tuned, as both transferrin-receptor and ferritin synthesis are coordinately and reciprocally regulated by iron concentration (Johnson et al., 1983; Klausner et al., 1993). When iron availability is low, TfR synthesis increases and ferritin synthesis decreases, with the reverse happening when iron availability is high. The mechanism by which this occurs is posttranscriptional and involves regions of the messenger RNA (mRNA) for ferritin and TfR able to bind a stem-loop region known as the iron-responsive element (IRE) located in the 5' and 3' regions, respectively. Specific iron-binding proteins that recognize these IREs, known as IRE-binding proteins (IRE-BP), are the effectors. The ferritin IRE-BP serves as a translational repressor of the ferritin gene (Leibold and Munro, 1988). That is, binding of the IRE-BP to the ferritin IRE blocks the translation of ferritin mRNA. The TfR IRE-BP operates by controlling mRNA half-life (Owen and Kuhn, 1987) via a more complex mechanism, involving the IREs and additional iron-independent "instability elements" affecting rapid degradation of the mRNA transcript (Harford and Klausner, 1990). When IRE-BP binds to the IRE, the instability element is inhibited, mRNA half-life increases, and TfR synthesis increases.

IRON ACQUISITION BY MICROBES

Because of the tightly regulated availability of iron in the human, microorganisms must compete with the host for iron, with a few exceptions (for example, *Lactobacillus* spp., which use manganese and cobalt instead) (Archibald, 1983). In fact, in most instances, microbes use systems of acquisition and transport of iron that are analogous to those of humans, because they too both require iron and a detoxification mechanism to prevent iron-mediated damage. These goals can be realized in several ways:

- Find another, less-toxic biocatalyst (e.g., *Lactobacilli*), which uses manganese and cobalt instead of iron.
- Make Fe^{+++} more soluble and easily transported by reduction to Fe^{++}, a strategy adopted by several organisms (*Bifidobacterium bifidum, Legionella pneumophila, Streptococcus mutans*, and *Streptomyces cerevisiae*).
- Produce chelators to bind ferric iron and transport proteins to safely obtain and use the metal, a solution adopted by most microbes.
- Produce receptors for iron protein that is bound by host in the form of transferrin, lactoferrin, or heme (e.g., pathogenic *Neisseria, Hemophilus influenzae, Helicobacter pylori, Vibrios*, and *Yersinia*).
- Develop multiple mechanisms to obtain and transport iron safely. These may be turned on in sequence as the conditions of iron restriction become more severe, thus allowing survival under different conditions of environmental stress conditions and protecting against mutational loss of the survival advantage.

A few organisms (for example, *Legionella pneumophila, Streptococcus mutans*, or the yeast *Saccharomyces cervisiae*) reduce ferric iron and transport the more soluble, less toxic ferrous form of the metal. Most, however, simply make ferric iron-specific, high-affinity chelators (siderophores) (Guerinot, 1994) that effectively remove iron from host iron-binding proteins, even from ferritin (Zahringer et al., 1976), which means that intracellular storage is not a safe strategy to withhold iron from intracellular pathogens. Moreover, in at least a few known cases, certain microorganisms obtain iron directly from host sources, for example *Neisseria meningiditis* or *N. gonorrhoea* and *Hemophilus influenzae*, which make human-like transferrin receptors to transport iron-transferrin just as the host cells do (Martinez et al., 1990).

The paradigm for iron acquisition and best-studied example is *Escherichia coli*. Under conditions of restricted iron availability, when a pathogen enters a human, the microbe rapidly and coordinately derepresses a set of genes responsible for the synthesis of iron acquisition and transport proteins that constitutes a system of iron chelators, outer membrane iron-siderophore receptors, and periplasmic and inner membrane transport proteins. This system is complex, involves multiple structural and regulatory genes and proteins, uses iron concentration as the signal, and is highly efficient (Neilands, 1995). It includes several types of chemically distinct siderophores (catechol enterobactins, hydroxamates such as aerobactin, and diverse molecules such as ferrichrome), all of which are characterized by an extremely high affinity for iron and a general similarity in the transport mechanisms. For example, the association constant of enterobactin for iron at neutral pH is, astoundingly, 10^{52}, which explains why it can strip iron from transferrin, for which the association constant is "only" 10^{36}. Certain Enterobacteriaceae can use siderophores made by other organisms, for example the fungal products ferrioxamine B and ferrichrome. In fact, the methane sulfonate salt of deferrated ferrioxamine B is used clinically as an iron chelator drug, Desferal, to treat iron overload states. Finally, when the iron-siderophore complex reaches the cytoplasm, iron is released from ferric enterochelin by an esterase or from aerobactin or citrate siderophores by reduction mediated through flavin reductases (ferri-siderophore reductase).

Some organisms produce and use several different siderophores. In some instances, there is a stepwise synthesis of distinct chelators of increasing affinity for iron as the iron concentration is reduced, which suggests a carefully evolved strategy of iron acquisition that may confer competitive advantages *in vivo* (Sevinc and Page, 1992). In contrast, in an anaerobic environment, a specialized system to solubilize iron may be unnecessary because reduced ferrous iron is both available and soluble. A ferrous iron transport gene, *feoAB*, has recently been cloned from *E. coli* (Kammler et al., 1993), suggesting that organisms with an anaerobic ecological niche may have specialized systems for taking up reduced iron. This assumption is consistent with the finding that *feo* mutants are worse colonizers of the mouse gut than the parental wild type *E. coli* (Stojiljkovic et al., 1993). Some organisms, for example pathogenic *Neisseria*, do not make siderophores, albeit they can use exogenously supplied chelators (West and Sparling, 1985; Yancey and Finkelstein, 1981). *N. gonorrhoeae* and *N. meningitidis* obtain iron from transferrin, whereas nonpathogenic strains are inhibited in the presence of transferrin (Michelsen and Sparling, 1981; Michelsen et al., 1982). These pathogens produce a transferrin receptor that specifically binds human transferrin and directly obtains iron in this manner (Schryners and Morris, 1988).

Many iron-regulated bacterial proteins are regulated at the transcriptional level by a common gene, *fur*, which encodes the iron-binding Fur protein. When iron is readily available, Fur binds the metal, which allows it to recognize a sequence with dyad symmetry in the promoter region of iron-regulated genes known as the "iron" or "Fur box." The iron-Fur complex acts as a repressor of the gene and stops the synthesis of the gene product. Under conditions of iron deprivation, Fur does not bind and the iron-regulated proteins are made. In this manner, the multiple genes involved in iron acquisition can be turned on together by this single mechanism. Fur proteins that recognize the consensus iron-box sequence have been sequenced from *Shigella* spp., *Yersinia pestis*, *Vibrio cholerae* and *V. vulnificus*, *Pseudomonas aeruginosa*, and *Neisseria* spp., and a similar protein in *Corynebacterium diphtheriae*, DtxR, plays a Fur-like role in this organism. It should be noted that the Fur system controls a number of proteins other than those involved in iron uptake, including carbon utilization pathway proteins, superoxide dismutase, acid adaptation responses, and others.

Iron regulation of gene transcription and translation is not just an *in vitro* phenomena; iron-regulated proteins are also made by bacteria growing *in vivo* in mammalian hosts, including clinical isolates obtained from human urinary and respiratory tract infections as well as from experimental animal infections using human pathogens (Camilli et al., 1994; Chart et al., 1988; Shand et al., 1985). Moreover, a number of virulence properties of microbes are iron regulated *in vitro* and are specifically turned on by low iron availability (Table 15-1). This mechanism is consistent with the generally held view that virulence genes are preferentially turned on *in vivo* in order to ensure biosynthetic economy of the organism. That is, to enhance the survival of pathogenic microbes outside of the host, the organism does not waste energy and substrate making things it does not need.

The clear evidence that pathogens adapt to low iron availability, that they have developed intricate iron acquisition mechanisms, and that they use iron levels as the signal for transcriptional regulation of these systems raises doubt about the validity of the iron-withholding hypothesis of nutritional immunity (Kontoghiorghies and Weinberg, 1995). Given the existence of these iron-regulated systems for iron acquisition, it may be reasonable to believe that iron deficiency or acute phase shifts of iron from the circulation to intracellular storage sites during infection will restrict microbial acquisition of iron *in vivo*. In the context of biologic regulation and the postulated role of iron in the

TABLE 15-1 Iron Regulated Bacterial Virulence Factors

Organism	Virulence Factor
Escherichia coli	Aerobactin, Shiga toxin-1, α-hemolysin
Shigella dysenteriae type	Shiga toxin
Serratia marcescens	Hemolysin
Vibrio cholerae	Iron-regulated gene A (IrgA)
Vibrio anguillarum	Anguibactin
Yersinia spp.	Iron-regulated outer membrane proteins
Neisseria gonorrhoeae	Transferrin-binding protein 1 and 2
Pseudomonas aeruginosa	Exotoxin A, elastase, protease
Corynebacterium diphtheriae	Diphtheria toxin

nutritional immunity hypothesis, iron is required by the host (as well as the microbe) and its uptake and distribution is so finely regulated by such a complex mechanism, that nature would chose a simple single solution (for example, iron withholding) as a major host defense against most infections.

EFFECTS OF IRON DEFICIENCY ON IMMUNE FUNCTION

Because iron is as essential for mammalian ribonucleotide reductase as it is for the microbial enzyme, it is not surprising that transferrin-iron is needed for clonal expansion of lymphocytes in immune responses (Kay and Benzie, 1986; Philips and Azari, 1975). In fact, iron uptake must precede DNA synthesis (Kronke et al., 1985), and therefore, transferrin receptors (CD71) must be expressed as T-lymphocytes become activated in response to interleukin (IL)-2/IL-2 receptor interactions (Brock and Rankin, 1981; Neckers and Cossman, 1983). Dependency on the uptake of transferrin iron has been reported for B-cell proliferation and the mixed lymphocyte reaction (Futran et al., 1989; Kemp et al., 1987). However, B-cells may have larger iron storage pools than T-cells and may be more resistant to iron-limiting conditions, for example in the presence of antitransferrin receptor antibody plus the iron chelator desferrioxamine (Kemp et al., 1987). Among T-cells, T-helper (Th)1 cells are much more sensitive than Th2 clones to the intracellular iron depletion produced by the combination of antitransferrin receptor antibody plus desferrioxamine (Thorson et al., 1991). Human peripheral blood mononuclear cells still respond to phytohemagglutinin (PHA) in iron-depleted medium (Taylor et al., 1988), and it is necessary to chelate intracellular iron with desferrioxamine to block this (Golding and Young, 1995), providing further evidence of iron stores and efficient uptake systems in activated lymphocytes. Chronic iron deficiency would deplete these stores, because a source of diferric-transferrin to replenish the intracellular iron pool is lacking. In humans with iron-deficiency anemia, a decrease in total CD3-positive and CD4-positive lymphocytes, B-lymphocytes, and K-cell activity has been reported, with a significant recovery of all but the K-cell activity with repletion of iron (Santos and Falcao, 1990). Similar findings are reported in mice that were made iron deficient, with reduced density of T-lymphocytes in the thymus and spleen, but no changes in lymphocyte subpopulation ratios (Kuvibidila et al., 1990). This study demonstrated no alteration in the serum or thymic concentration of the thymic hormone, thymulin, which is involved in T-lymphocyte differentiation.

Sufficient data exist to document that iron deficiency is associated with diminished, delayed-type skin test reactivity to recall antigens (Joynson et al., 1972; Krantman et al., 1982; Macdougall et al., 1975). *In vitro* mitogen-stimulated lymphocyte proliferation is also impaired (Fletcher et al., 1975; Sawitsky et al., 1976). Although some investigators have found no effects (Grosch-Warner et al., 1984; Gupta et al., 1982), negative *in vitro* studies could be confounded by rapid repletion of cellular iron from the culture medium. In contrast, B-cell number and function, measured by the antibody response to a strong protein antigen, tetanus toxoid, are normal (Chandra and Saraya, 1975). However, the kinetics of the response have not been studied. The critical role of iron metalloenzymes for DNA synthesis and cell proliferation makes it likely that iron deficiency can impair the speed of both T- and B-lymphocyte proliferative responses during activation. In fact, limited data in animals are consistent with the concept that antibody production is impaired in iron deficiency states (Kochanowski and Sherman, 1985). Because the rapidity with which host responses are mobilized *in vivo* plays an important role in determining whether or not exposure to an infectious agent results in illness, these effects of iron deficiency can have clinical significance.

Neutrophil myeloperoxidase, an iron metalloenzyme that generates reactive bactericidal halides during PMN phagocytosis, is reduced in iron deficiency states (Prasad, 1979; Turgeon-O'Brien et al., 1985; Yetgin et al., 1979). Myeloperoxidase-mediated killing is a redundant system; however, iron is also required for the production by phagocytic cells of reactive microbicidal oxygen species via the Fenton reaction (Fridovich, 1978). Impairment of this pathway in iron-deficient individuals is evidenced by the diminished ability of their PMNs to reduce the dye, nitroblue tetrazolium (NBT)[2] (Celada et al., 1979; Chandra, 1975). A modest diminution in *in vitro* intracellular bactericidal activity is also reported in some studies (Chandra, 1973; Moore and Humbert, 1984; Walter et al., 1986), although contradictory data also exist (Kulapongs et al., 1974; Van Heerden et al., 1981). Bactericidal assays are, however, not very sensitive to small changes in functional capacity and are most useful to detect profound defects. Other neutrophil functions, such as chemotaxis, phagocytosis, and degranulation, appear to be normal in iron deficiency, which suggests that the effects of iron deficiency are specific and related to the biological functions of the metal.

Macrophage functions, such as antigen presentation, have not been studied in iron-deficient subjects. Animal experiments have shown that clearance of polyvinylpyrrolidone and the generation of reactive oxygen species is impaired in iron-deficient mice (Kuvibidila and Wade, 1987; Thompson and Brock, 1986), and that IL-1 production is reduced in iron-deficient rat leukocytes (Heylar and Sherman, 1987).

Although it is difficult to extrapolate from *in vitro* studies of immune function to altered host susceptibility to infection, it can be concluded that iron deficiency is not going to enhance host immune responses. Whether or not delayed or diminished responses affect the course of the host-pathogen interaction at the clinical level remains to be conclusively shown. This, no doubt, differs from subject to subject and will relate to the severity of the iron

---

[2] The NBT test is used to detect the oxidative ability of PMN leukocytes by measuring the concomitant reduction of NBT, reflected in a measurable color change.

deficiency, the presence of concomitant nutritional defects, and the nature of the infecting organism.

EFFECTS OF IRON EXCESS ON IMMUNE FUNCTION

In developing the nutritional immunity concept, the evidence that iron promotes microbial growth while conditions characterized by iron excess impair immune function and increase susceptibility to infection has been used to support the argument that iron withholding protects the host. That is, if withholding iron protects, then excess iron will enhance infection (Weinberg, 1984). In fact, many examples exist in which the provision of exogenous iron or the addition of unsaturated iron-binding proteins to reduce iron availability correlates respectively with increased or diminished growth of organisms *in vitro* (Bullen et al., 1978; Chart and Griffiths, 1985). Furthermore, when microbial growth in complete medium is inhibited by the addition of apolactoferrin, this can be reversed by addition of excess iron.

Iron overload states, such as β-thalassemia or sickle-cell anemia with multiple transfusions, idiopathic hemochromatosis, or "Bantu" hemosiderosis due to grossly excessive oral iron loads are characterized by iron-saturated transferrin with the excess iron present as loose complexes of iron and albumin readily available to microorganisms (Hershko and Peto, 1987). In some of these disease states, the incidence of infection and fatal outcomes is increased (Barret-Connor, 1971; Buchanan, 1971). This association is supported by the increased mortality of infectious challenge of experimental animal hemochromatosis models compared with euferric states (Fletcher and Goldstein, 1970; Robins-Browne and Pripic, 1985). However, when the clinical parameters are reexamined to separate the effect of increased free iron from the effects due to damage of the liver and spleen and secondary diabetes, it becomes difficult to attribute increased susceptibility to iron itself rather than to damage to the reticuloendothelial system and cellular function as a consequence of iron-mediated oxidation/peroxidation effects (Hershko et al., 1988). Thus, while approximately 20 percent of deaths in β-thalassemia are attributed to infection, nearly all of these deaths occur in splenectomized patients. Similarly, the enhanced susceptibility to infection in sickle-cell patients occurs primarily in the young, before significant iron overload occurs. Clinical analysis thus suggests that it is not increased free iron availability in iron overload that is associated with increased incidence or severity of infection.

Because free iron is known to damage cells, iron excess is likely to impair immune function. PMNs from β-thalassemia or transfusion hemosiderosis patients produce less superoxide and hydrogen peroxide than controls (Flament et al., 1986; Martino et al., 1984; Waterlot et al., 1985), and NBT dye reduction is impaired as well (Cantinieaux et al., 1987; Tavo et al., 1977). Cells from thalassemia patients also show diminished chemotactic responses and reduced random migration (Khan et al., 1983). Peripheral blood monocytes from β-thalassemic patients are impaired in their microbicidal activity (Ballart et al., 1986; Van Asbeck et al., 1984a, b). Oxidative damage most likely impairs the functional responses of lymphocytes exposed to iron excess *in vitro*. For example, addition of increasing amounts of iron to normal T-lymphocytes diminishes cloning efficiency and reduces proliferative responses to mitogens (Good et al., 1988; Munn et al., 1981). Several studies report a reduction in the number and function of CD4 cells (Dwyer et al., 1987; Grady et al., 1985; Pardalos et al., 1987) and decreased natural killer (NK) cell activity (Akbar et al., 1986; Neri et al., 1984) in iron overload patients. Pokeweed mitogen-induced generation of immunoglobulin-producing cells is diminished in thalassemia major patients (Nualart et al., 1987). Co-culture with normal cells suggests that the defect resides at the Th-cell level. Some of these defects are corrected by iron chelation therapy, which suggests that they are due to the toxic effects of free iron.

CLINICAL DATA IN IRON DEFICIENCY AND IRON EXCESS

Published clinical studies to date that examined the effect of iron deficiency on susceptibility to infection are typically flawed in design, fail to include sufficient numbers of subjects to interpret the results, or do not account for confounders commonly encountered in field studies (Keusch and Farthing, 1986). Some studies have simply compared the hematological status of infants admitted to the hospital because of infection with that of another hospital control group. However, because inflammation results in shifts of iron and iron status markers, these studies cannot distinguish cause and effect. The most cited clinical studies of the past 70 years have involved a comparison of the morbidity among infants fed an iron-fortified formula and the same food without added iron (Andelman and Sered, 1966; Heresi et al., 1985; Hussein et al., 1985; MacKay, 1928). In general, the iron-fortified group was reported to experience fewer respiratory and intestinal infections. Unfortunately, the data are suspect because the controls were inadequate, and morbidity data were collected via recall interviews of the mothers, rather than active surveillance of illness by trained personnel. However, others reported no differences between unsupplemented and supplemented groups (Darsdaran et al., 1979; James and Combes, 1960), while some studies found an increased incidence of infections in the iron-treated subjects (Oppenheimer and Hendrickse, 1983). Although one study in adults suggested increased morbidity among iron-deficient adults compared with iron-supplemented adults (Basta et al., 1979), the clinical consequences of iron deficiency remain uncertain (Dhur et al., 1989; Strauss, 1978).

Nonetheless, there are a few examples where the association of iron overload and susceptibility to infection is related to the increased free iron available for the growth of pathogens that do not compete well for protein-bound iron *in vivo*. For example, low virulence *Yersinia enterocolitica*, which lack the *Yersinia* virulence plasmid encoding high-efficiency iron acquisition systems can use host free iron under conditions of iron overload, or even more efficiently, desferrioxamine chelated iron (Carniel et al., 1987, 1989). Life-threatening infections due to such strains in patients on chelation therapy (Blei and Puder, 1993; Green, 1992; Kelly et al., 1987; Rabson et al., 1975) or following massive oral ingestion of iron (Fakir et al., 1992; Melby et al., 1982; Mofenson et al., 1988) are described. In some instances, presentation with *Yersinia* sepsis has led to the discovery of an iron overload disease (Vadillo et al., 1994). *Vibrio vulnificus* also uses heme-iron or desferrioxamine-chelated iron (Helms et al., 1984; Wright et al., 1981), and infections are documented in iron overload patients (Blake et al., 1979). Other, less common associations between chelation therapy and sepsis include *Listeria* (Mossey and Sondheimer, 1985), and certain fungi, including pathogenic *Mucor* and *Rhizopus* species (Abe et al., 1990; Daly et al., 1989; Goodili and Abuelo, 1987). The effect of iron chelators may be dual, including serving as a source of iron and depressing host phagocytic and lymphocyte-mediated defenses (Autenrieth et al., 1994, 1995; Ewald et al., 1994).

Transient increases in free iron can result from parenteral administration of iron-polysaccharide complexes. Following the introduction of one such agent, iron-dextran, for rapid correction of neonatal iron deficiency in New Zealand, a striking increase in *E. coli* septicemia was detected (Barry and Reeve, 1973). The infections occurred shortly after the iron loading, which suggests that they were related to increased available iron. When this therapy was abandoned, the sepsis rate soon dropped by 10-fold (Barry and Reeve, 1977; Farmer and Becroft, 1976). Iron-sorbital-citrate, another loosely bound, low-molecular-weight iron complex for parenteral administration, rapidly saturates serum transferrin and is excreted in the urine. Use of this drug has been associated with increased pyuria in patients with chronic pyelonephritis, which suggests local exacerbation of infection (Briggs et al., 1963). This hypothesis is consistent with a report that this drug stimulates the growth of *E. coli* already present in the kidney in a model experimental murine pyelonephritis (Buchanan, 1971).

Several studies have shown an increase in malaria parasitemia in individuals given parenteral or oral iron (Masawe et al., 1974; Murray et al., 1978a). Although these reports are not entirely convincing because they lack appropriate placebo control groups, fail to control for the presence of protein energy malnutrition and associated reduced transferrin levels, and lack proper blinding, a recent, well-designed, double-blind study in Papua New Guinea confirms the observation (Oppenheimer et al., 1986a). Parenteral iron administration resulted in a 64 percent increase in parasitemia rate at both 6 and 12 months, along with a 20 to 40 percent increase in spleen rates[3] and significantly increased admissions to the hospital for malaria. In addition,

---

[3] In malaria endemic regions, repeated malarial infections and resulting hemolysis lead to splenomegaly in young children. Thus, the prevalence of splenomegaly ("spleen rate") reflects the frequency of clinical malaria.

admissions for measles, otitis media, and pneumonia were increased in the iron group as well (Oppenheimer et al., 1986b). The detrimental effects of the iron-dextran were most apparent in infants with the highest birth hemoglobin level and, therefore, the highest level of iron stores. Another careful study of total-dose, iron-dextran infusion in pregnant women in Papua New Guinea corroborated the increased risk of malaria parasitemia associated with the drug (Oppenheimer et al., 1986c). There are a number of explanations for this. Iron administration will increase erythropoiesis, and *Plasmodia* preferably invade young cells. Iron also increases hemoglobin synthesis, which is essential for parasite metabolism (Hershko and Peto, 1988), and provides the metal for growth rate-limiting iron-metalloenzymes (Scheibel, 1988; Scheibel and Sherman, 1988) (dihyroorotate dehydrogenase, phosphoenol pyruvate carboxykinase, cytochrome oxidase, and ribonucleotide reductase) necessary for parasite replication.

Hemolysis of any etiology is a known risk factor for *Salmonella* infection (Black et al., 1960; Jones et al., 1977), presumably related to the uptake of iron-hemoglobin by macrophages and secondary macrophage defects in phagocytosis and/or killing of the organism. In experimental murine models, hemolysis induced by *Plasmodium berghei* infection or phenylhydrazine dramatically increases the virulence of *Salmonella typhimurium*, whereas iron deficiency induced by bleeding did not (Kaye et al., 1967).

These data demonstrate that excess free iron may have a direct enhancing effect on a limited number of pathogens and that chronic iron overload results in oxidative and peroxidative damage to the immune system and impairs its function. The effects of iron overload cannot therefore be considered to be a continuum ranging from protection of the host due to iron withholding at one end to increased susceptibility due to iron excess at the other, as the nutritional immunity hypothesis presumes. Indeed, iron deficiency and iron excess both exert an adverse effect on host defenses but by entirely different mechanisms.

IMPLICATIONS OF IRON DEFICIENCY FOR THE MILITARY

The evidence reviewed suggests that iron deficiency offers little nonspecific protection against infections and that iron overload stimulates the growth of a very limited number of pathogens, but results in real damage of the immune system with more general effects on host defenses. At the same time, it is the parenteral administration of iron or the use of iron chelation therapy in iron overload diseases that have been associated with enhanced susceptibility to infections. However, no convincing data show that oral iron supplements for repletion of stores and treatment of iron-deficiency anemia have any adverse impact on infectious diseases.

Diminished iron stores among military personnel are most likely to be in women of child-bearing age. Screening for iron-deficiency anemia among recruits, and at regular examinations thereafter, represents an opportunity to prescribe iron for those in need who will benefit. This has two advantages to the military: first, improvement of physical fitness by correcting anemia and second, repletion of iron stores and optimization of immune function. There are no disadvantages and no risk of promoting infectious diseases. The major issue in compliance with supplemental iron is the intestinal side effects associated with oral iron, but this can be overcome by experimenting with the preparation used in a given patient and/or by lowering the daily dose.

REFERENCES

Abe, F., H. Inaba, T. Katoh, and M. Hotachi. 1990. Effects of iron and desferrioxamine on *Rhizopus* infection. Mycopathologia 110:87–91.

Akbar, A.N., P.A. Fitzgerald-Bocarsly, M. deSousa, P.J. Giardina, M.W. Hilgartner, and R.W. Grady. 1986. Decreased natural killer activity in thalassemia major: A possible consequence of iron overload. J. Immunol. 136:1635–1640.

Andelman, M.B., and B.R. Sered. 1966. Utilization of dietary iron by term infants: A study of 1,048 infants from a low socioeconomic population. Am. J. Dis. Child. 111:45–55.

Archibald, F. 1983. *Lactobacillus plantarum*, an organism not requiring iron. FEMS Microbiol. Lett. 19:29–32.

Autenrieth, I.B., E. Bohn, J.H. Ewald, and J. Heesemann. 1995. Deferoxamine B but not deferoxamine G1 inhibits cytokine production in murine bone marrow macrophages. J. Infect. Dis. 172:490–496.

Autenrieth, I.B., R. Reissbrodt, E. Saken, R. Berner, U. Vogel, W. Rabsch, and J. Heesemann. 1994. Desferrioxamine-promoted virulence of *Yersinia enterocolitica* in mice depends on both desferrioxamine type and mouse strain. J. Infect. Dis. 169:562–567.

Ballart, I.J., M.E. Estevez, L. Sen, R.A. Diez, J. Giuntoli, S.A. de Miani, and J. Penalver. 1986. Progressive dysfunction of monocytes associated with iron overload and age in patients with thalassemia major. Blood 67:105–109.

Barret-Connor, E.. 1971. Bacterial infection and sickle-cell anaemia. An analysis of 250 infections in 166 patients and a review of the literature. Medicine 50:97–112.

Barry, D.M.J., and A.W. Reeve. 1973. Iron injections and serious Gram negative infection in Polynesian newborn. N. Zeal. J. Med. 78:376.

Barry, D.M.J., and A.W. Reeve. 1977. Increased incidence of gram-negative neonatal sepsis with intramuscular iron administration. Pediatrics 60:908–912.

Basta, S.S., Soekirman, A. Karyadi, and N.S. Scrimshaw. 1979. Iron-deficiency anaemia and the productivity of adult males in Indonesia. Am. J. Clin. Nutr. 32:916–925.

Black, P.H., L.J. Kunz, and M.N. Swartz. 1960. Salmonellosis—a review of some usual aspects. N. Engl. J. Med. 262:811–817, 921–927.

Blake, P.A., M.H. Merson, R.E. Weaver, D.G. Hollis, and P.C. Heublein. 1979. Disease caused by a marine vibrio: Clinical characteristics and epidemiology. N. Engl. J. Med. 300:1–5.

Blei, F., and D.R. Puder. 1993. *Yersinia enterocolitica* bacteremia in a chronically transfused patient with sickle-cell anemia. Case report and review of the literature. Am. J. Pediatr. Hematol. Oncol. 15:430–434.

Bothwell, T.H.. 1995. Overview and mechanisms of iron regulation. Nutr. Rev. 53:237–245.

Briggs, J.D., C.A. Kennedy, and A. Goldberg. 1963. Urinary white cell excretion after iron-sorbitol-citric acid. Br. Med. J. ii:352–354.

Brock, J.H., and M.C. Rankin. 1981. Transferrin binding and iron uptake by mouse lymph-node cells during transformation in response to concanavalin A. Immunology 43:393–398.

Buchanan, W.M.. 1971. Shock in bantu siderosis. Am. J. Clin. Pathol. 55:401–406.

Bullen, J.J., and E. Griffiths, eds.. 1987. Iron and Infection. London: John Wiley & Sons.

Bullen, J.J., C.G. Ward, and S.N. Wallis. 1978. Virulence and the role of iron in Pseudomonas aeruginosa infection. Infect. Immun. 10:443–450.

Camilli, A., D. Beattie, and J.J. Mekalanos. 1994. Use of genetic recombination as a reporter of gene expression. Proc. Natl. Acad. Sci. USA 91:2634–2638.

Cantinieaux, B., C. Hariga, A. Ferster, E. de Maerterlaerre, M. Toppet, and P. Fondu. 1987. Neutrophil dysfunctions in thalassemia major: The role of iron overload. Eur. J. Haematol. 389:28–34.

Carniel, E., D. Mazigh, and H.H. Mollaret. 1987. Expression of iron-regulated proteins in Yersinia species and their relation to virulence. Infect. Immun. 55:277–280.

Carniel, E., O. Mercereau-Puijalon, and S. Bonnefoy. 1989. The gene coding for the 190,000-dalton iron-regulated protein of Yersinia species is present only in the highly pathogenic strains. Infect. Immun. 57:1211–1217.

Celada, A., V. Herreros, P. Pugin, and M. Rudolf. 1979. Reduced leukocyte alkaline phosphatase activity and decreased NBT reduction test in induced iron deficiency. Br. J. Haematol. 43:457–463.

Chandra, R.K. 1973. Reduced bactericidal capacity of polymorphs in iron deficiency. Arch. Dis. Child. 48:864–866.

Chandra, R.K. 1975. Impaired immunocompetence associated with iron deficiency. J. Pediatr. 86:899–902.

Chandra, R.K., and A.K. Saraya. 1975. Impaired immuno-competence associated with iron deficiency. J. Pediatr. 86:899–901.

Chart, H., and E. Griffiths. 1985. The availability of iron and the growth of Vibrio vulnificus in sera from patients with haemochromatosis. FEMS Microbiol. Lett. 26:227–231.

Chart, H., P. Stevenson, and E. Griffiths. 1988. Iron-regulated outer-membrane proteins of Escherichia coli strains associated with enteric or extraintestinal diseases of man and animals. J. Gen. Microbiol. 134:1549–1559.

Daly, A.L., L.A. Velazquez, S.F. Bradley, and C.A. Kauffman. 1989. Mucormycosis: Association with deferoxamine therapy. Am. J. Med. 87:468–471.

Damsdaran, M., A.N. Naidu, and K.V.R. Sarma. 1979. Anemia and morbidity in rural preschool children. Indian J. Med. Res. 69:448–456.

Dhur, A., P. Galan, and S. Hercberg. 1989. Iron status, immune capacity, and resistance to infections. Comp. Biochem. Physiol. 94A:11–19.

Dwyer, J., C. Wood, J. McNamara, A. Williams, W. Andiman, L. Rink, T. O'Connor, and H. Pearson. 1987. Abnormalities in the immune system of children with β-thalassemia. Clin. Exp. Immunol. 63:621–629.

Ewald, J.H., J. Heesemann, H. Rudiger, and I.B. Autenrieth. 1994. Interaction of polymorphonuclear leukocytes with Yersinia enterocolitica: Role of the Yersinia virulence plasmid and modulation by the iron-chelator desferrioxamine. Br. J. Infect. Dis. 170:140–150.

Fakir, M., C. Saison, T. Wong, B. Matta, and J.M. Hardin. 1992. Septicemia due to Yersinia enterocolitica in a hemodialyzed, iron-depleted patient receiving omeprazole and oral iron supplementation. Am. J. Kidney Dis. 19:282–284.

Farmer, K., and D.M.O. Becroft. 1976. Administration of parenteral iron to newborn infants [letter]. Arch. Dis. Child. 51:486.

Flament, J., M. Goldman, Y. Waterlot, E. Dupont, J. Wybran, and J.L. Vanherweghem. 1086. Impairment of phagocyte oxidative metabolism in hemodialysed patients with iron overload. Clin. Nephrol. 25:227–230.

Fletcher, J., and E. Goldstein. 1970. The effect of parenteral iron preparation on experimental pyelonephritis. Br. J. Exp. Pathol. 51:280–285.

Fletcher, J., J. Mather, M.J. Lewis, and G. Whiting. 1975. Mouth lesions in iron-deficiency anemia: Relationship to *Candida albicans* in saliva and to impairment of lymphocyte transformation. J. Infect. Dis. 131:44–50.

Fridovich, I.. 1978. The biology of oxygen radicals. Science 201:875–880.

Futran, J., J.D. Kemp, E.H. Field, A. Ora, and R.F. Ashman. 1989. Transferrin receptor synthesis is an early event in B-cell activation. J. Immunol. 143:787–792.

Golding, S., and S.P. Young. 1995. Iron requirements of human lymphocytes: Relative contributions of intra- and extracellular iron. Scand. J. Immunol. 41:229–236.

Good, M.F., L.W. Powell, and J.W. Halliday. 1988. Iron status and cellular immune competence. Blood Rev. 2:43–49.

Goodili, J.J., and J.G. Abuelo. 1987. Mucormycosis—a new risk of deferrioxamine therapy in dialysis patients with aluminum or iron overload? [letter] N. Engl. J. Med. 317:54.

Grady, R.W., A. Akbar, P.J. Giardina, M.W. Hilgartner, and M. deSousa. 1985. Disproportionate lymphoid cell subsets in thalassemia major: The relative contributions of transfusion and splenectomy. Br. J. Haematol. 72:361–367.

Green, N.S.. 1992. *Yersinia* infections in patients with homozygous β-thalassemia associated with iron overload and its treatment. Pediatric Hematol. Oncol. 9:247–254.

Griffiths, E.. 1987. Iron in biological systems. Pp. 1–25 in Iron and Infection, J.J. Bullen and E. Griffiths, eds. London: John Wiley & Sons.

Grosch-Warner, I., H. Grosse-Wilde, C. Bender-Gotze, and K.H. Schafer. 1984. Lymphozytenfunktionen bei kindern mit eisenmangel. Klin. Wochenschr. 62:1091–1093.

Guerinot, M.L.. 1994. Microbial iron transport. Ann. Rev. Microbiol. 48:743–772.

Gupta, K.K., P.S. Dhatt, and H. Singh. 1982. Cell-mediated immunity in children with iron-deficiency anemia. Indian J. Pediatr. 49:507–510.

Harford, J.B., and R.D. Klausner. 1990. Coordinate posttranscriptional regulation of ferritin and transferrin receptor expression: The role of regulated RNA-protein interaction. Enzyme 44:28–41.

Harford, J.B., J.L. Casey, D.M. Koeller, and R.D. Klausner. 1990. Structure, function, and regulation of the transferrin receptor: Insights from molecular biology. Pp. 302–334 in Intracellular Trafficking of Proteins, C.J. Steer and J.A. Hanover, eds. Cambridge: Cambridge University Press.

Helms, S.D., J.D. Oliver, and J.C. Travis. 1984. Role of heme compounds and haptoglobin in *Vibrio vulnificus* pathogenicity. Infect. Immun. 45:345–349.

Helyar, L., and A.R. Sherman. 1987. Iron deficiency and interleukin-1 production by rat leukocytes. Am. J. Clin. Nutr. 46:346–352.

Heresi, G., M. Olivaress, F. Pizarro, M. Cayazo, E. Hertrampf, E. Walter, and A. Stekel. 1985. Effect of iron fortification on infant morbidity [abstract]. XIII International Congress of Nutrition. Brighton, England, p 129.

Hershko, C., and T.E.A. Peto. 1987. Nontransferrin plasma iron. Br. J. Haematol. 66:149–151.

Hershko, C., and T.E.A. Peto. 1988. Deferoxamine inhibition of malaria is independent of host iron status. J. Exp. Med. 168:375–387.

Hershko, C., T.E.A. Peto, and D.J. Weatherall. 1988. Iron and infection. Br. Med. J. (Clin. Res. Ed.) 296(6623):660–664.

Hussein, M.A., M.A. Hassan, S. Salem, N. Scrimshaw, G. Keusch, and E. Pollit. 1985. Field work on the effects of iron supplementation [abstract]. XIII International Congress of Nutrition. Brighton, England, p. 129.

James, J.A., and M. Combes. 1960. Iron deficiency in the premature infant. Pediatrics 26:368–373.

Johnson, G., P. Jacobs, and L.R. Purves. 1983. Iron-binding proteins of iron-absorbing rat intestinal mucosa. J. Clin. Invest. 71:1467–1476.

Jones, R.L., C.M. Peterson, R.W. Grady, T. Kumbaraci, and A. Cerami. 1977. Effects of iron chelators and iron overload on *Salmonella* infection. Nature 267:63–64.

Joshi, J.G., and A. Zimmerman. 1988. Ferritin: An expanded role in metabolic regulation. Toxicology 48:21–29.

Joynson, D.H.M., A. Jacobs, D.M. Walker, and A.F. Dolby. 1972. Defect in cell-mediated immunity in patients with iron-deficiency anaemia. Lancet 2:1058–159.

Kammler, M., C. Schon, and K. Hantke. 1993. Characterization of the ferrous iron uptake system of *Escherichia coli*. J. Bacteriol. 175:6212–6219.

Kay, J.E., and C.R. Benzie. 1986. The role of the transferrin receptor in lymphocyte activation. Immunol. Lett. 12:55–58.

Kaye, D., F.A. Gill, and E.W. Hook. 1967. Factors influencing host resistance to *Salmonella* infections: The effects of hemolysis and erythrophagocytosis. Am. J. Med. Sci. 254:205–215.

Kelly, D.A., E. Price, V. Wright, M. Rossiter, and J.A. Walker-Smith. 1987. *Yersinia enterocolitica* in iron overload. J. Pediatr. Gastroenterol. Nutr. 6:643–645.

Kemp, J.D., J.A. Thorson, T. McAlmont, M. Horowitz, J.S. Cowdery, and Z.K. Ballas. 1987. Role of the transferrin receptor in lymphocyte growth: A rat IgG monoclonal antibody against the murine transferrin receptor produces highly selective inhibition of T- and B-cell activation protocols. J. Immunol. 138:2422–2426.

Keusch, G.T., and M.J.G. Farthing. 1986. Nutrition and infection. Ann. Rev. Nutr. 6:131–154.

Khan, A.J., C. Lee, J.A. Wolff, H. Chang, P. Khan, and H.E. Evans. 1983. Defects of neutrophil chemotaxis and random migration in thalassemia major. Pediatrics 60:349–351.

Klausner, R.D., T.A. Rouault, and J.B. Harford. 1993. Regulating the fate of mRNA: The control of cellular iron metabolism. Cell 72:19–28.

Kochanowski, B.A., and A.R. Sherman. 1985. Decreased antibody formation in iron-deficient rat pups—effect of iron repletion. Am. J. Clin. Nutr. 41:278–284.

Kontoghiorghies, G.J., and E.D. Weinberg. 1995. Iron: Mammalian defense systems, mechanisms of disease, and chelation therapy approaches. Blood Rev. 9:33–45.

Krantman, H.J., S.R. Young, B.J. Ank, C.M. O'Donnell, G.S. Rachelefsky, and E.R. Stiehm. 1982. Immune function in pure iron deficiency. Am. J. Dis. Child. 136:840–844.

Kronke, M., W.J. Leonard, J.M. Depper, and W.C. Greene. 1985. Sequential expression of genes involved in human T-lymphocyte growth and differentiation. J. Exp. Med. 161:1593–1598.

Kulapongs, P., V. Vithayasai, R. Suskind, and R.E. Olson. 1974. Cell-mediated immunity and phagocytosis and killing function in children with severe iron-deficiency anemia. Lancet 2:689–691.

Kuvibidila, S., and S. Wade. 1987. Macrophage function as studied by the clearance of ^{125}I-labeled polyvinylpyrrolidone in iron-deficient and iron replete mice. J. Nutr. 117:170–176.

Kuvibidila, S., M. Dardenne, W. Savino, and F. Lepault. 1990. Influence of iron-deficiency anemia on selected thymus functions in mice: Thymulin biological activity, T-cell subsets, and thymocyte proliferation. Am. J. Clin. Nutr. 51:228–232.

Leibold, E.A., and H.N. Munro. 1988. Cytoplasmic protein binds *in vitro* to a highly conserved sequence in the 5' untranslated region of ferritin heavy- and light-subunit mRNAs. Proc. Natl. Acad. Sci. USA 85:2171–2175.

Macdougall, L.G., R. Anderson, G.M. McNab, and J. Katz. 1975. The immune response in iron-deficient children: Impaired cellular defense mechanisms with altered humoral components. J. Pediatr. 86:833–843.

MacKay, H.M.. 1928. Anaemia in infancy: Its prevalence and prevention. Arch. Dis. Child. 3:117–147.

Martinez, J.L., A. Delgado Iribarren, and F. Baquero. 1990. Mechanisms of iron acquisition and bacterial virulence. FEMS Microbiol. Rev. 6:45–56.

Martino, M., M.E. Rossi, M. Resti, C. Vullo, and A. Vierucci. 1984. Changes in superoxide anion production in neutrophils from multitransfused β-thalassemia patients: Correlation with ferritin levels and liver damage. Acta Haematol. 71:289–298.

Masawe, A.E.J., J.M. Muindi, and G.B.R. Swai. 1974. Infections in iron deficiency and other types of anaemia in the tropics. Lancet 2:314–317.

Melby, K., S. Slordahl, T.J. Guttenberg, and S.A. Norbo. 1982. Septicemia due to *Yersinia enterocolitica* after oral overdoses of iron. Br. Med. J. (Clin. Res. Ed.) 285(6340):467–468.

Michelsen, P.A., and P.F. Sparling. 1981. Ability of *Neisseria gonorrhoeae, Neisseria meningitidis*, and commensal *Neisseria* species to obtain iron from transferrin and iron compounds. Infect. Immun. 33:555–564.

Michelsen, P.A., E. Blackman, and P.F. Sparling. 1982. Ability of *Neisseria gonorrhoeae, Neisseria meningitidis* and commensal *Neisseria* species to obtain iron from lactoferrin. Infect. Immun. 35:915–920.

Mofenson, H.C., T.R. Caraccio, and N. Sharieff. 1988. Iron sepsis: *Yersinia enterocolitica* septicemia possibly caused by an overdose of iron [letter]. N. Engl. J. Med. 316:1092–1093.

Moore, L.L., and J.R. Humbert. 1984. Neutrophil bactericidal dysfunction towards oxidant radical-sensitive microorganisms during experimental iron deficiency. Pediatr. Res. 18:684–689.

Mossey, R.T., and J. Sondheimer. 1985. Listeriosis in patients with long-term hemodialysis and transfusional iron overload. Am. J. Med. 79:397–399.

Munn, C.G., A.L. Markenson, A. Kapadia, and M. deSousa. 1981. Impaired T-cell mitogen responses in some patients with thalassemia intermedia. Thymus 3:119–128.

Murray, M.J., A.B. Murray, M.B. Murray, and C.J. Murray. 1978a. The adverse effect of iron repletion on the course of certain infections. Br. Med. J. 2(6145):1113–1115.

Neckers, L.M., and J. Cossman. 1983. Transferrin receptor induction in mitogen-stimulated human T-lymphocytes is required for DNA synthesis and cell division and is regulated by interleukin 2. Proc. Natl. Acad. Sci. USA 89:3494–3498.

Neilands, J.B.. 1995. Siderophores: Structure and function of microbial iron transport compounds. J. Biol. Chem. 270:26723–26726.

Neri, A., M. Brugiatelli, P. Iacopino, and F. Callea. 1984. Natural killer cell activity and T-cell subpopulations in thalassemia major. Acta Haematol. 71:263–269.

Nualart, P., M.E. Estevez, I.J. Ballart, S.A. deMiani, J. Penalver, and L. Sen. 1987. Effect of α-interferon on the altered T-B-cell immunoregulation in patients with thalassemia major. Am. J. Hematol. 24:151–159.

Oppenheimer, S.J., and R. Hendrickse. 1983. The clinical effects of iron deficiency and iron supplementation. Nutr. Abstr. Rev. 53:585–598.

Oppenheimer, S.J., F.D. Gibson, S.B. Macfarlane, J.B. Moody, C. Harrison, A. Spencer, and O. Bunari. 1986a. Iron supplementation increases prevalence and effects of malaria: Report on clinical studies in Papua New Guinea. Trans. R. Soc. Trop. Med. Hyg. 80:603–612.

Oppenheimer, S.J., S.B.J. Macfarlane, J.B. Moody, O. Bunari, and R.G. Hendrickse. 1986b. Effect of iron prophylaxis on morbidity due to infectious disease: Report on clinical studies in Papua New Guinea. Trans. R. Soc. Trop. Med. Hyg. 80:596–602.

Oppenheimer, S.J., S.B.J. Macfarlane, J.B. Moody, and C. Harrison. 1986c. Total dose iron infusion, malaria, and pregnancy in Papua New Guinea. Trans. R. Soc. Trop. Med. Hyg. 80:818–822.

Owen, D., and L.C. Kuhn. 1987. Noncoding 3' sequences of the transferrin receptor gene are required for mRNA regulation by iron. EMBO J. 6:1287–1293.

Pardalos, G., F. Kannakoudi-Tsakalidis, M. Malaka-Zafirin, H. Tsantali, and G. Papaevangelou. 1987. Iron-related disturbances of cell-mediated immunity in multitransfused children with thalassemia major. Clin. Exp. Immunol. 68:138–145.

Philips, J.L., and P. Azari. 1975. Effect of iron transferrin on nucleic acid synthesis in phytohaemagglutinin-stimulated human lymphocytes. Cell Immunol. 15:94–99.

Pollack, S. 1992. Receptor-mediated iron uptake and intracellular iron transport. Am. J. Hematol. 39:113–118.

Prasad, J.S.. 1979. Leukocyte function in iron-deficiency anemia. Am. J. Clin. Nutr. 32:550–552.

Rabson, A.R., A.F. Hallett, and H.J. Koornhof. 1975. Generalized *Yersinia enterocolitica* infection. J. Infect. Dis. 131:447–451.

Robins-Browne, R.M., and J.K. Pripic. 1985. Effects of iron and desferrioxamine on infections with *Yersinia enterocolitica*. Infect. Immun. 47:774–779.

Santos, P.C., and R.P. Falcao. 1990. Decreased lymphocyte subsets and K-cell activity in iron-deficiency anemia. Acta Haemtolog. 84:118–121.

Sawitsky, B., R. Kanter, and A. Sawitsky. 1976. Lymphocyte response to phytomitogens in iron deficiency. Am. J. Med. Sci. 272:153–160.

Scheibel, L.W. 1988. Plasmodial parasite biology: Carbohydrate metabolism and related organellar function during various stages of the life cycle. Pp. 171–217 in Malaria: Principles and Practice of Malariology, W. Wernsdorfer and I. McGregor, eds. Endinburgh: Churchill Livingstone.

Scheibel, L.W., and I.W. Sherman. 1988. Metabolism and organellar function during various stages of the life cycle: Proteins, lipids, nucleic acids, and vitamins. Pp. 219–252 in Malaria: Principles and Practice of Malariology, W. Wernsdorfer and I. McGregor, eds. Endinburgh: Churchill Livingstone.

Schryners, A.B., and J.L. Morris. 1988. Identification and characterization of the transferrin receptor from *Neisseria meningitidis*. Mol. Microbiol. 2:281–288.

Sevinc, M.S., and W.J. Page. 1992. Generation of *Azotobacter vinlandii* strains defective in siderophore production and characterization of a strain unable to produce known siderophores. J. Gen. Microbiol. 138:587–596.

Shand, G.H., H. Anwar, J. Kadurugamuwa, M.R.W. Brown, S.H. Silverman, and J. Melling. 1985. *In vivo* evidence that bacteria in urinary tract infection grow under iron-restricted conditions. Infect. Immun. 48:35–39.

Stojiljkovic, J., M. Cobeljic, and K. Hantke. 1993. *Escherichia coli* K-12 ferrous iron uptake mutants are impaired in their ability to colonize the mouse intestine. FEMS Microbiol. Lett. 108:111–116.

Strauss, R.G. 1978. Iron deficiency, infections, and immune function: A reassessment. Am. J. Clin. Nutr. 31:660–666.

Tavo, T.A., R. Minlero, and A. Ponsono. 1977. NBT test in thalassemia [letter]. J. Pediatr. 90:666.

Taylor, P.G., A. Soyano, E. Romano, and M. Layrisse. 1988. Iron and transferrin uptake by phytohaemagglutinin-stimulated human peripheral blood lymphocytes. Microbiol. Immunol. 32:945–955.

Theil, E.C.. 1987. Ferritin: Structure, gene regulation, and cellular function in animals, plants, and microorganisms. Ann. Rev. Biochem. 56:289–315.

Thompson, H.L., and J.H. Brock. 1986. The effect of iron and agar on production of hydrogen peroxide by stimulated and activated mouse peritoneal macrophages. FEBS Lett. 200:283–286.

Thorson, J.A., K.M. Smith, F. Gomez, P.W. Naumann, and J.D. Kemp. 1991. Role of iron in T-cell activation: Th1 clones differ from Th2 clones in their sensitivity to inhibition of DNA synthesis caused by IgG Mabs against the transferrin receptor and the iron chelator desferoxamine. Cell Immunol. 134:126–137.

Turgeon-O'Brien, H., J. Amiot, L. Lemieux, and J-C. Dillon. 1985. Myeloperoxidase activity of polymorphonuclear leukocytes in iron-deficiency anaemia and anaemia of chronic disorders. Acta Haematol 74:151–154.

Vadillo, M., X. Corbella, V. Pac, P. Fernandez-Viladrich, and R. Pujol. 1994. Multiple liver abscesses due to *Yersinia enterocolitica* discloses primary hemochromatosis: Three case reports and review. Clin. Infect. Dis. 18:938–941.

Van Asbeck, B.S., J.J.M. Marx, A. Struyvenberg, J.H. van Kats, and J. Verhoef. 1984a. Effect of iron (III) in the presence of various ligands on the phagocytic and metabolic activity of human polymorphonuclear leukocytes. J. Immunol. 132:851–856.

Van Asbeck, B.S., J.J.M. Marx, A. Struyvenberg, J.H. van Kats, and J. Verhoef. 1984b. Functional defects in phagocytic cells from patients with iron overload. J. Infect. 85:232–240.

Van Heerden, C., R. Oosthuizen, H. Van Wyk, P. Prinsloo, and P. Anderson. 1981. Evaluation of neutrophil and lymphocyte function in subjects with iron deficiency. S. Afr. Med. J. 24:111–113.

Walter, T., S. Arredondo, M. Arevalo, and A. Stekel. 1986. Effect of iron therapy on phagocytosis and bactericidal activity in neutrophils of iron-deficient infants. Am. J. Clin. Nutr. 44:877–882.

Waterlot, Y., B. Cantinieaux, C. Hariga-Mulier, E. de Maertelaere-Laurant, J.L. Vanherweghmen, and P. Fondu. 1985. Impairment of neutrophil phagocytosis in haemodialysed patients—the critical role of iron overload. Br. Med. J. 291:501–504.

Weinberg, E.D. 1984. Iron withholding: A defense against infection and neoplasia. Physiol. Rev. 64:65–102.

West, S.E.H., and P.F. Sparling. 1985. Response of *Neisseria gonorrheae* to iron limitation: Alteration in expression of membrane proteins without apparent siderophore production. Infect. Immun. 47:388–394.

Worwood, M. 1986. Serum ferritin. Clin. Sci. 70:215–220.

Wright, A.C., L.M. Simpson, and J.D. Oliver. 1981. Role of iron in the pathogenesis of *Vibrio vulnificus* infections. Infect. Immun. 34:503–507.

Yancey, R.J., and R.A. Finkelstein. 1981. Assimilation of iron by pathogenic *Neisseria* spp. Infect. Immun. 32:592–599.

Yetgin, S., C. Altay, G. Ciliv, and Y. Lalcli. 1979. Myeloperoxidase activity and bactericidal function of PMN in iron deficiency. Acta Haematol. 61:10–14.

Zahringer, J., B.S. Baliga, and H.S. Munro. 1976. Novel mechanism for translational control in regulation of ferritin synthesis by iron. Proc. Natl. Acad. Sci. USA 81:2752–2756.

DISCUSSION

PAUL ROATH: It seemed most of your talk centered on gram negatives. Is there any expectation of gram positives to have an iron uptake system because the membranes would conserve it differently?

GERALD KEUSCH: There are parallels in the gram positives. Most of the information has really come from the paradigm organism, *E. coli*. But *Corynelbactrerium diphtheriae* is a gram positive organism in which toxic production is closely regulated by iron. There is a good source of information on the gram positive bacteria and iron in the monograph *Iron and Infection*, edited by Bullen and Griffiths (1987).

Nutrition and Immune Function, 1999
Pp. 337–359. Washington, D.C.
National Academy Press

16

Trace Minerals, Immune Function, and Viral Evolution

Melinda A. Beck[1]

INTRODUCTION

A number of trace elements have been shown to be important for adequate functioning of the immune system, including copper, zinc, and selenium. Both deficiencies and luxus levels of trace elements can influence various parameters of the immune system, such as antibody responses, cell-mediated immunity ,and natural killer (NK) cell activity.

A functional immune system is required for the ability of the host to prevent or limit infections. This is particularly important for soldiers in the field, where exposure to novel infectious agents, as well as working in less-than-optimal hygienic conditions, is a real possibility. Clearly, the optimum level of trace elements and other nutrients for immune function needs to be included in any military diet.

[1] Melinda A. Beck, Department of Pediatrics and Nutrition, Frank Porter Graham Child Development Center, University of North Carolina at Chapel Hill, Chapel Hill, NC 27599-8180

In addition to the effect of trace elements on immune function, recent studies from Beck et al. (1995) have demonstrated that selenium (Se) levels can influence the genetics of a viral pathogen. Thus, trace element nutrition influences not only the host response to a pathogen but also the pathogen itself.

This paper reviews the effect of the trace minerals zinc (Zn), copper (Cu), and Se on immune function, as well as the effect of Se on a viral pathogen. Implications for soldiers in the field will also be discussed.

ZINC

Zn is perhaps one of the most studied trace elements with respect to its effect on the host immune system. Deficiencies in Zn have been classified into three syndromes by Henkin and Aamodt (1983): acute, chronic, and subacute deficiency. It has been suggested that subacute deficiency is the most common, affecting an estimated 4 million people in the United States (Walsh et al., 1994). Zn is obtained in the diet primarily from meat (50%), cereals and legumes (30%), and dairy products (20%) (USDA, 1986).

Zn deficiency has been noted to result in increased susceptibility to infectious disease (Bogden et al., 1988). In a mouse model of Zn deficiency (Fernandes et al., 1979; Fraker et al., 1978, 1986), a 30-d feeding period of suboptimal levels of Zn led to reduced thymus size and depleted macrophages and lymphocytes in the spleen. Suboptimal Zn status has also been associated with decreased T-cell function and antibody responses (Kruse-Jarres, 1989). If the Zn deficiency is corrected, immune status is restored (Walsh et al., 1994).

Excess levels of Zn have also been reported to be immunosuppressive, including decreased activities of polymorphonuclear leukocytes, decreased T-cell proliferation to mitogen, and decreased antibody production (Schlesinger et al., 1993). Thus, Zn status, both excess and deficient, adversely affects immune function.

Singh et al. (1994) found that supplemental Zn given prior to strenuous exercise reduced the amount of reactive oxygen species that occur post exercise. This antioxidant effect of Zn may be of importance to troops who are under chronic physical stress.

Driessen et al. (1995) found that, *in vitro*, lipopolysaccharide-stimulated peripheral blood mononuclear cell cultures exposed to 0.0125 mM Zn had elevated interleukin (IL)-1β levels that were 50 percent higher than cultures that were not supplemented with Zn. Secretion of interferon-gamma (INF-γ) increased 10-fold when cultures were supplemented with 0.1 mM Zn. However, monocyte stimulation by superantigens (staphylococcal enterotoxins A and E) was decreased in cultures supplemented with Zn. Thus, depending on the type of stimulus, supplemental Zn may exert different effects.

Zinc is a cofactor for a number of enzymes, including thymidine kinase, ribonuclease, and RNA and DNA polymerases. All of these enzymes are important for cell division. In addition, Zn is an essential cofactor for thymulin, a peptide hormone that plays a key role in T-cell maturation.

Thus, Zn has been shown in a number of studies to have an effect on immune function. However, depending on the type of immune stimulus and/or concentration of Zn present, the immune system can either be stimulated or suppressed. Further studies with Zn are required to clearly delineate the role of zinc in immune system functioning.

COPPER

Cu is an essential nutrient for humans, although Cu deficiency is rare. Cu-deficient animals are more susceptible to parasitic, bacterial, and viral infection (Newberne et al., 1968; Okmole and Onawunmi, 1979; Stabel et al. 1993). Children with Menkes syndrome, a genetic disease of Cu malabsorption, generally die from infectious bronchopneumonia (Prohaska and Failla, 1993).

Animal studies have demonstrated that Cu-deficient mice have impaired plaque formation to sheep blood red cells, demonstrating decreased B-cell activity, and decreased antibody responses to a number of antigens (Blakly and Hamilton, 1987; Failla et al., 1988; Koller, 1987; Prohaska and Lukasewycz, 1981, 1989, 1990; Vyas and Chandra, 1983).

Cell-mediated immunity has also been studied in Cu-deficient animals, with conflicting results. Jones (1984) reported delayed-type hypersensitivity (DTH) responses were enhanced in Cu-deficient mice, whereas Koller et al. (1987) reported normal DTH responses in Cu-deficient rats. However, T-cell proliferative responses to a variety of antigens are lower in Cu-deficient animals (Davis et al., 1987; Lukaswycz and Prohaska, 1983, 1985; Prohaska and Lukasewycz, 1981, 1989). NK cell activity is also decreased in Cu-deficient rats (Koller, 1987).

Lymphocyte subset populations are also altered in Cu-deficient animals. Higher numbers of B-cells and fewer T-helper (Th) cells are found in Cu-deficient animals as compared with animals with normal Cu nutriture.

In a human study, Kelley et al. (1995) fed healthy adult males a low copper diet for 66 days, followed by a period of normal Cu intake. Daily Cu intake was 0.66 mg/d for the first 24 days, 0.38 mg/d for the next 42 days, and 2.49 mg/d for the final 24 days of the study. A range of 1.5 to 3.0 mg/d of Cu is recommended for adults. Lymphoproliferative responses to mitogen were greatly reduced during the 0.38 mg/d feeding period, when compared with values at the start of the study, and were not restored within the 24 days of feeding the 2.49 mg/d Cu diet. Secretion of IL-2 receptor was also decreased. However, numbers of B-cells increased during the low Cu diet, although the numbers of total T-cells (CD3+) or T-cell subsets (CD4+, CD8+) did not change. Moreover, no changes were seen in neutrophil phagocytic function.

Although adequate Cu intake is important for immune function, the mechanism of action is not known. Cu has many biochemical activities, such as a cofactor for ferroxidase, cytochome c oxidase, and Zn-Cu superoxide dismutase, an enzyme that is important in limiting oxidative stress. Further research is necessary to delineate the role of Cu in immune system activities.

Cu-Zn Interactions

Zn and Cu are antagonistic with one another: Zn deficiency leads to an increase in Cu levels in liver and bone (Burch et al., 1975; Moses and Parker, 1964; Petering et al., 1971; Prasad et al. 1969). Conversely, excess Zn leads to Cu deficiency. Under certain conditions, Zn and Cu can inhibit one another's absorption. For example, Zn absorption in Zn-adequate rats is decreased with excess Cu, but not in Zn-deficient rats (Evans et al., 1974; Walsh et al., 1994). Both Cu and Zn absorption are increased with a Zn deficiency. However, only Cu absorption is increased with a Cu deficiency.

SELENIUM

Selenium (Se) is an essential component of glutathione peroxidase, an antioxidant enzyme that plays an important role in removing hydrogen peroxide and organic hydroperoxides (Chaudiere et al., 1984). A deficiency in Se can induce a state of oxidative stress in the host. Oxidative stress is a term used to describe the overabundance of the production of free radicals and other oxidants in comparison with antioxidant defenses. Thus, oxidative stress describes a situation in which prooxidants are favored over antioxidants. Oxidative stress can affect host cells in a number of ways. Beckman and Ames (1997) have suggested that oxygen free radicals damage on the order of 10,000 DNA bases per cell per day, of which a small percentage are not repaired. Membrane integrity of cells becomes impaired due to oxygen free radical-mediated lipid peroxidation, leading to the decrease or loss of cellular function. Proteins are also susceptible to free-radical damage. For example, hydroxy radicals modify amino acid residues at metal-binding sites of proteins (Stadtman, 1992). Oxidized proteins are more rapidly degraded than unoxidized proteins (Davies and Goldberg, 1987; Farber and Levine, 1982; Rivett, 1985). Oxidant stress also alters ion movement across cellular membranes by interfering with Na+ pumps and Na+K+Cl⁻ cotransporter activities (Elliott and Schilling, 1992).

Se deficiency has been associated with lower resistance to infection with *Pasturella multocida* and parainfluenza 3 virus (Chandra and Chandra, 1986; Dhur et al., 1990; Larsen, 1988; Larsen and Tollersund, 1981; Reffett et al., 1988; Sheffy and Schultz, 1979, Stable and Spears, 1993). The increased susceptibility to infectious pathogens in Se deficiency may be due to decreased antibody production and impaired lymphoproliferative responses (Chandra and Chandra, 1986).

Se deficiency has also been associated with an endemic cardiomyopathy in China known as Keshan disease. Keshan disease (KD) is characterized by acute or chronic heart conditions affecting heart function such as cardiac insufficiency, enlargement of the heart, arrhythmia, atrial fibrillation, and tachycardia (Li et al., 1985). Histologically, KD is characterized by multiple focal necrosis and myocardial parenchymatous degeneration (Gu, 1983). Epidemiologists in China found that the disease occurred only in areas with low Se soil content. Subsequently, it was found that individuals residing in KD endemic areas were of low Se status. Supplementation with Se to normal nutritional levels has prevented the widespread occurrence of KD in endemic areas of China. However, the Se deficiency alone did not explain all aspects of the disease. The seasonal and annual incidence of KD suggested that an infectious cofactor may play an etiological role in the development of the disease. Indeed, virologists in China have isolated several enterovirus strains from blood and tissue specimens of KD victims (Su et al., 1979). One of the enteroviruses, Coxsackievirus B4 (CVB4), recovered from a blood sample of a KD patient, caused a higher incidence and more severe myocarditis in neonatal mice born to Se-deficient dams than in neonates born to dams that were fed a diet containing adequate levels of Se (Bai et al., 1980; Ge et al., 1987).

Coxsackieviruses, and particularly CVB viruses, are etiological agents of viral-induced myocarditis and are suspected agents of dilated cardiomyopathy (DCM) (Fuster et al., 1981; Leslie, 1989). DCM is the second leading indication for heart transplantation in this country (O'Connell and Robinson, 1985), which suggests that infections with CVB viruses are responsible for a great deal of morbidity and mortality. Coxsackieviruses are nonenveloped RNA viruses in the Picornaviridae family, subgroup enterovirus (of which the most commonly known enterovirus is poliovirus). The genome consists of approximately 7,500 base pairs in an open reading frame, flanked by both 3' and 5' nontranslated regions.

With over 3 decades of research, the mouse model of CVB-induced myocarditis is widely accepted as an appropriate animal model for human myocarditis (Woodruff, 1980). Inoculation with Coxsackievirus B3 (CVB3) induces a myocardial inflammatory infiltrate 10 to 14 days later (Leslie, 1989), consisting primarily of both CD4+ and CD8+ T-cells, a pattern similar to that seen in human cases of myocarditis (Woodruff, 1980; Woodruff and Woodruff, 1974). Although the response is initiated by the viral infection, the heart pathology is widely believed to be due to an immunopathological process. Evidence for an immunopathological basis for enterovirus-induced cardiomyopathy is provided by the lack of or diminished disease in CVB3-infected athymic (nude) mice and lack of disease in gamma-irradiated adult mice that were not reconstituted with T-cells (Woodruff and Woodruff, 1974). In addition, at the peak period of cardiac inflammation, virus is not generally detectable in mouse heart tissue (Woodruff, 1980).

Although the immune system clearly contributes to the pathology, it also performs a protective function. Strains of mice that can clear virus from the heart more rapidly and rapidly produce neutralizing antibody develop only a mild myocarditis. However, strains of mice that have delayed viral clearance and delayed production of neutralizing antibody develop severe myocarditis (Herskovitz et al., 1985). In addition, hearts from severe combined-immunodeficient (SCID) mice inoculated with CVB3 develop severe cardiac necrosis (Chow et al., 1992). These effects have been attributed to direct viral lysis of cardiac myocytes due to the absence of a functioning immune system to clear the virus.

To investigate the role Coxsackieviruses may play in the development of KD, this laboratory utilized its well-characterized murine model of CVB3-induced myocarditis to study, in collaboration with Orville Levander at the U.S. Department of Agriculture, how a specific nutritional deficiency affects the host's response to a virus (Beck et al., 1994a,c, 1995).

C3H/HeJ male mice immediately postweaning were fed either a diet adequate or deficient in Se. Following 4 weeks of feeding the diets, mice were bled and serum glutathione peroxidase levels were analyzed as a biomarker of Se status. Mice fed the Se-deficient diet had serum glutathione peroxidase levels significantly depressed when compared with mice fed the Se-adequate diet (4.7 +/– 0.2 milliunits/mg protein vs. 50.8 +/– milliunits/mg protein). Mice were then inoculated with either CVB3/20, a myocarditic strain of CVB3, or CVB3/0, an amyocarditic strain.

As shown in Figure 16-1, hearts from CVB3/20 (myocarditic strain)-infected mice that were fed a Se-deficient diet had increased pathology at an earlier time point than infected mice that were fed a Se-adequate diet (Beck et al., 1994c). In the deficient mice, myocarditic lesions were larger, were more necrotic, and had a greater number of calcium deposits. Of particular interest, as shown in Figure 16-2, CVB3/0 (amyocarditic strain)-infected mice that were fed a Se-deficient diet developed a moderate level of myocarditis, in contrast to CVB3/0-infected mice that were fed a Se-adequate diet, which did not develop any heart inflammation (Beck et al., 1994a). Thus, a dietary deficiency in Se permitted a viral phenotype change: CVB3/20 developed enhanced virulence, and CVB3/0 changed from an avirulent virus to a virulent one.

Because some of the individuals living in KD endemic areas were also of marginal vitamin E status, and because Se and vitamin E can act synergistically and spare one another's nutritional requirements, additional studies were performed in this laboratory. To mimic this situation, mice were fed diets deficient in vitamin E and adequate in Se prior to infection with CVB3. Hearts from mice fed vitamin E-deficient diets, but diets adequate in Se, had increased pathology when infected with CVB3/20. CVB3/0 infection, which is normally benign, could now cause disease in mice fed a Se-adequate, vitamin E-deficient diet (Beck et al., 1994b).

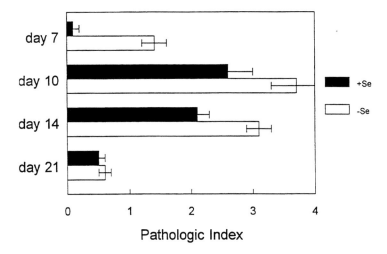

FIGURE 16-1 Histopathologic scores of CVB3/20 (myocarditic strain)-inoculated, selenium-adequate (+Se) or Se-deficient (–Se) mice at various times postinoculation. Scores: 0, no lesions; 1+, foci of mononuclear cell inflammation associated with myocardial cell reactive changes without myocardial cell necrosis; 2+, inflammatory foci clearly associated with myocardial cell reactive changes; 3+ – 4+, inflammatory foci clearly associated with myocardial cell necrosis and dystrophic calcification. Each bar represents the mean +/–SD of 10 mice.

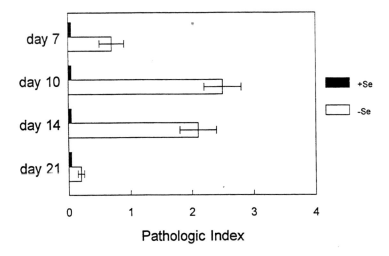

FIGURE 16-2 Histopathologic scores of CVB3/0 (amyocarditic strain)-inoculated, selenium-adequate (+Se) or Se-deficient (–Se) mice at various times postinoculation. Scores as for Figure 16-1. Each bar represents the mean +/–SD of 10 mice.

344   *MELINDA A. BECK*

Vitamin E also acts as an antioxidant, although by a very different mechanism from the antioxidant properties of Se. Thus, because either Se or vitamin E deficiency enhanced CVB3/20-induced myocarditis and allowed a normally benign CVB3/0 infection to become virulent, this author and colleagues proposed a common mechanism of oxidative stress.

Viral titers in various organs were examined to determine if viral replication patterns were altered as a result of replication in a nutritionally deficient animal. Altered patterns of replication may have been responsible for the increase in pathology seen in the deficient animals. As shown in Figure 16-3, cardiac virus titers were higher in the Se-deficient, CVB3/20-infected mice as compared with infected Se-adequate mice, although the kinetics of the response were identical. Thus, although the Se-deficiency enhanced viral replication, reflected in higher titers, the replication time did not change, as virus was detected at identical time points in both deficient and adequate mice. As shown in Figure 16-4, for mice infected with CVB3/0, higher virus cardiac titers were also detected in deficient animals. However, in contrast to infection with CVB3/20, virus persisted for approximately 1 week longer in the deficient mice. Similar results were obtained with infected vitamin E-deficient mice (data not shown).

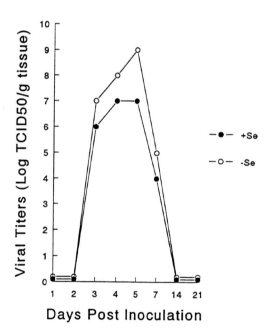

FIGURE 16-3 Heart virus titers from Se-adequate (+Se) or Se-deficient (–Se) mice infected with CVB3/20. Symbols represent the mean of 10 animals.

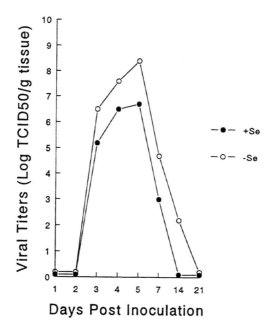

FIGURE 16-4 Heart virus titers from Se-adequate (+Se) or Se-deficient (–Se) mice infected with CVB3/0. Symbols represent the mean of 10 animals.

How does the increased oxidative stress affect either the host and/or the virus so that virulence is enhanced? Se and/or vitamin E deficiencies have a number of effects on immune function, including decreased proliferative responses to mitogen and reduced antibody production. For studies in this laboratory, several immune functions that are important in viral clearance mechanisms were examined: (1) B-cell function, measured by neutralizing antibody production, (2) T-cell proliferation against both antigen and mitogen, and (3) NK cell activity. In addition, mRNA was examined for IL-1, IL-6, and tumor necrosis factor-beta (TNF-β) in the hearts of deficient or adequate animals. All of these cytokines play critical roles in inflammatory processes.

No differences were found in neutralizing antibody titers between deficient and adequate mice (data not shown). However, spleen cell proliferative responses to both mitogen (Figure 16-5) and antigen (Figure 16-6) were decreased in Se-deficient mice when compared with Se-adequate mice. Mitogen responses were found to be much more depressed than antigen-specific responses. NK responses (data not shown) were also examined, as NK has been shown to be important in CVB3 clearance from normal animals (Gauntt et al., 1988). NK levels were only slightly depressed in Se-deficient mice, and this difference was not statistically significant.

346   MELINDA A. BECK

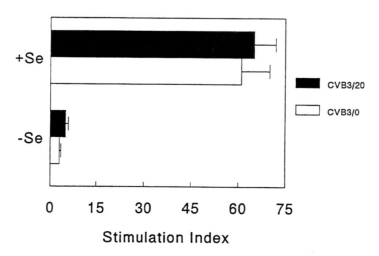

FIGURE 16-5 Mitogen-stimulated, spleen cell proliferative responses from Se-adequate (+Se) or Se-deficient (–Se) mice. Data expressed as stimulation indices calculated as ratio of counts per minute (cpm) in presence of mitogen over cpm in presence of medium (background). Each bar represents the mean +/–SD of 15 animals.

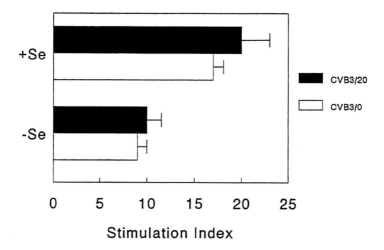

FIGURE 16-6 CVB3-antigen-specific-stimulated, spleen cell proliferative responses from Se-adequate (+Se) or Se-deficient (–Se) mice. Data expressed as stimulation indices calculated as ratio of counts per minute (cpm) in presence of antigen over cpm in presence of HeLa cell membranes (background). Each bar represents the mean +/–SD of 15 animals.

To examine cytokine production, heart tissue was isolated from CVB3/20-infected mice that were fed either Se-adequate or Se-deficient diets at various times post inoculation. Using reverse transcriptase-polymerase chain reaction (RT-PCR), PCR fragments were identified for IL-1, IL-6 and TNF-β. The fragments were normalized with α-tubulin and scanned using a laser densitometer. Figure 16-7 demonstrates the levels of mRNA for each sample isolated by measuring the area under the curve (AU) for each PCR fragment. As shown in Figure 16-7, mRNA levels for TNF-β and IL-6 are decreased in infected mice fed the Se-deficient diet as compared with mice fed the adequate diets. However, IL-1 levels were fairly similar between groups.

Levels of mRNA were also looked at for INF-γ in cultured spleen cells from infected mice with and without mitogen stimulation (10 days post-CVB3/20 inoculation, 48 hours in culture). As shown in Figure 16-8, INF-γ was produced by stimulated cells in both Se-deficient and Se-adequate mice, although no mRNA was found in the unstimulated cultures. Although exposure to mitogen could induce stimulation of INF-γ mRNA in cells from Se-deficient mice, it is not known if antigen stimulation of cells from CVB3-infected, Se-deficient mice can also stimulate mRNA for INF-γ. Thus, although neutralizing antibody and NK levels are unaffected, or slightly affected, under these conditions of nutriture, proliferation levels and mRNA for IL-6 and TNF-β are depressed in Se-deficient mice, which indicates that some immune dysfunction has occurred.

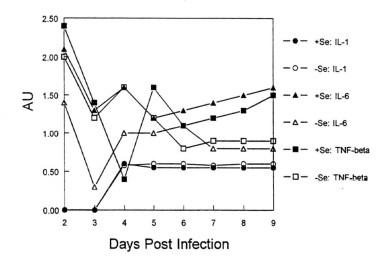

FIGURE 16-7 mRNA levels of cytokines in the hearts of Se-adequate or Se-deficient mice following infection with CVB3/20.

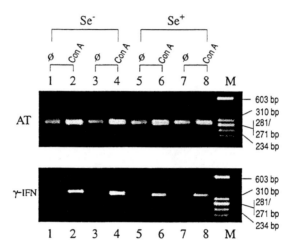

FIGURE 16-8 Agarose gel demonstrating cDNA fragments from RT-PCR of cultured spleen cells from four individual mice (two Se-adequate and two Se-deficient) with and without mitogen (Con A) stimulation. φ, control cultures with no added stimulation; Con A, concanavalin A; M, molecular weight markers (sizes noted on figure); AT, α-tubulin; γ-IFN, gamma-interferon.

These results may indicate a suppression of Th1 cells preferentially to Th2 cells. Th2 cells are necessary for providing B-cell help, secreting cytokines such as IL-4, IL-5, and IL-10. Th1 cells produce IL-2 and INF-γ. Because antibody responses were intact (suggesting that Th2 cells were functioning) and proliferation levels were decreased (suggesting a lack of IL-2 protein), the nutritional deficit may have affected Th1 activity.

The increased pathology seen in nutritionally deficient mice may have been due to changes in the host that allowed for the virus to cause increased damage, such as a decreased immune response or changes in heart cell physiology. A second possibility is that the virus itself changed as a consequence of replication in a Se-deficient host. To determine if this second possibility had occurred, virus obtained from Se- and vitamin E-deficient donors was passaged back into Se- or vitamin E-adequate recipients. The experiment was performed as follows: at 10 days postinoculation with either CVB3/20 or CVB3/0, hearts from mice that were fed either a Se-deficient or Se-adequate diet or a vitamin E-deficient or vitamin E-adequate diet were processed for virus isolation. The viruses recovered from the hearts were passaged onto HeLa cell monolayers, isolated, and titered. These viruses were then renamed to reflect the host from which they had been isolated. For example, CVB3/20 virus, which was isolated from a Se-adequate host, was designated CVB3/20Se+. Similarly, virus isolated from a Se-deficient host was designated CVB3/20Se⁻. The HeLa-passaged virus was then inoculated intraperitoneally at 1×10^5 TCID$_{50}$ in 100 µl medium into 7-week-old, male, *C3H/HeJ* mice fed a vitamin E- and Se-adequate diet. At 7 and 10 days postinoculation, mice were killed and their hearts examined for pathology and heart viral titers.

This laboratory was able to demonstrate that viruses from either Se- or vitamin E-deficient mice underwent a phenotypic change in the deficient animal, such that passage into a Se- and vitamin E-supplemented recipient also caused increased disease (Beck et al., 1994a, b, c). Not only did the Se deficiency enhance the virulence of the CVB3/20 myocarditic virus, the Se deficiency was also able to change the phenotype of the amyocarditic CVB3/0 virus from benign to virulent so that virus now caused damage even in a nutritionally adequate host (Beck et al., 1994c).

Was the phenotype change due to a change in virus genotype? To answer this question, four separate virus isolates obtained from CVB3/0-infected, Se-deficient mice and four separate isolates from CVB3/0-infected, Se-adequate mice were sequenced. The input virus was also sequenced for comparison (CVB3/0 is a cloned and sequenced virus). As shown in Table 16-1, it was found that six nucleotides in the viral genome had mutated in the virus recovered from the Se-deficient host. No virus mutations were found in the

TABLE 16-1 Nucleotide and Corresponding Amino Acid Differences between the Avirulent CVB3/0 and the Virulent CVB3/0Se– and Comparison with CVB3/20 (Virulent) Strain

Nucleotide Number (5'-3')	CVB3 Strain			Amino Acid Change
	CVB3/20[*]	CVB3/0[*]	CVB3/0Se–[†]	
234	T	C	T	Nontranslated region
788	A	G	A	Arg→Gly
2271	T	A	T	Phe→Tyr
2438	C	G	C	Gln→Glu
2690	A	G	G	None
3324	T	C	T	Val→Ala
7334	T	C	T	Nontranslated region

[*] CVB3/20 and CVB3/0 are cloned and sequenced strains of CVB3. The CVB3/0 preparation used to inoculate both Se-deficient and Se-adequate mice was sequenced.

[†] CVB3/0Se– virus was isolated from the heart of a Se-deficient mouse inoculated with CVB3/0. The same pattern of nucleotide changes was identified in three other virus isolates. These viruses are myocarditic when inoculated into Se-adequate mice.

isolates from the Se-adequate mice. Notably, all six nucleotides were identical to nucleotides found in the virulent CVB3/20 virus. Interestingly, one nucleotide, nt 2690, in the avirulent strain common to the cardiovirulent strain did not mutate. Thus, the CVB3/0Se- viruses were identical to each other and represented a hybrid between a known virulent strain and the avirulent input strain. To this author's knowledge, this is the first description of a specific host nutritional deficiency permitting an avirulent virus to develop virulence due to changes in the viral genotype (Beck et al., 1995).

Recently, this laboratory isolated virus from CVB3/0-infected, vitamin E-deficient mice. Identical nucleotide changes occurred in these viruses as well, suggesting that a common mechanism of oxidative stress leads to predictable nucleotide changes in the CVB3/0 genome, changing an avirulent virus to a virulent one (Beck et al., 1996).

Thus, the change in genotype in virus isolated from either Se- or vitamin E-deficient mice may be related to the virus' enhanced ability to replicate in deficient hosts. The most common causes of mutation in proliferating viruses are thought to be errors in polymerase transcription and endogenous damage to nucleic acid bases. Coxsackievirus is an RNA virus and therefore lacks the proofreading capability that is a feature of DNA replication. Because of the lack of RNA replicases with proofreading ability, RNA viruses are susceptible to high mutation rates. The high mutation rate of RNA viruses results in the continuous generation of virus mutants, producing a dynamic and changing viral population. Thus, any increase in viral replication may be expected to enhance the evolution of new viral mutants.

Two possibilities may account for the increased viral titers in the deficient mice. Virus may have escaped from normal immune clearance mechanisms, thus allowing a higher and more persistent degree of replication. A second alternative (although not mutually exclusive) is that cardiac cell membranes may have been compromised such that virus was able to replicate to higher titers in oxidatively stressed cardiac cells versus normal cardiac cells.

Another possible explanation for the change in viral genotype may be that the oxidative stress status of the host directly affected the virus. The reactive oxygen species (ROS) generated due to the nutritional deficiency may have damaged the viral RNA, which is similar to what occurs when ROS damages DNA. This damage may have resulted in the mutations. This possibility is currently being explored in this laboratory.

Thus, the work with Coxsackievirus and host Se deficiency demonstrates that not only can the nutritional deficiency affect the host, but effects on the pathogen must be considered as well. This work demonstrates that once the benign virus has mutated, as a result of replication in a nutritionally deficient host, it can now infect and cause disease even in mice of normal nutriture. The work has implications for troops deployed in the field. It may be possible that if a few soldiers are oxidatively stressed, as a result of a nutritional deficiency or severe physical activity, a viral pathogen could mutate into a potentially more virulent pathogen and infect other soldiers who may or may not be oxidatively stressed. It would seem prudent to ensure that any food products provided for the troops contain a balance of nutrients to limit oxidative stress.

AUTHOR'S SUMMARY AND CONCLUSIONS

Clearly, trace elements have been shown to be important for immune system functioning. A deficiency in Cu, Zn, or Se has immunosuppressive effects on the host, which can lead to increased susceptibility to infectious disease. The usual model for understanding the effect of nutrition on infectious disease is diagrammed as follows:

Inadequate host nutrition
↓
Inadequate immune response
↓
Increased susceptibility to infectious disease
↓
Illness

However, this author's work with Se and CVB3 demonstrates that host nutrition can affect not only the host but the pathogen as well. Therefore, the following model is proposed:

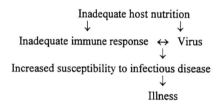

Inadequate host nutrition
↓   ↓
Inadequate immune response ↔ Virus
↓
Increased susceptibility to infectious disease
↓
Illness

This model takes into account not only the effect that host nutriture has on the immune response but also the effect of host nutriture on the viral pathogen. This model more accurately represents the relationship between nutrition and infectious disease.

A number of studies, many of which have been cited in this paper, have examined the effect of trace elements on immune function. These studies are important, in that they indicate which immune parameters are sensitive to these nutrients. However, these studies are limited in that most do not correlate immune dysfunction with an actual increase in illness. For example, if a mild deficiency in Zn decreases T-cell proliferative responses by 20 percent, is this enough to increase susceptibility to infectious disease? It is entirely possible that some of the immune changes induced by nutritional status will not result in increased incidence or duration of illness. The immune system has many redundant pathways, and measurements of one particular aspect of this system may not provide a true picture of the host's ability to respond to infection. The immune parameters that are examined need to be correlated with incidence and/or severity of infectious disease.

This author recommends that any food supplement tested in military personnel for its effect on immune function should also be ranked for protection against illness. Effects can be self-reported (although this is the least reliable measure) or medical personnel can record and monitor symptoms. Additionally, sampling of throat or nasal washes for common respiratory viruses could be obtained. Thus, a more "real world" indication of immune function—the ability to resist infection—can be determined.

REFERENCES

Bai, J., S. Wu, K. Ge, X. Deng, and C. Su. 1980. The combined effect of selenium deficiency and viral infection on the myocardium of mice. Acta Acad. Med. Sci. Sin. 2:29–31.

Beck, M.A., B.R. Blakly, and D.L. Hamilton. 1987. The effect of copper deficiency on the immune response in mice. Drug Nutr. Interact. 5:103–111.

Beck, M.A., P.C. Kolbeck, L.H. Rohr, Q. Shi, V.C. Morris, and O.A. Levander. 1994a. Benign human enterovirus becomes virulent in selenium-deficient mice. J. Med. Virol. 43:166–170.

Beck, M.A., P.C. Kolbeck, L.H. Rohr, Q. Shi, V.C. Morris, and O.A. Levander. 1994b. Vitamin E deficiency intensifies the myocardial injury of Coxsackievirus B3 infection of mice. J. Nutr. 124:345–358.

Beck, M.A., P.C. Kolbeck, Q. Shi, L.H. Rohr, V.C. Morris, and O.A. Levander. 1994c. Increased virulence of a human enterovirus (Coxsackievirus B3) in selenium-deficient mice. J. Infect. Dis. 170:351–357.

Beck, M.A., Q. Shi, V.C. Morris, and O.A. Levander. 1995. Rapid genomic evolution of a non-virulent Coxsackievirus B3 in selenium-deficient mice results in selection of identical virulent isolates. Nat. Med. 1:433–436.

Beck, M.A., Q. Shi, V.C. Morris, and O.A. Levander. 1996. From avirulent to virulent: Vitamin E deficiency in mice drives rapid genomic evolution of a CVB3 virus [abstract]. FASEB J. 10(3):A191.

Beckman, K.B., and B.N. Ames. 1997. Oxidative decay of DNA. J. Biol. Chem. 272:19633–19636.

Bogden, J.D., J.M. Oleske, M.A. Lavenhar, E.M. Munves, P.W. Kemp, K.S. Bruening, K.J. Holding, T.N. Denny, M.A. Guarino, L.M. Krieger, and B.K. Holland. 1988. Zinc and immunocompetence in elderly people: Effects of zinc supplementation for 3 months. Am. J. Clin. Nutr. 48:655–663.

Burch, R.E., R.V. Williams, H.K.J. Hahn, M.M. Jetton, and J.F. Sullivan. 1975. Serum and tissue enzyme activity and trace element content in response to zinc deficiency in the pig. Clin. Chem. 21:568–577.

Chandra, S., and R.K. Chandra. 1986. Nutrition, immune response, and outcome. Prog. Food Nutr. Sci. 10:1–7.

Chaudiere, J., E.C. Wilhelmsen, and A.L. Tappel. 1984. Mechanism of selenium-glutathione peroxidase and its inhibition by mercaptocaroxylic acids and other mercaptans. J. Biol. Chem. 259:1043–1050.

Chow, L.H., K.W. Beisel, and B.M. McManus. 1992. Enteroviral infection of mice with severe combined immunodeficieny. Evidence for direct viral pathogenesis of myocardial injury. Lab. Invest. 66:24–31.

Davies, K.J., and A.L. Goldberg. 1987. Proteins damaged by oxygen radicals are rapidly degraded in extracts of red blood cells. J. Biol. Chem. 262:8227–8231.

Davis, M.A., W.T. Johnson, M. Briske-Anderson, and T.R. Kramer. 1987. Lymphoid cell functions during copper deficiency. Nutr. Res. 7:211–222.

Dhur, A., P. Galan, and S. Hercberg. 1990. Relationship between selenium, immunity, and resistance against infection. Comp. Biochem. Physiol. 96C:271–280.

Driessen, C., K. Hirv, H. Kirchner, and L. Rink. 1995. Zinc regulates cytokine induction by superantigens and lipopolysaccharide. Immunology 84:272–277.

Elliott, S.J., and W.P. Schilling. 1992. Oxidant stress alters Na^+ pump and $Na^+K^+Cl^-$ cotransporter activities in vascular endothelial cells. Am. J. Physiol. 263:H96–H102.

Evans, G.W., C.I. Grace, and C. Han. 1974. The effect of copper and cadmium on ^{65}Zn absorption in zinc-deficient and zinc-supplemented rats. Bioinorg. Chem. 3:115–120.

Failla, M.L., U. Babu, and K.E. Seidel. 1988. Use of immunoresponsiveness to demonstrate that the dietary requirement for copper in young rats is greater with dietary fructose than dietary starch. J. Nutr. 118:487–496.

Farber, J.M., and R.L. Levine. 1982. Oxidative modification of the glutamine synthetase of *E. coli* enhances its susceptibility to proteolysis [abstract 3482]. Fed. Proc. 41:865.

Fernandes, G., M. Nair, K. Onoe, T. Tanaka, R. Gloyd, and R.A. Good. 1979. Impairment of cell-mediated functions by dietary zinc deficiency in mice. Proc. Natl. Acad. Sci. USA 76:457–461.

Fraker, P.J., P. DePasqual-Jardieu, C.M. Zwick, and R.W. Luecke. 1978. Regeneration of T-cell helper function in zinc-deficient adult mice. Proc. Natl. Acad. Sci. USA 75:5660–5664.

Fraker, P.J., M.E. Gershwin, R.A. Good, and A. Prasad. 1986. Interrelationships between zinc and immune function. Fed. Proc. 45:1474–1479.

Fuster, V., B.J. Gersh, E.R. Giuliani, A.J. Tajik, R.O. Brandenburg, and R.L. Frye. 1981. The natural history of idiopathic dilated cardiomyopathy. Am. J. Cardiol. 47:525–531.

Gauntt, C.J., E.K. Godeny, and C.W. Lutton. 1988. Host factors regulating viral clearance. Path. Immunol. Res. 7:251–265.

Ge, K.Y., J. Bai, X.J. Deng, S.Q. Wu, S.Q. Wang, A.N. Xue, and C.Q. Su. 1987. The protective effect of selenium against viral myocarditis in mice. Pp. 761–768 in Selenium in Biology and Medicine Part B, G.F. Combs, O.A. Levander, J.J. Spallholz, and J.E. Oldfield, eds. New York: Van Nostrand/Reinhold.

Gu, B.Q. 1983. Pathology of Keshan disease: A comprehensive review. Chinese Med. J. 96:251–261.

Henkin, R.I., and R.L. Aamodt. 1983. A redefinition of zinc deficiency. Pp. 83–105 in Nutritional Bioavailability of Zinc, G.E. Inglett, ed. Washington, D.C.: American Chemical Society.

Herskovitz, A., K.W. Beisel, L.J. Wolfgram, and N.R. Rose. 1985. Coxsackievirus B3 murine myocarditis: Wide pathologic spectrum in genetically defined inbred strains. Human Pathol. 16:671–673.

Jones, D.G. 1984. Effects of dietary copper depletion on acute and delayed inflammatory responses in mice. Res. Vet. Sci. 37:205–210.

Kelley, D.S., P.A. Daudu, P.C. Taylor, B.E. Mackeuy, and J.R. Turnland. 1995. Effects of low-copper diets on human immune response. Am. J. Clin. Nutr. 62:412–416.

Koller, L.D., S.A. Mulhern, N.C. Frankel, M.G. Steven, and J.R. Williams. 1987. Immune dysfunction in rats fed a diet deficient in copper. Am. J. Clin. Nutr. 45:997–1006.

Kruse-Jarres, J.D. 1989. The significance of zinc for humoral and cellular immunity. J. Trace Elem. Electrolytes Health Dis. 3:1–8.

Larsen, H.S. 1988. Effects of selenium on sheep lymphocyte responses to mitogens. Res. Vet. Sci. 45:11–18.

Larsen, J.H., and S. Tollersrund. 1981. Effects of dietary vitamin E and selenium on phytohemogglutinea response and pig lymphocytes. Res. Vet. Sci. 31:301–305.

Leslie, K. 1989. Clinical and experimental aspects of viral myocarditis. Clin. Microbiol. Rev. 2:191–197.

Li, G., F. Wang, D. Kang, and C. Li. 1985. Keshan disease: An endemic cardiomyopathy in China. Hum. Pathol. 16:602–609.

Lukasewycz, O.A., and J.R. Prohaska. 1983. Lymphocytes from copper-deficient mice exhibit decreased mitogen reactivity Nutr. Res. 3:335–341.

Lukasewycz, O.A., and J.R. Prohaska. 1985. Alterations in lymphocyte subpopulations in copper-deficient mice. Infect. Immun. 48:644–647.

Moses, H.A., and H.E. Parker. 1964. Influence of dietary zinc and age on the mineral content of rat tissues. Fed. Proc. 23:333–343.

Newberne, P.M., C.E. Hunt, and V.R. Young. 1968. The role of diet and reticuloendothelial system in the response of rats to Salmonella typhimurium infection. Br. J. Exp. Pathol. 49:448–457.

O'Connell, J., and J. Robinson. 1985. Coxsackie viral myocarditis. Postgrad. Med. J. 61:1127–1131.

Okmole, T.A., and O.A. Onawunmi. 1979. Effect of copper on growth and serum constituents of immunized and nonimmunized rabbits infected with Trypanosoma brucei. Ann. Parasitol. 54:495–506.

Petering, H.G., M.A. Johnson, and J.P. Horwitz. 1971. Studies of zinc metabolism in the rat. Arch. Environ. Health 23:93–101.

Prasad, A.S., D. Oberleas, P. Wolf, J.P. Horwitz, E.R. Miller, and R.W. Luecke. 1969. Changes in trace elements and enzyme activities in tissues of zinc-deficient pigs. Am. J. Clin. Nutr. 22:628–637.

Prohaska, J.R., and M.L. Failla. 1993. Copper and immunity. Pp. 309–332 in Nutrition and Immunology, D.M. Klurfeld, ed. New York: Plenum Press.

Prohaska, J.R., and O.A. Lukasewycz. 1981. Copper deficiency suppresses the immune response of mice. Science 213:559–561.

Prohaska, J.R., and O.A. Lukasewycz. 1989. Biochemical and immunological changes in mice following postweaning copper deficiency. Biol. Trace Elem. Res. 22:101–112.

Prohaska, J.R., and O.A. Lukasewycz. 1990. Effects of copper deficiency on the immune system. Adv. Exp. Med. Biol. 262:123–143.

Reffett, J.K., J.W. Spears, and T.T. Brown Jr. 1988. Effect of dietary selenium and vitamin E on the primary and secondary immune response in lambs challenged with parainfluenza 3 virus. J. Anim. Sci. 66:1520–1528.

Rivett, A.J. 1985. The effect of mixed-function oxidation of enzymes on their susceptibility to degradation by a nonlysosomal cysteine proteinase. Arch. Biochem. Biophys. 243:624–632.

Schlesinger, L., M. Arevalo, S. Arredondo, B. Lönnerdal, and A. Stekel. 1993. Zinc supplementation impairs monocyte function. Acta Paediatr. 82:734–738.

Sheffy, B.E., and R.D. Schultz. 1979. Influence of vitamin E and selenium on immune response mechanisms. Fed. Proc. 38:2139–2143.

Singh, A., M.L. Failla, and P.A. Deuster. 1994. Exercise-induced changes in immune function: Effects of zinc supplementation. J. Appl. Physiol. 76:2298–2303.

Stabel, J.R., and J.W. Spears. 1993. Role of selenium in immune responsiveness and disease resistance. Pp. 331–356 in Human Nutrition: A Comprehensive Treatise, D.M. Klureld, ed. New York: Plenum Press.

Stabel, J.R., J.W. Spears, and T.T. Brown Jr. 1993. Effect of copper deficiency on tissue, blood characteristics, and immune functions of calves challenged with infectious bovine Rhinotracheitis virus and *Pasteruella hemolytica*. J. Anim. Sci. 71:1247–1255.

Stadtman, E.R. 1992. Protein oxidation and aging. Science 257:1220–1224.

Su, C., C. Gong, J. Li, L. Chen, D. Zhou, and Q. Jin. 1979. Preliminary results of viral etiology of Keshan disease. Chin. J. Med. 59:466–472.

USDA (U.S. Department of Agriculture Nutrition Monitoring in the United States). 1986. A progress report from the Joint Nutrition Monitoring Evaluation Committee. DHHS publ. no. 1255. Hyattsville, Md.: USDA.

Vyas, D., and R.K. Chandra. 1983. Thymic factor activity, lymphocyte stimulation response and antibody producing cells in copper deficiency. Nutr. Res. 3:343–349.

Walsh, C.T., H.H. Sandstead, A.S. Prasad, P.M. Newberne, and P.J. Fraker. 1994. Zinc: Health effects and research priorities for the 1990s. Environ. Health Perspect. 102:5–46.

Woodruff, J.F. 1980. Viral myocarditis: A review. Am. J. Pathol. 101:427–482.

Woodruff, J.F., and J.J. Woodruff. 1974. Involvement of T-lymphocytes in the pathogenesis of Coxsackievirus B3 heart disease. J. Immunol. 113:17–26.

DISCUSSION

RONALD SHIPPEE: Maybe you mentioned this, and I missed it. When you are depleting selenium in mice, is there a food intake problem?

MELINDA BECK: No, but we did weigh the mice because we were worried about that.

RONALD SHIPPEE: You don't have to worry about feeding or anything like that?

MELINDA BECK: No.

GERALD KEUSCH: In the selenium-deficient model, in your initial experiments, did you refeed selenium-deficient animals at some time during the course of the infection and attenuate it?

MELINDA BECK: No, we haven't looked at that yet. That is one of those things that we are interested in doing.

GERALD KEUSCH: The second part of your presentation was instructive, and you had four separate isolates that you sequenced, and is it my understanding that all of them had undergone all of those changes?

MELINDA BECK: Right.

GERALD KEUSCH: So, you got multiple point mutations occurring?

MELINDA BECK: Right. What we think is happening is that the RNA viruses have a high mutation rate because they don't have repair mechanisms. So, when they replicate, if they make a mistake, they cannot fix it, and what I think is happening is we are driving the evolution of the virus by causing the immune deficiency.

So, the viruses replicate fast and they replicate to higher titers, which increases the chances for the mutations to occur, and because of the way we are doing the experiment, we are looking at the time of peak pathology and then taking those viruses out and sequencing them.

So, we are seeing the winners of the race, and, I think if we looked earlier, we might see fewer point mutations. If we look at day 3, for example, you might see three changes and then maybe at day 6 you see four changes, and by the time when we are looking, it is like, boom, here is the maximum number of changes that the virus can tolerate.

GERALD KEUSCH: Are you certain that the inoculum itself was not mixed inoculum, and you selected rather than ...

MELINDA BECK: Right, well, I mean with RNA viruses, you have a cloned virus, and a clone is never a clone when you are working with RNA viruses, because once I replicate it in cell culture, you are already introducing mutations.

What we are seeing is the consensus sequence of the dominant population. Nobody could ever say that what goes in is all the same sequence. So, you cannot do that.

GERALD KEUSCH: It is conceivable that it could be a selection of preexisting ...

MELINDA BECK: Right.

LEONARD KAPCALA: Would you speculate on how this may have any application or relevance to HIV?

MELINDA BECK: Yes, I think it has a lot of relevance to HIV because you know, you have a lot of quasi-species in a single individual with HIV, and I think that nutrition can be one mechanism for driving those changes. So, I think that is a strong possibility, and clearly people—I mean I am not an HIV expert, and you probably know better than I do—but I mean towards the end you see a lot of malnutrition and wasting-type syndromes in those people with HIV, and I think that can contribute to what we are seeing with the Coxsackievirus.

DAVID NIEMAN: I know this is an aside from what you are doing, but I think it is of importance to the military, especially the first couple of slides you showed, which is when animals are infected with the Coxsackievirus, depending on the strain, it can lead to infection of the heart and to mortality.

I know that there are some case reports in humans. In fact, there is one paper published on Air Force recruits in basic training where there were a number of deaths, and there was speculation in the paper that some of these—I think this was by Dr. Philips—may have been from infected recruits who exercised too heavily when they were infected.

Now, it is difficult for an individual to know if they are infected with the Coxsackievirus versus some other type of virus, but nonetheless, there are some cardiologists who are quite conservative on this and do recommend that there be no exercise at all during various respiratory types of infections, and I thought maybe you could give your opinion on this and maybe some of the military men in this room can talk to this because I doubt that when a ranger gets infected that they are allowed to rest. I think that that should be policy.

MELINDA BECK: I think you are right. I think that is a concern, and usually the types of instances where you see sudden death sorts of things other than anatomic problems with the heart is often when somebody has been exercising.

So, they are infected. They go out and they do strenuous exercising and they die, and like you said, it is difficult to know when do you have a rhinovirus and when is it a Coxsackievirus, and you shouldn't be out running around, and I mean I think it is a difficult problem.

I think the impression I get with the people in the Ranger course is if they get a sniffle or something they are certainly not going to go and complain about it. They are going to keep going.

DAVID NIEMAN: May I add to that, again, because I am sure you can answer this as well? I have a colleague at Ball State University who is the only researcher I know in the world who does this. They have rhinovirus number 16. As you know, there are more than 100 of them, but 16 is a moderate rhinovirus, and they spray this into the noses of the subjects whom they pay to do this, and then they exercise them to maximal exertion and look at whether or not the symptoms get worse, number 1, and number 2, whether or not their performance is affected, and they have found that there is no effect of a rhinovirus.

Now, my understanding though is Coxsackieviruses often feel like a bad cold, and so, rhinoviruses cause 40 percent of the common cold, and then there is a host of other viruses that cause similar symptoms.

So, the problem is going to be whether it is a benign virus like the rhinovirus or something more potent.

MELINDA BECK: I think even with Coxsackievirus—not every Coxsackievirus obviously is going to go on to infect the heart because there are many infections that people get and it doesn't go to the heart. So, I mean part of our research emphasis is to try to understand, you know, is it a difference in the virus or a difference in the person? Why person A when he gets a Coxsackievirus infection ends up with myocarditis and person B just gets a cold and it is fine?

RONALD SHIPPEE: As a nutritionist, this is fascinating. As someone who is working with the guys I am working with, it is scary, but you know, it even goes further because you cannot be sitting in a Ranger school in camp. You can have in 65 days, 72 hours in the clinic and that clock starts at day 1. So, if you go in for 4 or 5 hours of sick call, that is against your 72 hours. So, you are right, and these guys, there are notorious stories of guys walking around and finishing the course with broken toes, broken fingers, and they do. They suppress a lot, and this is fascinating.

DAVID NIEMAN: Look at Reggie Lewis(?).

RONALD SHIPPEE: Absolutely.

DAVID NIEMAN: It appears that he died from myocarditis, and he probably exercised too hard when he was infected.

RONALD SHIPPEE: Right, and you know, when Pål [Wiik] presented last night and this issue came up with his guys—they are going to finish this probably—but our guys, this is a career school, and if you are going to become a career officer in combat these days you are going to have a Ranger tab or Special Forces. So, when we go in to work with these folks and we do supplementation, we are messing around with their careers. So, that is the motivation there. This is fascinating.

G. RICHARD JANSEN: Is the converse true or have you tried the converse where the virulent strain could be transformed into a nonvirulent strain by passing through a selenium-adequate host?

MELINDA BECK: We have done the experiment where we pass it into a deficient host and made it like a super virus, and we haven't analyzed those sequences yet.

If you do multiple passages of ... We have done multiple passages, well, I haven't but the lab I came from has done multiple passages of both the 20 and the 0, and we have never seen any changes in the nucleotide.

So, just passing through adequate animals either doesn't attenuate or they don't acquire virulence either way. So, just normal passage doesn't seem to do it.

G. RICHARD JANSEN: I am talking about the virulent strain.

MELINDA BECK: Right, but if you do multiple passages of the 20, the virulent strain into normal animals, you don't see any attenuation.

VI

Health and Stress

Part VI begins with a description in Chapter 17 of the effects of both acute and long-term exercise on natural killer (NK) cells, neutrophils, macrophage/monocytes, and the lesser effects on T- and B-lymphocytes. In response to acute exercise, a rapid interchange of immune cells between lymphoid tissues and the circulation occurs. While the response depends on many factors, NK cells, neutrophils, and macrophages appear to be most responsive, both in terms of numbers and function. The only consistent finding to date with long-term exercise training is a significant increase in NK cell activity. Work performance tends to diminish with most systemic infections, and data suggest that increased severity of infection, relapse, and myocarditis may result when patients exercise vigorously.

Chapter 18 discusses the neuroendocrine consequences of systemic infection, emphasizing the primary role of the myriad polypeptide cytokines released into the circulation by lymphocytes, monocytes, macrophages, and endothelial cells. These pluripotent mediators induce the pathophysiological response termed the *acute phase reaction,* which is characterized by fever; nutrient catabolism; changes in protein, carbohydrate, and lipid metabolism; and profound changes in hepatic functions and in all components of the endocrine system.

Recent advances in identifying immune-neuroendocrine interactions are discussed in Chapter 19. The numerous interactions that have been characterized illustrate the important bi-directional communication between these two systems. Perhaps the most important interaction relates to immune activation of the hypothalamic-pituitary-adrenal axis via cytokines. Stimulation of this counter-regulatory response plays a critical role in preventing the host from mounting an excessive defense response against "inflammatory stress". Because of these interactions, regulatory relationships exist whereby behavioral stimuli and inflammatory stress can ultimately modulate the function of the immune system.

The influence of biological rhythms on the immune system is presented in Chapter 20. Biologic rhythmic behavior has been characterized in levels of circulating white blood cells and subsets of these cells, cytokines and their inhibitors, and in the humoral immune response, although circadian time dependence of human responses to vaccination is less well documented. Some of the rhythms affecting the immune system are genetically fixed, but in certain frequencies (e.g., circadian) the rhythm may be adjusted in its timing by periodic environmental factors such as light-darkness, activity-rest pattern, temperature, and for some parameters, the timing of food intake. Many of these rhythms have potential major significance to the military.

Finally, Chapter 21 provides a summary of the workshop presentations, identifying those issues of importance to the military and identifying the issues that the CMNR would consider in their report.

Nutrition and Immune Function, 1999
Pp. 363–389. Washington, D.C.
National Academy Press

17

Exercise, Infection, and Immunity: Practical Applications

David C. Nieman[1]

INTRODUCTION

Although publications on the topic of exercise immunology date from early in the twentieth century, not until the 1980s did a large number of investigators, worldwide, begin to dedicate their effort to this research area. Modern-day interest in the immunology of exercise coincided with a brief review article published in the *Journal of the American Medical Association* in 1984 (Simon). In this report, Simon urged that "there is no clear experimental or clinical evidence that exercise will alter the frequency or severity of human infections" (p. 2737). This was the same opinion registered more than 50 years earlier by Baetjer (1932), who complained that comparatively little experimental work had been done to test the relationship between exercise and infection.

During the past decade, a plethora of worldwide research has greatly increased understanding of the relationship among exercise, the immune system, and host protection. Although much more investigation is needed, enough high-quality exercise immunology data exist to provide athletes, military recruits, and

---

[1] David C. Nieman, Department of Health and Exercise Science, Appalachian State University, Boone, NC 28608

the general population with preliminary practical guidelines in the areas of exercise prescription, respiratory infection, aging, and athletic endeavor.

EXERCISE PRESCRIPTION AND THE IMMUNE RESPONSE TO ACUTE EXERCISE BOUTS

From early in this century, it has been regularly reported that during recovery from high-intensity, cardiorespiratory exercise, subjects experience a sustained neutrophilia and lymphocytopenia (Garrey and Bryan, 1935). Of all immune cells, natural killer (NK) cells, neutrophils, and macrophages (of the innate immune system[2]) appear to be most responsive to the effects of acute exercise, both in terms of numbers and function (Gabriel et al., 1992; Nieman and Nehlsen-Cannarella, 1994; Pyne, 1994). The longer and more intense the exercise bout (e.g., marathon race competition), the greater and more prolonged the response, with moderate exercise bouts (< 60% maximal aerobic power and < 60 minutes duration) evoking little change from resting levels (Nieman et al., 1989, 1991, 1993b, 1994).

Mechanisms Behind the Acute Immune Response to Exercise

Many mechanisms appear to be involved in the acute immune response to exercise, including exercise-induced changes in stress hormone and cytokine concentrations, body temperature changes, increases in blood flow, and dehydration (Brenner et al., 1995; Cupps and Fauci, 1982; Pedersen and Ullum, 1994).

Following prolonged running at high intensity, serum cortisol concentrations are significantly elevated above control levels for several hours (Nieman et al., 1995a) (Figure 17-1). Cortisol has been related to many of the immunosuppressive changes experienced during recovery (Cupps and Fauci, 1982). Glucocorticoids administered *in vivo* have been reported to cause neutrophilia, eosinopenia, lymphocytopenia, and a suppression of both NK and T-cell function, all of which occur during recovery from prolonged, high-intensity, cardiorespiratory exercise. Figure 17-2 demonstrates that a significant correlation exists between the change in serum cortisol and the change in the neutrophil/lymphocyte ratio following 2.5 to 3 hours of running (Nieman et al., 1995d). The neutrophil/lymphocyte ratio, which rises strongly after heavy, prolonged exertion, has been proposed as an excellent index of the physiologic stress on the immune system (Linden et al., 1991).

---

[2] Responses of this system are unaltered by repeated exposure to a given infectious agent.

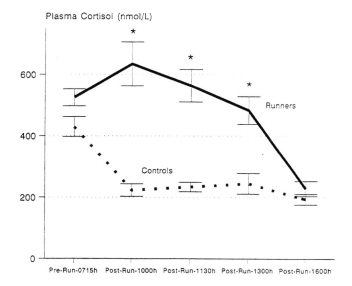

FIGURE 17-1 Serum cortisol response to 2.5 hours of running at approximately 75 percent $\dot{V}$ O$_2$max in marathon runners compared with values obtained from resting, sedentary controls. The pattern of change was significantly different between groups ($F[4,27] = 9.39$, $P < 0.001$). * $P < 0.0125$, between groups at given time point. SOURCE: Data from Nieman et al. (1995a).

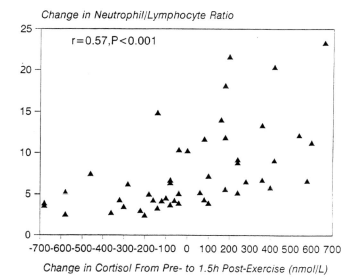

FIGURE 17-2 Correlation between change in cortisol and the neutrophil/lymphocyte ratio from pre- to 1.5-h postexercise in 50 marathon runners who ran 2.5 to 3 hours at 75.9 ± 0.9 percent $\dot{V}$ O$_2$max. SOURCE: Data taken from Nieman et al. (1995d) and unpublished data from author's laboratory.

Open Window of Decreased Host Protection

The following have all been reported to be suppressed for at least several hours during recovery from prolonged, intense endurance exercise: NK cell activity (Mackinnon et al., 1988; Nieman et al., 1993b, 1995a; Shinkai et al., 1993) (Figure 17-3), mitogen-induced lymphocyte proliferation (Eskola et al., 1978; Nieman et al., 1995d), upper airway neutrophil phagocytosis and blood neutrophil oxidative burst (Macha et al., 1990; Müns, 1993), and salivary IgA concentration (Mackinnon and Hooper, 1994; Mackinnon et al., 1987; Tomasi et al., 1982).

During this "window of decreased host protection," viruses and bacteria may gain a foothold, increasing the risk of subclinical and clinical infection (Pedersen and Bruunsgaard, 1995). This may be especially apparent when the athlete goes through repeated cycles of heavy exertion (Pyne, 1994).

Taken together, these data suggest that the immune system is suppressed and stressed following prolonged endurance exercise, which decreases host protection. Hoffman-Goetz and Pedersen (1994) have proposed that the immunological responses to acute exercise can be viewed as a subset of stress immunology. Other physical and mental stressors such as space travel (Barger et al., 1995), thermal and traumatic injury, surgery, acute myocardial infarction, and hemorrhagic shock have all been associated with immunosuppression (Pedersen et al., 1994). Prolonged mental stress and anxiety have been associated with immunosuppression and increased risk of infection (Cohen et al., 1991). Thus, it makes sense that physical exercise when performed at stressful levels may be related to the same outcomes.

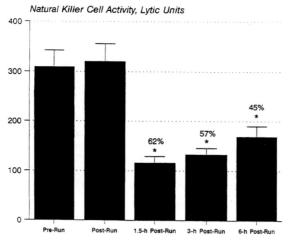

FIGURE 17-3 The pattern of change in natural killer cell activity over time in 50 marathon runners who ran 2.5 to 3 hours at 75.9 ± 0.9 percent $\dot{V} O_2 max$. * $P < 0.001$, comparison with pre-exercise. SOURCE: Data taken from Nieman et al. (1995a) and unpublished data from author's laboratory.

There are few convincing data at this time, however, supporting the notion that exercise-induced changes in immune function explain the increased risk of upper respiratory tract infection (URTI) seen among some athletes. In a small study of elite squash and hockey athletes, Mackinnon and coworkers (1993) have demonstrated that low salivary IgA concentrations precede URTI. However, exercise training-induced changes in T-cell or neutrophil function in two other studies (one in U.S. Air Force Academy cadets during basic training) have not been significantly associated with URTI (Lee et al., 1992; Pyne et al., 1995). Further research with larger groups of individuals is needed.

Practical Applications for Exercise Prescription

Nonetheless, in light of available data, it is prudent to advise the general public that exercise bouts of low-to-moderate intensity ($< 60\%$ $\dot{V}O_2max$) and duration (< 60 minutes/bout) exert less stress on the immune system than do prolonged sessions (> 90 minutes) of heavy exertion ($> 75\%$ $\dot{V}O_2max$). Moderate- versus high-intensity exercise results in a reduced stress hormone response, which has been associated with a more favorable immune response.

CHRONIC EXERCISE AND IMMUNITY

Ideally, to test the effect of regular physical activity on immune function, a large group of individuals randomly assigned to exercise and sedentary control groups would be followed for at least 1 year with multiple immune measures taken before, during, and after the study. This study, which has not yet been conducted, will require strong financial support before it becomes feasible. At present, only a few small longitudinal and cross-sectional studies (most comparing athletes and nonathletes) are available.

Cross-sectional comparisons of human endurance athletes and nonathletes for NK cell activity, neutrophil function (phagocytosis and oxidative burst), and lymphocyte proliferative response (T-cell function) have provided interesting but somewhat inconsistent data.

NK Cell Activity

Cross-Sectional Studies

The majority of cross-sectional studies support the finding of enhanced NK cell activity in athletes when compared with nonathletes, in both younger and older groups (Nieman et al., 1993a, 1995c; Pedersen et al., 1989; Tvede et al., 1991). In one study, NK cell activity was 57 percent higher in experienced marathon runners compared with sedentary controls (Nieman et al., 1995c) (Figure 17-4). The data of Tvede and coworkers (1991) support a higher NK

NK Cell Activity (Lytic Units / 10^7 Mononuclear Cells)

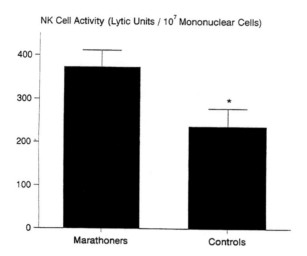

FIGURE 17-4 Natural killer (NK) cell cytotoxic activity was 57 percent higher in the marathon runners versus sedentary controls when expressed in lytic units per 107 mononuclear cells. * $P < 0.05$. SOURCE: Data from Nieman et al. (1995c).

cell activity in elite cyclists during the summer months (intensive training period) when compared with the winter (low training period). Not all studies, however, support the finding of a higher NK cell activity in athletes versus nonathletes (Nieman et al., 1995b).

Prospective Studies

Several prospective studies utilizing moderate endurance training regimens over 8 to 15 weeks have reported no significant elevation in NK cell activity relative to sedentary controls (Baslund et al., 1993; Nieman et al., 1990b, 1993a). Together, these data imply that endurance exercise may have to be engaged in for a prolonged time period (i.e., years) before NK cell activity is chronically elevated.

Neutrophil Function

The cross-sectional data on neutrophil function are in contrast to those for NK cell activity (both components of the innate immune system). No researcher has reported an elevation in neutrophil function (phagocytic and/or oxidative burst) among endurance athletes when compared with nonathletes (Baj et al.,

1994; Hack et al., 1992, 1994; Pyne et al., 1995; Smith et al., 1990). Instead, during periods of high-intensity training, neutrophil function has been reported to be suppressed in athletes. This is especially apparent in the studies by Hack and coworkers (1994) and Baj coworkers (1994), where neutrophil function in athletes was similar to controls during periods of low training workloads but significantly suppressed during the summer months of intensive training. Pyne and coworkers (1994, 1995) reported that elite swimmers undertaking intensive training had a significantly lower neutrophil oxidative activity at rest than did age- and sex-matched sedentary individuals and that function was further suppressed during periods of strenuous training prior to national-level competition.

Because neutrophils are considered the body's best phagocyte, suppression of neutrophil function during periods of heavy training is probably a significant factor explaining the increased URTI risk among athletes. Müns (1993) has reported that neutrophils in the upper airway passages of athletes have a decreased phagocytic capacity when compared with those of nonathletes and that following heavy exertion, a further suppression is experienced for 1 to 3 days afterwards.

Other data from Müns and coworkers (1989) have also shown that IgA concentration in nasal secretions is decreased by nearly 70 percent for at least 18 hours after individuals have raced 31 km. Following a marathon race, subjects' nasal mucociliary clearance is significantly slower for nearly a week compared with that of control subjects (Müns et al., 1995) These data suggest that host protection in the upper airway passages is significantly suppressed for a prolonged time after endurance running races. These data may be the most important evidence to date linking risk of respiratory infection with athletic endeavor. Repeated cycles of heavy exertion may thus put the athletes at increased risk of URTI.

T-Cell Function

Data on the mitogen-induced lymphocyte proliferative response (generally a measure of T-cell function) to athletic endeavor are less clear than for NK cells and neutrophils, but the data usually support no significant difference between athletes and nonathletes (Nieman et al., 1995c, d; Tvede et al., 1991). Baj and coworkers (1994) reported no difference between elite cyclists and nonathletes during low training periods (March) but increased levels in the athletes for PHA (phytohemagglutinin) and anti-CD3 mAb (monoclonal antibody to clonaldeterminant 3+ containing cells) (but not Con A [Concanavalin A] or PWM [pokeweed mitogen]) during intensive training. Interleukin (IL)-2 generation, however, was suppressed in the athletes versus controls during intensive training. These data contrast with that of Tvede and coworkers (1991) who found no difference between athletes and nonathletes during both low or high training periods.

Among highly conditioned elderly women (average age 73 years), PHA-induced lymphocyte proliferative response was reported to be 56 percent higher than among sedentary controls (Nieman et al., 1993a). Data from Japan also support enhanced T-cell function among trained elderly men versus untrained controls (Shinkai et al., 1995). These data are interesting because T-cell function tends to diminish with age (see section on "Exercise, Aging, and Immunity").

Other Measures of Immunity

Other components of immunity have been less well studied among human athletes and nonathletes. Tomasi and coworkers (1982) reported that resting salivary IgA levels were lower in elite cross-country skiers than in age-matched controls, but this was not confirmed in a follow-up study of elite cyclists (Mackinnon et al., 1987). As reviewed by Mackinnon and Hooper (1994), the secretory immune system of the mucosal tissues of the upper respiratory tract is considered the first barrier to colonization by pathogens, with IgA the major effector of host defense. Secretory IgA inhibits attachment and replication of pathogens, preventing their entry into the body. Although several studies have shown that salivary IgA concentration decreases after a single bout of intense endurance exercise, further research is needed to determine the overall chronic effect.

Practical Applications for Exercise Prescription

These data support the concept that the innate immune system responds differentially to the chronic stress of intensive exercise, with NK cell activity tending to be enhanced while neutrophil function is suppressed (especially during periods of heavy training). The adaptive immune system,[3] in general, seems to be largely unaffected (except perhaps in the highly trained elderly individuals), although the research data at present are mixed. Further research is needed with larger groups of athletes to allow a more definitive comparison.

Nonetheless, from a practical viewpoint, moderate amounts of exercise training (3–5 sessions/wk, 15–60 min/session, 40–60% $\dot{V}O_2max$) appear to have little if any chronic effect on immune function (when in a state of rest). Thus any positive effects on immunosurveillance and host protection that come with moderate exercise training are probably related to changes that occur during each exercise bout.

For athletes, periods of heavy training have been associated with suppression of neutrophil function. Neutrophils are an important component of

---

[3] That part of the immune system that responds in a manner that is (1) highly specific for a particular pathogen and (2) increased in intensity with each successive encounter with that pathogen.

the innate immune system, aiding in the phagocytosis of many bacterial and viral pathogens and in the release of immunomodulatory cytokines. Athletes should be made aware of this potential problem and urged to avoid overtraining (see "Practical Guidelines for Military Recruits and Athletes").

EXERCISE AND UPPER RESPIRATORY TRACT INFECTIONS

Among elite athletes and their coaches, a common perception is that heavy exertion lowers resistance and is a predisposing factor to URTI. There is also a common, contrasting belief among many individuals that regular exercise confers resistance against infection. For example, a survey of 750 masters athletes (ranging in age from 40 to 81 years) showed that 76 percent perceived themselves to be less vulnerable to viral illnesses than their sedentary peers (Shephard et al., 1995b).

Understanding the relationship between exercise and infection has potential implications for public health. For the athlete, it may mean the difference between being able to compete or performing at a subpar level or missing the event altogether because of illness.

The J Curve

Nieman (1994) has proposed that the relationship between exercise and URTI may be modeled in the form of a J curve (Figure 17-5). This model suggests that although the risk of URTI may decrease below that of a sedentary individual when one engages in moderate exercise training, risk may rise above average during periods of excessive amounts of high-intensity exercise. Much more research using larger subject pools and improved research designs is necessary before this model can be accepted or rejected.

Heavy Exertion and Risk of URTI

Several epidemiological reports suggest that athletes engaging in marathon-type events and/or very heavy training are at increased risk of URTI (Nieman et al., 1990a; Peters, 1990; Peters and Bateman, 1983; Peters et al., 1993) (Figure 17-6). URTI risk following a race event may depend on the distance, with an increased incidence conspicuous only following marathon or ultramarathon events. Among runners varying widely in training habits, the risk for URTI is slightly elevated for the highest distance runners, but only when several confounding factors (e.g., demographic and training variables, mental stress) are controlled (Nieman et al., 1990a).

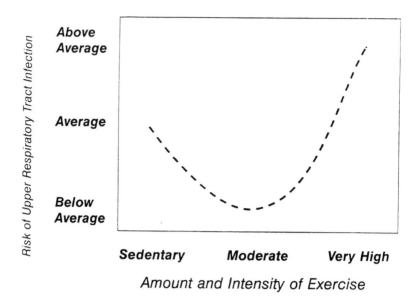

FIGURE 17-5 J-shaped model of relationship between varying amounts of exercise and risk of upper respiratory tract infection (URTI). This model suggests that moderate exercise may lower risk of URTI, while excessive amounts may increase the risk.

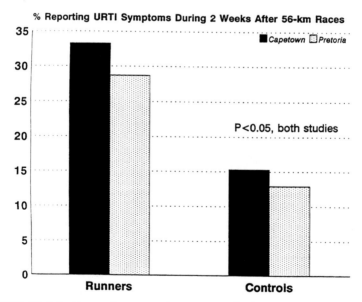

FIGURE 17-6 Incidence of upper respiratory tract infection was significantly higher in ultramarathon runners versus controls during the 2-wk period following the race event. SOURCE: Data from Peters (1990) and Peters and Bateman (1983).

Moderate Exercise and Risk of URTI

What about the common belief that moderate physical activity is beneficial in decreasing URTI risk? Very few studies have been carried out in this area, and more research is certainly warranted to investigate this interesting question. At present, there are no published epidemiological reports that have retrospectively or prospectively compared incidence of URTI in large groups of moderately active and sedentary individuals. Two randomized experimental trials using small numbers of subjects have provided important preliminary data in support of the viewpoint that moderate physical activity may reduce URTI symptomatology (Nieman et al., 1990b, 1993b).

In one randomized, controlled study of 36 women (mean age 35 years), exercise subjects walked briskly for 45 minutes, 5 days a week, and experienced one-half the number of days with URTI symptoms during the 15-wk period compared with that of the sedentary control group (5.1 ± 1.2 vs. 10.8 ± 2.3 days, $p = 0.039$) (Nieman et al., 1990b). In a study of elderly women, the incidence of the common cold during a 12-wk period in the autumn was observed to be lowest in highly conditioned, lean subjects who exercised moderately each day for about 1.5 hours (8%). Elderly subjects who walked 40 minutes, 5 times/wk had an incidence of 21 percent, as compared with 50 percent for the sedentary control group ($X = 6.36, p = 0.042$) (Nieman et al., 1993b).

Public Health Recommendations

Although public health recommendations must be considered tentative, the data on the relationship between moderate exercise and lowered risk of URTI are consistent with guidelines urging the general public to engage in near-daily brisk walking. For athletes engaging in long-endurance events, the risk of illness is high during the 1 to 2 week recovery time period, and several precautions to lower this risk are outlined in the last section of this paper.

INFECTION AND EXERCISE PERFORMANCE

It is well established that various measures of physical performance capability are reduced during most types of systemic infectious episodes (Daniels et al., 1985; Friman et al., 1991, 1985; Roberts, 1985,1986). Although causes are debated, muscle protein catabolism, circulatory deregulation, and mitochondrial abnormalities have been reported (Ilbäck et al., 1991).

Several case histories have been published demonstrating that in some individuals sudden and unexplained deterioration in athletic performance can be traced to either recent URTI or subclinical viral infections that run a protracted course (Roberts, 1985; Sharp, 1989). In some athletes, a viral infection may lead to a severely debilitating state known as post-viral fatigue syndrome (PVFS)

(Maffulli et al., 1993). The symptoms can persist for several months and include lethargy, atypical depression, excessive sleep, night sweats, easy fatiguability (made worse by exercise), and myalgia.

Exercise Recommendations during Infection

Endurance athletes are often uncertain of whether they should exercise or rest during an infectious episode. Few data are available in humans to provide definitive answers. Most clinical authorities in this area recommend that if the athlete has symptoms of a common cold with no constitutional involvement, regular training may be safely resumed a few days after the resolution of symptoms (Sharp, 1989). Mild exercise during illness with a common cold does not appear to be contraindicated, but more research in this area is needed. In one study, nasal injection with rhinovirus 16 (leading to common cold symptoms) had no effect on exercise performance (Personal communication, T. Weidner, Ball State University, Muncie, Ind., 1995). Clinicians recommend, however, if there are symptoms of systemic involvement (e.g., fever, extreme tiredness, muscle aches, swollen lymph glands), 2 to 4 weeks should probably be allowed before resumption of intensive training (Roberts, 1985; Sharp, 1989).

These recommendations are speculative, however, and are primarily based on animal studies and some case reports of humans who died following bouts of vigorous exercise during an acute viral illness. Depending on the pathogen (with some more affected by exercise than others), animal studies generally support the finding that one or two periods of exhaustive exercise following inoculation of the animal leads to a more frequent appearance of infection and a higher fatality rate (Cannon, 1993). The problem is that most individuals are unaware of the pathogen with which they are infected, which necessitates a conservative approach to prevent relapse, a worsening of the disease, myocarditis, or other types of injury. In general, if the symptoms are from the neck up, moderate exercise is probably acceptable, while bed rest and a gradual progression to normal training are recommended when the illness is systemic.

EXERCISE AND HIV INFECTION

Pertinent questions have been raised regarding HIV transmission during sports that require close physical contact. Most patients diagnosed with active AIDS are acutely and chronically ill and are not likely to participate in athletic endeavors. For each patient with clinically apparent AIDS, however, there are many more who are HIV infected and free of clinical manifestations who may be capable of normal participation in sports (Calabrese and LaPerriere, 1993).

Routine social or community contact with an HIV-infected person carries no risk of transmission; only sexual exposure and exposure to blood or tissues carry a risk. Although HIV has been found in saliva, tears, urine, and bronchial secretions, there is no evidence that the virus can be transmitted after contact with these secretions.

Several situations exist, however, in which the transmission of HIV is of concern in athletic settings (Goldsmith, 1992). During sport activities in which athletes can be cut, such as boxing or wrestling, or in other contact sports such as football, basketball, and baseball, risk of HIV transmission exists when the mucous membranes of a healthy athlete are exposed to the blood of an infected athlete. Currently, the testing of all athletes prior to sports participation is thought to be impractical, unethical, and unrealistic (Brown et al., 1994). Therefore, the team physician and athletic trainer are urged to provide information about the transmission of HIV, recommended behavior to reduce risks, and referral for care or diagnosis.

Can exercise training be used as a method to delay the progression from HIV infection to AIDS? Few investigators have published results in this area (LaPerriere et al., 1991; MacArthur et al., 1993; Rigsby et al., 1992). Rigsby and colleagues (1992) studied the effects of an exercise program (three 1-h sessions per week of strength training and aerobic exercise) on 37 HIV-infected subjects who spanned the range of HIV disease progression from asymptomatic to a diagnosis of AIDS (CD4 counts ranged from 9 to 804 cells/mm3). Subjects were randomly assigned to either a 12-week exercise training or a counseling control group. Although exercise training had the expected effect of improving both strength and cardiorespiratory fitness in exercise subjects, no significant change in CD4 cell counts or the CD4/CD8 ratio was found for either condition. These results are similar to those of LaPerriere and coworkers (1991).

This increase in strength with weight training, which has also been reported by Spence and coworkers (1990) in AIDS subjects, is noteworthy in that muscle atrophy and nervous system disorders are common among ARC (AIDS-related complex) and AIDS patients. Weight training may provide one means of retarding the wasting syndrome that accompanies AIDS and improving the quality of life for these individuals.

Practical Recommendations

One tentative conclusion that can be made from these studies is that appropriately supervised exercise training does not appear to affect HIV-infected individuals adversely (Lawless et al., 1995). Several potential benefits of both aerobic and strength training by HIV-infected individuals, especially when initiated early in the disease state, include improvement in psychological coping, maintenance of health and physical function for a longer period, and attenuation of negative immune system changes. Improved quality of life is perhaps the chief benefit of regular exercise by HIV-infected patients.

It is recommended that exercise prescriptions for all HIV-infected individuals be made on an individual basis, with appropriate initial screening.

The exercise prescription should emphasize both cardiorespiratory and musculoskeletal training components.

EXERCISE, AGING, AND IMMUNITY

Immune senescence or age-associated immune deficiency appears to be partly responsible for the afflictions of old age (Nieman and Henson, 1994). Elderly persons are more susceptible to many infections, autoimmune disorders, and cancers when compared with younger adults. Death rates from pneumonia and influenza, for example, are much higher among the very old (≥ 85 years) as compared to adults of late middle age (55–59 years) (1,361 deaths/100,000 vs. 18/100,000, respectively). Death rates for cancer also climb steeply with increasing age.

A new and growing area of research is the study of the relationship between certain lifestyle factors (in particular, physical activity and diet) and immune senescence. Regarding physical activity, national surveys have shown that older adults exercise less and have lower levels of cardiorespiratory fitness than do younger adults. Could regular physical activity attenuate the decrease in immune function with increase in age?

Very few studies have been conducted in this area (Nasrullah and Mazzeo, 1992; Nieman et al., 1993a). The most interesting results come from cross-sectional studies of highly active and lean elderly subjects and their sedentary peers (Nieman et al., 1993a; Shinkai et al., 1995). As shown in Figure 17-7, NK

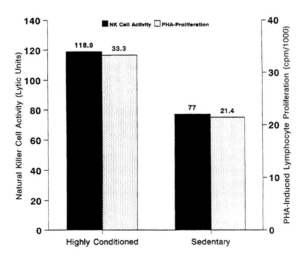

FIGURE 17-7 Natural killer (NK) cell activity was 54 percent higher and PHA (phytohemagglutinin)-induced lymphocyte proliferation 56 percent higher in trained versus untrained elderly females. * $P < 0.05$. SOURCE: Data from Nieman et al. (1993a).

cell activity and PHA-induced lymphocyte proliferation were significantly higher in elderly athletes versus sedentary controls (Nieman et al., 1993a). This finding has also been confirmed in a cross-sectional study of trained and untrained elderly subjects in Japan (Shinkai et al., 1993). In a randomized study of elderly women, however, 12 weeks of moderate cardiorespiratory exercise training did not result in any improvement in NK- or T-cell function relative to sedentary controls (Nieman et al., 1993a).

Although the relative importance of high volumes of physical activity, nutrient intake, self-selection, and other confounders is impossible to determine, the data taken together do suggest that exercise training may need to be long-term (i.e., for multiple years) and of sufficient volume to induce changes in body weight and fitness before any change in immunity can be expected in old age (Nieman and Henson, 1994). In other words, because the aging process is so dominant in old age, long-term physical activity combined with leanness and other positive lifestyle habits may be necessary before immune function is enhanced.

PRACTICAL GUIDELINES FOR MILITARY RECRUITS AND ATHLETES

For military recruits and athletes who may be undergoing heavy exercise stress in preparation for combat or competition, several precautions may help them reduce their risk of URTI. Considerable evidence indicates that two other environmental factors, improper nutrition (Chandra, 1991) and psychological stress (Cohen et al., 1991) can compound the negative influence of heavy exertion on the immune system. Based on current understanding, the athlete is urged to eat a well-balanced diet, keep other life stresses to a minimum, avoid overtraining and chronic fatigue, obtain adequate sleep, and space vigorous workouts and race events as far apart as possible.

Possible indicators of overtraining include immunosuppression with loss of motivation for training and competition, depression, poor performance, and muscle soreness. However, at this time, there are no practical markers of immunosuppression (other than infection) that coaches and clinicians can use to indicate that the athlete is overtrained.

Immune system function appears to be suppressed during periods of low caloric intake and weight reduction (Kono et al., 1988; Nieman et al., 1996), so when necessary, the athlete is advised to lose weight slowly during noncompetitive training phases. Cold viruses are spread by both personal contact and breathing the air near sick people. Therefore, if at all possible, athletes should avoid being around sick people before and after important events. If the athlete is competing during the winter months, a flu shot is recommended.

Some preliminary data support that various immunomodulator drugs may afford athletes some protection against infection during competitive cycles

(Ghighineishvili et al., 1992). Much more research is needed before any of these drugs can be recommended. Indomethacin, which inhibits prostaglandin production, has been administered to athletes prior to exercise or used *in vitro* to determine whether the drop in NK cell activity can be countered (Nieman et al., 1995a; Pedersen et al., 1990). Following 2.5 hours of intensive running, indomethacin had no effect in countering the steep drop in NK cell activity (Nieman et al., 1995a). Other medications such as aspirin or ibuprofen are currently being studied for their effects on the immune system following heavy exertion.

Should athletes use nutrient supplements to decrease their risk of immunosuppression and infection? Glutamine is an important fuel for lymphocytes and monocytes, but glutamine supplementation *in vitro* has not been found capable of negating the exercise-induced decrease in T-cell function after exercise (Rohde et al., 1995).

Peters and coworkers (1993) have published data that support the use of vitamin C supplementation prior to ultramarathon race events to lower the incidence of URTI during the 2-wk recovery period. In this study, 68 percent of runners reported the development of symptoms of URTI within 2 weeks after the 90 km Comrades Ultramarathon. The incidence of URTI was greatest among the runners who trained the hardest coming into the race (85% vs. 45% of the low- or medium-training status runners). Using a double-blind placebo research design, it was also determined that only 33 percent of all runners taking a 600 mg vitamin C supplement daily for 3 weeks prior to the race developed URTI symptoms. The authors suggested that because heavy exertion enhances the production of free oxygen radicals, vitamin C, which has antioxidant properties, may be required in increased quantities. This is an interesting finding, and further research will help to determine if this finding also applies to runners racing shorter distances (for example, a typical marathon of 42.2 km). Vitamin C supplementation (double blind, placebo controlled) in a study conducted in the author's laboratory was shown to have no effect on the immune response to 2.5 hours of intense treadmill running (Nieman et al., 1997a).

Supplementation with *N*-acetylcysteine, a pro-glutathione free radical scavenger, has been associated with a reduction in the formation of reactive oxygen species by granulocytes following maximal graded exercise (Huupponen et al., 1995). Although antioxidant supplementation may attenuate oxidative stress following prolonged and strenuous exertion, the effect this attenuation may have on altering the exercise-induced immune response is uncertain.

The effects of electrolyte- and carbohydrate-containing solutions have also been tested. A recent double-blind, placebo, randomized study investigated the effect of drinking Gatorade on the immune response to 2.5 hours of running (Nieman et al., 1997b). In prior research, carbohydrate versus water ingestion during prolonged endurance exercise had been associated with an attenuated cortisol and epinephrine response through its effect on the blood glucose. On the test day, following a blood sample at 0700 hours in a 12-h fasted state, subjects drank 750 ml of either Gatorade or a placebo solution. At 0730 hours, subjects began running at 75 to 80 percent $\dot{V}O_2$max for 2.5 hours, and ingested 250 ml Gatorade or placebo every 15 minutes. Immediately after the 2.5-h run (1000 hours), another blood sample was taken, followed by 1.5-, 3-, and 6-h recovery samples. Subjects drank 500 ml/h of Gatorade or placebo during the first 1.5 hours of recovery and then 250 ml/h during the last 4.5 hours of recovery.

Gatorade ingestion before, during, and after 2.5 hours of running attenuated the rise in both cortisol and the neutrophil/lymphocyte ratio. Blood glucose concentrations were significantly higher in the Gatorade versus placebo group. Recovery Con A- and PHA-induced proliferation tended to be lower in the placebo group (interaction effect, $P = 0.147$, $P = 0.195$, respectively). These data suggest that carbohydrate ingestion before, during, and after prolonged endurance exercise may help to lessen the stress on the immune system.

AUTHOR'S CONCLUSIONS AND RECOMMENDATIONS

During the last 95 years, 629 papers (60% in the 1990s) dealing specifically with exercise and immunology have been published. Major findings of practical importance in terms of public health and human performance include:

• In response to acute exercise (the most frequently studied area of exercise immunology), a rapid interchange of immune cells between peripheral lymphoid tissues and the circulation occurs. The response depends on many factors, including the intensity, duration, and mode of exercise; concentrations of hormones and cytokines; and change in body temperature, blood flow, hydration status, and body position. Of all immune cells, NK cells, neutrophils, and macrophages (of the innate immune system) appear to be most responsive to the effects of acute exercise, both in terms of numbers and function. In general, acute exercise bouts of moderate duration (< 60 minutes) and intensity (< 60% $\dot{V}O_2$max) are associated with fewer perturbations and less stress to the immune system than are prolonged, high-intensity sessions.

• In response to long-term exercise training, the only finding to date reported with some congruity between investigators is a significant elevation in NK cell activity. Changes in the function of neutrophils, macrophages, and T- and B-cells in response to training have been reported inconsistently, but there is some indication that neutrophil function is suppressed during periods of heavy training.

• Limited data suggest that unusually heavy, acute, or chronic exercise may increase the risk of URTI, while regular moderate physical activity may reduce URTI symptomatology.

• Work performance tends to diminish with most systemic infections, and clinical case studies and animal data suggest that increased infection severity, relapse, and myocarditis may result when patients exercise vigorously. Military recruits with systemic infections such as influenza should not exercise vigorously until 2 weeks after symptoms have diminished.

• Although regular exercise has many benefits for HIV-infected individuals, helper T-cell counts and other immune measures are not enhanced significantly.

• As individuals age, they experience a decline in most cell-mediated and humoral immune responses. Two human studies suggest that immune function is superior in highly conditioned versus sedentary elderly subjects.

• Mental stress, undernourishment, quick weight loss, and improper hygiene have each been associated with impaired immunity. Military recruits who are undergoing heavy training regimens should realize that each of these factors has the potential to compound the effect of exercise stress on their immune systems.

REFERENCES

Baetjer, A.M. 1932. The effect of muscular fatigue upon resistance. Physiol. Rev. 12:453–468.

Baj, Z., J. Kantorski, E. Majewska, K. Zeman, L. Pokoca, E. Fornalczyk, H. Tchorzewski, Z.Sulowska, and R. Lewicki. 1994. Immunological status of competitive cyclists before and after the training season. Int. J. Sports Med. 15:319–324.

Barger, L.K., J.E. Greenleaf, F. Baldini, and D. Huff. 1995. Effects of space missions on the human immune system: A meta-analysis. Sports Med. Train. Rehabil. 5:293–310.

Baslund, B., K. Lyngberg, V. Andersen, J. Halkjaer-Kristensen, M. Hansen, M. Klokker, and B.K. Pedersen. 1993. Effect of 8 weeks of bicycle training on the immune system of patients with rheumatoid arthritis. J. Appl. Physiol. 75:1691–1695.

Brenner, I.K.M., P.N. Shek, and R.J. Shephard. 1995. Heat exposure and immune function: Potential contribution to the exercise response. Exerc. Immunol. Rev. 1:49–80.

Brown, L.S., R.Y. Phillips, C.L. Brown, D. Knowlan, L. Castle, and J. Moyer. 1994. HIV/AIDS policies and sports: The National Football League. Med. Sci. Sports Exerc. 26:403–407.

Calabrese, L.H., and A. LaPerriere. 1993.. Human immunodeficiency virus infection, exercise and athletics. Sports Med. 15:6–13.

Cannon, J.G. 1993. Exercise and resistance to infection. J. Appl. Physiol. 74:973–981.

Chandra, R.K. 1991. 1990 McCollum award lecture. Nutrition and immunity: Lessons from the past and new insights into the future. Am. J. Clin. Nutr. 53:1087–1101.

Cohen, S., D.A. Tyrrell, and A.P. Smith. 1991. Psychological stress and susceptibility to the common cold. N. Engl. J. Med. 325:606–612.

Cupps, T.R., and A.S. Fauci. 1982. Corticosteroid-mediated immunoregulation in man. Immunol. Rev. 65:133–155.

Daniels, W.L., D.S. Sharp, J.E. Wright, J.A. Vogel, G. Friman, W.R. Beisel, and J.J. Knapik. 1985. Effects of virus infection on physical performance in man. Milit. Med. 150:8–14.

Eskola J., O. Ruuskanen, E. Soppi, M.K. Viljanen, H. Järvinen, H. Toivonen, and K. Kouvalainen. 1978. Effect of sport stress on lymphocyte transformation and antibody formation. Clin. Exp. Immunol. 32:339–345.

Friman, G., N.G. Ilbäck, D.J. Crawford, and H.A. Neufeld. 1991. Metabolic responses to swimming exercise in *Streptococcus pneumoniae* infected rats. Med. Sci. Sports Exerc. 23:415–421.

Friman, G., J.E. Wright, N.G. Ilbäck, W.R. Beisel, J.D. White, D.S. Sharp, E.L. Stephen, W.L. Daniels, and J.A. Vogel. 1985. Does fever or myalgia indicate reduced physical performance capacity in viral infections? Acta. Med. Scand. 217:353–361.

Gabriel, H., L. Schwarz, P. Born, and W. Kindermann. 1992. Differential mobilization of leukocyte and lymphocyte subpopulations into the circulation during endurance exercise. Eur. J. Appl. Physiol. 65:529–534.

Garrey, W.E., and W.R. Bryan. 1935. Variations in white blood cell counts. Physiol. Rev. 15:597–638.

Ghighineishvili, G.R., V.V. Nicolaeva, A.J. Belousov, P.G. Sirtori, V. Balsamo, A. Miani, R. Franceschini, M. Ripani, M. Crosina, and G. Cosenza. 1992. Correction by physiotherapy of immune disorders in high-grade athletes. Clin. Ter. 140:545–550.

Goldsmith, M.F. 1992. World health organization consensus statement. Consultation on AIDS and sports. J. Am. Med. Assoc. 267:1312–1314.

Hack, V., G. Strobel, J-P. Rau, and H. Weicker. 1992. The effect of maximal exercise on the activity of neutrophil granulocytes in highly trained athletes in a moderate training period. Eur. J. Appl. Physiol. 65:520–524.

Hack, V., G. Strobel, M. Weiss, and H. Weicker. 1994. PMN cell counts and phagocytic activity of highly trained athletes depend on training period. J. Appl. Physiol. 77:1731–1735.

Hoffman-Goetz, L., and B.K. Pedersen. 1994. Exercise and the immune system: A model of the stress response? Immunol. Today 15:382–387.

Huupponen, M.R.H., L.H. Mäkinen, P.M. Hyvönen, C.K. Sen, T. Rankinen, S. Väisänen, and R. Rauramaa. 1995. The effect of *N*-acetylcysteine on exercise-induced priming of human neutrophils. Int. J. Sports Med. 16:399–403.

Ilbäck, N.G., G. Friman, D.J. Crawford, and H.A. Neufeld. 1991. Effects of training on metabolic responses and performance capacity in *Streptococcus pneumoniae* infected rats. Med. Sci. Sports Exerc. 23:422–427.

Kono, I., H. Kitao, M. Matsuda, S. Haga, H. Fukushima, and H. Kashiwagi. 1988. Weight reduction in athletes may adversely affect the phagocytic function of monocytes. Physician Sportsmed. 16(7):56–65.

LaPerriere, A.R., M.A. Fletcher, M.H. Antoni, N.G. Klimas, G. Ironson, and N. Schneiderman. 1991. Aerobic exercise training in an AIDS risk group. Int. J. Sports Med. 12(suppl. 1):S53–S57.

Lawless, D., C.G.R. Jackson, and J.E. Greenleaf. 1995. Exercise and human immunodeficiency virus (HIV-1) infection. Sports Med. 19:235–239.

Lee, D.J., R.T. Meehan, C. Robinson, T.R. Mabry, and M.L. Smith. 1992. Immune responsiveness and risk of illness in U.S. Air Force Academy cadets during basic cadet training. Aviat. Space Environ. Med. 63:517–523.

Linden, A., T. Art, H. Amory, A.M. Massart, C. Burvenich, and P. Lekeux. 1991. Quantitative buffy coat analysis related to adrenocortical function in horses during a three-day event competition. Zentralbl. Veterinärmed. 38:376–382.

MacArthur, R.D., S.D. Levine, and T.J. Birk. 1993. Supervised exercise training improves cardiopulmonary fitness in HIV-infected persons. Med. Sci. Sports Exerc. 25:684–688.

Macha, M., M. Shlafer, and M.J. Kluger. 1990. Human neutrophil hydrogen peroxide generation following physical exercise. J. Sports Med. Phys. Fitness 30:412–419.

Mackinnon, L.T., and S. Hooper. 1994. Mucosal (secretory) immune system responses to exercise of varying intensity and during overtraining. Int. J. Sports Med. 15:S179–S183.

Mackinnon, L.T., T.W. Chick, A. Van As, and T.B. Tomasi. 1987. The effect of exercise on secretory and natural immunity. Adv. Exp. Med. Biol. 216A:869–876.

Mackinnon, L.T., T.W. Chick, A. Van As, and T.B. Tomasi. 1988. Effects of prolonged intense exercise on natural killer cell number and function. Exerc. Physiol.: Current Selected Research 3:77–89.

Mackinnon, L.T., E.M. Ginn, and G.J. Seymour. 1993. Temporal relationship between decreased salivary IgA and upper respiratory tract infection in elite athletes. Aust. J. Sci. Med. Sport 25:94–99.

Maffulli, N., V. Testa, and G. Capasso. 1993. Post-viral fatigue syndrome. A longitudinal assessment in varsity athletes. J. Sports Med. Phys. Fitness 33:392–399.

Müns, G. 1993. Effect of long-distance running on polymorphonuclear neutrophil phagocytic function of the upper airways. Int. J. Sports Med. 15:96–99.

Müns, G., H. Liesen, H. Riedel, and K-Ch. Bergmann. 1989. Einfluá von langstreckenlauf auf den IgA-gehalt in nasensekret und speichel. Deutsche Zeitschr. Sportmed. 40:63–65.

Müns, G., P. Singer, F. Wolf, and I. Rubinstein. 1995. Impaired nasal mucociliary clearance in long-distance runners. Int. J. Sports Med. 16:209–213.

Nasrullah, I., and R.S. Mazzeo. 1992. Age-related immunosenescence in Fischer 344 rats: Influence of exercise training. J. Appl. Physiol. 73:1932–1938.

Nieman, D.C. 1994b. Exercise, upper respiratory tract infection, and the immune system. Med. Sci. Sports Exerc. 26:128–139.

Nieman, D.C., and D.A. Henson. 1994. Role of endurance exercise in immune senescence. Med. Sci. Sports Exerc. 26:172–181.

Nieman, D.C., and S.L. Nehlsen-Cannarella. 1994. The immune response to exercise. Semin. Hematol. 31:166–179.

Nieman, D.C., J.C. Ahle, D.A. Henson, B.J. Warren, J. Suttles, J.M. Davis, K.S. Buckley, S. Simandle, D.E. Butterworth, O.R. Fagoaga, and S.L. Nehlsen-Cannarella. 1995a. Indomethacin does not alter natural killer cell response to 2.5 hours of running. J. Appl. Physiol. 79:748–755.

Nieman, D.C., L.S. Berk, M. Simpson-Westerberg, K. Arabatzis, W. Youngberg, S.A. Tan, and W.C. Eby. 1989. Effects of long endurance running on immune system parameters and lymphocyte function in experienced marathoners. Int. J. Sports Med. 10:317–323.

Nieman, D.C., D. Brendle, D.A. Henson, J. Suttles, V.D. Cook, B.J. Warren, D.E. Butterworth, O.R. Fagoaga, and S.L. Nehlsen-Cannarella. 1995b. Immune function in athletes versus nonathletes. Int. J. Sports Med. 16:329–333.

Nieman, D.C., K.S. Buckley, D.A. Henson, B.J. Warren, J. Suttles, J.C. Ahle, S. Simandle, O.R. Fagoaga, and S.L. Nehlsen-Cannarella. 1995c. Immune function in marathon runners versus sedentary controls. Med. Sci. Sports Exerc. 27:986–992.

Nieman, D.C., D.A. Henson, D.E. Butterworth, B.J. Warren, J.M. Davis, O.R. Fagoaga, and S.L. Nehlsen-Cannarella. 1997a. Vitamin C supplementation does not alter the immune response to 2.5 hours of running. Int. J. Sport Nutr. 7:173–184.

Nieman, D.C., D.A. Henson, E.B. Garner, D.E. Butterworth, B.J. Warren, A. Utter, J.M. Davis, O.R. Fagoaga, and S.L. Nehlsen-Cannarella. 1997b. Carbohydrate affects natural killer cell redistribution but not activity after running. Med. Sci. Sports Exerc. 29:1318–1324.

Nieman, D.C., D.A. Henson, G. Gusewitch, B.J. Warren, R.C. Dotson, D.E. Butterworth, and S.L. Nehlsen-Cannarella. 1993a. Physical activity and immune function in elderly women. Med. Sci. Sports Exerc. 25:823–831.

Nieman, D.C., L.M. Johanssen, J.W. Lee, and K. Arabatzis. 1990a. Infectious episodes in runners before and after the Los Angeles Marathon. J. Sports Med. Phys. Fitness 30:316–328.

Nieman, D.C., A.R. Miller, D.A. Henson, B.J. Warren, G. Gusewitch, R.L. Johnson, J.M. Davis, D.E. Butterworth, J.L. Herring, and S.L. Nehlsen-Cannarella. 1994. Effects of high- versus moderate-intensity exercise on lymphocyte subpopulations and proliferative response. Int. J. Sports Med. 15:199–206.

Nieman, D.C., A.R. Miller, D.A. Henson, B.J. Warren, G. Gusewitch, R.L. Johnson, J.M. Davis, D.E. Butterworth, and S.L. Nehlsen-Cannarella. 1993b. The effects of high-versus moderate-intensity exercise on natural killer cell cytotoxic activity. Med. Sci. Sports Exerc. 25:1126–1134.

Nieman, D.C., S.L. Nehlsen-Cannarella, K.M. Donohue, D.B.W. Chritton, B.L. Haddock, R.W. Stout, and J.W. Lee. 1991. The effects of acute moderate exercise on leukocyte and lymphocyte subpopulations. Med. Sci. Sports Exerc. 23:578–585.

Nieman, D.C., S.L. Nehlsen-Cannarella, D.A. Henson, D.E. Butterworth, O.R. Fagoaga, B.J. Warren, and M.K. Rainwater. 1996. Immune response to obesity and moderate weight loss. Int. J. Obesity Relat. Metab. Disord. 20:353–360.

Nieman, D.C., S.L. Nehlsen-Cannarella, P.A. Markoff, A.J. Balk-Lamberton, H. Yang, D.B.W. Chritton, J.W. Lee, and K. Arabatzis. 1990b. The effects of moderate exercise training on natural killer cells and acute upper respiratory tract infections. Int. J. Sports Med. 11:467–473.

Nieman, D.C., S. Simandle, D.A. Henson, B.J. Warren, J. Suttles, J.M. Davis, K.S. Buckley, J.C. Ahle, D.E. Butterworth, O.R. Fagoaga, and S.L. Nehlsen-Cannarella. 1995d. Lymphocyte proliferation response to 2.5 hours of running. Int. J. Sports Med. 16:404–408.

Pedersen, B.K., and H. Bruunsgaard. 1995. How physical exercise influences the establishment of infections. Sports Med. 19:393–400.

Pedersen, B.K., and H. Ullum. 1994. NK cell response to physical activity: Possible mechanisms of action. Med. Sci. Sports Exerc. 26:140–146.

Pedersen, B.K., M. Kappel, M. Klokker, H.B. Nielsen, and N.H. Secher. 1994. The immune system during exposure to extreme physiologic conditions. Int. J. Sports Med. 15:S116–S121.

Pedersen, B.K., N. Tvede, L.D. Christensen, K. Klarlund, S. Kragbak, and J. Halkjaer-Kristensen. 1989. Natural killer cell activity in peripheral blood of highly trained and untrained persons. Int. J. Sports Med. 10:129–131.

Pedersen, B.K., N. Tvede, K. Klarlund, L.D. Christensen, F.R. Hansen, H. Galbo, A. Kharazmi, and J. Halkjaer-Kristensen. 1990. Indomethacin *in vitro* and *in vivo* abolishes post-exercise suppression of natural killer cell activity in peripheral blood. Int. J. Sports Med. 11:127–131.

Peters, E.M. 1990. Altitude fails to increase susceptibility of ultramarathon runners to post-race upper respiratory tract infections. S. Afr. J. Sports Med. 5:4–8.

Peters, E.M. 1997. Exercise, immunology, and upper respiratory tract infections. Int. J. Sports Med. 18 (suppl. 1):S69–S77.

Peters, E.M., and E.D. Bateman. 1983. Respiratory tract infections: An epidemiological survey. S. Afr. Med. J. 64:582–584.

Peters, E.M., J.M. Goetzsche, B. Grobbelaar, and T.D. Noakes. 1993. Vitamin C supplementation reduces the incidence of postrace symptoms of upper respiratory tract infection in ultramarathon runners. Am. J. Clin. Nutr. 57:170–174.

Pyne, D.B. 1994. Regulation of neutrophil function during exercise. Sports Med. 17:245–258.

Pyne, D.B., M.S. Baker, P.A. Fricker, W.A. McDonald, and W.J. Nelson. 1995. Effects of an intensive 12-wk training program by elite swimmers on neutrophil oxidative activity. Med. Sci. Sports Exerc. 27:536–542.

Rigsby, L.W., R.K. Dishman, A.W. Jackson, G.S. Maclean, and P.B. Raven. 1992. Effects of exercise training on men seropositive for the human immunodeficiency virus-1. Med. Sci. Sports Exerc. 24:6–12.

Roberts. J.A. 1985. Loss of form in young athletes due to viral infection. Br. J. Med. 290:357–358.

Roberts J.A. 1986. Viral illnesses and sports performance. Sports Med. 3:296–303.

Rohde, T., H. Ullum, J.P. Rasmussen, J.H. Kristensen, E. Newsholme, and B.K. Pedersen. 1995. Effects of glutamine on the immune system: Influence of muscular exercise and HIV infection. J. Appl. Physiol. 79:146–150.

Sharp, J.C.M. 1989. Viruses and the athlete. Br. J. Sports Med. 23:47–48.

Shephard, R.J., T. Kavanagh, D.J. Mertens, S. Qureshi, and M. Clark. 1995b. Personal health benefits of masters athletics competition. Br. J. Sport Med. 29:35–40.

Shinkai, S., H. Kohno, K. Kimura, T. Komura, H. Asai, R. Inai, K. Oka, Y. Kurokawa, and R.J. Shephard. 1995. Physical activity and immunosenescence in elderly men. Med. Sci. Sports Exerc. 27:1516–1526.

Shinkai, S., Y. Kurokawa, S. Hino, M. Hirose, J. Torii, S. Watanabe, S. Watanabe, S. Shiraishi, K. Oka, and T. Watanabe. 1993. Triathlon competition induced a transient immunosuppressive change in the peripheral blood of athletes. J. Sports Med. Phys. Fitness 33:70–78.

Simon, H.B. 1984. The immunology of exercise: A brief review. J. Am. Med. Assoc. 252:2735–2738.

Smith, J.A., R.D. Telford, I.B. Mason, and M.J. Weidemann. 1990. Exercise, training and neutrophil microbicidal activity. Int. J. Sports Med. 11:179–187.

Spence, D.W., M.L.A. Galantino, K.A. Mossberg, and S.O. Zimmerman. 1990. Progressive resistance exercise: Effect on muscle function and anthropometry of a select AIDS population. Arch. Phys. Med. Rehabil. 71:644–648.

Tomasi, T.B., F.B. Trudeau, D. Czerwinski, and S. Erredge. 1982. Immune parameters in athletes before and after strenuous exercise. J. Clin. Immunol. 2:173–178.

Tvede, N., J. Steensberg, B. Baslund, J. Halkjaer-Kristensen, and B.K. Pedersen. 1991. Cellular immunity in highly-trained elite racing cyclists and controls during periods of training with high and low intensity. Scand. J. Sports Med. 1:163–166.

DISCUSSION

SUSANNA CUNNINGHAM-RUNDLES: Does the natural killer cell assay use separated cells or whole blood?

DAVID NIEMAN: We are using separate cells. However, we are in transition to a whole blood flow cytometry assay, which is tricky. So we are sticking to the chromium-51 release assay until we get that under control.

HELLEN GREENBLATT: You had mentioned two factors when you mentioned vitamin C. First, you showed data that vitamin C supplementation reduced upper respiratory tract infections by about 50 percent. But then you showed data that vitamin C did not affect cortisol levels. I was wondering if those were temporal effects where you really cannot compare those studies, or whether those are long-term effects that are more important than short-term?

DAVID NIEMAN: Well, she is asking about, first of all, the epidemiologic research by Edith Peters (Peters et al., 1993) in South Africa, where she showed that vitamin C supplementation would reduce the infection rate during the 2-wk period after an ultramarathon. Now, Edith Peters and I are good friends. She has followed that study up with another, showing the same thing (Peters, 1997). She has found, by the way, that β-carotene has no effect on infection rates. She also found that vitamin E has no effect. It is only with the vitamin C that she has found an effect. So, in light of her research, we conducted a double-blind placebo study where, for 1 week, runners were supplemented with 1,000 mg of vitamin C a day for 8 days prior to coming into the lab, and then we measured cortisol and immune response. I did not show the other slides. But we have measured every key cell of the immune system: neutrophils, monocytes, natural killer cells, B-cells, and T-cells. None of the immune cells were affected by the vitamin C relative to placebo (Nieman et al., 1997a).

Now, Edith Peters, who is an epidemiologist and does not work in the lab with the assays, has her epidemiology showing that vitamin C helps with the infection rates of ultramarathons. In the lab, we are showing it has no effect on the immune response to a simulated marathon. Well, she says that they are doing an ultramarathon and we are doing only a marathon. They are looking at epidemiology, we are looking at immune response. So we are just going to have to sort these things out. She feels that, if we would run the athletes for 5, 6 hours like hers, that maybe vitamin C would have an effect—that the vitamin C pools in the body may be sufficient to keep the immune cells operating at the proper level until you get out there to the ultra-marathon distances. That is her interpretation of the data thus far. But, so far, that is all of the research we have. So it is all speculation right now.

STEVE GAFFIN: I just wanted to mention one other piece of information, and that is that in epidemiological work in the United States, Schwartz and Weiss have shown that lung function is related to vitamin C status in normal individuals—that those individuals in the U.S. population, as part of the NHANES study, had better forced respiratory volume when they were consuming a relatively modest amount of vitamin C, 178 mg, compared with 60 mg. So maybe immune function is not the proper assay to use to look at what is happening in the respiratory area when it comes to viral infections. Maybe there are other assays that need to be looked at.

DAVID NIEMAN: Dr. Munck does these nasal lavages. He feels that if it is an upper respiratory tract problem, so then that is what he studies. I showed you three of his studies showing that there is a marked suppression of immunity in that area. So the question would be would vitamin C help that area? We will have to see. I am not a supplement person. I fight it as much as possible. I am hard to convince that it has an effect. Maybe when you get out to ultramarathon distances, it may become more important in that arena.

WILLIAM BEISEL: It would be nice to find a unifying theory. One thing that cortisol does is it is a very important hormone for gluconeogenesis. In these heavy activities, the only fuel you are going to have is neutrophil production. So it would be interesting to make certain or see that the mechanism for the cortisol is just purely a way to mobilize the fuel rather than being a component of a stress response that is not due to a cytokine. Because it would then suggest that that would be the mechanism to deal with it. It is purely just a mobilization or substrate line.

There was some earlier work with vitamin C and upper respiratory infections (URIs) with nonexercising individuals. Are you using as an index for infection just symptoms of URIs or actual infections . . .

DAVID NIEMAN: Self-report symptoms.

WILLIAM BEISEL: Self-report symptoms? There is good evidence that vitamin C will reduce self-reported symptoms. There is no evidence that I am aware of, though, that it actually reduces infection.

DAVID NIEMAN: I agree with you on that part.

WILLIAM BEISEL: I think when you start talking about "immune" you really should make certain of your definition because, if vitamin C does not prevent infection, then reduction in immunity may not be a factor. The decrease in symptoms may have an entirely different etiology.

DAVID NIEMAN: I agree with you 100 percent. When we are at the epidemiology level, it takes many more years of research to figure it out.

Now, I do want to respond to the first question there, which was on the mechanism of a carbohydrate supplement. There have now been a growing number of both animal and human studies showing very carefully that the stress hormone response carefully tracks the blood glucose response to exercise. So we feel that anything that can keep the blood glucose response at a near flat-line level, should attenuate the stress hormone response and then, in our hands, we have shown that then the immune system is less suppressed. So everything is multifactorial. But the data thus far point towards a blood glucose response.

WILLIAM BEISEL: You are saying it is very important to define that. I would certainly measure that. But I would also measure the other major hormones for gluconeogenesis, which under that setting would be glucagon, and see whether the glucagon levels are also reproducible during this period of time.

DAVID NIEMAN: Dr. John Smith from Australia has looked at glucagon. Indeed, it has the same lessened response with the carbohydrate.

WILLIAM BEISEL: Because what it [measuring glucagon] would then do for you is it would indicate whether this is a separate phenomenon from what we would need to look at if people started talking about lymphocytes causing the release of IL-1 and so forth, which also causes cortisol release. But it is that cortisol release in that setting, which has a very, very different implication.

RANJIT CHANDRA: My question relates to the data on chronic exercise on resting immune responses. I feel that it partly depends on the subject at issue. For instance, if you are dealing with young individuals, with near normal responses to begin with, then you do not expect them to enhance that, even though they are sedentary to begin with. If you deal with, say, a population of elderly individuals who for a variety of reasons, including a sedentary lifestyle, have reduced immune responses, then chronic exercise for 4 to 6 months, regular exercise does have a partial or significant effect on resting immune responses and on the incident of common infection.

DAVID NIEMAN: Yes.

RANJIT CHANDRA: The question I have is whether in the studies that you have done or reviewed, coincident with chronic exercise, nutrient intakes were measured?

DAVID NIEMAN: Yes.

RANJIT CHANDRA: You did refer to one study where mood changes and other psychological indices were looked at. Both of those factors, among others, may have an effect on the immune response.

DAVID NIEMAN: Yes. We have conducted three randomized, controlled training studies for 12 to 15 weeks, one with elderly women and now two with women in their 30s and 40s, who are overweight. In all of those studies, we measured psychological mood changes and dietary intake, along with immunity and infection. Even with the elderly women, 12 weeks of walking 40 minutes 5 days a week, was an insufficient stimulus to do anything to resting immunity. It had no effect whatsoever. But, when we compared those highly conditioned, lean elderly women with their sedentary peers, where the $\dot{V}O_2$max of the highly conditioned group was 67 percent higher, which is a huge separation, then we found the natural killer cell activity was elevated. We feel that the natural killer cell activity is only elevated in the most extreme comparisons [of highly active vs. sedentary individuals] and that, as soon as you get into the middle there is nothing.

ROBERT NESHEIM: We will have one last question, and then we could continue the discussion at the end of the afternoon's program. We will take one more and then we will move on.

GERALD KEUSCH: I want to focus in on one issue. It gets at the functional significance of some of these measurements, the neutrophil. You measured neutrophil number and circulation under circumstances in which the hormonal environment had altered the number of circulating neutrophils. Those of us who come from a background of infectious disease do not believe that the neutrophil does anything in circulation. It acts on the surface or within tissue. So changes in the number do not mean anything to me without knowing what the redistribution is unless there is an activation event that has altered the functional capacity of those cells. Measuring the number alone is not a marker to me of anything of importance, although I believe the changes are obviously real.

It might be worthwhile to try and focus on things that you could measure in the circulation like primary and secondary granular products. You can measure lactoferrin in the circulation. There should not be very much there under normal circumstances; but if you are activating the neutrophils in a way that is altering their functional capacity, you might find elevations in lactoferrin or elastase or something of that nature.

I think that just looking at the number is not going to get us very far in understanding what is going on. Under no circumstances do I believe that the changes in neutrophils would have anything to do with viral infection.

DAVID NIEMAN: Well, we agree 100 percent. You see, with the neutrophil/lymphocyte ratio, trainers of race horses have used that index as a simple way to see how stressed the animal is. Because of the pretty good correlation between rises in cortisol and that ratio, it is used as an index of the stress that the animal or the human is going through. So that is the only purpose there.

Now, I did not show slides. We have measured neutrophil and monocyte phagocytic function and oxidative burst activity in response to 2½ hours of running. The phagocytic response goes way up, 85 percent elevation in phagocytic response of *Staphylococcus aureus* bacteria using flow cytometry. Whereas, the oxidative burst activity is significantly reduced. So we personally feel that this represents the inflammatory response.

At the same time, IL-6, which we have measured, goes up sixfold. So the IL-6 is way up. The phagocytic response is way up. Oxidative burst activity is down. We feel that that is just representing the inflammatory response that is going on.

Nutrition and Immune Function, 1999
Pp. 391–407. Washington, D.C.
National Academy Press

18

Neuroendocrine Consequences of Systemic Inflammation

Seymour Reichlin[1]

INTRODUCTION

Bacterial and viral infections, bacterial toxins, and severe tissue injury induce a relatively stereotypical pathophysiologic response manifested by fever, catabolism, and sickness behavior. If mild, sickness behavior is manifested by anorexia, drowsiness, and impaired cognition; if severe, delirium, stupor, and coma can supervene. All organ systems are altered by acute and chronic inflammatory states. The dramatic changes in liver function, termed the *acute-phase response* include suppression of synthesis of albumin, transthyretin, transferrin, and ceruloplasmin, and increase in synthesis of several proteins including fibrinogen, β-2 microglobulin, serum amyloid antecedent (SAA), and C-reactive protein (Dinarello and Wolff, 1993). Chronic inflammation, such as that seen in rheumatoid arthritis, induces a less severe and persistent version of

---

[1] Seymour Reichlin, University of Arizona Health Sciences Center, Tucson, AZ 85724-5099

Work from the author's laboratory that is cited in this paper was supported by NIH Grant 16684.

the acute-phase response. When the acute-phase response is mild, functional capacity is suppressed; when severe, prostration and death can occur.

These changes are mediated by a flood of polypeptide molecules, the inflammatory cytokines, which are released into the circulation by lymphocytes, monocytes, macrophages, and endothelial cells and are produced locally in tissues by resident macrophages and several other types of parenchymal cells. Among the most important of the cytokines released during inflammatory stress are interleukin (IL)-1, IL-2, IL-6, tumor necrosis factor-alpha (TNF-α), interferon-gamma (INF-γ), and several cytokines with intrinsic anti-inflammatory activity, including IL-1 receptor antagonist (IL-1ra), transforming growth factor-β, and soluble TNF receptor (Dinarello, 1994; Dinarello and Wolff, 1993). Cytokines are highly synergistic, and highly potent (Figure 18-1).

Are cytokine responses helpful to survival? That is certainly the case in experimental sepsis in animals where the cytokine effects can be neutralized early in infection. In humans, preliminary studies of extremely sick septic patients showed improved survival after blockade of IL-1 (with IL-1ra) (Fisher et al., 1994b), but in a larger study with patients of varying severity of sepsis, there was no benefit overall (Fisher et al., 1994a). However, subgroup analysis of the larger study suggests that IL-1ra may have been of benefit in a subgroup of the most severely sick individuals (Fisher et al., 1994a). The possible usefulness of the TNF component of response has been reviewed (van der Poll and Lowry, 1995).

Many neuroendocrine functions are profoundly altered during states of inflammatory disease (Reichlin, 1993, 1994, 1995; Sternberg, 1992; Wilder, 1995) (Table 18-1). Some have positive homeostatic value, while others may contribute to the deleterious impact of inflammation. This chapter focuses on changes in the pituitary and in pituitary target hormones; abnormalities in the pancreas, bone, and brain (all of which occur in sepsis or after exposure to inflammatory cytokines) are not considered further. Many of the endocrine responses observed in inflammation are due in part to the associated decrease in nutrient consumption. These are pointed out in sections below.

HYPOTHALAMIC-PITUITARY-ADRENAL ACTIVATION

The classical pituitary-adrenal response to stress can be induced by infection or by the injection of bacterial toxin (Kimball et al., 1968; Michie et al., 1990) (Figures 18-1, 18-2). Lipopolysaccharides (LPS) (and other toxins) act on pituitary-adrenal function by stimulating cytokine release. IL-1, IL-2, IL-6, and TNF-α are all capable of activating corticotropin-releasing hormone (CRH) secretion (Kakuscska et al., 1993; Sapolsky et al., 1987). Systemic LPS is also capable of activating central IL-1 neuronal pathways (Breder et al., 1988; Lechan et al., 1990). Toxin-induced cytokine release stimulates secretion of the hypothalamic neuropeptides, CRH, and vasopressin (VP), which synergize at

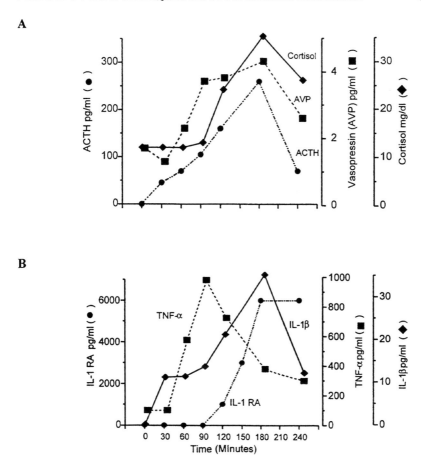

FIGURE 18-1 Composite diagram to illustrate the response of acute-phase cytokines, pituitary-adrenal, and neurohypophysial hormones to the injection of *Escherichia coli* endotoxin. SOURCE: Figure reprinted from Reichlin (1998) with permission. (A) Changes in adrenocorticotrophic hormone (ACTH) cortisol, and arginine vasopressin (AVP) following injection of *E. coli* endotoxin. Both ACTH and AVP are activated within 30 minutes, followed approximately 30 minutes later by increased cortisol secretion. As discussed in the text, endotoxin acts by mobilizing peripheral release of inflammatory cytokines, tumor necrosis factor (TNF), and interleukin (IL)-1, which act directly and indirectly on the hypothalamus. Figure was redrawn from the published data of Michie et al. (1990). (B) Time course of appearance in the blood of IL-1β, TNF-α, and IL-receptor antagonist (ra) following intramuscular injection of *E. coli* endotoxin. Redrawn from the published data of Dinarello and Wolff (1993) and Granowitz et al. (1993). Note that TNF-α appears first and then rapidly falls, that IL-1β next appears, which is then followed approximately 90 minutes later by IL-1ra. The concentration of IL-1ra is approximately 100 times greater than that of IL-1, giving a molar ratio sufficient to ensure that IL-1 effects are fully neutralized.

TABLE 18-1 Neuroendocrine and Endocrine Consequences of Inflammatory Disease

Pituitary-adrenal activation

Syndrome of inappropriate ADH secretion (SIADH)

Sick euthyroid syndrome

Sick gonad syndrome

Growth hormone increase/decrease

Impaired insulin secretion, insulin resistance

Sick bone syndrome

Sick brain syndrome

the pituitary level to increase the secretion of adrenocorticotrophic hormone (ACTH). Toxin can also act less directly through stimulation of vagal afferents in the liver bed and elsewhere in the abdomen (Watkins et al., 1995b). The vagal afferent system, which acts through chemosensory vagal paraganglia is especially vulnerable to toxic products arising in the abdomen viscera. Central activation of CRH neurons leads to stimulation of the peripheral autonomic nervous system (Irwin et al., 1990) with enhanced release of epinephrine from the adrenal medulla and of norepinephrine from sympathetic nerve endings. Epinephrine synergizes with CRH and VP in stimulating ACTH release.

The consequent release of glucocorticoids in turn modulates the intensity of the acute response, virtually all of whose components are inhibited by glucocorticoids (Munck et al., 1984). These include inhibition of cytokine secretion by immunocompetent cells and the consequent loss of lymphocyte reactions that are secondary to cytokine actions. Among the factors that are inhibited are INF-γ, granulocyte-monocyte stimulating factor, IL-1, IL-2, IL-3, IL-6, and TNF-α. The secretion of many inflammatory mediators by activated lymphocytes and macrophages is also inhibited. These include bradykinin, serotonin, and histamine and the tissue-destructive enzymes collagenase, elastase, plasminogen activator, and prostaglandins. Natural killer (NK) cell activity is also suppressed by glucocorticoids (Callawaert et al., 1991).

Although these anti-inflammatory effects of glucocorticoids are the basis of its widespread clinical use to treat immune disorders, they were for many years looked on as pharmacological side effects and not relevant to physiological function. However, in one view of Munck and colleagues (1984), the pituitary-adrenal response to stress evolved as a mechanism to suppress and modulate an overexuberant inflammatory response to toxins, antigens, and invading organisms. Intense mobilization of cytokines and inflammatory mediators may be fatal.

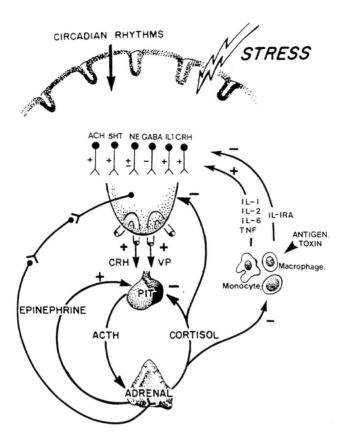

FIGURE 18-2 Schematic outline of the neuroendocrine factors that regulate the secretion of the adrenal cortex. SOURCE: Figure reprinted from Reichlin (1998) with permission. Adrenocorticotrophic hormone (ACTH) release from the pituitary is stimulated by corticotropin-releasing hormone (CRH) and vasopressin (VP) acting synergistically. Circulating epinephrine (the response of the activated sympathetic nervous system) is also synergistic for ACTH release. The secretion of ACTH is inhibited at the pituitary level by circulating glucocorticoids, and at the hypothalamic level, CRH and VP are also under negative feedback control by glucocorticoids. VP and CRH neurons are in turn subject to a wide range of influences—circulating cytokines, prostaglandins, and many neurotransmitters. Some such as acetylcholine (ACH) are stimulatory, and others such as γ-amino butyric acid (GABA) are inhibitory. Interacting with the hypothalamic-pituitary-adrenal axis is the peripheral immune system (as well as endothelia and other structures), which releases cytokines into the blood which then can activate the adrenal. Each of the major inflammatory cytokines, interleukin (IL)-1 (α or β), IL-2, IL-6, and tumor necrosis factor (TNF)-α are capable of activating ACTH release. The peripheral immune system provides a chemosensory system by which the presence of foreign molecules can be communicated to the brain and can induce an appropriate response, a model of "bidirectional communication between the brain and the immune system" Blalock (1989).

An excellent example of the validity of the Munck hypothesis has come from the study of immune responses in the Lewis strain of rats, which have a genetic defect in hypothalamic CRH synthesis (Chrousos, 1995; Sternberg, 1992; Wilder, 1995). Rats of the Lewis strain develop acute arthritis when injected with streptococcal cell wall suspensions, whereas rats of the Fischer strain do not. Lewis rats are susceptible to many other forms of induced autoimmune disease. Lewis rats differ from Fischer rats in that Lewis rats do not show increased adrenal glucocorticoid release when challenged with antigen and do not increase their hypothalamic content of mRNA coding for CRH as do Fischer rats. Measures that inhibit pituitary-adrenal function in the Fischer rat convert their immune responses to those resembling the Lewis (susceptible) strain. Clinical studies have tested this hypothesis in patients with established rheumatoid arthritis (Chikanza et al., 1992), chronic fatigue syndrome (Demitrack, 1994; Goldenberg, 1993; Manu et al., 1992), and fibromyalgia (Crofford et al., 1994; Goldenberg, 1993; Griep et al., 1993). Studies in rheumatoid arthritis (RA) patients are the most convincing; patients with RA undergoing major joint surgery have a lower or absent glucocorticoid response as compared with patients with osteoarthritis undergoing the same procedure. Moreover, patients with RA have a higher IL-1 response to the surgical procedure, which suggests that glucocorticoids are not damping their stress response. Results of studies of patients with chronic fatigue syndrome or fibromyalgia are ambiguous, though they do suggest some impaired adrenal function in some patients. Whether or not there is a pituitary-adrenocortical deficit in patients with these disorders, current studies do not distinguish whether they arise as secondary or primary abnormalities.

Although it is well established that patients with adrenal deficiency are more likely to die during sepsis than those with normal adrenal function, most studies show that treatment of sepsis with glucocorticoids in patients with normal adrenal function does not improve survival, and in fact, it may increase mortality (Sheagren, 1991). These observations suggest that otherwise healthy individuals respond to sepsis with an appropriate pituitary-adrenal response.

SYNDROME OF INAPPROPRIATE ANTIDIURETIC HORMONE SECRETION

Characteristic of the response to sepsis is an increase in secretion of VP (antidiuretic hormone, ADH). Lobar pneumonia has been shown to be accompanied by elevated VP levels and by impaired water excretion (Dreyfuss et al., 1988), changes that are secondary to activation of central vasopressinergic pathways. These insights are not new. It has been known since the introduction of serum chloride measurements into clinical chemistry that serum chloride levels in patients with bacterial pneumonia are reduced (secondary to hemodilution) and that the crisis of recovery in lobar pneumonia (in the preantibiotic era) was heralded by a sudden increase in serum chloride concentration ("chloride shift"). A possible homeostatic value of VP is its ability to inhibit the pyrogenic effects of bacterial toxin (Naylor et al., 1987). There is a downside to the VP response because it stimulates the kidney to delay water excretion, which in septic and elderly individuals enhances the vulnerability to overhydration.

PITUITARY-THYROID REGULATION IN
INFLAMMATORY DISEASE

The sick euthyroid syndrome is the most common form of thyroid abnormality encountered in populations of acute and chronically ill individuals. It is characterized by low circulating levels of triiodothyronine (T3), low or low normal blood levels of thyroxine (T4), and depressed thyroid hormone binding proteins (Wartofsky and Burman, 1982). Concentrations of thyroid hormones in tissues obtained at autopsy from patients dying with the sick euthyroid syndrome are lower than those of individuals who died suddenly (Arem et al., 1993). The most striking neuroendocrine feature of this disorder (and the one most useful in clinical differentiation from primary thyroid abnormalities) is that the low circulating thyroid hormones do not induce elevation of plasma thyroid-stimulating hormone (TSH) levels as would normally be the case through the operation of the hypothalamic-pituitary thyroid negative feedback system.

The syndrome can be reproduced to a degree in rats by injections of bacterial toxin, IL-1, or TNF-α (Pang et al., 1989) and in humans by injections of TNF-α (van der Poll and Lowry, 1995; van der Poll et al., 1990). In a detailed analysis of the cytokine etiology of the sick euthyroid state in the mouse, none of the cytokines tested individually (TNF-α, IL-1α, IL-6, and INF-γ) were as potent as bacterial toxin in inducing the disorder. Nor were these cytokines as potent when tested together (Boelen et al., 1995). In sick euthyroid humans, depression of the T3 level was proportional to circulating levels of TNF (Mooradian et al., 1990) and was a function of serum IL-6 concentration only in very severely ill individuals (Boelen et al., 1993). Blockade of IL-1 effects with one Il-1 receptor antagonist did not prevent the effects of endotoxin or pituitary-thryoid function (van der Poll et al., 1995). This observation suggests that a number of other cytokines are involved in the diagnosis.

Sick euthyroidism comes about through cytokine-induced alterations at every level of the pituitary-thyroid axis: hypothalamic, pituitary, thyroid gland itself, and peripheral thyroid metabolism (Reichlin, 1993, 1994). In the hypothalamus, thyrotropin-releasing hormone (TRH) synthesis is inhibited (Kakuscska et al., 1994), and somatostatin synthesis enhanced (Scarborough et al., 1989). Within the pituitary, IL-1 is induced in a subpopulation of thyrotrope cells (Koenig et al., 1990) and exerts autocrine and paracrine inhibition of responsiveness to TRH (Sumita et al., 1994). In the thyroid, a number of metabolic abnormalities are induced—impaired peroxidation and impaired cAMP responsiveness, which leads to reduced TRH responsiveness—while in the periphery, reduced conversion of T4 to T3 and reduced hepatic synthesis of transthyretin and albumin lead to the characteristic low T3 and, in severe cases, low T4 levels (Reichlin, 1993). Starvation contributes to the abnormal T4 to T3 conversion; in uninfected individuals, fasting by itself is sufficient to decrease T4 to T3 conversion with restoration by carbohydrate supplementation (Vagenakis et al., 1975). In septic patients with low serum T3 values, hyperalimentation restored T3 values to normal (Richmand et al., 1980).

In contrast to other chronic inflammatory diseases, patients with AIDS manifest elevation of thyroxine-binding globulin as the disease progresses, and the low T3 syndrome does not appear until patients approach a terminal state when malnutrition and cachexia dominate the clinical picture (Lambert, 1994).

Still unsettled is whether these decreases in thyroid function are homeostatically valuable. In experimental streptococcal pneumonia in the rat, low thyroid levels were associated with reduced mortality, whereas high levels increased vulnerability (Reichlin and Glaser, 1958). In another model of sepsis, pulmonary surfactant levels were restored to normal by T3 supplementation (Dulchavsky et al., 1995). Studies in the human are limited. Thyroid hormone treatment had no benefit (nor did harm) to a relatively small number of septic individuals with the sick euthyroid syndrome (Brent and Hershman, 1986), but in volunteers whose T3 levels were reduced by a period of fasting, T3 supplementation increased the magnitude of negative nitrogen balance (Gardner et al., 1979). These studies are admittedly difficult to carry out, and the results are less than convincing. At this time, there is no evidence that thyroid supplementation is beneficial in patients with sick euthyroid disease, but the question has not been resolved definitively.

PITUITARY-GONADAL REGULATION

Burns and severe inflammatory illness induce a dramatic fall in sex steroids (Dong et al., 1992). TNF-α also inhibits gonadal secretion (van der Poll et al., 1993). As in the case of pituitary-thyroid dysfunction in sepsis, cytokine suppression of pituitary-gonad function is exerted at many levels. IL-1 reaching the gonads through the circulation, or released from Leydig cells within the testis as an autocrine-paracrine secretion, inhibits steroidogenesis and other cell functions (Syed et al., 1993). In the ovary, intrinsic cytokines, IL-6, TNF-α, and IL-1 regulate steroidogenesis, maturation, atresia, and apoptosis of ovarian cells. Indeed, cytokine-induced apoptosis of granulosa cells is the triggering event that culminates in follicular atresia. At the level of the hypothalamus, IL-1 inhibits pulsatile secretion of gonadotropin-releasing hormone (GnRH), which leads to low gonadotropin secretion and low levels of sex steroids (Rivest and Rivier, 1995; Shalts et al., 1991). These effects are probably mediated at the hypothalamic level by the induction of CRH and/or VP (Rivest and Rivier, 1995; Shalts et al., 1991).

Currently, no useful data exist to indicate that low gonadotropin-sex steroid secretion is homeostatically valuable or harmful in the human or in other species. One could argue that testosterone deficiency might be harmful in that it would increase wasting of muscle mass, but suitable studies of anabolic steroid treatment in sepsis have not been published.

Starvation, in the absence of sepsis is also capable of inhibiting gonadal function in both men (Samuels and Kramer, 1996) and women (Olson et al., 1995). Short-term starvation reduces the magnitude of pulsatile gonadotropin release in both sexes but the degree of gonadotropin suppression is greater in men than in women.

GROWTH HORMONE IN SEPSIS

In humans, a single injection of LPS induces a sharp increase in growth hormone (GH) (Kimball et al., 1968; Wagner et al., 1975), while in rats, cytokines in low dosage stimulate (Payne et al., 1992) and in large doses, suppress GH (Payne et al., 1992; Peisen et al., 1995; Wada et al., 1995) . Severe sepsis is associated with elevated GH levels (Bentham et al., 1993) or normal levels (Voerman et al., 1992a, 1993), and in one particular chronic inflammatory illness, RA, daily GH secretion was reduced (Rall et al., 1996).

However, GH levels alone may not reflect actual GH effects as expressed at the tissue level. GH effects on protein metabolism are mediated through the secretion of somatomedin C (insulin-like growth factor I), a liver-derived protein whose secretion is dependent both on GH stimulation and on the availability of metabolic substrate. For example, in states of nutritional deficiency (protein-calorie malnutrition, kwashiorkor, anorexia nervosa), blood levels of GH are markedly elevated, but somatomedin C concentrations are low, which suggests that tissue "effective" levels of GH are low.

In humans with sepsis, somatomedin C levels are low and can be restored to normal by hyperalimentation (Bentham et al., 1993) or by GH treatment (Voerman et al., 1992b). In what may be an analogous situation—the catabolic state associated with large burns—blood GH levels are elevated, somatomedin values are low, but the administration of additional amounts of GH appear to improve survival and graft healing and to shorten the duration of hospitalization (Knox et al., 1995; Nguyen et al., 1996). One conclusion therefore is that the elevated GH seen in sepsis is homeostatically valuable but that the normal response is suboptimal. Hepatic somatomedin-C response to GH is probably reduced in burns and sepsis; for this reason, somatomedin C (which would bypass the liver) may possibly be a more useful agent than GH in this setting. In a murine model of sepsis, both GH and somatomedin C enhanced host defense (Inoue et al., 1995).

AUTHOR'S SUMMARY AND CONCLUSIONS

Activation of inflammatory cytokines by toxins or products of cell injury (as in burns and physical trauma) leads to a variety of metabolic and endocrine changes, mediated in part by the direct action of cytokines on tissue function and by changes in pituitary-endocrine end organ function. Some of the endocrine responses, such as pituitary-adrenal activation and GH hypersecretion, are homeostatically valuable and promote survival or healing. Other responses may be harmful. Increased VP secretion may modulate fever but create water intolerance and susceptibility to hypo-osmolar states. Loss of gonadal activity has possible catabolic consequences. Reduced supply of the active form of thyroid hormone to tissues may conserve metabolic demand but could interfere with some normal thyroid hormone-dependent functions. Cytokine-driven responses of the neuroendocrine system resemble those seen in starvation: reduced thyroid function, reduced levels of GH-dependent peptides, and suppression of gonadal function.

Areas for possible additional study in soldiers under stress include the use of gonadal steroids or anabolic steroids and the use of GH and/or somatomedin C. Newly developed devices the size of a fountain pen make injections feasible under field conditions. Glucocorticoid treatment will be unlikely to help manage stress in individuals whose underlying adrenal reserve is normal. Studies designed specifically to evaluate thyroid status under field conditions of stress and malnutrition would be of value, but on the basis of the limited information on treatment of sick euthyroid patients with thyroid hormone, it is unlikely that this form of therapy will be helpful. Cytokine-mediated changes in neuroendocrine activity interacting with poor nutrition could well impair immunological function and overall resistance to stress.

REFERENCES

Arem, R., G.J. Wiener, S.G. Kaplan, H.S. Kim, S. Reichlin, and M.M. Kaplan. 1993. Reduced tissue thyroid hormone levels in fatal illness. Metab. Clin. Exp. 42:1102–1108.

Bentham, J., J. Rodriguez-Arnao, and R.J. Ross. 1993. Acquired growth hormone resistance in patients with hypercatabolism. Horm. Res. 40:87–91.

Blalock, J.E. 1989. A molecular basis for bidirectional communication between the immune and neuroendocrine systems. Physiol. Rev. 69:1–32.

Boelen, A., M.C. Platvoet-Ter Schiphorst, O. Bakker, and W.M. Wiersinga. 1995. The role of cytokines in the lipopolysaccharide-induced sick euthyroid syndrome in mice. J. Endocrinol. 146:475–483.

Boelen, A., M.C. Platvoet-Ter Schiphorst, and W.M. Wiersinga. 1993. Association between serum interleukin-6 and serum 3,5,3'-triiodothyronine in nonthyroidal illness. J. Clin. Endocrinol. Metab. 77:1695–1699.

Breder, C.D., C.D. Dinarello, and C.B. Saper. 1988. Interleukin-1 immunoreactive innervation of the human hypothalamus. Science 240:321–324.

Brent, G.A., and J.M. Hershman. 1986. Thyroxine therapy in patients with severe nonthyroidal illnesses and low serum thyroxine concentration. J. Clin. Endocrinol. Metab. 63:1–8.

Callewaert, D.M., V.K. Moudgil, G. Radcliff, and R. Waite. 1991. Hormone specific regulation of natural killer cells by cortisol: Direct inactivation of the cytotoxic function of cloned human NK cells without an effect on cellular proliferation. FEBS Lett. 285:108 015–110.

Chikanza, I.C., P. Petrou, G. Kingsley, G. Chrousos, and G.S. Panayi. 1992. Defective hypothalamic response to immune and inflammatory stimuli in patients with rheumatoid arthritis. Arthritis Rheum. 35:1281–1288.

Chrousos, G.P. 1995. The hypothalamic-pituitary-adrenal axis and immune-mediated inflammation. N. Engl. J. Med. 332:1351–1362.

Crofford, L.J., S.R. Pillemer, K.T. Kalogeras, J.M. Cash, D. Michelson, M.A. Kling, E.M. Sternberg, P.W. Gold, G.P. Chrousos, and R.L. Wilder. 1994. Hypothalamic-pituitary-adrenal axis perturbations in patients with fibromyalgia. Arthritis Rheum. 37:1583–1592.

Demitrack, M.A. 1994. Chronic fatigue syndrome a disease of the hypothalamic-pituitary-adrenal axis? Ann. Med. 26:1–5.

Dinarello, C.A. 1994. The biological properties of interleukin-1. Euro. Cytokine Netw. 5:517–531.

Dinarello, C.A., and S.M. Wolff. 1993. The role of Interleukin-1 in disease. New Engl. J. Med. 328:106–113.

Dong, Q., F. Hawker, D. McWilliam, M. Bangah, H. Bureger, and D.J. Handelsman. 1992. Circulating immunoreactive inhibin and testosterone levels in men with critical illness. Clin. Endocrinol. 36:399–404.

Dreyfuss, D., F. Leviel, M. Paillard, J. Rahmani, and I. Coste. 1988. Acute infectious pneumonia is accompanied by a latent vasopressin-dependent impairment of renal water excretion. Am. Rev. Resp. Dis. 138:583–585.

Dulchavsky, S.A., S.M. Ksenzenko, A.A. Saba, and L.N. Diebel. 1995. Triiodothyronine (T3) supplementation maintains surfactant biochemical integrity during sepsis. J. Trauma 39:53–57.

Fisher, Jr., C.J., J.F. Dhainaut, S.M. Opal, J.P. Pribble, R.A. Balk, G.J. Slotman, T.J. Iberti, E.C. Rackow, M.J. Shapiro, R.L. Greenman et al. 1994a. Recombinant human interleukin 1 receptor antagonist in the treatment of patients with sepsis syndrome. Results from a randomized, double-blind, placebo-controlled trial. Phase III rhIL-1ra Sepsis Syndrome Study group. J. Am. Med. Assoc. 271:1836–1843.

Fisher, Jr., C.J., G.J. Slotman, S.M. Opal, J.P. Pribble, R.C. Bone, G. Emmanuel, D. Ng, D.C. Bloedow, and M.A. Catalano. 1994b. Initial evaluation of human recombinant interleukin-1 receptor antagonist in the treatment of sepsis syndrome: A randomized, open-label, placebo-controlled multicenter trial. The IL-1RA Sepsis Syndrome Study Group. Crit Care Med. 22:12–21.

Gardner, D.F., M.M. Kaplan, C.A. Stanley, and R.D. Utiger. 1979. Effect of triiodothyronine replacement on the metabolic and pituitary responses to starvation. N. Engl. J. Med. 300:579–584.

Goldenberg, D.L. 1993. Fibromyalgia, chronic fatigue syndrome, and myofascial pain syndrome. Curr. Opin. Rheumatol. 5:199–208.

Granowitz, E.V., R. Porat, J.W. Mier, S.F. Orencole, M.V. Callahan, J.G. Cannon, E.A. Lynch, K. Ye, D.D. Poutsiaka, E. Vannier et al. 1993. Hematologic and immunomodulatory effects of an interleukin-1 receptor antagonist coinfusion during low-dose endotoxemia in healthy adults. Blood 82:2985–2990.

Griep, E.N., J.W. Boersma, and E.R. de Kloet. 1993. Altered reactivity of the hypothalamic-pituitary-adrenal axis in the primary fibromyalgia syndrome. J. Rheumatol. 20:469–474.

Inoue, T., H. Saito, R. Fukushima, T. Inaba, M.T. Lin, K. Fukatsu, and T. Muto. 1995. Growth hormone and insulin-like growth factor I enhance host defense in a murine sepsis model. Arch. Surg. 130:1115–1122.

Irwin, M.T., R.L. Hauger, L. Jones, M. Provencio, and K.T. Britton. 1990. Sympathetic nervous system mediates central corticotropin-releasing factor induced suppression of natural killer cytotoxicity. J. Pharmacol. Exp. Ther. 255:101–107.

Kakucska, I., L.I. Romero, B.D. Clark, J.M. Rondeel, Y. Qi, S. Alex, C.H. Emerson, and R.M. Lechan. 1994. Suppression of thyrotropin-releasing hormone gene expression by interleukin-1β in the rat: Implications for nonthyroidal illness. Neuroendocrinology 59:129–137.

Kakuscska, I., Y. Qi, B.D. Clark, and R.M. Lechan. 1993. Endotoxin-induced corticotropin-releasing hormone gene expression in the hypothalamic paraventricular nucleus is mediated centrally by interleukin-1. Endocrinology 133:815–821.

Kimball, H.R., M.B. Lipsett, W.D. Odell, and S.M. Wolff. 1968. Comparison of the effects of the pyrogens, etiocholanolone and bacterial endotoxin on plasma cortisol and growth hormone in man. J. Clin. Endocrinol. Metab. 28:337–342

Knox, J., R. Demling, D. Wilmore, P. Sarraf, and A. Santos. 1995. Increased survival after major thermal injury: The effect of growth hormone therapy in adults. J. Trauma 39:526–530.

Koenig, J.I., K. Snow, B.D. Clark, R. Toni, J.G. Cannon, A.R. Shaw, C.A. Dinarello, S. Reichlin, S.L. Lee, and R.M. Lechan. 1990. Intrinsic pituitary interleukin-1β is induced by bacterial lipopolysaccharide. Endocrinology 127:3053–3058.

Lambert, M. 1994. Thyroid dysfunction in HIV infection. Baillieres Clin. Endocrinol. Metab. 8:825–835.

Lechan, R.M., R. Toni, B.D. Clark, J.G. Cannon, A.R. Shaw, C.A. Dinarello, and S. Reichlin. 1990. Immunoreactive interleukin-1β localization in the rat forebrain. Brain Res. 514:135–140.

Manu, P., T.J. Lane, and D.A. Matthews. 1992. The pathophysiology of chronic fatigue syndrome: Confirmations, contradictions, and conjectures. Int. J. Psychol. Med. 22:397–408.

Michie, H.R., J.A. Majzoub, S.T. O'Dwyer, A. Revhaug, and D.W. Wilmore. 1990. Both cyclooxygenase-dependent and cyclooxygenase-independent pathways mediate the neuroendocrine response in humans. Surgery 108:254–259.

Mooradian, A.D., R.L. Reed, D. Osterweil, R. Schiffman, and P. Scuderi. 1990. Decreased serum triiodothyronine is associated with increased concentrations of tumor necrosis factor. J. Clin. Endocrinol. Metab. 71:1239–1242.

Munck, A., P.M. Guyre, and N.J. Holbrook. 1984. Physiological functions of glucocorticoids in stress and their relation to pharmacological actions. Endocrinol. Rev. 5:25–44.

Naylor, A.M., K.E. Cooper, and W.L. Veale. 1987. Vasopressin and fever: Evidence supporting the existence of an endogenous antipyretic system in the brain. Can. J. Physiol. Pharm. 65:1333–1338.

Nguyen, T.T., D.A. Gilpin, N.A. Meyer, and D.N. Herndon. 1996. Current treatment of severely burned patients. Ann. Surg. 223:14–25.

Olson, B.R., T. Cartledge, N. Sebring, R. Defensor, and L. Nieman. 1995. Short-term fasting effects luteinizing hormone secretory dynamics but not reproductive function in normal-weight sedentary women. J. Clin. Endocrinol. Metab. 80:1187–1193.

Pang, X.P., J.M. Hershman, C.J. Mirell, and A.E. Pekary. 1989. Impairment of hypothalamic-pituitary-thyroid function in rats treated with human recombinant tumor necrosis factor-α (cachectin). Endocrinology 125:76–84.

Payne, L.C., F. Obal, Jr., M.R. Opp, and J.M. Krueger. 1992. Stimulation and inhibition of growth hormone secretion by interleukin-1β: The involvement of growth hormone-releasing hormone. Neuroendocrinology 56:118–123.

Peisen, J.N., K.J. McDonnell, S.E. Mulroney, and M.D. Lumpkin. 1995. Endotoxin-induced suppression of the somatotropic axis is mediated by interleukin-1β and corticotropin-releasing factor in the juvenile rat. Endocrinology 136:3378–3390.

Rall, L.C., N.T. Lundgren, S. Reichlin, J.D. Veldhuis, and R. Roubenoff. 1996. Growth hormone (GH) kinetics in aging and chronic inflammation. FASEB J. 10:A754.

Reichlin, S. 1993. Neuroendocrine-immune interactions. N. Engl. J. Med. 329:1246–1253.

Reichlin, S. 1994. Neuroendocrine consequences of systemic inflammation. Pp. 83–96 in Advances in Endocrinology and Metabolism, E.L. Mazzaferri, R.S. Bar, and R.A. Kreisberg, eds. St. Louis: Mosby.

Reichlin, S. 1995. Endocrine-Immune Interaction. Pp. 2964–3012 in Endocrinology, L.J. DeGroot, ed. Philadelphia: W.B. Saunders Company.

Reichlin, S. 1998. Neuroendocrinology. In William's Textbook of Endocrinology, 9th ed. [in press], J.D. Wilson, D. Foster, P.R. Larsen, and H. Kronenberg, eds. Philadelphia: W.B. Saunders Company.

Reichlin, S., and R.J. Glaser. 1958. Thyroid function in experimental streptococcal pneumonia in the rat. J. Exp. Med. 107:219–236.

Richmand, D.A., M.E. Molitch, and T.F. O'Donnell. 1980. Altered thyroid hormone levels in bacterial sepsis: The role of nutritional adequacy. Metab. Clin. Exp. 29:936–942.

Rivest, S., and C. Rivier. 1995. The role of corticotropin-releasing factor and interleukin-1 in the regulation of neurons controlling reproductive functions. Endocr. Rev. 16:177–199.

Romero, L.I., J.B. Tatro, J.A. Field, and S. Reichlin. 1996. Roles of IL-1 and TNF-α in endotoxin-induced activation of nitric oxide synthase in cultured rat brain cells. Am. J. Physiol. 270:R326–R332.

Samuels, M.H., and P. Kramer. 1996. Differential effects of short-term fasting on pulsatile thyrotropin, gondotropin, and α-subunit secretion in healthy men—a clinical research center study. J. Clin. Endocrinol. Metab. 81:32–36.

Sapolsky, R., C. Rivier, G. Yamamoto, P. Plotsky, and W. Vale. 1987. Interleukin-1 stimulates the secretion of hypothalamic corticotropin-releasing factor. Science 238:522–524.

Scarborough, D.E., S.L. Lee, C.A. Dinarello, and S. Reichlin. 1989. Interleukin-1 stimulates somatostatin biosynthesis in primary cultures of fetal rat brain. Endocrinology 126:3053–3058.

Shalts, E., Y-J. Feng, and M. Ferrin. 1991. Vasopressin mediates the interleukin-1a-induced reduced decrease in luteinizing hormone secretion in the ovariectomized rhesus monkey. Endocrinology 131:153–158.

Sheagren, J.N. 1991. Corticosteroids for the treatment of septic shock. Infect. Dis. Clin. North Am. 5:875–882.

Sternberg, E.M. 1992. The stress response and the regulation of inflammatory disease. Ann. Int. Med. 117:854–866.

Syed, V., N. Gérard, and A. Kaipia. 1993. Identification of an interleukin-6 like factor in rat seminiferous tubule. Endocrinology 132:293–299.

Sumita, S., Y. Ujike, A. Namiki, H. Watanabe, M. Kawamata, A. Watanabe, and O. Satoh 1994. Suppression of the thyrotropin response to thyrotropin-releasing hormone and its association with severity of critical illness. Crit. Care Med. 22:1603–1609.

Vagenakis, A.G., A. Burger, G.I. Portnoy, M. Rudolph, J.R. O'Brian, F. Azzizi, R.A. Arky, P. Nicod, S.H. Ingbar, and L.E. Braverman. 1975. Diversion of peripheral thyroxine metabolism from activating to inactivating pathways during complete fasting. J. Clin. Endocrinol. Metab. 41:191–194.

van der Poll, T., and S.F. Lowry. 1995. Tumor necrosis factor in sepsis: Mediator of multiple organ failure or essential part of host defense? Shock 3:1–12.

van der Poll, T., J.A. Romijn, E. Endert, and H.P. Sauerwein. 1993. Effects of tumor necrosis factor on the hypothalamic-pituitary-testicular axis in healthy men. Metabolism 42:303–307.

van der Poll, T., J.A. Romijn, W.M. Wiersinga, and H.P. Sauerwein. 1990. Tumor necrosis factor: A putative mediator of the sick euthyroid syndrome in man. J. Clin. Endocrinol. Metab. 71:1567–1572.

van der Poll, T., K.J. Van Zee, E. Endert, S.M. Coyle, D.M. Stiles, J.P. Pribble, M.A. Catalano, L.L. Moldawer, and S.F. Lowry. 1995. Interleukin-1 receptor blockade does not affect endotoxin-induced changes in plasma thyroid hormone and thyrotropin concentrations in man. J. Clin. Endocrinol. Metab. 80:1341–1346.

Voerman, H.J., A.B. Groenveld, H. de Boer, R.J. Strack van Schijndel, J.P. Nauta, E.A. van der Veen, and L.G. Thijs. 1993. Time course and variability of the endocrine and metabolic response to severe sepsis. Surgery 114:951–959.

Voerman, H.J., R.J. Strack van Scijndel, A.P. Groenevelkd, H. de Boer, J.P. Nauta, and L.G. Thijs. 1992a. Pulsatile hormone secretion during severe sepsis: Accuracy of different blood sampling regimens. Metabolism 41:934–940.

Voerman, H.J., R.J. van Schijndel, A.B. Groeneveld, H. de Boer, J.P. Nauta, E.A. van der Veen, and L.G. Thijs. 1992b. Effects of recombinant human growth hormone in patients with severe sepsis. Ann. Surg. 216:648–655

Wada, T., M. Sato, M. Niimi, M. Tamaki, T. Ishida, and J. Takahara. 1995. Inhibitory effects of interleukin-1 on growth hormone secretion in conscious male rats. Endocrinology 136:3936–3941.

Wagner, H., E. Zierden, and W.H. Hauss. 1975. Effects of synthetic somatostatin on endotoxin-induced changes of growth hormone, cortisol and insulin in plasma, blood sugar and blood leukocytes in man. Klin. Wochenschr. 53:539–541.

Wartofsky, L. and K.D. Burman. 1982. Alterations in thyroid function in patients with systemic illness: the "euthyroid sick syndrome." Endocr. Rev. 3(2):164–217.

Watkins, L.R., S.F. Maier, and L.E. Goehler. 1995b. Cytokine-to-brain communication: A review and analysis of alternative mechanisms. Life Sciences 57:1011–1026.

Wilder, R.L. 1995. Neuroendocrine-immune system interactions and autoimmunity. Ann. Rev. Immunol. 13:307–338.

DISCUSSION

LEONARD KAPCALA: In the IL-1 receptor antagonist studies in which no benefits were demonstrated, I wonder whether their treatment may be too late.

SEYMOUR REICHLIN: That is a very good point. First of all, in several species of experimental animals, IL-1 receptor antagonist has really very excellent effects in preventing death, so that if you inject the material prior to challenge, it is effective.

Secondly, in the preliminary studies with a small number of patients treated with IL-1 receptor antagonist, very, very sick patients were used, and these patients did have a beneficial effect. Then when the study was expanded, individuals were included who were less septic than the original series, and in that group the interleukin receptor antagonist had no effect. In that study, those in the subgroup who were very, very sick had a beneficial effect. What that means to me is that under most circumstances, you make about as much IL-1 as you need, and that the extreme septic people make too much, but you would have to know that at the time you make the diagnosis, and also if the acute illness had gone on for 2 days it may be too late to do anything.

I think that is the practical point.

WILLIAM BEISEL: I was certainly glad to hear your presentation, to hear the interpretations of modern-day cytokinology by a classic endocrinologist. It was a delightful presentation.

SEYMOUR REICHLIN: Thank you. I have to tell you that Dr. Beisel was an endocrinologist in his former life.

WILLIAM BEISEL: I want to point out the committee interest in many of these cytokines—or my personal interest in what I call cytokine-induced malnutrition. This is the acute problem of loss of nitrogen and loss of vitamins and loss of minerals such as zinc, sequestration of iron and zinc. All of those metabolic effects have acute effects on the soldier in a short period of time, and so, in addition to all their beneficial effects and their deleterious effects that can lead to death, I think for the mild infections that our committee is concerned mostly about, how many nutrients are lost and what this has done . . .

SEYMOUR REICHLIN: I would underline what Dr. Beisel said, that in addition to a metabolic disturbance caused by neuroendocrine effects, several of the cytokines, particularly TNF-α have profound direct metabolic effects at the tissue level.

They produce profound catabolic disturbance, which may actually be more important than the effects that are mediated through the classical endocrine system. I would definitely emphasize the cachectin type of responses.

NED BERNTON: I have a question and a comment. Dr. Beisel many years ago worked in volunteers with the spread of infections. Since blood draws in major studies have always been done in the morning, it is very hard to get a feel for what is going on in the circadian rhythm of cortisol secretion, and if indeed that reflects a systemic inflammatory response, and we did some preliminary studies with salivary cortisol that suggested that in some of the subjects, the circadian rhythm was lost, but measuring salivary cortisol levels may be a very interesting way to gain data tracking the circadian rhythm, which would make a lot more sense. And my other question is as IGF [insulin-like growth factor]-I is decreased by malnutrition and infection, would IGF (as a marker of GH secretion that is not subject to the pulsatile variation of GH) possibly give a useful indication of what was purely nutritional and what was due to hypothalamic-pituitary functional changes?

SEYMOUR REICHLIN: Dr. Bernton's point here I think is extremely valuable. Because of the problems of sampling, you don't really get a clear picture of the changes in circadian rhythm. As a matter of fact, I have been unable to find any studies of melatonin rhythms in the conditions of severe stress such as combat training.

The second question you raised, I think is also important. Somatomedin C levels should be measured. Treatment with this hormone may be beneficial. Is it reasonable to consider genetic hormone treatment under these conditions?

The Genentech Company now sells a fountain pen-size syringe for injecting growth hormone in kids with dwarfism that you can just put in your pocket and give yourself a shot once a day.

DOUGLAS WILMORE: Sy, I wonder if you and Jeff [Rossio] could help the committee and talk about both cytokine and endocrine responses in patients fed different types of nutrients or people who are underfed? A classic beginning would be taking fish oil and not seeing IL-1 elaboration from monocytes, but I wonder if you could expand on that because that is really what we are charged with, it seems to me, to think about how we can modulate nutrient intake and maybe in fact modulate these effector messages.

SEYMOUR REICHLIN: I want to make one comment and turn it over to Jeff, because this is a field I really don't know enough about, but in the study of sick euchyroidism that Mark Molitch (Richmand, O'Donnell, and Molitch), they repleted the patients with hyperalimentation.

They found that carbohydrate replacement in sick euthyroid patients reversed the low T3 levels. It would be, from my point of view, extremely important to look at the other side of the coin, that is, the effect of nutritional status on cytokine production. I don't think there is anything on that, is there?

JEFFREY ROSSIO: I am not aware of anything. You did a study with Charles Dinarello, didn't you, where you gave fish oil supplements and showed that there was a lower IL-1 response?

SEYMOUR REICHLIN: I wasn't involved in that study, but Dinarello did it.

JEFFREY ROSSIO: But wasn't that with your material?

SEYMOUR REICHLIN: It was in collaboration with Sheldon Wolff. That is a very relevant experiment. I don't think that has been done.

JONATHAN KUSHNER: I had a question along the same line until you pointed out the similarities between starvation and inflammation on pituitary secretion. Do you think that in pure starvation any of those effects are cytokine mediated, or do you know?

SEYMOUR REICHLIN: Many of the changes we are talking about can be induced by starvation. Some are hypogonadism, sick euthyroid, increased cortisol, decreased IGF-I. For sure, those three, at least are identical, and there is a starvation component even in those who are infected.

LEONARD KAPCALA: Relevant to that, there are a lot of data showing that insulin can limit the hypogonadism but the insulin only acts centrally. If you administer it peripherally, you don't get that effect, suggesting that insulin acting locally is required for the induction of IL-1 in the brain.

SEYMOUR REICHLIN: Dr. Kapcala is making a point I would like to emphasize. We have done a lot of work—which I didn't show—comparing interleukin with toxins. And LPS, which is a paradigm toxin, is much more potent on most of these reactions than is interleukin or any single interleukin that is available or in combination. Also, effects that we observed with LPS can be blocked only partially with TNF-α, soluble receptor, and IL-1 receptor antagonist (Romero et al., 1996).

The effects of bacterial toxin are mediated by many factors. There are probably some mediators that we still don't even recognize, there are receptors for LPS itself, and there is a direct effect of LPS as a cytokine.

Nutrition and Immune Function, 1999
Pp. 409–436. Washington, D.C.
National Academy Press

19

Inflammatory Stress and the Immune System

Leonard P. Kapcala[1]

INTRODUCTION

During the last several years, it has become apparent that important "bidirectional" communication occurs between the neuroendocrine and immune systems. More precisely this cross-talk occurs among the immune, endocrine, and central nervous systems and relates to perturbations in any of these systems (Besedovsky and del Ray, 1996). Communication is mediated by a variety of molecules, including neuropeptides, neurotransmitters, hormones, and cytokines which are contained within these systems along with their respective receptors. Learning about these interactions has particularly been made possible based on the discovery and characterization of cytokines (Besedovsky and del Ray, 1996). Cytokines are glycoproteins/proteins produced by many cell types, including macrophages and monocytes, B- and T-lymphocytes, endothelial cells, fibroblasts, neurons, glia (microglia and astrocytes), and some epithelial cells. Cytokines act on many cell types, exert redundant actions, induce the

---

[1] Leonard P. Kapcala, Department of Medicine and Department of Physiology, Division of Endocrinology, University of Maryland School of Medicine and Baltimore Veterans Administration Medical Center, Baltimore, MD 21201. *Currently affiliated with* the Department of Physiology, University of Maryland School of Medicine.

production and secretion of other cytokines (e.g., stimulate a cascade of many cytokines), and often synergize with other cytokines to potentiate their actions.

One immune-neuroendocrine interaction that has been extensively investigated pertains to cytokine regulation of the hypothalamic-pituitary-adrenal axis (HPAA) (Bateman et al., 1989; Besedovsky and del Ray, 1996; Chrousos, 1995; Gaillard, 1994; Harbuz and Lightman, 1992; Koenig, 1991; Lilly and Gann, 1992; Reichlin, 1993; Rivier, 1995; Tilders et al., 1994). Although many cytokines appear to modulate HPAA activation, the most important cytokines involved in this regulation are interleukin (IL)-1, IL-6, and tumor necrosis factor-α (TNF-α). Major biochemical components in this neuroendocrine axis (Figure 19-1) include hypothalamic corticotropin-releasing hormone (CRH) and arginine vasopressin (AVP), anterior pituitary adrenocorticotropin (ACTH), and adrenal glucocorticoids (cortisol in humans; corticosterone [CORT] in rodents) (Chrousos, 1995). In response to stress, HPAA activation occurs primarily by increased release of hypothalamic CRH and AVP (Harbuz and Lightman, 1992). Whereas AVP, a relatively weak secretagogue for ACTH secretion, markedly potentiates CRH stimulation and may be a critical factor in facilitating responses to recurrent stress (Harbuz and

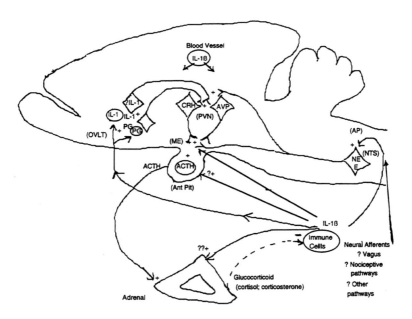

FIGURE 19-1 Schematic model of potential regulatory relationships between cytokines (using interleukin [IL]-1 as prototype) and the hypothalamic-pituitary-adrenal axis (HPAA) in the rat. AP, area postrema; AVP, arginine vasopressin; CRH, corticotropin-releasing hormone; E, epinephrine; ME, median eminence; NE, norepinephrine; NTS, nucleus tractus solitarius; OVLT, organum vasculosum of lamina terminalis; PG, prostaglandin; PVN, paraventricular nucleus. SOURCE: Adapted from Kapcala et al. (1995).

Lightman, 1992), CRH is the major stimulator of ACTH release. Stimulated ACTH secretion subsequently stimulates adrenocorticosteroid (CS, particularly glucocorticoid) secretion. Glucocorticoids in turn modulate and inhibit HPAA activation via negative feedback effects at suprahypothalamic, hypothalamic, and pituitary levels (Harbuz and Lightman, 1992).

Why does the HPAA become activated during various immune, inflammatory, and infectious insults? According to a hypothesis proposed by Munck and colleagues (1984) several years ago, such activation of the HPAA occurs so that glucocorticoids can suppress immune and inflammatory responses initiated by cytokines and thereby can modulate and dampen immune system activation. This dampening of immune system activation prevents more severe and excessive catabolic effects, including the ultimate deleterious effect, death. Consequently, immune system activation of the HPAA appears to occur to modulate excessive, deleterious effects of cytokines after they have produced their initial, beneficial effects (Urbaschek and Urbaschek, 1987; Vogel and Hogan, 1990) in facilitating an inflammatory response. A fine balance occurs relative to the level of cytokine activity. In general, relatively low levels of specific cytokines promote beneficial protective effects in helping the host respond to a perturbing immune, inflammatory, or infectious challenge. In contrast, uncontrolled production of specific cytokines resulting in relatively high circulating levels often results in severe pathological consequences, such as hypotension and lethal shock. Although responses to specific inflammatory, immune, or infectious insults are not necessarily identical, they provoke a similar central neuroendocrine response via the generation of similar cytokines and thus can all be viewed as "inflammatory stress." For purposes of discussion, these environmental perturbations can be viewed similarly not only because they induce a similar counterregulatory response (i.e., HPAA activation) but also because the consequences of this response expose the organism to similar immunosuppressive and anti-inflammatory actions following the initial induction of immune potentiating and inflammatory effects (Besedovsky and del Ray, 1996). These actions are aimed at controlling the disruption of homeostasis produced by the offending agent or stimulus.

IMMUNE REGULATION OF THE HPAA BY CYTOKINES

IL-1, TNF-α, and IL-6 are the most important cytokines for stimulating the HPAA (Chrousos, 1995; Gaillard, 1994; Reichlin, 1993). Because IL-1 is the most potent (on a molar basis) cytokine that activates the HPAA, and the most frequently studied relative to the HPAA, stimulation of the HPAA by IL-1 is often viewed as a prototypical model for immune activation of the HPAA. Additional complexity is added by the fact that IL-1 exists in two forms (α, which is primarily membrane-associated, and β, which is primarily secreted); that there are at least two IL-1 receptors; and that IL-1 actions can be counterregulated by an endogenous receptor antagonist (IL-1ra) (Dinarello,

1992; Pruitt et al., 1995; Schöbitz et al., 1994). IL-1 effects may also be diminished by soluble receptors or a "decoy" receptor that is not coupled to a signal transduction message. Furthermore, IL-1 can exert a positive auto-feedback whereby it stimulates its own expression in the periphery (Dinarello et al., 1987) and brain (Gao et al., 1996; He et al., 1996) and stimulates hypothalamic transcription of its type 1 receptor (Gao et al., 1996, based on inhibition of an IL-1 stimulated increase in mRNA by a pharmacological inhibitor of transcription). Under acute circumstances, cytokines are thought to act centrally to stimulate hypothalamic CRH and perhaps AVP release (Bateman et al., 1989; Chrousos, 1995; Gaillard, 1994; Harbuz and Lightman, 1992; Lilly and Gann, 1992; Reichlin, 1993; Rivier, 1995), and subsequently ACTH and glucocorticoid secretion are stimulated.

Other studies suggest the possibility that direct stimulation of IL-1 at the pituitary level may also occur, but that stimulation at this level develops primarily during more prolonged cytokine activation (Chrousos, 1995; Gaillard, 1994; Koenig, 1991; Kehrer et al., 1988). However, it is not clear whether such stimulation is related to circulating cytokines or induction of IL-1, other cytokines, or other events within the pituitary via paracrine effects (Koenig et al., 1990). In addition, direct stimulation of IL-1 at the level of the adrenal has been suggested based on *in vitro* and *in vivo* studies (Andreis et al., 1991; Bateman et al., 1989; Chrousos, 1995; Gaillard, 1994; Gwosdow et al., 1992). This stimulation also appears to require prolonged exposure to IL-1. If such cytokine stimulation at these other levels of the axis are of physiological import, these mechanisms could be particularly significant during prolonged immune/cytokine system stimulation.

The major mechanism (Figure 19-1) mediating acute stimulation of ACTH secretion by IL-1 appears to involve CRH release (Bateman et al., 1989; Chrousos, 1995; Matta et al., 1990; Rivier, 1995; Sapolsky et al., 1987) and possibly AVP release (Nakatsuru et al., 1991; Watanobe and Takebe, 1994; Whitnall et al., 1992) from terminals at the median eminence. Based on many studies, it appears that the potency of the immune stimulus is directly related to the magnitude and duration of HPAA activation. This phenomenon of prolonged activation is manifested by higher levels of circulating ACTH or glucocorticoid for longer periods. IL-1 administered peripherally in relatively high doses or centrally also increases CRH mRNA (Brady et al., 1994; Ericsson et al., 1994; Harbuz et al., 1992b; Rivier, 1995; Suda et al., 1990) and immunocytochemical CRH (Ju et al., 1991; Rivest et al., 1992) in some parvocellular paraventricular nuclear (PVN) neurons, which are involved in stimulating the HPAA. Furthermore, IL-1 stimulates expression of mRNA and protein of an immediate-early gene (c-*fos*) in PVN and several other brain sites (Brady et al., 1994; Chang et al., 1993; Ericsson et al., 1994; Ju et al., 1991; Rivest et al., 1992; Veening et al., 1993). Together, these studies illustrate activation of the CRH perikaryon (i.e., cell body); however, the relationship between IL-1-induced c-*fos* production and activation of CRH gene expression is not clear. Nevertheless, it appears that stimulation of perikarya producing CRH in PVN results in enhanced CRH synthesis when a sufficiently strong immune stimulus above a certain threshold induces significant cytokine production and secretion. Augmented CRH synthesis could maintain increased CRH release and therefore facilitate prolonged HPAA activation. In addition, centrally administered IL-1 increased AVP mRNA in PVN (Lee and Rivier, 1994), and it was found that endotoxin/lipopolysaccharide (LPS), which induces the production of cytokines, increased AVP mRNA in PVN when administered peripherally in a high dose (Kapcala et al., 1995). Increased release of AVP into the pituitary portal circulation has also been found in an animal model of inflammatory arthritis (Harbuz et al., 1992a), raising the possibility that different mechanisms may be involved in facilitating chronic activation of the HPAA in response to a chronic inflammatory stimulus.

Central Actions of IL-1

Although it is clear that peripherally generated cytokines activate the HPAA centrally, precise mechanisms by which this occurs have not been clearly established. Recognizing the presence of IL-1 receptors in many sites throughout the brain (Cunningham and DeSouza, 1994), including circumventricular organs, there are several putative mechanisms by which peripherally generated cytokines may communicate with the brain and more specifically regulate the HPAA (Figure 19-1). Although IL-1 transport into the brain has been described (Banks et al., 1991), stimulation via this mechanism is not widely held because IL-1 does not easily cross the blood-brain barrier (Coceani et al., 1988) under normal circumstances. However, with increased levels of circulating cytokines, the blood-brain barrier may be made more permeable to macromolecules such as cytokines (Burrought et al., 1992; Saija et al., 1995) and permit some cytokine entry into brain. Alternatively, a peripheral cytokine such as IL-1 might transduce brain signaling by stimulating endothelial IL-1 receptors (Cunningham and DeSouza, 1994; Dinarello, 1992; Tilders et al., 1994). Subsequently, a cytokine signal may spread throughout brain parenchyma (Breder et al., 1994; van Dam et al., 1995) by mechanisms that remain to be elucidated. Actions at circumventricular organs (e.g., the organum vasculosum of lamina terminalis [OVLT], median eminence, and area postrema—brain regions where a normal blood-brain barrier is not intact) could be important. This concept is consistent with stimulating CRH secretion from the median eminence (Matta et al., 1990) via IL-1 receptor stimulation of catecholamine release from axon terminals in this location. Additional evidence suggests peripheral IL-1 signaling of the brain and the HPAA particularly at the OVLT (Gaillard, 1994; Katsuura et al., 1990; Tilders et al., 1994). More specifically, it has been proposed (Katsuura et al., 1990) that IL-1 enters the OVLT and stimulates cells such as astrocytes to synthesize and release prostaglandins, which stimulate neuronal circuits that ultimately activate CRH and AVP neurons in the PVN. Stimulation of presumably transcription of an immediate early gene such as c-*fos* in the nucleus tractus solitarius of the medulla, which sends noradrenergic projections to the median eminence and PVN, could reflect neuronal activation by IL-1 and would support peripheral IL-1 stimulation of the brain via the nearby area postrema. In consonance with this view, neuroanatomical cuts caudal to hypothalamus inhibit HPAA activation by intravenous (iv) IL-1β (Sawchenko et al., 1996).

Brain signaling by peripheral cytokines may also involve stimulation of afferent sensory circuits such as the vagus or peripheral nociceptive (pain-transmitting) neural pathways (Dantzer et al., 1994; Donnerer et al., 1992; Lilly and Gann, 1992; Wan et al., 1994). Subdiaphragmatic vagotomy inhibits the induction of many central effects produced by IL-1 or LPS particularly when administered intraperitoneally (Bluthe et al., 1994; Laye et al., 1995; Maier et al., 1993; Wan et al., 1994; Watkins et al., 1994a, b, 1995a). Of interest to the focus here, vagotomy inhibits stimulation of ACTH by intraperitoneal (ip) IL-1β (Kapcala et al., 1996) and LPS (Gaykema et al., 1995) and stimulation of CORT (Fleshner et al., 1995) secretion by ip IL-1β. Treatment with capsaicin (an alkaloid derivative of red pepper that inhibits the function of peripheral sensory afferents, including those mediating nociception) inhibits stimulation of plasma ACTH and CORT by iv IL-1 (Watanobe et al., 1994). Thus peripheral afferents may also play an important role in brain signaling by peripheral cytokines. Finally, it is also possible that invoking different mechanisms may not necessarily be mutually exclusive. Different mechanisms for brain signaling by peripheral cytokines may operate simultaneously or under specific circumstances depending on the body compartment in which the primary cytokine stimulus arises.

The Role of the Locus of Origin of IL-1

Increasingly, a consensus has been developing among researchers in the field that many mechanisms may be responsible for cytokine stimulation of the HPAA by an inflammatory, infectious, or immune stress and that the body compartment in which the stimulus originates may primarily dictate the main mechanism involved. Experimental corollaries of this view are that the administration of a cytokine such as IL-1 by a different route (e.g., iv, ip, intracerebroventricular [icv]) may result in the utilization of different mechanisms of activation of the HPAA (Rivier, 1995; Tilders et al., 1994).

Different modulatory effects of various regulatory factors on IL-1 activation of the HPAA have been reported depending on the route of IL-1 administration. Whereas inhibition of prostaglandin synthesis does not consistently and potently inhibit stimulation of ACTH or CORT by ip IL-1, this treatment virtually abolishes stimulation by iv IL-1 (Dunn and Chuluyan, 1992; Rivier, 1993). Lesioning of central noradrenergic pathways that modulate activity of the HPAA has different effects on stimulation of the HPAA depending on whether IL-1 is administered centrally or peripherally (e.g., intra-arterially) (Barbanel et al., 1993). Removal of CS negative feedback by adrenalectomy abolished IL-1 stimulation of ACTH secretion when IL-1 was given centrally (Weidenfield et al., 1989), but did not diminish stimulation when IL-1 was given peripherally (iv or ip) (Selmanoff et al., 1996). Finally, peripherally (ip or iv) administered IL-1 in doses that potently stimulated ACTH and CORT secretion did not stimulate gene expression of CRH and AVP in PVN as did centrally administered IL-1 (Lee and Rivier, 1994). Altogether, these observations support the likelihood of a developing overview that cytokine activation of the HPAA is quite complex and involves a multiplicity of mechanisms.

Use of LPS to Elucidate the Effects of IL-1

LPS, derived from the cell wall of gram-negative bacteria, induces the septic shock syndrome and is often used as a model for studying the sepsis syndrome in experimental animals or conditions associated with marked induction of cytokines. Not surprisingly, LPS is a potent activator of the HPAA, which has been recognized for many years. This action occurs via its stimulation of the production and release of cytokines (Bateman et al., 1989; Chrousos, 1995; 1993; Dunn, 1992; Ebisui et al., 1994; Perlstein et al., 1993; Vogel and Hogan, 1990), particularly IL-1 and TNF, but also perhaps IL-6. It has been proposed that LPS activates the HPAA mainly via generation of IL-1 (Rivier et al., 1989; Schotanus et al., 1993). It has also been proposed that induction of septic shock (Ohlsson et al., 1990; Pruitt et al., 1995; Russell and Tucker, 1995; Wakabayashi et al., 1991) by LPS may also be highly dependent on IL-1 because antagonism of IL-1 with IL-1ra was therapeutic. The level of circulating LPS, and correspondingly, the level of cytokines generated by LPS may also be important for determining the mechanism of HPAA stimulation. One study showed that low doses of LPS activated the HPAA mainly via TNF but that higher doses invoked an important role for IL-1 (Ebisui et al., 1994), suggesting that a different intensity of immune stimulation by the same factor may operate through different mechanisms. Other studies showed that macrophage depletion (DeRijk et al., 1991) and blockade of IL-6 actions (Perlstein et al., 1993) selectively attenuated relatively low-dose LPS stimulation. These results also support different mechanisms of HPAA stimulation depending on the magnitude of stimulation by LPS.

Despite beliefs that LPS stimulates the HPAA via induction of cytokines that acutely act primarily centrally, it seems likely that LPS may also stimulate ACTH and glucocorticoid secretion by generating cytokines that act directly on the anterior pituitary and possibly on the adrenal cortex. A variety of studies show that rats with hypothalamic resection, lesions, deafferentation, and pituitary stalk section (Elenkov et al., 1992; Makara et al., 1970, 1971) were still able to increase plasma CORT after LPS. Consequently, it appears that immune stimulation of the stress axis may operate through several fail-safe mechanisms that facilitate at least a partial activation of this critically important response.

The Role of IL-1β

Expression of the IL-1β gene in brain can be induced by various stimuli including LPS, immobilization stress, ischemia, mechanical injury, and various pharmacological treatments (Ban et al., 1992; Dantzer et al., 1994; Higgins and Olschowka, 1991; Laye et al., 1995; Minami et al., 1991, 1992; Takao et al., 1993; van Dam et al., 1992, 1995; Yan et al., 1992). Although IL-1β mRNA has been reported to be present throughout several rat brain regions in the basal state (Bandtlow et al., 1990), and immunocytochemical IL-1β has been found in rat brain (Lechan et al., 1990), after central colchicine administration and in human brain (Breder et al., 1988) at autopsy, a consensus view among many investigators is that expression of brain IL-1 or IL-1β mRNA is minimal under basal, unstimulated conditions (Ban et al., 1992; Dantzer et al., 1994; Higgins and Olschowka, 1991; Laye et al., 1995; Minami et al., 1991, 1992; Takao et al., 1993; van Dam et al., 1992, 1995; Yan et al., 1992). Consistent with this perspective, this author (He et al., 1996) has found that peripherally (ip) administered LPS potently stimulates expression of IL-1β mRNA in specific brain regions including circumventricular organs (OVLT, median eminence, subfornical organ, area postrema) and parenchymal sites (PVN, arcuate-peri-arcuate region, vagal nucleus) that do not normally express this mRNA in the unstimulated state. Although peripherally administered IL-1β also induced IL-1β mRNA in these same regions, the intensity of stimulation was much weaker than LPS based on the number of cells expressing the mRNA and the signal intensity per cell. Considering that these stimuli activate the HPAA and that extremely small doses of centrally administered IL-1 potently activate the HPAA (Kapcala et al., 1995), induction of brain IL-1 expression particularly in hypothalamus by cytokines originating in the periphery has been considered as a potential mechanism by which amplification of immune activation of the HPAA could occur (Tilders et al., 1994) especially as a mechanism to prolong HPAA activation.

IMMUNE SYSTEM ACTIVATION OF THE HPAA COUNTERREGULATES CYTOKINES AND PROTECTS AGAINST AN EXCESSIVE HOST RESPONSE TO INFLAMMATORY, IMMUNE, AND INFECTIOUS INSULTS

Lethality of IL-1 in Adrenalectomized or Hypophysectomized Animals

It has been proposed that CS secretion (Munck et al., 1984) protects against potentially deleterious, catabolic effects of cytokines produced during immune, infectious, or inflammatory processes by downmodulating the production, release, and actions of cytokines. In support of this hypothesis is the markedly increased sensitivity to lethal effects in animals with a defective HPAA or surgically induced compromise of the HPAA (Table 19–1) after exposure to LPS, various inflammatory conditions that stimulate cytokine production, and cytokines themselves (Bertini et al., 1988; Butler et al., 1989; Harbuz et al., 1993; MacPhee et al., 1989; Nakano et al., 1987; Sternberg et al., 1989). Glucocorticoid treatment administered in some of these studies (Bertini et al., 1988; Butler et al., 1989; MacPhee et al., 1989; Nakano et al., 1987) protected against lethal effects (Table 19-1), which strongly suggests that the HPAA plays a protective role against immune or inflammatory stimuli.

Adrenalectomy (ADX) or hypophysectomy (HYPOX) (removal of the pituitary) also results in LPS stimulation of higher serum levels of IL-1 and TNF for longer periods, which indicates a modulatory role of the endogenous HPAA (Butler et al., 1989, Zuckerman et al., 1989). Increased sensitivity to lethal effects of IL-1 has been described in mice following ADX or HYPOX (Bertini et al., 1988; Butler et al., 1989), and enhanced lethal sensitivity to LPS has been reported in the rat (Nakano et al., 1987) (perhaps the most commonly studied

TABLE 19-1 Conditions Producing Lethal Effects in Animals with an Abnormal Hypothalamic-Pituitary-Adrenal Axis (HPAA)

Condition[*]	Animal	Abnormal HPAA	Glucocorticoid Rx	Reference
IL-1β, TNF-α, LPS	Mouse	ADX	DEX 30 mg/kg	Bertini et al., 1988
IL-1β, TNF-α, LPS	Mouse	ADX, HYPOX	DEX 10 mg/kg CORT 100 mg/kg	Butler et al., 1989
LPS	Rat	ADX	DEX 0.05 mg/kg CORT 5 mg/kg	Nakano et al., 1987
Encephalitis (allergic)	Rat	ADX	CORT 50 mg pellet	MacPhee et al., 1989
Arthritis (streptococcal cell wall)	Rat (Lewis)	Central (CRH) hypoadrenalism		Sternberg et al., 1989
Arthritis (adjuvant)	Rat	ADX		Harbuz et al., 1993

NOTE: Rx, treatment; IL, interleukin; TNF, tumor necrosis factor; ADX, adrenalectomy; HYPOX, hypophysectomy; DEX, dexamethasone; CORT, corticosterone

[*] Various doses of LPS, IL-1, or TNF were studied.

SOURCE: Adapted from Kapcala et al. (1995).

laboratory animal) following ADX. However, this author was not aware that lethal effects of IL-1 had been reported in rats or in any other species (rabbits, monkeys) treated with relatively high doses of IL-1. Questions about the significance of lethal effects of IL-1 in isolated mouse studies were raised because mice show variable susceptibility to experimentally induced inflammatory conditions as a function of their genetic composition and activity of their HPAA (Mason et al., 1990) and can also exhibit idiosyncratic responses to specific stimuli that are not necessarily observed in other species. This laboratory was interested in determining whether lethality induced by IL-1 was a species-specific response exhibited solely in mice. Thus, rats were studied to place into perspective the physiological importance of immune activation of the HPAA and particularly to determine whether the increased sensitivity to lethal effects of IL-1 in mice is a general phenomenon associated with compromised CS secretion. The focus on IL-1 was especially influenced by the central role that IL-1 is thought to play in facilitating various immune, infectious, and inflammatory disorders (Dinarello and Wolff, 1993; Pruitt et al., 1995). This laboratory was additionally interested in determining the physiological significance of protection from lethality by glucocorticoid treatment because previous studies (Bertini et al., 1988; Butler et al., 1989) had shown protection against lethal effects of IL-1 only when pharmacological quantities of glucocorticoid were used.

The effects of ADX on lethal responses to IL-1β were studied in adult Sprague-Dawley rats and compared to effects of LPS. ADX rats exhibited dose-dependent lethality after IL-1β (generously provided by Janet Kerr and Maryanne Covington at DuPont-Merck) and ultimately 100 percent mortality at the highest dose studied (Table 19-2) (Kapcala et al., 1995). In contrast, rats with an intact HPAA did not show any lethal responses after similar doses of IL-1β. The treatment time after adrenal removal did not affect the lethal response to IL-1β based on studying rats at different times (2–23 days) after ADX. These results demonstrated that lethal effects produced by IL-1 in ADX mice were not species specific nor idiosyncratic to mice and clearly illustrated that IL-1β could be lethal to rats when CS secretion is compromised. Similar responses were seen after LPS. Rats with an intact HPAA tolerated a range of relatively high doses (4–40 mg/kg ip) of LPS during monitoring over 12 hours (Table 19-2). However, ADX rats were exquisitely sensitive to lethal effects of LPS (Table 19-2) and exhibited at least a 200-fold increased sensitivity.

Glucocorticoid Treatment in Adrenalectomized Animals

This laboratory also wanted to determine whether glucocorticoid treatment in physiological quantities reflecting stress-stimulated CS secretion could protect rats against cytokines, as does an intact HPAA. Treatment of ADX rats with CORT or dexamethasone in doses estimated to be equivalent to a physiological stress response was protective against lethal effects of IL-1β and

LPS (Table 19–2). Normal CORT replacement in the rat is approximately 2 to 3 mg/kg (Akana et al., 1985). Thus, it was estimated that CORT treatment would approximate a nearly maximal (10-fold increase of CORT secretion) stress response and that the dexamethasone dose would be the glucocorticoid equivalent of at least a moderate stress response and might possibly be equivalent to a maximal stress response. Conceivably, the lack of complete protection by CORT may have been related to the fact that the treatment was not optimized with CORT to mimic the normal kinetics of the CORT response shown by rats with an intact HPAA. Complete protection by treatment with dexamethasone compared with CORT may have been due to the longer plasma and biological half-life of dexamethasone. These unique observations clearly demonstrated that complete protection against lethality induced by IL-1β was afforded by glucocorticoid treatment in quantities approximating stress physiological CS secretion. Not only did these results show the lethal capability of a cytokine such as IL-1β in the face of a compromised HPAA, they also supported the hypothesis that physiological activation of the HPAA by immune-inflammatory response stimuli is a general means across species for counterregulating cytokine actions, modulating host defense immune-inflammatory reactions and ultimately protecting against potentially lethal actions of cytokines.

TABLE 19-2 Effects of IL-1β and Endotoxin/Lipopolysaccharide (LPS) on Percent Survival in Adrenalectomized or Hypophysectomized Rats (n = 4 to 5 rats per group)

Condition	IL-1β (60 µg/kg ip)	LPS (4 mg/kg ip)
Sham ADX	100	100
ADX	0	0
ADX + DEX (0.2 mg/kg)	100	100
ADX + CORT (24 mg/kg)	75	67[*]
Sham HYPOX	100	100
HYPOX	50[†]	100

NOTE: ip, intraperitoneal; ADX, adrenalectomy; DEX, dexamethasone; CORT, corticosterone; HYPOX, hypophysectomy.

[*] n = 3 in this group only.

[†] Identical survival rate as ADX rats given same dose in this experiment. DEX or CORT were administered ip 1 hour prior to recombinant human IL-1β (DuPont-Merck) or LPS (*E. coli* serotype 055:B5).

SOURCE: Adapted from Kapcala et al. (1995).

Hypophysectomy and IL-1 Lethality

This laboratory next sought to determine the importance of the pituitary gland by studying lethal effects of IL-1β and LPS in HYPOX rats. HYPOX had been performed on the day prior to study to ensure that the adrenal cortex of HYPOX rats would still be responsive to direct stimulation as was observed in some rats stimulated with a biologically potent analogue of ACTH, $ACTH_{1-24}$. Hypox rats also typically showed low basal CORT levels (< 8 μg/dl). HYPOX rats exhibited an increased sensitivity to lethal effects of IL-1β and LPS, similar to ADX rats (Table 19–2). These responses confirmed the importance of the pituitary component of the stress axis for modulating the immune-inflammatory response and protecting the organism from excessive host defensive responses that could ultimately be fatal. Regardless that *in vitro* studies (Andreis et al., 1991; Bateman et al., 1989; Gaillard, 1994; Gwosdow et al., 1992) had shown that IL-1 could directly stimulate CORT secretion from the adrenal after prolonged exposure, lethal responses to IL-1β in HYPOX rats suggested that direct stimulation of CORT secretion from the adrenal cortex by IL-1β was not sufficient *in vivo* to protect against lethal actions by IL-1β, and supported the idea that cytokine actions directly at the level of the adrenal were not physiologically important.

Earlier in this chapter, it was outlined that many studies (Bateman et al., 1989; Besedovsky and del Ray, 1996; Chrousos, 1995; Gaillard, 1994; Harbuz and Lightman, 1992; Rivier, 1995; Tilders et al., 1994) clearly illustrate that the primary locus of cytokine action for activating the HPAA occurs acutely at the level of the hypothalamus. However, given that cytokine effects on the pituitary (Chrousos, 1995; Gaillard, 1994; Kehrer et al., 1988; Koenig, 1991) have been described, the importance of the brain in facilitating a glucocorticoid stress response which protects organisms against deleterious host defense responses induced by immune-inflammatory stimuli was questioned. Therefore, this laboratory assessed the importance of the brain's influence, particularly the hypothalamic component of the HPAA for mediating a critical, protective stress response to immune-inflammatory stimuli. Rats which had undergone acute pituitary stalk section (PSS), and thereby disconnection of the hypothalamus from the pituitary, were tested to determine their ability to tolerate an LPS challenge. PSS rats treated with a relatively high dose of LPS (20 mg/kg) showed approximately a 25 percent lethality rate (Kapcala et al., 1995). PSS rats pretreated with a stress equivalent dose of glucocorticoid (0.2 mg/kg dexamethasone) were completely protected against the lethal effects of LPS. These results suggested that activation of at least the pituitary-adrenal axis by LPS may result in significant protection against potentially lethal effects of cytokines.

Protection provided by an intact pituitary-adrenal axis without the influence of the hypothalamus was not as complete as that produced by an intact HPAA. Nevertheless, it was remarkable and noteworthy that significant protection occurred. These results indicate a functional significance to earlier reports in which LPS stimulated CORT secretion in rats with hypothalamic resection, lesions, deafferentation, and PSS (Elenkov et al., 1992; Makara et al., 1970, 1971). Several potential mechanisms for stimulating the pituitary can be postulated based on previous investigations (DeSouza et al., 1993; Kehrer et al., 1988; Koenig et al., 1990). It is recognized that presumed stimulation of a pituitary-adrenal axis (without hypothalamic regulation) may not result in circulating glucocorticoid levels generated as rapidly or as high as those produced by an intact HPAA. Nevertheless, this stimulatory mechanism may still be important for counterregulation against immune, infectious, or inflammatory stress and can still provide a significant level of protection. Considering the vital importance of glucocorticoid secretion and the protection derived from such secretion, it seems teleologically reasonable that the stress axis might operate in a fail-safe, redundant manner with multiple back-up mechanisms for ultimately stimulating glucocorticoid secretion.

INFLAMMATORY, IMMUNE, AND INFECTIOUS STRESS INDUCES PERIPHERAL IMMUNOSUPPRESSION AND ANTI-INFLAMMATORY EFFECTS

Immune-neuroendocrine interactions and putative mechanisms mediating a protective neuroendocrine response against inflammatory, immune, or infectious stress have been described. Protection by the host against an excessive cytokine response is related to suppression of the immune system and modulation of cytokine responses by immune-inflammatory cells. Induction of related counterregulatory responses are believed to play an important role in modulating susceptibility to inflammatory disorders (Mason et al., 1990; Sternberg and Licinio, 1995; Sternberg et al., 1992; Wick et al., 1993). For general purposes of discussion, peripheral anti-inflammatory and immunosuppressive effects will be broadly considered without distinction. This stress-induced peripheral immunosuppression (Friedman and Irwin, 1995; Sternberg and Licinio, 1995; Sternberg et al., 1992) optimally develops via central mechanisms stimulating hypothalamic CRH neurons. Stimulation of CRH-producing neurons and related HPAA activation ultimately increases secretion of CS, which plays a pivotal role in this immunosuppression. Immune activation of central CRH neurons also stimulates the sympathetic nervous system, and this action produces additional peripheral immunosuppression independent of CS (Friedman and Irwin, 1995; Sundar et al., 1990). Although it is clear that the CS-dependent mechanism plays a critical role in suppressing and modulating the host's cytokine response, the physiological significance of the CS-independent immunosuppression remains to be more precisely determined.

Protective Role of Glucocorticoids

What mechanisms are involved in CS protection against an excessive inflammatory-immune response by the host and a potentially lethal result? CSs via their glucocorticoid potency exert anti-inflammatory actions on many cell types at many sites via multiple mechanisms. Glucocorticoids are potent inhibitors (Dinarello, 1992; Knudsen et al., 1987; Lee et al., 1988; Munck et al., 1984; Peretti et al., 1989; Pruitt et al., 1995; Staruch and Wood, 1985) of the production, secretion, and actions of cytokines and a variety of other mediators (e.g., prostaglandins, leukotrienes, platelet-activating factor, complement, histamine, and small peptides such as bradykinin, substance P), which participate in inflammatory and immune reactions (Munck et al., 1984; Williams and Yarwood, 1990). These molecules facilitate many inflammatory actions such as increasing vascular permeability, influx of leukocytes, and generation of other mediators that enhance the inflammatory cascade of events. Important targets on which glucocorticoids exert anti-inflammatory effects include (1) macrophages and monocytes, which produce many cytokines and mediate antigen presentation to immune cells; (2) B-lymphocytes, which produce antibodies and primarily mediate humoral immunity, and T-lymphocytes, which primarily facilitate cell-mediated immunity; and (3) endothelial cells, which produce cytokines, eicosanoids, and nitric oxide, a key molecule that mediates several features of LPS-induced septic shock.

Glucocorticoids inhibit the transcription of IL-1β mRNA, decrease mRNA stability, and diminish the efficiency of cytokine mRNA translation (Dinarello, 1992; Knudsen et al., 1987; Lee et al., 1988; Marx, 1995; Munck et al., 1984). Another mechanism that mediates counterregulatory effects of glucocorticoids involves lipocortins (Perretti, 1994; Pruitt et al., 1995; Williams and Yarwood, 1990). Lipocortins are a family of proteins that inhibit phospholipase A$_2$ and thereby inhibit the release of arachidonic acid. This inhibition prevents the formation of important inflammatory mediators such as prostaglandins and thromboxanes via the cyclo-oxygenase pathway and leukotrienes via the lipoxygenase pathway (Perretti, 1994; Pruitt et al., 1995; Williams and Yarwood, 1990).

The significance of increased glucocorticoid secretion induced by LPS administration has also been investigated from a pathophysiological perspective by antagonizing glucocorticoid actions with RU 486 (a competitive glucocorticoid receptor antagonist). Treatment with RU 486 resulted in more severe hypotension and pathological changes in multiple organs and more striking elevations of phospholipase A$_2$ activity and lipoperoxide (Fan et al., 1994), which implies that glucocorticoid secretion counterregulated these effects. In another study (Szabo et al., 1994), RU 486 treatment enhanced a pathological cardiovascular response (i.e., hypotension and vascular hyporeactivity to vasoconstriction by norepinephrine) to LPS and augmented the induction of nitric oxide synthase by LPS. Nitric oxide synthase produces nitric oxide, which is intimately involved in mediating many cardiovascular effects of septic shock. Moreover, Szabo and colleagues (1994) suggested that glucocorticoids may play a key role in promoting endotoxin tolerance and protecting against the deleterious effects of excessive nitric oxide production that may occur in chronic inflammatory conditions.

Glucocorticoid treatment of dogs and nonhuman primates (baboons) dramatically improves survival (Hinshaw et al., 1982) when given prior to administration of LPS or gram-negative bacteria (*E. coli*) or shortly thereafter. Yet, in large studies of humans, a clear benefit of glucocorticoids for decreasing mortality in septic patients (Veterans Cooperative Group, 1987) has not been demonstrated. Although it had been questioned (Veterans Cooperative Group, 1987) whether glucocorticoids may benefit a subset of septic patients, if this is so, it is still not clear which septic patients should receive glucocorticoids, in what doses, and at what time. Considering that baboon studies (Hinshaw et al., 1982) clearly show that glucocorticoids enhance survival during the sepsis syndrome only when administered during a relatively narrow window of opportunity, it is likely that by the time the diagnosis of the sepsis syndrome has been made in humans, sepsis may have progressed too far for exogenous glucocorticoids to be of any significant benefit.

Protective Role of Sympathoadrenal Responses

Stress activation of hypothalamic CRH neurons can also produce peripheral immunosuppression independent of glucocorticoids via stimulation of the sympathoadrenomedullary system (Friedman and Irwin, 1995) (Figure 19-2). It has long been recognized that CRH regulates autonomic activity via axon terminals from the hypothalamus that project to the locus coeruleus, and that stimulation of these neurons increases peripheral sympathetic activity and adrenomedullary secretion resulting in increased plasma epinephrine levels (Besedovsky and del Ray, 1996; Friedman and Irwin, 1995). Peripheral immunosuppression occurs via neurohormonal modulation of immune cells in lymphoid organs and the circulation (Besedovsky and del Ray, 1996; Friedman and Irwin, 1995). This modulation is related to the presence of β-adrenergic receptors on immune cells and innervation of lymphoid organs such as spleen, thymus, lymph nodes, and bone marrow by sympathetic noradrenergic neurons.

Central administration of IL-1 decreases a humoral immune response as reflected by reduced antibody production in response to an antigen and also a cell-mediated immune response as reflected by reduced natural killer cell cytotoxicity, and mitogen-induced lymphocyte proliferation and IL-2 production (Saperstein et al., 1992; Sundar et al., 1990; Weiss et al., 1994). This central effect of IL-1 is mediated by CRH because it is blocked by antagonizing CRH (Saperstein et al., 1992) and can be replicated by central administration of CRH (Friedman and Irwin, 1995). That a significant component of this immunosuppressive effect is independent of glucocorticoid is demonstrated

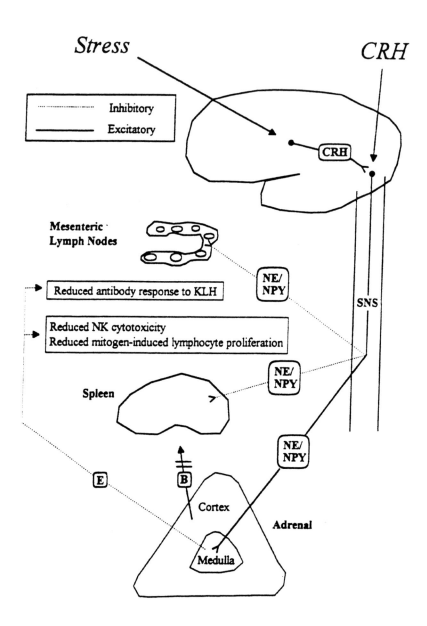

FIGURE 19-2 Proposed model for stress-induced modulation of immune function by corticotropin-releasing hormone (CRH) and the sympathetic nervous system. B, corticosterone; E, epinephrine NE, norepinephrine; NPY, neuropeptide Y; SNS, sympathetic nervous system. SOURCE: Friedman and Irwin (1995), used with permission.

by the fact that it can still be induced after ADX (Sundar et al., 1990). Its dependence on the sympathetic nervous system is further illustrated by pharmacologically inhibiting the effect via blockade of sympathetic activity (Sundar et al., 1990). Central administration of LPS can also reproduce this peripheral immunosuppression, which is associated with an increase in central IL-1 activity (Weiss et al., 1994). Although the immunosuppressive actions of glucocorticoids are well known, the immunosuppressive effects mediated by the sympathoadrenomedullary system are not nearly as well recognized. Neither is the general concept appreciated that central effects mediating alterations in brain function can produce peripheral immunosuppression and anti-inflammatory actions.

AUTHOR'S CONCLUSIONS AND RECOMMENDATIONS

During recent years, an increasing number of immune-neuroendocrine interactions have been identified and characterized that illustrate important bidirectional communication between these systems (Besedovsky and del Ray, 1996). Perhaps the most important interaction relates to immune system activation of the HPAA via cytokines. Stimulation of this counterregulatory response is believed to play a critical role in preventing the host from mounting an excessive defense response involving cytokines against "inflammatory stress," such as inflammatory, immune, and infectious insults. Because of these interactions, which have become appreciated relatively recently, regulatory relationships exist whereby behavioral stimuli and inflammatory stress can ultimately modulate the function of the immune system. Conversely, immune-inflammatory stimuli can ultimately modify behavioral output.

One interesting consequence of these interactions has been observed in animal studies but has not been investigated in humans. This phenomenon relates to the observation that pretreatment of animals with low doses of a cytokine or LPS, which induces cytokines, can diminish or abolish lethal or toxic effects of subsequent inflammatory-immune stimulation with a cytokine, LPS, radiation, or infectious agent (Evans et al., 1991; Morrissey et al., 1995; Neta et al., 1992, 1993; Shalaby et al., 1991; Sheppard and Norton, 1991). Mechanisms mediating these beneficial and protective effects are not clear. Conceivably, some beneficial effect may be related to stimulation of hypothalamic CRH neurons and subsequent activation of glucocorticoid-dependent and glucocorticoid-independent (sympathoadrenomedullary) anti-inflammatory-immunosuppressive mechanisms. Additional investigation of these observations, derived from animal studies, and understanding of mechanisms involved might ultimately lead toward developing treatment regimens that would protect humans against inflammatory, immune, or infectious insults under specific circumstances. Investigative studies utilizing pretreatment regimens with specific cytokines, LPS, or nontoxic immune stimulation could potentially be extremely valuable in designing novel therapeutic approaches to minimize deleterious consequences of inflammatory, immune, or infectious insults.

Based on the information that has been accumulated and presented, major recommendations include the following:

• Continue to investigate and characterize interactions among the immune, endocrine, and nervous systems and learn about mechanisms mediating these interactions.
• Determine and characterize effects of nutritional abnormalities on interactions among the immune, endocrine, and nervous systems and whether nutritional supplements can beneficially enhance the organism's response to inflammatory stress.
• Investigate and determine protective mechanisms afforded by pretreatment of animals with LPS or a cytokine against lethal or toxic effects of inflammatory stress produced by an inflammatory (e.g., traumatic injury or radiation exposure), immune, or infectious insult.
• Investigate in humans whether pretreatment with a specific regimen (based on specific doses and times) with a cytokine, LPS, or immunotherapy can temporarily modulate the immune system in a beneficially, protective manner against detrimental effects of inflammatory stress induced by inflammatory, immune, or infectious insults.
• Determine whether pretreatment with a specific regimen of a cytokine, LPS, or immunotherapy can temporarily modulate the immune system in a beneficial manner to counterregulate the potentially detrimental effects of immunosuppression induced by stress (e.g., combat stress).

ACKNOWLEDGMENTS

Grateful appreciation is extended to Drs. Lee Eiden, Thierry Chautard, and Robert Eskay for their contributions and participation in the lethality studies and to Connie Mack for secretarial assistance.

REFERENCES

Akana, S.F., C.S. Cascio, J. Shinsako, and M.F. Dallman. 1985. Corticosterone: Narrow range required for normal body and thymus weight and ACTH. Am. J. Physiol. 249:R527–R532.
Andreis, P.G., G. Neri, A.S. Belloni, M. Giuseppina, A. Kasprzak, and L.G.G. Nussdorfer. 1991. Interleukin-1β enhances corticosterone secretion by acting directly on the rat adrenal gland. Endocrinology 129:53–57.
Ban, E., F. Haour, and R. Lenstra. 1992. Brain interleukin-1 gene expression induced by peripheral lipopolysaccharide administration. Cytokine 4:48–54.
Bandtlow, C.E., M. Meyer, D. Lindholm, M. Spranger, R. Heumann, and H. Thoenen. 1990. Regional and cellular codistribution of interleukin-1β and nerve growth factor

mRNA in the adult rat brain: Possible relationship to the regulation of nerve growth factor synthesis. J. Cell Biol. 111:1701–1711.

Banks, W.A., L. Ortiz, S.R. Plotkin, and A.J. Kastin. 1991. Human interleukin (IL)-1 (IL-1α) and murine IL-1β are transported from blood to brain in the mouse by a shared saturable mechanism. J. Pharm. Exp. Ther. 259:988–996.

Barbanel, G., S. Gaillet, M. Mekaouche, L. Givalois, G. Ixtart, P. Siaud, A. Szafarczyk, F. Malaral, and I. Assenmacher. 1993. Complex catecholaminergic modulation of the stimulatory effect of interleukin-1β on the corticotropic axis. Brain Res. 626:31–36.

Bateman, A., A. Singh, R. Kral, and S. Solomon. 1989. The immune-hypothalamic-pituitary-adrenal axis. Endocr. Rev. 10:92–112.

Bertini, R., M. Bianchi, and P. Ghezzi. 1988. Adrenalectomy sensitizes mice to the lethal effects of interleukin-1 and tumor necrosis factor. J. Exp. Med. 167:1708–1712.

Besedovsky, H.O., and A. del Rey. 1996. Immune-neuro-endocrine interactions: Facts and hypotheses. Endocr. Rev. 17(1):64–102.

Bluthe, R.M., V. Walter, P. Parnet, S. Laye, J. Lestage, D. Verrier, S. Poole, B.E. Stenning, K.W. Kelley, and R. Dantzer. 1994. Lipopolysaccharide induces sickness behavior in rats by a vagal mediated mechanism. C.R. Acad. Sci. Paris, Sciences de la via/Life sciences. 317:499–503.

Brady, L.S., A.B. Lynn, M. Herkenham, and Z. Gottesfeld. 1994. Systemic interleukin-1 induces early and late patterns of c-*fos* mRNA expression in brain. J. Neurosci. 14:4951–4964.

Breder, C.D., C.A. Dinarello, and C.B. Saper. 1988. Interleukin-1 immunoreactive innervation of the human hypothalamus. Science 240:321–324.

Breder, C.D., C. Hazuka, T. Ghayur, C. Klug, M. Huginin, K.Yasuda, M. Teng, and C.B. Saper. 1994. Regional induction of TNF-α expression in the mouse brain after systemic lipopolysaccharide administration. Proc. Nat. Acad. Sci. USA 91:11393–11397.

Burrought, M., C. Cabellos, S. Prasad, and E. Tuomanen. 1992. Bacterial components and the pathophysiology of injury to the blood-brain barrier: Does cell wall add to the effects of endotoxin in gram-negative meningitis? J. Infect. Dis. 165 (suppl. 1):S82–S85.

Butler, L.D., N.K. Layman, P.E. Riedl, R.L. Cain, and J. Shellhaas. 1989. Neuroendocrine regulation of *in vivo* cytokine production and effects: I. *In vivo* regulatory networks involving the neuroendocrine system, interleukin-1 and tumor necrosis factor-α. J. Neuroimmunol. 24:143–153.

Chang, S.L., T. Ren, and J.E. Zadina. 1993. Interleukin-1 activation of *fos* proto-oncogene protein in the rat hypothalamus. Brain Res. 617:123–130.

Chrousos, G.P. 1995. The hypothalamic-pituitary-adrenal axis and immune-mediated inflammation. N. Engl. J. Med. 332:1351–1362.

Coceani, F., J. Lees, and C. A. Dinarello. 1988. Occurrence of interleukin-1 in cerebrospinal fluid of the conscious cat. Brain Res. 446:245–250.

Cunningham, E.T., and E. DeSouza. 1994. Interleukin 1 receptors in the brain and endocrine tissues. Immunol. Today 14:161–176.

Dantzer, R., R.M. Bluthe, J.L. Bret-Dibat, S. Laye, R. Parnet, J. Lestage, D. Verrier, S. Poole, B. E. Stenning, and K.W. Kelley. 1994. The neuroimmune basis of sickness behavior [abstract]. P. 41 in Proceedings of the 25th Congress of the International Society for Psychoneuroendocrinology.

DeRijk, R., N. Van Rooijen, F.J.H. Tilders, H.O. Besedovsky, A. Del Rey, and F. Berkenbosch. 1991. Selective depletion of macrophages prevents pituitary-adrenal activation in response to subpyrogenic, but not to pyrogenic, doses of bacterial endotoxin in rats. Endocrinology 129:330–338.

DeSouza, E.B. 1993. Corticotropin-releasing factor and interleukin-1 receptors in the brain-endocrine-immune axis. Ann. N.Y. Acad. Sci. 697:9–27.

Dinarello, C.A. 1992. The biology of interleukin-1. Mol. Biol. Immunol. 51:1–32.

Dinarello, C.A., and S.M. Wolff. 1993. The role of interleukin-1 in disease. N. Engl. J. Med. 328:106–113.

Dinarello, C.A., T. Ikejima, S.J.C. Warner, S.F. Orencole, and G. Lonnemann. 1987. Interleukin-1 induces interleukin-1. I. Induction of circulating interleukin-1 in rabbits in vivo and in human mononuclear cells in vitro. J. Immunol. 139:1902–1910.

Donnerer, J., R. Amann, G. Skofitsch, and F. Lembeck. 1992. Substance P afferents regulate ACTH-corticosterone release. Ann. N.Y. Acad. Sci. 632:296–303.

Dunn, A.J. 1992. The role of interleukin-1 and tumor necrosis factor-α in the neurochemical and neuroendocrine responses to endotoxin. Brain Res. Bull. 29:807–812.

Dunn, A.J., and H.E. Chuluyan. 1992. The role of cyclo-oxygenase and lipoxygenase in the interleukin-1-induced activation of HPA axis. Life Sci. 51:219–225.

Ebisui, O., J. Fukata, N. Murakami, H. Kobayashi, H. Segawa, S. Muro, I. Hanaoka, Y. Naito, Y. Masui, Y. Ohmmoto, H. Imura, and K. Nakao. 1994. Effects of IL-1 receptor antagonist and antiserum to TNF-α on LPS-induced plasma ACTH and corticosterone rise in rats. Am. J. Physiol. 29:E986–E992.

Elenkov, I.J., K. Kovacs, J. Kiss, L. Bertok, and E. S. Vizi. 1992. Lipopolysaccharide is able to bypass corticotrophin-releasing factor in affecting plasma ACTH and corticosterone levels: Evidence from rats with lesions of the paraventricular nucleus. J. Endocrinol. 133:231–236.

Ericsson, A., K.J. Kovacs, and P.E. Sawchenko. 1994. A functional anatomical analysis of central pathways subserving the effects of interleukin-1 on stress-related neuroendocrine neurons. J. Neurosci. 14:897–913.

Evans. M.J., C.J. Kovacs, J.M. Gooya, and J.P. Harrell. 1991. Interleukin-1α protects against the toxicity associated with combined radiation and drug therapy. Int. J. Radiat. Oncol. Biol. Phys. 20:303–306.

Fan, J., X. Gong, J. Wu, Y. Zhang, and R. Xu. 1994. Effect of glucocorticoid receptor (GR) blockade on endotoxemia in rats. Circ. Shock 42:76–82.

Fleshner, M., L.E. Goehler, J. Hermann, J.K. Relton, S.F. Maier, and L.R. Watkins. 1995. Interleukin-1β induced corticosterone elevation and hypothalamic NE depletion is vagally mediated. Brain Res. Bull. 37:605–610.

Friedman, E.M., and M.R. Irwin. 1995. A role for CRH and the sympathetic nervous system in stress-induced immunosuppression. Ann. N.Y. Acad. Sci. 771:396–418.

Gaillard, R.C. 1994. Neuroendocrine-immune system interactions. Trends in Endocrinology and Metabolism 7:303–309.

Gao, Y., J.R. He, and L.P. Kapcala. 1996. Interleukin-1β and lipopolysaccharide regulation of interleukin-1β and interleukin-1 type 1 receptor in hypothalamic neurons and glia [abstract 336.3]. Soc. Neurosci. 21.

Gaykema, R.P.A., I. Dijkstra, and F.J.H. Tilders. 1995. Subdiaphragmatic vagotomy suppresses endotoxin-induced activation of hypothalamic corticotropin-releasing hormone neurons and ACTH secretion. Endocrinology 136:4717–4770.

Gwosdow, A.R., N.A. O'Connell, J.A. Spencer, and M.S.A. Kuman. 1992. Interleukin-1-induced corticosterone release occurs by an adrenergic mechanism from rat adrenal gland. Am. J. Physiol. 263:E461–E466.

Harbuz, M.S., and S.L. Lightman. 1992. Stress and the hypothalamo-pituitary-adrenal axis: Acute, chronic, and immunological activation. J. Endocrinol. 134:327–339.

Harbuz, M.S., R.G. Rees, D. Eckland, D.S. Jessop, D. Brewerton, and S.L. Lightman. 1992a. Paradoxical responses of hypothalamic corticotropin-releasing factor (CRF) messenger ribonucleic acid (mRNA) and CRF-41 peptide and adenohypophysial proopiomelanocortin mRNA during chronic inflammatory stress. Endocrinology. 130:1394–1400.

Harbuz, M.S., R.G. Rees, and S.L. Lightman. 1993. HPA axis responses to acute stress and adrenalectomy during adjuvant-induced arthritis in the rat. Am. J. Physiol. 264:R179–R185.

Harbuz, M.S., A. Stephanou, N. Sarlis, and S.L. Lightman. 1992b. The effects of recombinant human interleukin (IL)-1α, IL-1β, or IL-6 on hypothalamo-pituitary-adrenal axis activation. J. Endocrinol. 133:349–355.

He, J.R., Y. Gao, and L.P. Kapcala. 1996. Induction of interleukin-1β gene expression in specific brain sites by peripheral interleukin-1β and lipopolysaccharide [abstract 336.1]. Soc. Neurosci. 21.

Higgins, G.A., and J.A. Olschowka. 1991. Induction of interleukin-1β mRNA in adult rat brain. Mol. Brain Res. 9:143–148.

Hinshaw, L.B., B.K. Beller-Todd, and L.T. Archer. 1982. Current management of the septic shock patient: Experimental basis for treatment. Circ. Shock 9:543–553.

Ju, G., X. Zhang, B.Q. Jin, and C.S. Huang. 1991. Activation of corticotropin-releasing factor containing neurons in the paraventricular nucleus of the hypothalamus by interleukin-1 in the rat. Neurosci. Lett. 132:151–154.

Kapcala, L.P., T. Chautard, and R.L. Eskay. 1995. The protective role of the hypothalamic-pituitary-adrenal axis against lethality produced by immune, infectious, and inflammatory stress. Ann. N.Y. Acad. Sci. 771:419–437.

Kapcala, L.P., J.R. He, Y. Gao, J.O. Pieper, and L.J. DeTolla. 1996. Subdiaphragmatic vagotomy inhibits intra-abdominal interleukin-1β stimulation of adrenocorticotropin secretion. Brain Res. 728:247–254.

Katsuura, G., A. Arimura, K. Koves, and P.E. Gottschall. 1990. Involvement of organum vasculosum of lamina terminalis and preoptic area in interleukin 1β-induced ACTH release. Am. J. Physiol. 258:E163–E173.

Kehrer, P., D. Turnill, J.M. Dayer, A.F. Muller, and R.C. Gaillard. 1988. Human recombinant interleukin-1β and -α, but not recombinant tumor necrosis factor-α, stimulate ACTH release from rat anterior pituitary cells *in vitro* in a prostaglandin E$_2$ and cAMP independent manner. Neuroendocrinology 48:160–166.

Knudsen, P.J., C.A. Dinarello, and T.B. Strom. 1987. Glucocorticoids inhibit transcriptional and post-transcriptional expression of IL-1 in U93F cells. J. Immunol. 139:4129–4134.

Koenig, J.I. 1991. Presence of cytokines in the hypothalamic-pituitary axis. Prog. Neuroendocrin. Immunol. 4:143–153.

Koenig, J.I., K. Snow, B.D. Clark, R. Toni, J.G. Cannon, A.R. Shaw, C.A. Dinarello, S. Reichlin, and S.L. Lee. 1990. Intrinsic pituitary interleukin-1β is induced by bacterial lipopolysaccharide. Endocrinology 126(6):3053–3058.

Laye, S., R.M. Bluthe, S. Kent, C. Combe, C. Medina, P. Parnet, K. Kelly, and R. Dantzer. 1995. Subdiaphragmatic vagotomy blocks induction of IL-1β mRNA in mice brain in response to peripheral LPS. Am. J. Physiol. 268:R1327–R1331.

Lechan, R.M., R. Toni, B.D. Clark, J.G. Cannon, A.R. Shaw, C.A. Dinarello, and S. Reichlin. 1990. Immunoreactive IL-1β localization in rat forebrain. Brain Res. 514:135–140.

Lee, S., and C. Rivier. 1994. Hypophysiotropic role and hypothalamic gene expression of corticotropin-releasing factor and vasopressin in rats injected with interleukin-1 systemically or into the brain ventricles. Neuroendocrinology 6:217–224.

Lee, S.W., A.P. Tsou, H. Chan, J. Thomas, K. Petrie, E.M. Eugui, and A.C. Allison. 1988. Glucocorticoids selectively inhibit the transcription of the interleukin-1β gene and decrease the stability of interleukin-1β mRNA. Proc. Natl. Acad. Sci. USA 85:1204–1208.

Lilly, M.P., and D.S. Gann. 1992. The hypothalamic-pituitary-adrenal-immune axis. Arch. Surg. 127:1463–1474.

MacPhee, I.A., F.A. Antoni, and D.W. Mason. 1989. Spontaneous recovery of rats from experimental allergic encephalomyelitis is dependent on regulation of the immune system by endogenous adrenal corticosteroids. J. Exp. Med. 169:431–445.

Maier, S.F., E.P. Wiertelak, D. Martin, and L.R. Watkins. 1993. Interleukin-1 mediates the behavioral hyperalgesia produced by lithium chloride and endotoxin. Brain Res. 632:321–324.

Makara, G.B., E. Stark, and T. Meszaros. 1971. Corticotrophin release induced by E. coli endotoxin after removal of the medial hypothalamus. Endocrinology 88:412–414.

Makara, G.B., E. Stark, and M. Palkovits. 1970. Afferent pathways of stressful stimuli: Corticotrophin release after hypothalamic deafferentation. J. Endocrinol. 47:411–416.

Marx, J. 1995. How the glucocorticoids suppress immunity. Science 270:232–233.

Mason, D.I., I.A. MacPhee, and F.A. Antoni. 1990. The role of the neuroendocrine system in determining genetic susceptibility to experimental allergic encephalomyelitis and implications for human inflammatory disease. Immunology 70:1–5.

Matta, S.G., J. Singh, R. Newton, and B.M. Sharp. 1990. The adrenocorticotropin response to interleukin-1β instilled into the rat median eminence depends on the local release of catecholamines. Endocrinology 127:2175–2182.

Minami, M., Y. Kuraishi, T. Yamaguchi, S. Nakai, Y. Hirai, and M. Satoh. 1991. Immobilization stress induces interleukin-1β mRNA in the rat hypothalamus. Neurosci. Lett. 123:254–256.

Minami, M., Y. Kuraishi, T. Yamaguchi, K. Yabuuchi, A. Yamazaki, and M. Satoh. 1992. Induction of Interleukin-1β mRNA in rat brain after transient forebrain ischemia. J. Neurochem. 58:390–392.

Morrissey, P.J., K. Charrier, and S.N. Vogel. 1995. Exogenous tumor necrosis factor-α and interleukin-1α increase resistance to Salmonella typhimurium: Efficacy is influenced by the Ity and LPs loci. Infect. Immun. 63:3196–3198.

Munck, A., P.M. Guyre, and N.J. Holbrook. 1984. Physiological functions of glucocorticoids in stress and their relation to pharmacological actions. Endocr. Rev. 5:25–44.

Nakano, K., S. Suzuki, and C. Oh. 1987. Significance of increased secretion of glucocorticoids in mice and rats injected with bacterial endotoxin. Brain Behav. Immun. 1:159–172.

Nakatsuru, K., S. Ohgo, Y. Oki, and S. Matsukura. 1991. Interleukin-1 (IL-1) stimulates arginine vasopressin (AVP) release from superfused rat hypothalamo-neurohypophyseal complexes independently of cholinergic mechanism. Brain Res. 554:38–45.

Neta, R., R. Perlstein, S.N. Vogel, G.D. Ledney, and J. Abrams. 1992. Role of interleukin 6 (IL-6) in protection from lethal irradiation and in endocrine responses to IL-1 and tumor necrosis factor. J. Exp. Med. 175:689–694.

Neta R., D. Williams, F. Selzer, and J. Abrams. 1993. Inhibition of c-kit ligand/steel factor by antibodies reduces survival of lethally irradiated mice. Blood 81(2):324–327.

Ohlsson, K., P. Bjork, M. Bergenfeldt, R. Hageman, and R.C. Thompson. 1990. Interleukin-1 receptor antagonist reduces mortality from endotoxin shock. Nature 348:550–552.

Perlstein R.S., M.H. Whitnall, J.S. Abrams, E.H. Mougey, and R. Neta. 1993. Synergistic roles of interleukin-6, interleukin-1, and tumor necrosis factor in adrenocorticotropin response to bacterial lipopolysaccharide in vivo. Endocrinology 132:946–952.

Perretti, M. 1994. Lipocortin-derived peptides. Biochem. Pharmacol. 47(6):931–938.

Perretti, M., C. Becherucci, G. Scapigliati, and L. Parente. 1989. The effect of adrenalectomy on interleukin-1 release in vitro and in vivo. Br. J. Pharmacol. 98:1137–1142.

Pruitt J.H., E.M. Copeland, and L.L. Moldawer. 1995. Interleukin-1 and interleukin-1 antagonism in sepsis, systemic inflammatory response syndrome, and septic shock. Shock 3(4):235–251.

Reichlin, S. 1993. Neuroendocrine-immune interactions [review article]. New Engl. J. Med. 329(17):1246–1253.

Rivest, S., G. Torres, and C. Rivier. 1992. Differential effects of central and peripheral injection of interleukin-1β on brain c-fos expression and neuroendocrine functions. Brain Res. 587:13–23.

Rivier, C. 1993. Effect of peripheral and central cytokines on the hypothalamic–pituitary-adrenal axis of the rat. Ann. N.Y. Acad. Sci. 697:97–105.

Rivier, C. 1995. Influence of immune signals on the hypothalamic-pituitary axis of the rodent. Front. Neuroendocrinol. 16:151–182.

Rivier, C., R. Chizzonite, and W. Vale. 1989. In the mouse, the activation of the hypothalamic-pituitary-adrenal axis by a lipopolysaccharide (endotoxin) is mediated through interleukin-1. Endocrinology 125:2800–2805.

Russell, D.A., and K. K. Tucker. 1995. Combined inhibition of interleukin-1 and tumor necrosis factor in rodent endotoxemia: Improved survival and organ function. J. Infect. Dis. 171:1528–1538.

Saija, A., P. Princi, M. Lanza, M. Scalese, E. Aramnejad, and A. De Sarro. 1995. Systemic cytokine administration can affect blood-brain barrier permeability in the rat. Life Sci. 56:775–784.

Saperstein, A., H. Brand, T. Audhya, D. Nabriski, B. Hutchinson, S. Rosenzweig, and C. S. Hollander. 1992. Interleukin 1β mediates stress-induced immunosuppression via corticotropin-releasing factor. Endocrinology 130:152–158.

Sapolsky, R., C. Rivier, G. Yamamoto, P. Plotsky, and W. Vale. 1987. IL-1 stimulates the secretion of hypothalamic CRF. Science 238:522–524.

Sawchenko, P.E., E.R. Brown, R.K.W. Chan, A. Ericsson, H.-Y. Li, B.L. Roland, and K.J. Kovács. 1996. The paraventricular nucleus of the hypothalamus and the functional neuroanatomy of visceromotor responses to stress. Pp. 201–222 in The Emotional Motor System, G. Holstege, R. Bandler, and C.B. Saper, eds. Progress in Brain Research, vol. 107. Amsterdam: Elsevier.

Schöbitz, B., E.R. De Kloet, and F. Holsboer. 1994. Gene expression and function of interleukin-1, interleukin-6, and tumor necrosis factor in the brain. Prog. Neurobiol. 44:397–432.

Schotanus, K., F. Tilders, and F. Berkenbosch. 1993. Human interleukin-1 receptor antagonist prevents adrenocorticotropin, but not interleukin-6 response to bacterial endotoxin in rats. Endocrinology 132:1569–1576.

Selmanoff, M.K., L.P. Kapcala, J.R. He, Y. Gao, D.N. Darlington, and D.E. Carlson. 1996. Adrenocorticosteroid feedback is not necessary for adrenocorticotropin stimulation by peripheral interleukin-1β. Soc. Neurosci. 21:336.4.

Shalaby, M.R., J. Halgunset, O.A. Haugen, H. Aarset, L. Aarden, A. Waage, K. Matsushima, H. Kvithyll, D. Boraschi, J. Lamvik, and T. Espevid. 1991. Cytokine-associated tissue injury and lethality in mice: A comparative study. Clin. Immunol. Immunopathol. 61:69–82.

Sheppard, B.C., , and J.A. Norton. 1991. Tumor necrosis factor and interleukin-1 protection against lethal effects of tumor necrosis factor. Surgery 109:698–705.

Staruch, M.J., and D.D. Wood. 1985. Reduction of serum interleukin-1-like activity after treatment with dexamethasone. J. Leukocyte Biol. 37:193–207.

Sternberg, E.M., and J. Licinio. 1995. Overview of neuroimmune stress interactions: Implications for susceptibility to inflammatory disease. Ann. N.Y. Acad. Sci. 771:364–371.

Sternberg, E.M., G.P. Chrousos, R.L. Wilder, and P.W. Gold. 1992. The stress response and the regulation of inflammatory disease. Ann. Int. Med. 117:854–866.

Sternberg, E.M., J.M. Hill, G.P. Chrousos, T. Kamilaris, S.J. Listwak, P.W. Gold, and R. Wilder. 1989. Inflammatory mediator-induced hypothalamic-pituitary-adrenal axis activation is defective in streptococcal cell wall arthritis-susceptible Lewis rats. Proc Natl. Acad. Sci. USA 86:2374–2378.

Suda, T., F. Tozawa, T. Ushiyama, T. Sumitomo, M. Yamada, and H. Demura. 1990. Interleukin-1 stimulates corticotropin-releasing factor gene expression in rat hypothalamus. Endocrinology 126:1223–1228.

Sundar, S.K., M.A. Cierpial, C. Kilts, J.C. Ritchie, and J.M. Weiss. 1990. Brain IL-1-induced immunosuppression occurs through activation of both pituitary-adrenal axis and sympathetic nervous system by corticotropin-releasing factor. J. Neurosci. 10:3701–3706.

Szabo, C., C. Thiemermann, C. Wu, M. Perretti, and J.R. Vane. 1994. Attenuation of the induction of nitric oxide synthase by endogenous glucocorticoids accounts for endotoxin tolerance in vivo. Proc. Natl. Acad. Sci. USA 91:271–275.

Takao, T., S.G. Culp, and E.B. DeSouza. 1993. Reciprocal modulation of interleukin-1β (IL-1β) and IL-1 receptors by lipopolysaccharide (endotoxin) treatment in the mouse brain-endocrine-immune axis. Endocrinology 132:1497–1504.

Tilders, F.J.H., R.H. DeRijk, A.M. vanDam, K. Schotanus, and T.H.A. Persoons. 1994. Activation of the hypothalamic-pituitary-adrenal axis by bacterial endotoxins: Routes and intermediate signals. Psychoneuroendocrinology 19:209–232.

Urbaschek, R., and B. Urbaschek. 1987. Tumor necrosis factor and interleukin-1 as mediators of endotoxin-induced beneficial effects. Rev. Infect. Dis. 9 (suppl. 5):S607–S615.

van Dam, A., M. Bauer, F.J.H. Tilders, and F. Berkenbosch. 1995. Endotoxin-induced appearance of immunoreactive interleukin-1β in ramified microglia in rat brain: A light and electron microscopic study. Neuroscience 65(3):815–826.

van Dam, A., M. Brouns, S. Louisse, and F. Berkenbosch. 1992. Appearance of interleukin-1 in macrophages and in ramified microglia in the brain of endotoxin-treated rats: A pathway for the induction of non-specific symptoms of sickness? Brain Res. 588:291–296.

Veening, J.G., M.J.M. van der Meer, H. Joosten, A.R.M.M. Hermus, C.E.M. Rijnnkels, L.M. Geeraedts, and C.G. Sweep. 1993. Intravenous administration of interleukin-1β induces fos-like immunoreactivity in corticotropin-releasing hormone neurons in the paraventricular hypothalamic nucleus of the rat. J. Chem. Neuroanat. 6:391–397.

Veterans Cooperative Group. 1987. Effect of high-dose glucocorticoid therapy on mortality in patients with clinical signs of systemic sepsis. N. Engl. J. Med. 317:659–665.

Vogel, S.N., and M.M. Hogan. 1990. Role of cytokines in endotoxin-mediated host responses. Pp. 238–258 in Immunophysiology, The Role of Cells and Cytokines in Immunity and Inflammation, J. Oppenheim and E. M. Shevach, eds. New York: Oxford University Press.

Wakabayashi, G., J.A. Gelfand, J. F. Burke, R.C. Thompson, and C.A. Dinarello. 1991. A specific receptor antagonist for interleukin-1 prevents Escherichia coli-induced shock in rabbits. FASEB J. 5:338–343.

Wan, W., L. Wetmore, C.M. Sorensen, A.H. Greenberg, and D.M. Nance. 1994. Neural and biochemical mediators of endotoxin and stress-induced c-fos expression in the rat brain. Brain Res. Bull. 34:7–14.

Watanobe, H., and K. Takebe. 1994. Effects of intravenous administration of interleukin-1β on the release of prostaglandin E_2, corticotropin-releasing factor, and arginine vasopressin in several hypothalamic areas of freely moving rat: Estimation by push-pull perfusion. Neuroendocrinology 60:8–15.

Watanobe, T., A. Morimoto, N. Tan, T. Makisumi, S.G. Shimuda, T. Nakamori, and N. Murakami. 1994. ACTH response induced in capsaicin-desensitized rats by intravenous injection of interleukin-1 or prostaglandin. Eur. J. Physiol. 475:139–145.

Watkins, L.R., L.E. Goehler, J.K. Relton, N. Tartaglia, L. Silbert, D. Martin, and S.F. Maier. 1995a. Blockade of interleukin-1 induced hyperthermia by subdiaphragmatic vagotomy: Evidence for vagal mediation of immune-brain communication. Neurosci. Lett. 183:27–31.

Watkins, L.R., E.P. Wiertelak, L.E. Goehler, K. Mooney-Heiberger, J. Martinez, L. Furness, K.P. Smith, and S.F. Maier. 1994a. Neurocircuitry of illness-induced hyperalgesia. Brain Res. 639:283–299.

Watkins, L.R., E.P. Wiertelak, L.E. Goehler, K.P. Smith, D. Martin, and S.F. Maier. 1994b. Characterization of cytokine-induced hyperalgesia. Brain Res. 654:15–26.

Weidenfeld, J., O. Abramsky, and H. Ovadia. 1989. Effect of interleukin-1 on ACTH and corticosterone secretion in dexamethasone and adrenalectomized pretreated male rats. Neuroendocrinology 50:650–654.

Weiss, J.M., N. Quan, and S.K. Sundar. 1994. Widespread activation and consequences of interleukin-1 in the brain. Ann. N.Y. Acad. Sci. 741:338–357.

Whitnall, M.H., R.S. Perlstein, E.H. Mougey, and R. Neta. 1992. Effects of interleukin-1 on the stress-responsive and -nonresponsive subtypes of corticotropin-releasing hormone neurosecretory axons. Endocrinology 131:37–44.

Wick, G., Y. Hu, and G. Krooemer. 1993. Immunoendocrine communication via the hypothalamic-pituitary adrenal axis in autoimmune diseases Endocr. Rev. 14:539–563.

Williams, T.J., and H. Yarwood. 1990. Effect of glucocorticosteroids on microvascular permeability. Am. Rev. Respir. Dis. 141:S39–S43.

Yan, H.Q., M.A. Banos, P. Herregodts, and E.L. Hooghe. 1992. Expression of interleukin (IL)-1β, IL-6, and their respective receptors in the normal rat brain and after injury. Eur. J. Immunol. 22:2963–2971.

Zuckerman, S.H., J. Shellhaas, and L.D. Butler. 1989. Differential regulation of lipopolysaccharide-induced interleukin-1 and tumor necrosis factor synthesis: Effects of endogenous and exogenous glucocorticoids and the role of the pituitary-adrenal axis. Eur. J. Immunol. 19:301–305.

DISCUSSION

ROBERT NESHEIM: Thank you, Dr. Kapcala. Questions? This has been a very interesting, in some ways, elucidating and, in some ways, confusing discussion.

DOUGLAS WILMORE: I enjoyed your presentation. It pretty much I think, in balance, mimics sort of Selye's point of view about the need for the adrenal gland in the stress response. I would just like to offer some other evidence that may indicate that this response may not be as important as we always thought.

First of all, there are knock-out animals. If you look at knock-out animals, all you need steroids for are to mature their lungs when they are born. It is awfully hard to make those animals die any more than any other animals when they do not have adrenal gland function. You can do swimming and running and all sorts of other things that relate to that.

LEONARD KAPCALA: I think the important thing to keep in mind is that those are stressors that would not necessarily be inducing a lot of cytokines. So what I think is important is, if you take animals that have a subnormal HPA-axis, I believe you can show increased susceptibility to severe illness and even the lethal effects, if you have enough of a cytokine challenge.

DOUGLAS WILMORE: Yes. If you have enough of a cytokine challenge, you can kill anything.

LEONARD KAPCALA: Right. But, as you can see, the intact animals survive tremendous cytokine challenges. So what we are looking at is a sensitivity. It is not an all-or-nothing phenomenon. If you have got enough of a challenge or an immune or inflammatory stimulus that comes along, a subnormal axis will put you at increased risk of dying. I think that that is the concept to keep in mind, not necessarily that animals will die in the basal state.

DOUGLAS WILMORE: Yes. Along with that same point of view is that, for example, in modern anesthesia [comment off mike] will turn off steroid stimulation to cortisol responses. That is really practiced all around the world now. It used to be that we always thought that people who had adrenal suppression needed high doses of stress steroids to go through an operative procedure. That in fact is not right.

What is right, however, is that a basal level of steroid administered through a general kind of response is needed—not a big peak response, but a basal steroid dose is needed.

We have done experiments where we put IL-1 into the head and looked at the catabolic response. There is a very nice catabolic-response model. You can get rodents, for example, to be catabolic for a week or so. Our thesis was very much like yours, that we could adrenalectomize those animals and do away with the response, because we were working down through the HPA-axis. The fact of the matter is that when we did adrenalectomize those animals, we gave them low-dose maintenance steroids at the same time. Those animals still had their stress response, still responded the same way, and it appeared to us that the redundancy of the system somehow had now turned on other mediators to do this. It particularly has to do with some of the brain work that you have done to show that the sympathetic nervous system is now being turned on and other hormonal regulation is coming to the fore.

So the only reason for the comment is that I think that we need to move ahead with sort of the view that we have to have an adrenal gland and a big adrenal response to function. I would be very interested, for example, to take some of your runners and suppress their adrenal elaboration and take them up to 80 percent $\dot{V}O_2max$ and see whether in fact you would get the same immunosuppression or not. Because I think that will help elucidate some of these mechanisms.

LEONARD KAPCALA: At the end of some of these studies where you give these small cytokine challenges or endotoxin, and you boost the immune response to a lethal subsequent dose, it would be interesting to study them [small cytokine changes] in, say, animals that had undergone a stalk section because then you might be inhibiting a corticosterone response, but you would still allow the CRH sympathetic response and might be able to determine how much of that component might be important. I think that probably you would get the maximal response when you have both components working. But when you have at least the sympatho-adrenal system functioning, that component gives you some protection.

DOUGLAS WILMORE: I think it is worth pointing out that Bill Beisel directed work here back in the 1960s or 1970s, if I remember the reference right—maybe the early 1970s—when IL-1 was really put into the head at a dose of about one-four hundredth of what had to be put into the systemic circulation to get a comparable kind of fever response.

The business of brain IL-1 cytokine responses, I think, is a tremendously important thing. There are a number of us in this room—Bruce [Bistrian], Joe [Cannon], myself, and others—who have worked until we are blue in the face to try to find these circulating factors in the blood stream, and they are awfully hard to recover. The business of stuff circulating through the blood stream and going to the brain and creating signals and looking for those specific cytokines has not been a real fruitful area unless you are terribly, terribly sick with infectious disease.

Other mediators, such as complement, and other sorts of inflammatory mediators, may well turn on central cytokines to then add these outflow kinds of responses. So I think we still have an awful lot to learn about the picture, and I just do not want us to get locked into the stereotypic Selye model of response.

WILLIAM BEISEL: When the steroid drugs were first introduced into medicine in about 1949 or thereabouts, every infectious disease on the books was used as a model to see if these corticosteroids would help in the treatment. The concept then was Selye's adrenal-response model. The thousands of papers published, unfortunately, showed that steroids in megadoses did not help that much in the treatment of infectious diseases in people. Still, the clinical value of corticosteroids just did not appear to be present. When we began actually measuring the amount of the adrenal response in human volunteers in this building, who were being infected with various microorganisms, we were surprised that the adrenal response was minuscule compared to the immune response of surgical patients.

We did some of the same type of studies in animals that Dr. Wilmore just talked about. We found that a permissive effect of the steroids was necessary for a lot of responses by the animal and in adrenalectomized animals—the guy with the stress of just a small permissive dose would keep those animals going. I am still not convinced the large doses of steroids are of any protective value at all.

LEONARD KAPCALA: When our studies were performed, basically, what we were trying to do was to mimic what a maximal stress was, just showing that because, as you saw, the HPA axis of intact animals was completely protected so that these animals could tolerate very large doses.

I would just like to make one other comment. I know, in the medical literature right now, the pendulum has gone back and forth in terms of sepsis, and whether or not to give steroids. Right now it is in the camp that steroids have not been shown to be beneficial. I would just add one caveat though. I think that pharmacological steroids might be beneficial if they were given early enough because by the time you make the diagnosis, sepsis has advanced to a certain stage, and it is already too late, because animal models such as baboons, given sublethal or lethal doses of endotoxin can be protected. So I think the problem is that with humans, we just cannot really do that study. By the time we say this person is undergoing sepsis it is already too late, and the cytokine cascade has gone too far.

I would agree with your point about the importance of the permissive action of glucocorticoid in a certain situation such as the basal state. I think one reason we see relatively low cytokine levels in the basal, unstimulated state is because glucocorticoids are modulating some cytokine production and secretion. It has been shown that adrenalectomized animals will show an increased expression of cytokines just basally so that that is an important concept: that you do not necessarily need large amounts, but you do need larger amounts when the cytokine challenge becomes more significant.

Nutrition and Immune Function, 1999
Pp. 437–496. Washington, D.C.
National Academy Press

20

Chronobiology of the Immune System

Erhard Haus[1]

INTRODUCTION

The human organism at all levels of biologic organization shows an intricate time structure consisting of rhythmic variations in multiple frequencies of most biologic variables studied, which are superimposed on trends like development and aging. Many of the rhythms are genetically fixed. The inheritance of rhythm characteristics and genes and gene products determining the occurrence, the extent, and the timing of the rhythmic variations have been described (Feldmann, 1985; Konopka, 1979; Lakatua, 1994; Lee et al., 1996; Myers et al., 1996; Peleg et al., 1989; Reinberg et al., 1985; Rensing, 1997; Young, 1993; Young et al., 1985). Biologic rhythms of various frequencies were found in single cells and in cell organ cultures removed from the organism and studied *in vitro* (Edmunds, 1994; Milos et al., 1990; Morse et al., 1989; Schweiger et al., 1986). *In vivo*, these numerous oscillators are adjusted within the organism in their timing by pacemakers through humoral and/or neural

[1] Erhard Haus, Regions Hospital, Health Partners Research Foundation, St. Paul, MN, 55101-2595, University of Minnesota, Minneapolis, MN 55455

messages synchronizing the target cells or organs. In turn, many target cells provide feedback information in the form of humoral signals, for example, through cytokines or polypeptide hormones and neurotransmitters that act on the superimposed neuroendocrine structures and modify their response (Blalock, 1992, 1994). The interactions of the neuroendocrine and immune system are time dependent and follow rhythmic patterns in multiple frequencies. In some frequencies, the rhythms are adjusted in time (externally synchronized) by periodic environmental factors like light-darkness, social routine, the work schedule, and to some extent the time of food uptake. The spontaneous rhythms encountered are complemented by reactive, rhythmic response patterns to environmental stimuli, some of which may equally be genetically fixed (endogenous) in nature. Such rhythmic response patterns can be triggered by single stimuli (e.g., the introduction of an antigen) and in their timing relate to the time of stimulation and not to environmental rhythms, for example, the calendar week. Environmental stimuli may also change some rhythm parameters like timing or amplitude transiently for only as long as the environmental stimulus persists ("masking" the rhythm).

The complexity of the human time structure and its adaptation to changing environmental conditions, presumably including geophysical factors (Breus et al., 1989; Lipa et al., 1976; Sitar, 1991), make it necessary to qualify the assumption that sampling at a fixed time of the day, the week, and/or the season will "control" rhythmic variables, and that the need for the observation of rhythms could be avoided.

The rhythmically changing physiologic state of the organism determines the response to environmental stimuli like physical exercise, pain perception, mental stress, toxic substances, bacterial and viral infections, antigenic stimulation, and drugs used in clinical medicine. The state of the host organism at the time of stimulation often determines critically the response to a stimulus in extent, and in some instances, in direction. This is shown dramatically in the response of mice to the injection of *Escherichia coli* endotoxin (Figure 20-1). Death or survival can be made experimentally a function of the time when the agent is injected.

The development of an immune response involves a series of interactions between lymphocytes and other mononuclear cells that may include cell-to-cell communication; generation of immunoreactive molecules; immunoglobulin synthesis and secretion; expression of cell surface markers that are not generally found on resting cells or changes in their receptor density and activity; and finally cell proliferation of immunocompetent cells. An effective immune response requires a balance in the function of lymphocyte subsets (e.g., helper and cytotoxic T-cells, and antibody-producing B-cell lymphocytes), macrophages, and natural killer (NK) cells, and a balance in the production of enhancing or inhibiting soluble factors or cytokines as expressed in the Th1 or Th2 response to immune stimulation. Each of these factors is directly or indirectly under the influence of neuroendocrine rhythmic variables directing

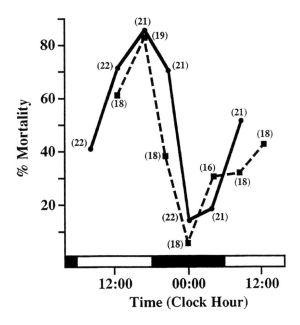

FIGURE 20-1 Circadian rhythm in susceptibility of *Balb/C* mice to intaperitoneal (i.p.) injection of *Escherichia coli* endotoxin. The same dose injected at different circadian stages into subgroups of comparable animals kept at a lighting regimen of Light-Dark (LD) 12:12 leads to dramatic differences in response (two studies show high degree of reproducibility). SOURCE: Adapted from Halberg et al. (1960) and Haus et al. (1974b).

components of the immune response and in turn provides signals to other immunocompetent cells or to the superimposed neuroendocrine centers via feedback regulation. Rhythmic variations in several frequencies are found in every step of the development of an immune response in the humoral as well as the cellular arm of the immune system. Rhythmic variations of the immune response in its different aspects have been studied most extensively in the circadian frequency range. Circadian rhythmic variations in hormone secretion or in the effect of humoral messengers on the target tissue caused by changes at the receptor level (Lakatna et al., 1986) or the interaction with other humoral factors can increase or decrease the number and functional activity of the immune-competent cells in the peripheral blood and/or in lymphoid and other tissues. These changes lead to differences in the immune response during certain stages of the circadian cycle, which may be of importance both for the response to a primary antigenic stimulation or to a challenge of the immunized organism. Disturbances of the usual temporal pattern in the function of the different cells of the immune system are found in disturbances in the immune response (e.g., in states of immunodeficiency) or may lead to autoantibody production with the development of a chronic autoimmune disease.

More recently, rhythms of about 7-day duration (circaseptan rhythms), synchronized or not by the environmental social week, have been recognized for their importance in the human time structure (Cornélissen et al., 1993; Levi and Halberg, 1982). Some of them appear to be endogenous in nature and may be found free running from known environmental time cues (Halberg and Hamburger, 1964). In addition to the spontaneously occurring circaseptan rhythms, a circaseptan response pattern characterizes the mammalian organism. After exposure to an environmental load, for example, to anoxic kidney damage (Hübner, 1967) or the exposure to an antigen (DeVecchi et al., 1981) or treatment with immunosuppressive agents (Hrushesky and März, 1994; Many and Schwartz, 1971), the response of the organism occurs in a rhythmic fashion with approximate (but not always exactly) 7-d periods. This response pattern is unrelated to the calendar day of the week but is triggered by the one-point stimulation at the time of exposure to the stimulus (e.g., the introduction of an antigen).

Seasonal variations as they are observed in the immune response may be due to environmental factors like differences in the length of the daily light span, temperature differences, and differences in exposure to a variety of antigens, including microorganisms. The environmental effects on the immune system may be mediated by seasonal changes in the function of the pineal gland (light-dark related), the thyroid gland (temperature related), or prolactin (PRL) (Arendt, 1994; Haus et al., 1980, 1988; Nicolau and Haus, 1994). However, rhythms of approximate duration of 1 year may in certain functions also be endogenous and presumably genetically fixed (so-called circannual rhythms). Circannual rhythms have been observed experimentally in animals, who for generations were kept under light- and temperature-controlled experimental laboratory conditions and have never been exposed to variations in day length or temperature (Haus et al., 1984, 1997; Haus M. et al., 1984). Figure 20-2 shows the circannual variations in cell proliferation as measured by the ^{3}H-thymidine uptake in DNA of lymphatic organs and of the hematopoietic and lymphatic cells in the bone marrow in mice subgroups of which were studied over 2 years and measured during each season over a 24-h span with the circadian mean plotted in the figure. It is of interest that there appear to be phase differences between different lymphatic organs and the bone marrow. Other evidence about the endogenous nature of circannual variations is the observation of free-running circannual rhythms of body functions in human subjects (Haus and Touitou, 1994a).

The intricate web of neuroendocrine-immune regulation makes a separate discussion of some of its components artificial. However, experimental design and clinical studies can follow only a limited number of variables and end points. In presenting the results of studies of the time structure of certain parts of this complex system, it must be realized that each observation has to be understood in the context of its role within the framework of the system as a whole.

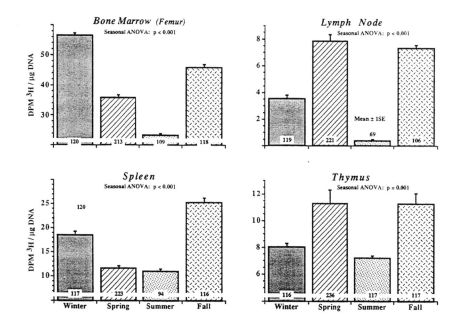

FIGURE 20-2 Circannual rhythm of ^{3}H-thymidine uptake into DNA of lymphoid tissues and bone marrow of *BDF₁* male mice kept for several generations on artificial lighting (LD 12:12), under controlled temperatures, and fed the same mouse chow. The animals were studied over an entire 24-h span (six sampling times at 4-h intervals) in several studies per season during 2 consecutive years (results pooled). A circannual rhythm is found as a group phenomenon without known environmental seasonal variations. Note phase difference among organs. SOURCE: Adapted from Haus et al. (1997).

BIOLOGIC RHYTHMS IN THE NUMBER AND FUNCTION OF CIRCULATING WHITE BLOOD CELLS

The numbers of circulating white blood cells involved in the defense of the human body show high-amplitude circadian variations. Regularity, timing, and amplitude of these rhythms vary among the different cell types, and among different age groups and populations examined (e.g., Haus, 1959, 1994, 1996; Haus et al., 1983, 1988; Swoyer et al., 1989). In the peripheral blood, the periodic changes in the number of circulating leukocytes may be the result of multiple factors, such as distribution between the circulating and the marginal cell compartments, distribution among different tissues and organs of the body, influx from storage sites, proliferation of cells, release of newly formed cells into the circulation, and cell destruction and removal. Several or all of these factors may contribute to the number of circulating white blood cells, and these factors will vary in their importance from one cell type to the other, which may lead to differences in timing and amplitude of each circadian (or other) rhythm. In considering the relative importance of the number of circulating immune-competent cells for defense reactions and the immune response of the body, it must be realized that with some cell types, only a very small percentage of the cells is circulating. For example, in lymphocytes, the circulating cells are fewer than 1 percent. The much larger fraction is found in the lymphatic organs, bone marrow, and other tissues (e.g., the lamina propria and submucosa of the intestinal and respiratory tract).

Figure 20-3 shows the circadian rhythms of the circulating white blood cells and platelets in 150 clinically healthy young adults (24 ± 10 years of age) following a diurnal activity pattern with rest during the night from approximately 23:00 to 06:30.

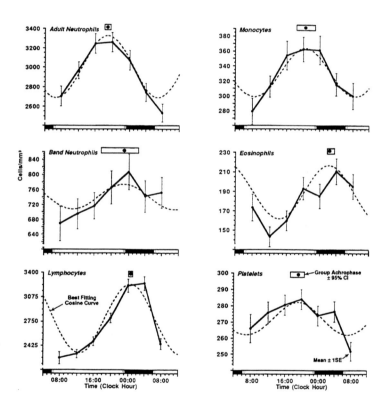

FIGURE 20-3 Circadian rhythm in circulating white blood cells in 150 clinically healthy adult subjects. Each subject sampled six times over a 24-h span. Data are shown with best fitting cosinor curve and circadian group-acrophase derived from cosinor analysis (Nelson et al., 1979). The small 95 percent confidence interval of the acrophase is due to group size and hides a substantial degree of individual variability. SOURCE: Adapted from Haus (1994, 1996); Haus et al. (1983, 1988).

The circadian variations in circulating white blood cells are consistent and highly reproducible as group phenomena. However, there is a substantial individual variation and in some of the 150 apparently clinically healthy subjects summarized as a group in Figure 20-3, the peak or trough of the values measured could be found at any clock hour of the day (Haus, 1996). The regularity and timing of the rhythms also varies by cell type. In neutrophil leukocytes, the location of the trough values is more consistent and reproducible than that of the peak values. Lymphocytes show a very regular rhythm with both peak and trough equally conspicuous. Circulating monocytes and eosinophils show more variability within and between individuals.

The circadian rhythm in circulating eosinophil leukocytes shows an apparent relation to the circadian rhythm in corticosteroid concentration, and exogenous corticosteroids and stress suppress the number of circulating eosinophils (Haus, 1959). The circadian change in the number of circulating eosinophils (rather than the absolute value) has been used in the past for the assessment of adrenal cortical function (Halberg and Stephens, 1959; Halberg et al., 1958; Haus, 1959), and the change in their number under stress conditions may still be of some interest, as an indicator (at least in part) of the peripheral response of a target tissue to corticosteroids.

TABLE 20-1 Peak-Trough Difference and Range of Change in Circulating Leukocytes (173 subjects) and Platelets (87 subjects) over a 24-h Span in Clinically Healthy Subjects

	Peak-Trough Difference (cells/mm^3)		% Range of Change [(highest − lowest/lowest) × 100]	
	Mean ± Standard Deviation	Range	Mean ± Standard Deviation	Range
Total white blood cells	2,400 ± 1,000	400–6,100	41 ± 18	7–133
Total neutrophils	1,840 ± 1,028	480–7,168	66 ± 42	20–346
Adult neutrophils	1,567 ± 856	330–6,347	72 ± 43	18–344
Bands	563 ± 350	56–1,790	152 ± 114	15–780
Lymphocytes	1,616 ± 770	331–5,556	84 ± 41	14–234
Monocytes	366 ± 167	80–974	277 ± 221	30–1,560
Eosinophils	230 ±110	40–816	292 ± 190	64–1,031
Basophils	105 ± 57	0–390	315 ± 175	27–658
Platelets (× 10^3)	54 ± 32	12–198	23 ± 15	3–83

The extent of the circadian variation encountered in 173 apparently clinically healthy subjects (irrespective of timing in each individual) is shown in Table 20-1. The within-day (circadian) peak-trough difference is expressed in absolute numbers at the left and as percent range of change at the right (the extent of change expressed in percent of the trough value). Also in the extent of the rhythms, there are very marked individual variations in an apparently clinically healthy population following a regular routine without known unusual stress or infection.

The variability in the absolute number of cells, and in the timing of peak, and trough, and extent of the circadian variation suggest a clinical usefulness for time-qualified reference values for the evaluation of single cell counts mainly in circulating lymphocytes (Figure 20-4). The reference value for the number of circulating lympocytes in blood drawn early in the morning is different from that in blood drawn at noon. However, the extent of change in the different cell types, which can occur spontaneously in a given individual within a 24-h span must be kept in mind for the evaluation of consecutive measurements in the same patient. Circadian periodicity has to be taken into account in studies in which circulating cell numbers serve as end points.

In clinically healthy subjects, the circadian rhythm in the number of circulating lymphocytes is a very regular and highly reproducible phenomenon. The peak values occur in most diurnally active human subjects during the night

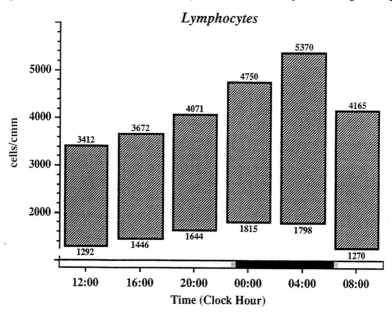

FIGURE 20-4 Circadian variation in usual range (expressed as fifth and ninety-fifth percentile) of numbers of circulating lymphocytes in 150 clinically healthy subjects studied over a 24-h span. SOURCE: Adapted from Haus (1994, 1996) and Haus et al. (1983).

proportion as part of the total circulating lymphocyte population. The most consistent variations were found in the CD3+ (mature T-cells) and CD4+ hours, with the highest values found between midnight and 01:00. Also the subsets of lymphocytes show a circadian rhythm in their number and/or their (helper inducer cells), while in the CD8+ (suppresser cytotoxic cells) some investigators reported no significant circadian rhythm as a group phenomenon (Ritchie et al., 1983) or a 12-h rhythm only (Levi et al., 1985, 1988a). In this author's laboratory, a prominent circadian rhythm was evident also in the CD8+ cells, with an additional shorter frequency apparent in the men (Haus, 1994) (Figure 20-5). The circadian variation in the number of circulating lymphocytes persisted under conditions of sleep deprivation (Ritchie et al., 1983). A circadian rhythm in E-rosette-forming (T) cells was found *in vitro* in aliquots of

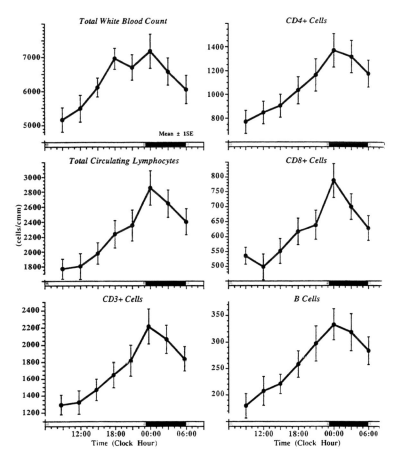

FIGURE 20-5 Circadian variation in lymphocyte subtypes in 10 clinically healthy subjects. (The double peak in "total white blood count" is due to the earlier circadian peak of neutrophils.)

blood samples studied over 24 hours and was reported to continue in 4-d-old cell cultures (Gamaleya et al., 1988). These *in vitro* studies suggest that the rhythmic fluctuations in at least some subpopulations of blood lymphocytes depend on circadian changes in the cells (a cellular oscillator) rather than on extracellular factors such as the circadian rhythm in plasma cortisol. However, cortisol may act as a synchronizer, or if given exogenously, it can transiently alter (mask) the circadian rhythm.

Not only the number of circulating lymphocytes but also several aspects of lymphocyte function show circadian periodicity. Circadian periodic variations in the response to external stimuli were recognized experimentally in changes of the number of cells in the peripheral blood (Figure 20-6) and bone marrow (Figure 20-7). In some studies, the T-cell response to phytohemagglutinin (PHA) was found to be circadian periodic with a remarkably large amplitude (Haus et al., 1974a, 1983; Tavadia et al., 1975) (Figure 20-8). However, there appears to be some variability in circadian timing of this rhythm, possibly due to seasonal or other factors that may not allow one to recognize a rhythm if sampling does not occur at the "right" times, for example, if only two time points are selected according to clock hour rather than according to the stage of the rhythm. Mixed lymphocyte reactions (MLRs) in PHA-activated T-cells and autologous non-T-cell activation showed statistically significant circadian variations with proliferation response of T-cells in both types of autologous MLRs, but with an apparent phase difference between them. The difference in timing of the two types of autologous MLRs may be due to the different types of cells responding (Damle and Gupta, 1982).

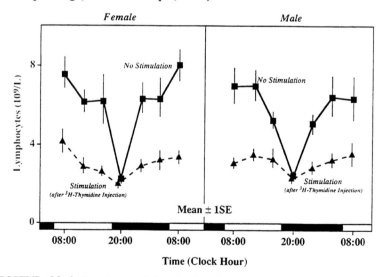

FIGURE 20-6 Circadian variation in lymphocytopenic response to handling and intraperitoneal injection of ^{3}H-thymidine (1 μc ^{3}H-thy in 0.2 ml saline/20 g body weight) in male and female *Balb/C* mice (sampling 2 hours after treatment).

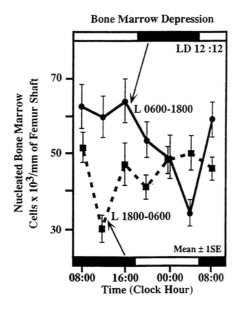

FIGURE 20-7 Circadian rhythm in sensitivity of nucleated cells in the bone marrow of *Balb/C* mice. Subgroups of mice were exposed at different circadian stages to 350 rad whole body x-irradiation. Half of the animals were kept on a lighting regimen of LD 12:12 with light from 06:00 to 18:00 , the other half for 3 weeks prior to the study on LD 12:12 with light from 18:00 to 06:00. SOURCE: Adapted from Haus et al. (1974b, 1983).

For some investigators, the predominant B-cell activation by pokeweed mitogen (PWM) showed a circadian variation (Haus et al., 1983; Moldofsky et al., 1986), while for other investigators it did not (Indiveri et al., 1985). It appears that seasonal (Canon et al., 1986; Gamaleya et al., 1988) and perhaps other rhythmic and nonrhythmic variations may play a role in the modification of lymphocyte functions. Sleep deprivation of 40 hours led to a phase alteration of the circadian rhythm in the lymphocyte response to PWM but not to PHA (Moldofsky et al., 1989).

A circadian rhythm was reported for urinary neopterin excretion (Auzeby et al., 1988) which indicates T-cell activation (Huber et al., 1984). The peak of urinary neopterin (06:30) followed that of the circulating lymphocytes in the same clinically healthy subjects by about 2 hours (Levi et al., 1988a). Figure 20-9 shows the circadian rhythm in serum neopterin in patients with rheumatoid arthritis.

In a study that took samples at two time points, the frequency of sister chromatin exchange in human blood lymphocytes was significantly less at 09:00 than at 21:00 which suggests a circadian variation of this parameter (Slozina and Golovachev, 1986). This variation may be of importance for the lymphocyte

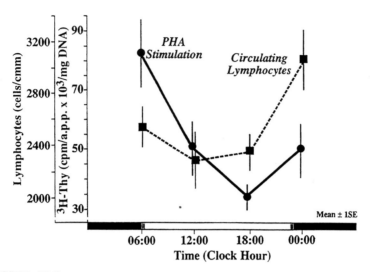

FIGURE 20-8 Circadian rhythm of lymphocytes in response to phytohemagglutinin (PHA). Lymphocyte cultures containing 1 to 2×10^6 cells/2 ml culture were set up with a 1:100 dilution of PHA. Five hours before the end of the 48-h incubation span, 50 λ (approximately 20 μCi, 1.9 Ci/μmole) ^{3}H-thymidine was added to each culture tube. After 5 hours, the reaction was terminated and DNA was measured colorimetrically in triplicate cultures. An aliquot of the same sonicate was counted in a liquid scintillation counter. Counts per minute of acid-precipitable protein (a.p.p.) were adjusted for 1.0×10^6 of inoculated cells. NOTE: The rhythm in PHA response is out of phase with rhythm in the number of circulating lymphocytes. SOURCE: Adapted from Haus et al. (1983).

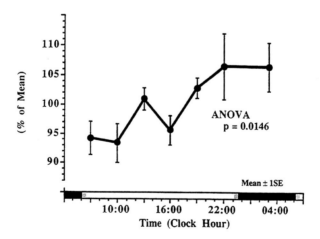

FIGURE 20-9 Circadian variation in serum neopterin concentration in 29 patients with rheumatoid arthritis. SOURCE: Adapted from Suteanu et al. (1995).

response to damage caused by a number of environmental stimuli, including radiation and certain carcinogenic agents.

Circadian variations in lymphocyte adrenoreceptor density were reported, with peak values around noon and a trough around midnight (Pangerl et al., 1986). Circannual variations of the same variable were found with high values in spring and summer and low values during winter (Haen et al., 1988; Pangerl et al., 1986). Disturbances in the expression and function of adrenoreceptors are thought to play a role in the pathobiology of, for example, hypertension and bronchial asthma (Pangerl et al., 1986), both of which show circadian and circannual chronopathology in their disease manifestations.

A circadian variation in the glucocorticoid receptor content of lymphocytes was reported with the values at 23:00 being 38 percent higher than at 08:00. The receptor affinity did not change over the 24-h span, and there was no seasonal variation in number and affinity of glucocorticoid receptors (Homo-Delarche, 1984).

The NK cell activity in the peripheral blood of clinically healthy adult subjects shows a reproducible circadian rhythm, with the activity being high in the early morning and declining to a minimum during the night hours (Abo et al., 1981; Angeli et al., 1992; Gatti et al., 1986, 1988; Moldofsky et al., 1986, 1989; Williams, et al. 1979). The NK cell activity is out of phase with the number of circulating lymphocytes of most other subtypes. There was a circadian rhythm in the response of NK cell activity to stimulation with interferon-gamma (INF-γ), which was synchronous with the spontaneous NK cell activity (acrophase[2] around 04:00) (Angeli et al., 1992; Gatti et al., 1988). Corticosteroids are potent inhibitors of NK cell activity (Herberman and Callewaert, 1985; Richtsmeier, 1985). The maximum inhibitory effect by glucocorticosteroids was found earlier during the night preceding the peak in spontaneous NK cell activity (Angeli et al., 1992; Gatti et al., 1987).

The chronic administration of melatonin leads to a substantial increase in spontaneous NK cell activity and in the responsiveness of those cells to INF-γ (Angeli et al., 1992; Gatti et al., 1990). The decrease in melatonin production during aging may also contribute through this mechanism to the lower immunocompetence of the elderly. Investigations by Gatti et al. (1988) were suggestive of a seasonal (circannual) variation of NK cell activity.

Alterations of the circadian periodicity of human lymphocytes have been reported in patients with lymphoid tumors (Swoyer et al., 1975). Infection with the lymphotrophic human immunodeficiency virus (HIV) leads to alterations in the circadian rhythm of the circulating lymphocytes as an early event in the development of the AIDS related complex (ARC) and AIDS (Bourin et al., 1989; Martini et al., 1988a,b; Swoyer et al., 1990). Circadian periodicity in hemoglobin, hematocrit, and the number of circulating red blood cells is maintained with comparable timing, but with significantly lower amplitude in

---

[2] Peak time of cosine curve best fitting to the data

HIV-infected patients (Swoyer et al., 1990). No day-night synchronized circadian rhythm was demonstrable as a group phenomenon in the HIV-infected patients in the number of circulating neutrophils, monocytes, total lymphocytes, CD3+, CD8+, and B1+ lymphocytes or in platelets. However, in individual HIV-infected patients, marked variations in the numbers of the circulating leukocytes over the 24-h span did persist but without the usual environmental synchronization (Haus, 1994, 1996; Swoyer et al., 1990). In the same patients, the circadian rhythm in circulating cortisol was maintained as a group phenomenon, with the circadian mean serum concentration and amplitude comparable to those of healthy controls (Haus, 1994, 1996). The circadian rhythm alterations in polymorphonuclear leukocytes and monocytes in HIV-infected subjects indicate a wider disturbance of the hematopoietic system than just in the lymphocyte series. Although the rhythm disturbances are more pronounced in the more severely affected patients, circadian rhythm disturbances appear to be an early consequence of HIV infection.

Circaseptan about 7-day variations have been found in many immune-related parameters (for reviews, see Haus and Touitou, 1994a, b; Haus et al., 1983, 1988; Levi and Halberg, 1982) and seem to represent a genetically fixed response pattern of the humoral as well as of the cell-bound immune system to an immunologic stimulus. Treatment with an immunosuppressive agent, melphalan, was shown to trigger a cyclic response pattern (with slightly longer than 7 day period) of immune regeneration in mice (Many and Schwartz, 1971). This response to a single stimulus points to the endogenous nature of the circaseptan organization of the immune system. Circaseptan rhythms are found in hematologic recovery after partial bone marrow suppression (Morley et al., 1970) and thus may develop during cancer chemotherapy. Circaseptan susceptibility rhythms of rodents to chemotherapeutic agents have been described (Bixby et al., 1982; Liu et al., 1986), but they need to be studied further in humans. Circaseptan variations in the numbers of circulating T- and B-cells were observed during the development of an antigenically triggered encephalomyelitis in guinea pigs. In this animal model, the peak in the number of circulating T-cells occurred at the time of the trough in the number of B-cells. The relapse occurred when the number of circulating T-cell lymphocytes was low (Raine et al., 1978). Nonimmunological stressors (such as a high salt diet in rats) can also lead to circaseptan response patterns (Uezono et al., 1987).

Circannual variations in the relative number of circulating T- and B-lymphocytes as determined by a bacterial adhesion test were described in clinically healthy human subjects, with the peak of the T-cells in late fall and of the B-cells in winter. The circannual variation was apparent in the subtypes only; the total number of lymphocytes in this study showed no statistically significant circannual variation (Bratescu and Teodorescu, 1981). Levi et al. (1988b) described circannual changes in the number and circadian rhythm characteristics of circulating total lymphocytes (with circannual acrophase of the circadian mean in November), Pan-T-cells (acrophase in March), suppressor-cytotoxic T-cells (acrophase in December), and NK cells (acrophase in October).

Seasonal variations in the response of human (Shifrine et al., 1982a) and canine (Shifrine et al., 1980, 1982b) lymphocytes to PHA-induced transformation suggest a circannual cycle in cell-mediated immunity. The peak in PHA response was found during summer and the low response during winter.

Phase adaptation of hematologic rhythms is seen in human subjects after changes in their sleep-wakefulness pattern and their activity-rest cycles as encountered in shift workers or in subjects exposed to transmeridian flights over several time zones (Haus, 1994; Haus et al., 1988; Sharp, 1960). However, there is a considerable interindividual variation in shift-work adaptation. The phase adaptation to a 12-h difference in shift (e.g., change from night shift to day shift) may in some subjects require several weeks to adapt the timing of the circadian rhythms in plasma cortisol and in circulating lymphocytes to the changed light-dark and activity-rest schedule serving as environmental synchronizer (Haus and Touitou, 1994 a,b; Reinberg and Sindensky, 1994). A full-phase adaptation to the shift schedule may not occur at all in nonpermanent shift workers or in permanent shift workers if the subjects do not fully change their living habits during the week and return to a diurnal activity pattern on weekends (Haus et al., 1984).

The susceptibility-resistance cycles of the hematopoietic cells to agents used in the treatment of human malignancies including leukemia and solid tumors, are of considerable interest (Bjarnason and Hrushesky, 1994; Haus and Halberg, 1978; Haus et al., 1972, 1983; Hrushesky and März, 1994; Levi, 1994, 1996a, 1997; Levi et al., 1986, 1994; Rivard et al., 1993). Many chemotherapeutic agents are immunosuppressive, and circadian cycles of susceptibility and resistance to these toxic agents are also found in the immune system. A circadian rhythm of sensitivity of mice to whole body irradiation could be shown to parallel the number of surviving nucleated cells in the bone marrow studied 4 days after exposure to a single dose of 350 rads x-irradiation (Haus et al., 1974a, 1983) (Figure 20-7). In the same study, a phase alteration in the timing of maximum and minimum sensitivity could be obtained by a change in lighting regimen, which, however, after 2 weeks of exposure to the altered lighting regimen was not complete, indicating a longer time required to accomplish a phase shift of this nature. The myelotoxicity of recombinant human INF-α in mice, measured by a decrease in the number of white blood cells and the number of bone marrow myeloid precursors, was lowest when the agent was administered in the middle of the rest span. In contrast, the least toxicity of murine INF-γ was found during the mid-activity span (Koren and Fleischmann, 1993). Thus, different forms of interferon show a remarkable difference in the circadian timing of their effects. The susceptibility-resistance cycles to a large number of chemotherapeutic agents have been documented in nocturnal rodents with characteristic timing of the acrophase for various agents (Levi et al., 1986). For human application on a purely empirical basis, a 12-h time difference was chosen as a guideline for the timing of chemotherapy in diurnally active human subjects. Thus far, this seems to have been successful, although the animal data on circadian timing in peripheral blood and bone marrow are sometimes at variance with the simplified assumption of a 12-h time difference (Haus et al., 1983).

BIOLOGIC RHYTHMS IN CYTOKINES AND THEIR INHIBITORS

The central nervous system (CNS), endocrine, and immune systems respond to physiological and pharmacological stimuli in a coordinated manner with bidirectional communication between the systems (Beneviste, 1992; Blalock, 1992, 1994; Rivier and Rivest, 1993; Smith, 1992). The immune-competent cells recognize and respond to the introduction of antigens, to exposure to bacterial and other toxins, and to other tissue damage and initiate the appropriate defense. Signaling among the diverse forms of cells, including lymphocytes, macrophages, fibroblasts, and vascular endothelia, occurs through locally produced substances, including hormones and cytokines.

Cytokines are relatively small proteins or glycoproteins, most of which are characteristically multifunctional and exert their biologic activity in an autocrine and paracrine fashion in or close to the cells of origin. In addition, some cytokines are released into the circulation and exert endocrine effects on target tissues remote from the cell of origin, for example, on cells of the hematopoietic and immune systems, cells involved in inflammatory reactions, and a variety of mesenchymal (e.g., bone forming) and epithelial tissues (e.g., in breast, prostate). These circulating cytokines also act on certain hypothalamic centers and on cells of endocrine glands that in turn regulate cytokine production (Besedovsky and Del Rey, 1996; Spangelo and Gorospe, 1995).

The close interaction between cytokines and the neuroendocrine system leads, in some instances, to feedback regulation, for example, between the pro-inflammatory cytokines (especially interleukin [IL]-1), which are produced at the site of tissue injury, and the strongly anti-inflammatory response elicited in response to cytokine action on hypothalamic centers through the production and release of corticotropin-releasing factor (CRF), adrenocorticotrophic hormone (ACTH), and corticosteroids. Intravenous doses of IL-6 result in a dose-dependent increase in plasma ACTH levels. Antibodies to CRF block the rise in plasma ACTH induced by IL-1 and IL-6 (Naitoh et al., 1988). The increased release of hormones such as ACTH and corticosteroids in the course of immune challenges is considered important as a regulatory mechanism that provides negative feedback in response to overproduction of interleukins (Besedovsky and Del Rey, 1992; Rivier and Rivest, 1993). The immune system serves, through the production of cytokines, as a sensory organ that signals the exposure to antigen (e.g., bacterial or viral invasion, bacterial toxins) to the CNS and endocrine system, which then respond to the challenge and provide for the body's defense but at the same time limit the inflammatory and related responses and prevent damage by overshoot of the inflammatory and immune defenses, leading to a balanced host response to environmental stimuli.

The circadian stage and the temporal sequence in which cytokines reach the hypothalamic oscillators in the CNS and/or endocrine organs may in part determine the particular response elicited and/or the alterations in the immune and endocrine systems as they are observed in some autoimmune diseases (Berczi et al., 1993). Little is known about rhythms in the auto- and paracrine action of cytokines at the sites of ongoing immune reactions, although in view of the multifrequency periodicities of the neuroendocrine regulation of inflammatory and immune reactions, and the periodicity found at the cellular level, rhythmic variations of these variables have to be assumed.

The circadian periodicity in the various components of the immune system also leads to circadian rhythmicity of cytokines and some of their soluble receptors or receptor antagonists released into circulation (Bourin et al., 1990; Sothern et al., 1995; Suteanu et al., 1995; Young et al., 1995). A circadian rhythm in IL-1 concentration was found in the serum of clinically healthy subjects (Bourin et al., 1990). Cytokines, including IL-1β and tumor necrosis factor (TNF), may be involved in the physiologic alternation of sleep and wakefulness (Krueger, 1990). Higher values of IL-1β and IL-6 were reported in clinically healthy subjects during nighttime sleep (Covelli et al., 1992; Gudewill et al., 1992). Peaks in serum IL-1 and IL-2-like activity occur shortly after sleep onset in healthy human subjects (Gudewill et al., 1992; Moldofsky et al., 1986).

A circadian rhythm has been described for the responsiveness of T-cells to IL-2 (Levi et al., 1991). In a whole blood assay, there was a large-amplitude circadian variation in tetanus toxoid and purified protein derivative of tuberculin (PPD)-stimulated production of INF-γ with highest values during the evening and nighttime (Petrovsky et al., 1994), which was about 12 ± 1 hours out of phase (by cosinor analysis) with the circadian variation in plasma cortisol. A seasonal variation of INF-γ production by mitogen-stimulated T-cells has also been reported (Katila et al., 1993).

IL-6 is a multifunctional cytokine that is produced by various types of lymphoid and nonlymphoid cells and that plays a central role in host defense mechanisms and in inflammation and immune responses (Mackiewicz et al., 1995) and exerts a protective role against lipopolysaccharide-induced (TNF-γ and IL-1 mediated) shock (Barton and Jackson, 1993), the mortality from which in animal experiments shows a very large amplitude circadian rhythm (Halberg et al., 1960; Haus et al., 1974a). The serum concentrations of IL-6 show a circadian rhythm in clinically healthy men, with high values during the night with a peak around 01:00 and a trough around 10:00. The range of change from the lowest to the highest value during a 24-h span ranged from 120 to 531 percent (Sothern et al., 1995). In the same subjects, Young et al. (1995) found a circadian rhythm in IL-2 with a peak during midday (12:48) and a range of change between 31 and 1,367 percent. In contrast, two daily peaks were observed for IL-10 (07:30 and 19:30; range of change between 8 and 266%) for granulocyte macrophage-colony stimulating factor (GM-CSF) (13:30 and 19:30; range of change between 32 and 12,684%), and TNF-γ (07:30 and 13:30 with a range of change between 16 and 131%). Spontaneous *in vitro* secretion of IL-1, IL-6, and TNF-γ was higher when the lymphocytes were collected during the day (Zabel et al., 1990, 1993).

A circadian rhythm in soluble IL-2 receptor was found in clinically healthy subjects, with a peak value around 12:30 and a trough value around 04:15 (Lemmer et al., 1992). In patients with rheumatoid arthritis, circadian rhythms were found in IL-6 (Arvidson et al., 1994; Suteanu et al., 1995) and neopterin, a product of T-cell activation (Suteanu et al., 1995). Statistically significant within-day variation, presumably representing ultradian rhythms, were found in patients with rheumatoid arthritis in soluble IL-2 receptor, IL-1β, TNF-γ, and soluble TNF receptors I and II (Suteanu et al., 1995).

Human peripheral leukocytes infected by virus or treated with endotoxin will synthesize immunoreactive corticotropin and endorphins in addition to cytokines. The immunoreactive ACTH produced by the immunocompetent cells appears to be identical to pituitary ACTH, and appears to act on the same receptors in the target tissues and shows a steroidogenic response in mice. The production of ACTH both by pituitary cells and leukocytes in response to synthetic CRF is suppressed by dexamethasone *in vitro* and *in vivo*, which suggests that the production of ACTH and endorphins by leukocytes is controlled by CRF (Smith et al., 1986).

BIOLOGIC RHYTHMICITY OF THE HUMORAL IMMUNE RESPONSE

Both the time of exposure of immunocompetent cells to an antigen (Fernandes et al., 1977, 1980; Pownall et al., 1979) and the response to challenge of the immunized organism after reintroduction of the antigen show circadian periodic variations in human subjects and in animals (Cove-Smith et al., 1978; Fernandes et al., 1976, 1977, 1980; Lee et al., 1977; Pownall et al., 1979). In animal experiments, the instensity of the humoral immune response to T-cell-dependent and independent antigens shows circadian periodicity (Fernandes et al., 1974, 1976; Pownall and Knapp, 1980). After immunization, circadian periodic variations in antibody titer and in the number of plaque-forming cells (PFC) were found in mice in response to sheep red blood cell (SRBC) antigen (Fernandes et al., 1974). The fewest PFC were seen when the antigen was injected close to the daily dark span, corresponding to the time of the highest corticosterone concentrations in nocturnal rodents (Calderon and Thomas, 1980; Fernandes et al., 1976).

The concentrations of serum proteins that are important for immune function, including the immunoglobulins and several other components of serum proteins, undergo circadian periodic changes (Halberg et al., 1977; Haus et al., 1983, 1988; Hayashi and Kikuchi, 1982; Reinberg et al., 1979; Scheving et al., 1968, 1977). In clinically healthy subjects, the peak concentrations of all three major classes of immunoglobulins occurred in the early to late afternoon (e.g., Reinberg et al., 1979).

In patients with some clinical conditions, alterations in the circadian rhythms of the humoral immune system have been detected. In patients with allergic asthma, Cricchio et al. (1979) found statistically significant circadian rhythms only in immunoglobulins G (IgG) and M (IgM) with peak concentrations occurring at the same time as in clinically healthy subjects. In patients with allergic rhinitis, circadian rhythms were detected in all three immunoglobulins with a 3-h delay in the peaks of IgG and IgM as compared with healthy subjects (Cricchio et al., 1979) (Figure 20-10).

Surface IgA in the nasal secretions, a primary immune defense in the respiratory tract, shows a circadian rhythm (Hughes et al., 1977) that was found to be phase shifted in shift workers. Although peak and trough of the circadian rhythm in nasal secretory IgA (SIgA) coincide in diurnally active human subjects with those of plasma cortisol, suppression of the daily rise in plasma cortisol by a dexamethasone suppression test does not alter the concentration or the rhythm of SIgA (Menzio et al., 1980).

A circadian rhythm of serum IgE concentrations has been reported by some (Cricchio et al., 1978; Nye et al., 1975) but was not found by others (DeLeonardis and Brandi, 1984). Gaultier et al. (1987) compared the circadian

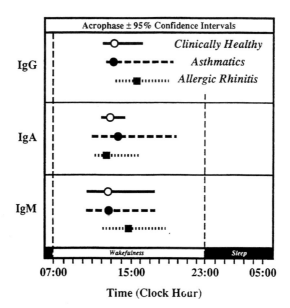

FIGURE 20-10 Circadian acrophase with 95 percent confidence interval of serum immunoglobulins in clinically healthy subjects and patients with allergic asthma or rhinitis. SOURCE: Adapted from Cricchio et al. (1979).

variations in serum total IgE in clinically healthy children with that in asthmatic patients. No statistically significant circadian rhythm was validated ·in the healthy children, who showed low levels of IgE. In contrast, the asthmatic children who had substantially higher serum IgE concentrations showed a large-amplitude circadian rhythm with a double peak during daytime (presumably representing a 12-h rhythm) and a nocturnal trough.

Circadian variations in complement components, and in the activation of the alternate pathway in the complement response, were reported (Haus et al., 1983; Hoopes and McCall, 1977; Kim et al., 1980). The timing of the circadian rhythms of properdin was altered during starvation (Kim et al., 1980). In disease states like systemic lupus and rheumatoid arthritis, circulating immune complexes show circadian variations that may be of clinical importance (Isenberg et al., 1981).

Periodicities and/or response patterns that are not circadian are prominent in humoral immune phenomena. Rhythms with about 7-d periods (circaseptan rhythms) or longer (most frequently in multiples of the 7-d cycle, e.g., 14 or 21 days) occur in the function of several components of the immune system, for example, in the formation of antibodies in different experimental systems in a large number of animal species. Circaseptan rhythms in antibody-forming cells or antibody blood levels and in the hemagglutination response of rodents after immunization against sheep red blood cells or allogenic thymic cells have been reported by Britton and Moller (1968), Grossman et al. (1980), Romball and Weigle (1973, 1976), Stimpfling and Richardson (1967), Weigle (1975), and others (for review, see Levi and Halberg, 1982).

Seasonal variations or circannual rhythms in serum immunoglobulins were reported in clinically healthy subjects with peak levels of IgG, IgA, and IgM occurring during midsummer to midautumn (Lu et al., 1979; Reinberg et al., 1979). In patients with atopic diseases, there were some differences in phase, with slightly earlier values for IgG and IgA but with a substantially different timing for IgM, which showed a peak in February.

BIOLOGIC RHYTHMS IN RESPONSE TO VACCINATION

Circadian time dependency of the human response to inoculation with antigens is less well documented. Pöllman and Pöllman (1988) found a statistically significant lower antibody titer in subjects inoculated with hepatitis B antigen during the morning hours (07:00–09:00) as compared with subjects immunized during the afternoon (13:00–15:00). Also the side effects (pain and swelling around the injection site) were less after inoculation in the morning. The question was raised if these differences may be due to differences in the plasma cortisol concentration, which are higher in the morning and which already in physiologic concentrations show recognizable effects upon monocytes and T-lymphocytes.

Feigin et al. (1967a) gave attenuated Venezuelan equine encephalomyelitis (VEE) vaccine at 08:00 or at 20:00 to 40 healthy young men (20 at each time). A significant serologic response verifying infection was demonstrated in each subject. The number of subjects immunized at 08:00. who became ill was not statistically different from those immunized at 20:00, and there was no difference in the duration or severity of illness between the two groups (Alevizatos et al., 1967). However, the number of virus particles present in white blood cells reached its peak on day 2 after immunization at 08:00 and was delayed until day 6 in the subjects inoculated at 20:00.

There was a marked alteration in the circadian rhythm of whole blood amino acids (Feigin et al., 1967a, b) in all subjects sampled irrespective of time of inoculation. However, the rhythm alteration was apparent during days 1 through 4 in the group immunized at 08:00 and during days 2 through 8 in the group immunized at 20:00. Thus, both the disappearance of the virus particles from the circulating white blood cells and the disturbance of amino acid circadian periodicity occurred later after inoculation at 20:00 as compared with the inoculation at 8:00 A.M. These observations suggest that the effect of an infectious microorganism on the human host may depend to some degree on the time of exposure (Feigin et al., 1967a).

Langlois et al. (1995) reported data from two field trials of influenza vaccine (one conducted during summer, the other during fall). The vaccine given in both studies contained three antigens (A/Chile/83, A/Philippines 82, and B/USSR/83). The vaccine was administered to over 800 different patients between 08:30 and 17:00. Injection time-dependent differences in antibody response were detected in first-time inoculated subjects only in one of these studies and only for the A/Philippines antigen. The antibody response to this antigen was considerably larger than the response to the two others, which may explain these differences. However, the difference between the two studies could also be due to seasonal variations in the antibody response. Seasonal variations in the immune system have been reported in human subjects (Levi et al., 1988b; Shifrine et al., 1982a) and in experimental animals (Fernandes, 1994; Shifrine et al., 1982b).

The systemic reactions noted after first vaccination in these studies showed no circadian variation in occurrence or severity. In contrast, the local side effects after revaccination showed a statistically significant circadian variation even after correction for all known potentially confounding factors including age. The local reactions at the injection site (redness, hardness, and soreness) were most pronounced when the immunization took place around midafternoon. This finding was consistent in both studies and is in agreement with the observations by Pöllman and Pöllman (1988) using a different antigen (HB vaccine).

Effects of immunization on the circadian time structure of the immunized subjects were also observed. Westaway et al. (1995) studied the urinary excretion of cortisol in infants before and after immunization against diphtheria;

tetanus; pertussis; and haemophilus influenzae, type B. The immunization produced a significant increase of rectal temperature during the following night in all infants. Body temperature failed to fall during the night, although febrile levels were rarely obtained. Infants without an adult-like circadian body temperature pattern showed a significant increase in urinary cortisol excretion during the night and the morning after immunization. After an adult-like body temperature pattern had developed, immunization no longer significantly raised urinary cortisol output.

No such correlation was observed between the extent of temperature disturbance and the excretion of cortisol after the second immunization. These observations suggest significant developmental changes in the cortisol response to immunization. The change in the hypothalamic-pituitary-adrenal (HPA) axis from responding to not responding to the vaccines appeared to be more strongly related to the development of an adult-like body temperature pattern than to age. Since adult-like body temperature patterns develop at considerably different ages in different babies, it appears that some infants will remain in an infantile stage of their immunological development as far as cortisol excretion is concerned for much longer than others. The developing infant seems to undergo a series of changes that may radically affect the way in which it copes with infection. Individual differences in this developmental process may underlie differences in vulnerability among infants.

Data thus far available on the response of human subjects to vaccination support the following conclusions:

• Differences in immune response as a function of the circadian time of the introduction of antigen may occur as indicated by differences in antibody titer in clinically healthy subjects. These differences may be limited to certain antigens and/or to a certain degree of immune response and may also depend on other factors (such as seasonal variations), which at this time have not been systematically studied.

• Higher antibody titers can be achieved by vaccinating during midday or afternoon. However, the circadian differences described are quantitative in nature and all subjects studied achieved some degree of immunity irrespective of the time of vaccination.

• The circadian rhythms in antibody response described conceivably will be of some importance for the success of vaccinations, especially in subjects with poor antibody formation (Fletscher, 1993).

• Vaccination leads to a disturbance of the circadian rhythms of clinical (e.g., body temperature), endocrine (cortisol), and metabolic (e.g., blood amino acids) variables, which differ as a function of the time of inoculation and, in infants, as a function of the maturity of the circadian time structure.

• The most consistent findings of rhythmicity of the effects of antigen exposure in human subjects are the more pronounced local side effects after antigen inoculation at noon and during the afternoon in a previously sensitized individual.

• Vaccination response patterns other than those with circadian rhythmicity (e.g., circaseptan or circannual) have thus far not been explored.

CHRONOBIOLOGY IN CELL-MEDIATED IMMUNITY, INCLUDING ALLOGRAFT REJECTION

The development of cell-mediated immunity and the response to challenge, including the elimination of immunologically incompatible cells as seen in allograft rejection, is a complex process involving macrophages, cytotoxic T-cells, NK cells, cytokines, and other factors. Several of these factors are circadian periodic. In addition, many cell-mediated immune phenomena (e.g., rejection of tissue allografts) also show infradian (mostly circaseptan) response patterns.

The development of cell-mediated immunity and the response to reintroduced or persisting antigen are modified both by the time when the antigen is first encountered and by the time of challenge. In oxazolone-sensitized, light-dark synchronized rats, the ear swelling after challenge with this agent showed a large-amplitude circadian rhythmicity. The mean response to challenge during the daily rest span of the animals was more than 8 times that seen in rats challenged at the time of onset of the daily activity (Knapp et al., 1981). A reversed light-dark cycle did reverse the timing of the peak and trough of the response to antigen challenge (Pownall et al., 1979).

Clinically healthy, diurnally active human subjects testing positive for PPD (due largely to BCG[3] vaccination) showed, when injected intradermally with PPD during different circadian stages, a circadian variation in response with a maximum at 07:00 and a minimum at 22:00. The asymmetric biphasic pattern in this study suggests a superimposed ultradian rhythmicity (Cove-Smith et al., 1978).

In allograft rejection, although the immune-incompatible cells remain inside the host organism during development of the immune response, the time of the first encounter with the antigen modifies the intensity of the ensuing immune reaction. For example, the rejection of allogenic skin in mice and of kidney grafts in rats was delayed significantly by grafting during the early dark span, the activity period of the animals that corresponds to the time of the circadian peak in serum corticosterone (Halberg et al., 1974; Ratté et al., 1973).

The more marked local response to PPD administered to sensitized human subjects during the early morning hours and the more frequent manifestation of the signs of renal allograft rejection at that time (Knapp et al., 1981) (the peak in both variables found to be around 07:00) suggests that the cell-mediated immune response is more vigorous during the late night and early morning

---

[3] Bacillus Calmette-Guerin, used for tuberculosis vaccination.

hours. This rhythm may be of interest for treatment with immunosuppressive agents that are given in current medical practice without chronotherapeutic considerations mainly during daytime. Sinusoidal infusions of cyclosporin with the maximal dose of the drug given at certain times of the day showed in dogs carrying kidney allografts (in comparison with a treatment with equal doses given throughout the 24-h span) a statistically significant circadian rhythm in response. Similarly, cyclosporin chronotherapy of pancreas-allotransplanted rats revealed circadian stage dependence of the dosing time to obtain an optimal gain in graft function (Liu et al., 1986).

Transplant studies in human subjects have shown, in addition to the circadian rhythm in the onset of the functional manifestations of renal transplant rejection, a circaseptan rhythm in the rejection of kidney allografts (DeVecchi et al., 1981). In 157 patients with kidney transplants, rejection episodes were clinically diagnosed when one of the biochemical variables of primary interest as a criterion of rejection (i.e., blood creatinine, blood urea, proteinuria) began to change. The occurrence of rejection episodes during a 2-mo observation after transplantation followed an infradian rhythm with a period longer than precisely 7 days (8.1 days). The fact that the period found in these patients is slightly but consistently different from the 7 days of the social week suggests that this period is endogenous in origin. The apparent 8.1-d periodicity was also different from the changes in corticosteroid regimen in those patients, which occurred at precisely 7-d intervals. Similar findings in human studies as well as in animal experiments have been reported also for heart and pancreas allografts (Liu et al., 1986).

The circaseptan rhythm in allograft rejection is of clinical interest since it appears to provide an opportunity to optimize antirejection therapy, both along the circaseptan and the circadian time scales. The timing of the best antirejection treatment schedule in diurnally active human subjects, with the maximal dose given during the dark span, is of interest in view of a similar timing found for the optimal cyclosporine effects in nocturnal rats bearing heart or pancreas allografts (Liu et al., 1986). A similarity of timing of duration of circadian rhythms in diurnally active humans and nocturnal rodents is found also in the circadian rhythm of melatonin and of some red cell parameters in the peripheral blood (Haus et al., 1983).

TIME-DEPENDENT CHANGES IN CUTANEOUS ALLERGY AND ALLERGIC ASTHMA

The cutaneous response to histamine and to the antigens of ragweed, grass pollen antigen, and house dust, varies in a circadian rhythmic fashion. The greatest sensitivity is found 3 to 6 hours prior to the middle of the patient's sleep span, which in diurnally active human subjects usually corresponds to the hours between 18:00 and 23:00. The area of a reaction from a skin test carried out during this time is on the average about 2 to 3 times larger than that found for an identical test on the same patient during the time of low reactivity (between 07:00 and 11:00) (Lee et al., 1977; Reinberg, 1967; Reinberg et al., 1965). In the application to patients with allergic diseases, testing with antigens or substances like histamine or acetylcholine early in the day may result in false negatives. In repeated testing of allergic patients, it is important to apply the antigen or other stimuli during the same circadian stage of cutaneous or bronchial reactivity. Only standardization of the time of testing in relation to the activity-rest pattern of the patient will yield reproducible results that are comparable from one test to the other (Reinberg and Sidi, 1966).

In bronchial asthma, the circadian times of the peak and trough of the hyperreactivity of the bronchial tree to histamine (DeVries et al., 1962) are almost identical with those found for the circadian rhythm in cutaneous reactivity to intradermal injections with histamine or skin allergens (Lee et al., 1977; Reinberg, 1967; Reinberg et al., 1963, 1965). A similar circadian rhythm was found in the hyperactivity of the bronchial response to the inhalation of acetylcholine (Reinberg et al., 1971). The time when asthmatics are exposed to a specific triggering agent appears to be almost as important as the quantitative aspects of the exposure. Asthmatic attacks, including deaths from severe asthmatic attacks, occur predominantly during the night hours primarily between 02:00 and 07:00, with peak incidence between 04:00 and 05:00 (Benatar, 1986; Dethlefsen and Repges, 1985; Hetzel et al., 1977; Turner-Warwick, 1988).

It appears that these rhythms are predominantly an expression of host sensitivity and are determined by endogenous circadian bioperiodicities in relationship to changes in the external environment during the 24-h day (Barnes, 1984a, b; Smolensky et al., 1981, 1986a, b). The times of greatest susceptibility to asthmatic attacks and the highest cutaneous sensitivity to antigen coincide with the trough of the circadian rhythm in the excretion of adrenocorticosteroids (Reinberg et al., 1963) and also coincide with the trough of the circadian rhythm in plasma catecholamines. Assumption of a causal relationship between the manifestations of cutaneous and bronchial allergy and the circadian rhythms in cortisol and catecholamines appears tempting. Although the circadian rhythms in plasma cortisol and catecholamines do not seem to be the only factor responsible for the nocturnal exacerbation of the chronic inflammatory processes, it could conceivably contribute to the day-night difference in sensitivity and thus be related to the risk and the frequency of asthma attacks. In addition to the inflammatory component of the disease, the bronchial tone is also strongly regulated by adrenergic mechanisms.

The circadian rhythm in serum IgE may also be related to the periodicity of allergic manifestations. Gaultier et al. (1987) found a fivefold greater mean concentration of IgE in asthmatics than in clinically healthy children, with a high-amplitude circadian rhythm equal to 30 percent of the 24-h mean in asthmatics, which was absent in the healthy subjects (Figure 20-11). In

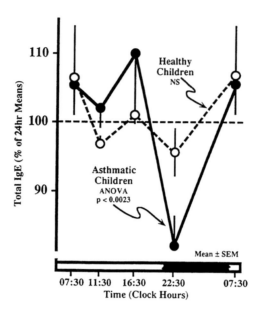

FIGURE 20-11 Circadian rhythm in serum immunoglobulin E (IgE) in children with allergic asthma is not evident in clinically healthy subjects. SOURCE Adapted from Gaultier et al. (1987).

asthmatics, the highest serum IgE levels occur around midday, and the lowest levels occur at night (Kunkel and Jusuf, 1984).

Successful management of asthmatic patients requires an understanding of the circadian features of the disease to achieve an effective chronotherapy for antiasthmatic medications (Reinberg, 1989; Reinberg et al., 1988a,b; Smolensky and D'Alonzo, 1994, 1997; Smolensky et al., 1986b, 1987).

THE RHYTHMS OF SLEEP AND IMMUNITY

The alternation of sleep-wakefulness is a fundamental part of the human circadian time structure and coordinates numerous other neuroendocrine variables. Several immunologically active hormones and peptides influence the sleep-wake cycle of the brain and are involved in a bidirectional or multidirectional communication among neuroendocrine, immune, and CNS functions (Table 20-2). Most of them show circadian rhythmicity, and some are influenced by environmental factors acting as synchronizers or as masking agents. IL-1 and other cytokines play a regulatory role on the sleep-wake cycle (Opp et al., 1992) and interact in this process with various immunologically active neuroendocrine substances (Krueger, 1990). The physiologic regulation

TABLE 20–2 Immunologically Active Variables Affecting Sleep and/or Wakefulness

Promoting Sleep	Reference
Stimulating IL-1 and Sleep	
Insulin	Krueger, 1990
Growth hormone	Krueger, 1990
Growth hormone releasing factor	Krueger, 1990
Melatonin	Krueger, 1990
Somatostatin	Krueger, 1990
Immunologically Active Peptides	
Interleukin-1 (IL-1)	Krueger et al., 1983, 1984; Tobler et al., 1984
Interleukin-2 (IL-2)	De Sarro et al., 1990
Interferon-α	De Sarro et al., 1990
Tumor necrosis factor	Shoham et al., 1987
Factor S	Krueger et al., 1982
Muramyl peptides	Krueger et al., 1984; Masek and Kadlec, 1983; Pappenheimer, 1983
Vasoactive intestinal peptide	Jouvet, 1984; O'Dorisio et al., 1984
Delta sleep-inducing peptide	Graf and Kastin, 1984; Yehuda et al., 1987

Promoting Wakefulness	Reference
Inhibiting IL-1 and Sleep	
Corticotropin-releasing factor	Krueger, 1990
ACTH	Krueger, 1990
α-MSH	Krueger, 1990
Glucocorticoids	Krueger, 1990

of the sleep-wakefulness rhythm requires a specific constellation of multiple natural sleep-promoting or wakefulness-promoting substances which are, in part, determined by their circadian rhythms and in part by environmental and behavioral conditions (Moldofsky, 1994). Periods of predisposition to sleepiness are separated by periods of resistance to sleep (Lavie and Weller, 1989).

Numerous immunologic variables are influenced by the sleep-wakefulness pattern and may be altered at times of environmentally enforced sleep irregularities and especially by sleep deprivation. For example, NK cell activity is related to sleep and declines during nocturnal (or other) sleep periods (Shahal et al., 1992). Sleep deprivation in experimental animals and in human subjects leads to an impairment of immune functions, which if prolonged, will lead to the death of the animals (Everson, 1993) and to the fatal familial insomnia syndrome of human subjects (Portaluppi et al., 1994). However, even much shorter periods of sleep deprivation lead to rhythm alterations and to marked impairment of immune function. In human subjects, Moldofsky et al. (1989) found during a single night of sleep deprivation increased plasma IL-1 and IL-2 concentrations with an alteration in the PMW response of B-lymphocytes and a depression or absence of the nocturnal decline in NK cell activity. The response to PHA remained unchanged. These changes appeared to be unrelated to the circadian rhythm in plasma cortisol. After 48 hours of sleep deprivation, Palmblad et al. (1979) also found a reduced PHA mitogen response. After 72 hours of sleep deprivation, there was an increase in plasma cortisol, an increase in interferon production by lymphocytes, and reduced phagocytosis by polymorphonuclear leukocytes (Palmblad et al., 1976).

The effect of sleep deprivation on the ability to respond to the introduction of an antigen has been studied in mice. Mice immunized against influenza virus were challenged, followed by a 7-h span of sleep deprivation. Whereas normally sleeping, immunized mice were able to clear the virus from the respiratory tract within 3 days of challenge, in immunized, sleep-deprived animals, the extent of viral recovery was almost the same as in nonimmunized animals (Figure 20-12) (Brown et al., 1989; Husband, 1993).

Phase shifts, as they are encountered in shift workers or after transmeridian flights, or rhythm disturbances in people under grossly irregular work schedules lead to internal desynchronization of immune-related circadian rhythms and to impairment of immune functions. In rats, weekly inversion of a light:dark (LD) 12:12 lighting regimen led after 2 months to a decreased cellular immune response as measured by mitogen stimulation with concanavalin A (ConA) and by a popliteal lymph node assay (Kort and Weijma, 1982). A rather severe immune impairment was found after 33 weeks of weekly phase shifting. Spot checks of adrenal function in these animals, measured *in vitro* and *in vivo* at a single time point only, did not reveal substantial changes. The latter result has to be qualified since single time point sampling does not allow an evaluation of the adrenal cycle. In studies of shift workers, Nakano et al. (1982) reported lower proliferative responses in lymphocytes as compared with regular daytime workers. Since shift work is often accompanied by a certain degree of sleep deprivation, it is unclear whether the impaired immune function in shift workers is a consequence of circadian desynchronization, sleep deprivation, or both.

CHANGES IN IMMUNE SYSTEM-RELATED VARIABLES DURING THE MENSTRUAL CYCLE

Gonadal steroids contribute to the regulation of immune function (Da Silva and Hall, 1992; H. S. Fox, 1995b; Hasty et al., 1994; Mortin and Courchay, 1994; Schuurs and Verheul, 1990). Receptors for steroid hormones are present in circulating lymphocytes (Bellido et al., 1993; Daniel et al., 1983; Stimson,

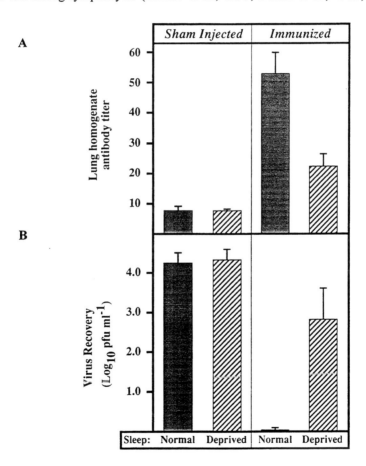

FIGURE 20-12 Effect of sleep deprivation on ability to respond to challenge with antigen (influenza virus) in immunized mice. Challenge followed by 7 hours of sleep deprivation. Sleep deprivation leads to impairment of antibody response (A) and of elimination of antigen (B). SOURCE: Adapted from Brown et al. (1989).

1988). No or only minor changes in the number of circulating blood cells were reported during the menstrual cycle (Eichler and Keiling, 1988; Fox et al., 1991). In a comparison between day 6 and day 22 of the menstrual cycle, there were no consistent changes in the proportion of lymphocyte subtypes, nor were there any significant changes in the absolute numbers or in the circadian rhythmicity in total white blood cell count, granulocytes, lymphocytes, T- and B-cells, T-helper and suppressor cells, and NK cells (Dixon-Northern et al., 1994). The only apparent difference as a function of the day of the menstrual cycle was found in the circadian periodicity of monocytes, for which the trough was found at 12 noon for day 6 and at midnight for day 22 (Dixon-Northern et al., 1994). The limited sampling and the small number of subjects in these studies do not allow the drawing of final conclusions.

In contrast, the plasma IL-1 activity (Cannon and Dinarello, 1985) is consistently increased after ovulation in the luteal phase of the menstrual cycle simultaneously with the elevation in body temperature. In view of the thermogenic effect of IL-1, this may be related and may also be consistent with the observation that progesterone and estrogen increase the macrophage production of IL-1 (Olsen and Kovacs, 1996).

Related to differences in the human immune response during different stages of the menstrual cycle may be the clinical observation of a greatly reduced overall and recurrence-free survival in women with breast cancer who were operated on during days 3 to 12 after onset of menstruation as compared with women operated on between days 0 through 2 or days 13 through 32 (Badwe et al., 1991; Hrushesky and März, 1994; Senie et al., 1991).

SEASONAL CHANGES AND/OR CIRCANNUAL VARIATIONS IN IMMUNE RESPONSE

Changes of immune-related variables during different seasons may be caused by climatic differences, including day length, temperature, and related factors such as exposure to allergens and microorganisms, but they may also be the consequence of endogenous circannual rhythms that may or may not be synchronized by environmental (climatic and other) stimuli (Haus and Touitou, 1994b). Circannual rhythms have been demonstrated in animals kept for their entire life, and in some instances for generations, in environments with a standardized lighting regimen and constant temperature (Figure 20-12) (Brock, 1983, 1991; Haus et al., 1974a, 1984, 1997; Haus M. et al., 1984), and free-running circannual rhythms have been described in human subjects (Haus and Touitou, 1994a). The seasonal rhythmicity in lymphocyte blastogenic response persists in young mice kept in a constant environment (Brock, 1983). Mortality in the young animals varied in a circannual fashion, with the peak occurring when the proliferation rates of both T- and B-cells were low (Brock, 1987). In contrast in old animals, the amplitude of the circannual rhythm of T- and B-cells was markedly decreased, and mortality was consistently higher throughout the year (Brock, 1987, 1991).

Levi et al. (1988b) found seasonal modulation of the circadian rhythms of circulating T-and NK-lymphocyte subsets in healthy volunteers. These studies suggested a rhythm with a period of about 6 months for circulating T-helper cells. There appeared to be circadian desynchronization of circulating lymphocytes during spring, which corresponded in its timing to the peak incidence of viral infections and of Hodgkin's disease (Levi et al., 1988b). Pati et al. (1987) described in mice a 6-mo rhythm in the proliferative mitogen response of splenic B-lymphocytes and a circannual rhythm for NK cell activity. Shifrine et al. (1980, 1982a, b) found seasonal variations in cell-mediated immunity in dogs and in humans. Studying the whole-blood, lectin-induced, lymphocyte mitogen response, they observed a peak in summer and poor response to mitogens in winter.

A circannual variation of rubella antibody titer was noted in a large number of patients who were followed for 7 years (Rosenblatt et al., 1982). In Finland, a country with marked climatic differences between the seasons, Katila et al. (1993) found a seasonal variation in the interferon-producing capacity of leukocytes from clinically healthy subjects, with low values during the summer months. In contrast, no seasonal differences in this variable were found in Japan (Kishida et al., 1987), a country with lesser seasonal climatic changes.

Deficiency in erythrocyte adenosine aminohydrolase activity has been reported in patients with severe combined immunodeficiency disease (Giblett et al., 1972), and alterations in the activity of this enzyme have been associated with immunologic loads (Tritsch et al., 1975) and with neoplasia (Zimmer et al., 1975). In a study extending over 2 years, Nechaev et al. (1977) showed a circannual variation of erythrocyte adenosine aminohydrolase in healthy subjects and in patients with a variety of neoplastic diseases of various stages and treated with a variety of chemotherapeutic agents. In healthy subjects and in patients with cancer, the circannual variation resulted in relatively low enzyme levels between April and June and higher levels between October and February.

Seasonal modifications in immune response must be considered in clinical trials and in the planning of immunotherapeutic treatment strategies for various diseases.

MODIFICATION OF IMMUNE-RELATED RHYTHMS BY EXERCISE

Physical exercise alters the circadian periodicity of several components of the immune system and of related neuroendocrine variables (Shephard et al., 1995; Winget et al., 1994). With moderate exercise, these changes are short in duration and may only transiently mask the circadian rhythm of, for example, catecholamines, the numbers of polymorphonuclear leukocytes, and lymphocytes. Physical performance and performance tolerance vary rhythmically. Maximal performance (e.g., in grip strength or diverse sport activities) is reached in diurnally active human subjects during the late afternoon (Lundeen et al., 1990; Winget et al., 1994).

Exercise induces changes in the T-cell number, in the relation of CD4+ cells to CD8+ cells, the sensitivity of T-cell β-adrenoceptors, NK cell activity, interleukin production, and cell proliferation. While moderate physical exercise and training may improve certain immune functions, severe and exhaustive exercise is immunosuppressive (for review, see Shephard et al., 1995). Severe and exhaustive exercise can also mark many of the neuroendocrine rhythms that are instrumental in regulating the rhythmicity and, to some degree, the integrity of the immune system (Opstad, 1991, 1992). However, no investigations of the effects of circadian and other periodicities in performance on the response of the immune system to exercise have been found in the available literature. Investigations of the periodicity in exercise effects (acute strenuous as well as endurance) on the neuroendocrine-immune system network might be of considerable interest for military and sports medicine.

MODIFICATION OF IMMUNE-RELATED RHYTHMS BY TIME OF FOOD UPTAKE

The activity-rest and sleep-wakefulness pattern is not the only synchronizer acting on the mammalian circadian system. If a large proportion of the daily caloric intake is taken as one major meal at a certain circadian phase, the timing of food uptake may mask the circadian rhythms. If such intake persists for a prolonged time, it may become the dominant synchronizer of some circadian periodic functions. In animal studies, many circadian rhythms related directly or indirectly to immune functions can be adjusted in their timing by time-restricted meal feeding at certain circadian stages (Halberg and Stephens, 1959; Lakatua et al., 1983; Nelson et al., 1975; Scheving et al., 1976). Other rhythms, however, will remain synchronized to the light-dark regimen in experimental animals or to the activity-rest pattern in humans. A number of endocrine and hematologic rhythms may show, under the influence of the "competing" synchronizers, some changes in their usual timing without the apparent predominance of either synchronizer.

In human subjects, time adaptation of rhythms by timed food uptake is much less pronounced and can be achieved only by exposure to rigorous feeding schedules that would be uncommon in everyday life. Clinically healthy, young adult volunteers following a diurnal activity pattern with sleep during the night (typically between 23:00 and 06:30) who received all their calories in the form of a single meal as breakfast or as dinner were studied over a 24-h span at the end of 3 weeks on that regimen. The circadian rhythms of plasma insulin, serum iron, and blood urea nitrogen concentration had adapted their timing to the time of food uptake, irrespective of the activity pattern of the subjects. In contrast, the timing of the circadian rhythms in growth hormone (GH), plasma cortisol, serum chlorides, and total leukocyte count had shifted only slightly, while the rhythm in circulating lymphocytes was not statistically significantly different between the (same) subjects studied on both dietary regimens and on a three-meal eating schedule (Halberg et al., 1995; Haus et al., 1984, 1988). In a shorter study in which all calories were given either as breakfast or as dinner, Sensi et al. (1984) found after only 3 days, marked phase shifts in the circadian rhythms of respiratory quotient and variables related to carbohydrate metabolism and lipid oxidation. In urinary catecholamines, the evening meal-only schedule delayed the circadian peak for over 5 hours. Cortisol did not seem to be influenced by the short period of meal timing, and sodium and potassium excretion did not show consistent differences between the two diet regimens. After 18 days on the altered schedule of calorie uptake, plasma cortisol and thyroid-stimulating hormone (TSH) circadian rhythms were similar, as seen with a three-meal diet. The circadian rhythm in PRL was detectable when the single daily meal was given at 18:00 but disappeared when the meal was given at 10:00.

From these and other studies in human subjects (Goetz et al., 1976; Sensi et al., 1984) and in animals (Lakatua et al., 1983; Scheving et al., 1976), it appears that for the circadian rhythms related to digestive and metabolic functions, including those of the endocrine and exocrine pancreas and of the gastrointestinal tract epithelia, the time of food uptake acts as the dominant synchronizer. Also the circadian rhythms of many liver enzymes are synchronized primarily by the time of food uptake (Fuller and Snoddy, 1968). In human subjects, some of the most stable rhythms (such as plasma cortisol and circulating lymphocytes), which directly relate to the regulation of immune functions, are apparently synchronized predominantly by the activity-rest schedule and the related light-dark regimen. However, with prolonged exposure to unusual feeding schedules, the changes observed in GH and insulin may well lead to changes in the timing of certain immune-related variables, although experimental evidence for such a relationship is thus far lacking.

It appears that the phase adaptation of a number of circadian rhythms of physiologic importance in shift workers can be reinforced, delayed, or even prevented by the timing of food uptake in relation to the activity-rest pattern. Internal desynchronization brought about by the independent alteration of two competing synchronizers may lead to functional or even organic disturbances, as has been suggested by a variety of problems, including the appearance of gastric ulcers in shift workers exposed to physiologically unacceptable alterations of their activity-rest pattern and the time of food uptake (Carandente and Halberg, 1976; Gibinski et al., 1979; Tarquini, 1980).

BIOLOGIC RHYTHMICITY IN NEUROENDOCRINE-IMMUNE INTERACTIONS

The rhythmicity observed in the immune system is in part regulated by the multifrequency neuroendocrine rhythms that characterize the mammalian time structure and in some frequencies are environmentally synchronized (for reviews, see, e.g., Touitou and Haus, 1994; Van Cauter and Turek, 1995). Interactions between the endocrine and the immune system are found at every level from the hypothalamic nuclei to the receptors in the cells of the target organs (for reviews, see Auernhammer and Strasburger, 1995; Besedovsky and Del Rey, 1996; Blalock, 1992; Daynes et al., 1995; Fabris et al., 1995; Maestroni, 1993; Murphy et al., 1995; Olsen and Kovacs, 1996; Weigent and Blalock, 1995; Wilder, 1995).

Neuroendocrine hormones that act as immune modulators include CRF, ACTH, cortisol, dehydroepiandrosterone (DHEA), and DHEA-sulfate (-S), estrogen, progesterone, testosterone, melatonin, PRL, GH, vasopressin, β-endorphin, and other proopiomelanocortin (POMC) peptides, thyrotropin-releasing hormone (TRH), and TSH (Blalock, 1989, 1992; Weigent and Blalock, 1995).

Immune competent cells, including both T- and B-lymphocytes, carry high-affinity receptors for the POMC peptides including ACTH (Clarke and Bost, 1989) and opioid peptides (Carr, 1991). The same classes of receptors as found in neural tissue have been identified on cells of the immune system (Carr, 1991). ACTH and endorphins inhibit antibody production (Johnson et al., 1982) and modulate many aspects of immune cell function (Carr, 1992; Johnson et al., 1982, 1992).

In turn, mouse and human lymphocytes produce POMC-derived peptides, including ACTH, which are biologically active (Blalock, 1992, 1994), as shown by the rise in corticosterone found in hypophysectomized animals exposed to infectious agents (Bayle et al., 1991; Smith et al., 1982). This effect was abolished in chicken if B-lymphocytes were deleted by bursectomy (Bayle et al., 1991). Although the lymphocyte-produced hormones usually do not reach concentrations in the circulation that allow their measurement, their local production in an auto- or paracrine manner by cells of the immune system at the site of an immune process or inflammation can lead to immunomodulation (Johnson et al., 1992). At the present time, no information is available on the periodicity of hormone production by activated cells of the immune system, although some of these cells seem to respond to humoral neuroendocrine controls like CRF or ACTH.

Glucocorticoids exert their powerful anti-inflammatory actions in part by downregulating the transcription of inflammatory mediators (Russo, 1992), including the cytokines IL-1 (Kern et al., 1988), IL-2 (Kelso and Munck, 1984), IL-3 (Homo-Delarche et al., 1991), IL-6 (Besedovsky and Del Rey, 1996), IL-8 (Mukaida et al., 1993), GM-CSF, TNF-α (Homo-Delarche et al., 1991), and

INF-γ (Kelso and Munck, 1984). The large-amplitude circadian rhythm in plasma cortisol concentration in humans with peak values in the early morning hours in diurnally active subjects has been related to changes in immune response, with the minimum in response corresponding to the peak in cortisol concentrations (Lee et al., 1997; Reinberg et al., 1963). This same association has been observed for the circadian rhythm in plasma corticosterone in nocturnal rodents, which exhibit peak corticosterone values at the end of the daily light span and the beginning of the dark span.

The anti-inflammatory action of cortisol is balanced at any one time by the immunostimulatory hormones, including GH, PRL, and melatonin (Hooghe et al., 1993; Maestroni et al., 1986), which all peak during the night hours. The circadian rhythmicity in immune response appears to be, to a large extent, the net result of the balance at any one time between the immunosuppressive effect of glucocorticoids and the effect of immunostimulant hormones modulated by cytokine feedback and peripheral hormone production by cells of the immune system (Weigent and Blalock, 1995).

Immunomodulation also occurs at the target tissue level with selectivity of hormone effects and temporal variations due to the activity of specific enzyme systems metabolizing and transforming hormones at the level of the target cells. This seems to be the case for the formation of DHEA from its prehormone DHEA-S in lymphoid tissues (Daynes et al., 1995). DHEA modulates the immune response in lymphoid tissue after antigen exposure (Daynes et al., 1995). Its decreased production (e.g., with aging or the decreased liberation from its prehormone DHEA-S) leads to immunosenescence, which can be overcome by the administration of DHEA. The poor response of immunosenescent elderly subjects to vaccination (Schwab et al., 1989) is thought to be a consequence of the decrease in production of DHEA (Daynes et al., 1995). When aged animals were given oral supplementation with DHEA-S, the usual mature adult pattern of inducible T-cell lymphokines was restored, and a solid humoral immune response was obtained (Daynes and Araneo, 1992; Garg and Bondada, 1993). Similarly, the direct incorporation of DHEA or DHEA-S into a protein vaccine formulation was found to promote the development of a strong immune response in age-compromised hosts (Araneo et al., 1993). There is a high-amplitude circadian rhythm of DHEA, which in its timing is comparable to that of cortisol (Haus et al., 1995). In contrast, DHEA-S in humans characteristically shows a more flat circadian variation, with a peak later during the day (Haus et al., 1988, 1995). DHEA-S also shows a circannual rhythm, which in its amplitude may be equal to or higher than that of the circadian rhythm (Haus et al., 1988; Nicolau et al., 1984). No data are available relating these rhythmic variations in adrenal androgens to circadian or circannual changes in the immune system.

The serum PRL concentration shows a large-amplitude circadian rhythm, with peak values during the night hours (Haus et al., 1980). This rhythm is modulated by a marked seasonal variation found in women but not in men

(Haus et al., 1980, 1988; Touitou et al., 1983). Also ethnic-geographic differences in the circadian and circannual amplitudes of PRL concentrations have been reported (Haus et al., 1980). The circadian variation in plasma PRL concentrations is modulated by sleep but to a lesser degree than that of growth hormone (hGH).

PRL is a major immunoregulating hormone. CD4+ and CD8+ cells and macrophages express PRL receptors (Gala and Shevach, 1993). Nuclear PRL receptors play an important role in IL-2 induced T-cell proliferation *in vitro* (Clevenger et al., 1990), which can be inhibited by PRL antibodies (Hartmann et al., 1989). Lymphocytes and macrophages also seem to produce PRL or a "PRL-like" factor (Gala and Shevach, 1994), and PRL has been suggested as a growth factor for lymphoid cell proliferation (Russell et al., 1988).

In animal experiments, hypophysectomy or suppression of PRL secretion by the dihydroxyphenylalanine (DOPA) agonist bromocryptine leads to a state of immunodeficiency with decreased resistance to infection, which can be reversed by treatment with PRL (Bernton et al., 1988; Nagy et al., 1983). Cyclosporine, an immunosuppressive fungal peptide, inhibits PRL binding to T-lymphocytes (Hiestand et al., 1986), competing in a dose-dependent fashion for receptor sites. Stimulation of PRL secretion can reverse the immunosuppression induced by cyclosporine (Hiestand et al., 1986), suggesting that the immunosuppressive effect of cyclosporine, which in its extent is circadian, circaseptan, and circannual periodic, may be mediated by the displacement of PRL from binding sites on lymphocytes (Liu et al., 1986).

The unbalanced prevalence of proinflammatory hormones like PRL and GH over the anti-inflammatory regulators like the hormones of the HPA axis is thought to favor the development of chronic inflammatory and autoimmune diseases like rheumatoid arthritis (Berczi et al., 1993). Improvement of autoimmune uveitis occurred in patients treated (for unrelated conditions) with bromocryptine (Hedner and Bynke, 1985), an observation that seemed to be supported by observations in an animal model (Palestine et al., 1987). The relapse in patients with rheumatoid arthritis often seen after childbirth may be related to the high serum PRL concentrations encountered at this time (Wilder, 1995). Events that affect PRL secretion, like chronic stress and sleep deprivation as experienced in military situations, and also the administration of many pharmacotherapeutic agents that are known to alter the secretion of PRL (e.g., phenothiazines, opiates, neuroleptics, L-DOPA, and bromocryptine) may alter immunologic function and show undesirable and sometimes unexpected side effects.

GH shows a marked circadian rhythm that is largely but not exclusively related to sleep, with a major spike in hormone secretion after sleep onset and a decrease in peak height reported during aging. Sleep deprivation and irregular sleep-wakefulness patterns alter this rhythm through the "masking" effect of sleep. Receptors for GH have been found on immunocompetent cells, many of which also show receptors for growth hormone-releasing hormone (GHRH) (for review, see Auernhammer and Strasburger, 1995); GHRH in low (but not in high) concentrations enhances PHA-stimulated lymphocyte proliferation, IL-2 production in human peripheral blood mononuclear cells (PBMC) (Valtora et al., 1991), and antigen responses (Mercola et al., 1981). Conversely, *in vitro* stimulation of human PBMC by the T-cell mitogens PHA and ConA or by IL-2 produces a marked rise in GH secreted by PBMC (Hattori et al., 1990; Varma et al., 1993), which suggests bidirectional interactions within a somatotropic immune axis (Walker, 1994). Many of the effects of GH on the immune system are not direct, but they may be mediated through insulin-like growth factor (IGF)-I or may be due to high-affinity binding of GH to the PRL receptor. IGF-I shows a low-amplitude circadian rhythm (Haus et al., 1988) and exerts proliferative effects both on T-cells (Clark et al., 1993) and on B-cell progenitors (Gibson et al., 1993; Landreth et al., 1992). Both GH and IGF-I induce immunoglobulin production and proliferation of human plasma cell lines (Kimata and Yoshida, 1994). The local production of hGH and IGF-I, with the autocrine and paracrine effects of these factors on the immune system, may be at least as important as the circulating hormone concentrations.

Melatonin acts as messenger providing information on environmental light and darkness and shows a high-amplitude circadian variation that depends to a large extent on the presence and/or absence of photic stimulation. Melatonin represents an important endogenous immunomodulating agent (Maestroni, 1993) that has been shown to amplify the immune effects of IL-2 and reduce its toxicity (Lissoni et al., 1994) and to modulate TNF toxicity and biologic activity (for review, see Kopp et al., 1994). Melatonin activates human monocytes and induces their cytotoxic properties along with IL-1 secretion (Morrey et al., 1994). The immunostimulating properties of melatonin depend on activated CD4+ cells, which upon melatonin stimulation, show an increased synthesis and/or release of opioid peptides, IL-2 and IL-4, and INF-γ (Maestroni, 1993, 1995). Especially the Th2 variant of T-helper cells is a target of the circadian melatonin signal. Th2 cells are sensitive to INF-γ, which selectively inhibits their proliferative response (Del Prete et al., 1994). INF-γ in turn stimulates melatonin production in the pineal gland (Withyachumnarnkul et al., 1990), while IL-4 inhibits INF-γ production by activated T-cells (Banchereau, 1991), contributing to the balance of pro- and anti-inflammatory and immunostimulating factors. Immune competent cells like macrophages and their predecessors, monocytes, can also synthesize melatonin and serotonin from tryptophan in peripheral blood and tissues (Finocchiaro et al., 1988, 1991), forming a peripheral immunomodulary circuit also involving INF-γ (Finocchiaro et al., 1988). This bidirectional interaction leads to a complex pineal-immune axis, in which melatonin-induced Th2 cytokines, such as IL-4, exert a feedback on Th1 cytokines, such as INF-γ, and restrain their immunostimulating effect on melatonin synthesis. The pineal-immune axis helps to maintain the Th1-Th2 balance, which is instrumental in developing a successful and balanced immune response.

Pinealectomy or functional pinealectomy by constant light or by the β-adrenergic blocker propanolol leads to a decreased ability to mount a primary antibody response (Maestroni and Pierpaoli, 1981). Melatonin can augment the immune response and correct these immunodeficiency states and those that may follow acute stress, viral diseases, or immunosuppressive drug treatment and those found during the process of aging (Maestroni and Conti, 1993). In experimental autoimmune disorders, melatonin acts as an immune stimulant during the development of the disease and accentuates its severity (Hansson et al., 1992; Mattsson et al., 1994).

The effects of melatonin and of drugs acting on melatonin synthesis are strictly circadian time dependent. In animal experiments, the immune suppression by the β-adrenergic blocker propanolol occurred only after evening administration, but not after morning administration of the drug, and could be reversed only by evening administration of melatonin (Maestroni et al., 1987a). Similarly, immune enhancement by melatonin in intact animals was found only when melatonin was injected during the late afternoon or evening (Maestroni et al., 1988). Melatonin given in the morning was either ineffective or even immunosuppressive (Maestroni et al., 1987b).

TSH shows a high-amplitude circadian rhythm and seasonal variation, presumably at least in part as a response to environmental temperature (Haus et al., 1988). Both TRH and TSH interact with the immune system. TSH was reported to augment both T-dependent and T-independent antibody production (Blalock, 1992), to increase the proliferative response of mouse lymphocytes to lectin mitogens, and to stimulate IL-2-induced NK cell activity (Provinciali et al., 1992), apparently acting on both T- and B-cells. TRH induces TSH production by lymphocytes and its effect on the immune system may be mediated by this mechanism (Kruger et al., 1989).

Prolonged, hard, physical exercise combined with sleep and energy deprivation as experienced, for example, during military training courses may lead to rhythm alterations of numerous neuroendocrine variables interacting with the immune system (Opstad, 1991, 1992). Severe physical exercise together with sleep deprivation maintained throughout a span of 5 days leads to partial and, for some of the neuroendocrine variables, complete disappearance of circadian rhythmicity as a group phenomenon (Opstad, 1994). This observation may be due to actual disappearance of a recognizable circadian rhythm due to the severe stress (masking) or due to a desynchronization among the members of the group studied. Some changes (e.g., in the circadian mean of plasma cortisol) were still present 4 to 5 days after termination of the exposure to the combined-exercise sleep deprivation stress. Since optimal function in the human body depends on the "right" sequence of events as expressed by a certain phase relation ("internal timing") of the biologic rhythms within a frequency range, a disruption of this sequence that results in the right metabolite not being provided at the right time may lead to malfunction and immune deficiencies, as seen during exposures to phase shift, sleep deprivation, severe stress, and other factors. Some of these exposures may be unavoidable in a military setting, but they should be recognized as a problem for soldiers and should be included, wherever feasible, in the planning for military deployment and action.

CHRONOPHARMACOLOGY AND CHRONOTHERAPEUTICS

The rhythmicity of events in the immune system and in related functions provides an opportunity to predict the time when certain events are most likely to occur and allows the recognition of transient risk states for immune-related phenomena (e.g., the circadian peak in sensitivity to allergen exposure or the circaseptan response pattern in allograft rejection). The prediction of such risk states allows one to initiate preventive measures or to treat an immune-related disorder at a time when optimal effects can be obtained. Both the time-dependent changes in the pharmacokinetics of an agent (chronopharmacokinetics) and the time-dependent changes in the host response (chronopharmacodynamics) must be considered in the design of a chronotherapeutic treatment schedule (Wood and Hrushesky, 1994). Timing of treatment with INF-α, according to the circadian rhythm in susceptibility and/or tolerance of the patient, has led to improved therapeutic effects and decreased toxicity (Depres-Brummer et al., 1991). Timing of treatment with cytokines and/or their inhibitors (including soluble receptors and receptor antagonists) is also expected to be effective in the immunotherapy of cancer (Kopp et al., 1994; Lissoni et al., 1990, 1993, 1995; Soiffer et al., 1996), in preventing allograft rejection in several forms of critical illness (Souba, 1994), in the treatment of rheumatoid arthritis (Breedveld, 1994; D. A. Fox, 1995a; Maini et al., 1994; Rankin et al., 1995; Wendling et al., 1993), and for numerous other conditions.

Immunosuppression by corticosteroids in patients with kidney allografts was most effective and accompanied by the fewest side effects if the dosing occurred in the morning, as compared with groups of patients taking the drug in the evening or throughout the day (Knapp et al., 1980). The toxic effects of immunosuppressive drugs are still a major obstacle for use in human subjects (Shaw et al., 1996). If a treatment with immunotoxic agents must be used, for example, in cancer chemotherapy, the time of maximal resistance of the relevant rhythm in the immune system of the host can be chosen to achieve the therapeutic effect with a minimum of undesirable side effects (for reviews, see Hrushesky, 1994; Hrushesky and März, 1994; Lemmer, 1989; Levi, 1996b; Levi et al., 1988a; Reinberg et al., 1991).

Seasonal as well as circadian variations in the toxicity of chemotherapeutic agents were found for epirubicin and for doxorubicin (Mormont et al., 1988), THP (4'-0-tetrahydropyranyladriamycin) (Levi et al., 1988a), and other agents (Hrushesky and März, 1994). Manipulation of the feeding schedule in mice was shown to alter the circadian rhythm in toxicity of adriamycin (Halberg, 1974) and of the immunosuppressant chemotherapeutic agent, methotrexate (Song et al., 1993) regardless of the light-dark regimen.

In animal experiments, the timing of cyclosporine treatment, according to the circadian, circaseptan, and circannual rhythm of the toxicity of this agent, led to a substantial improvement of the toxic-therapeutic ratio and of the survival of the allografted animals (Liu et al., 1986). In human subjects, cyclosporine shows a circadian rhythm in its pharmacokinetics after oral dosing (Ohlman et al., 1993; Sabate et al., 1990; Venkataramanan et al., 1986) and during continuing infusion (Heifets et al., 1995; Ohlman et al., 1993). Peak plasma concentrations were found in the early morning hours, between 03:30 07:30, and the lowest values between 15:30 and 19:30 (Heifets et al., 1995). The lowest rate of drug clearance occurred early in the morning, and the highest rate occurred in the afternoon. Monitoring of drug levels was recommended during the morning hours (around 07:00–08:00), which correspond to the nadir phase of the circadian variation of drug effect (Heifets et al., 1995). The importance of these findings for the therapeutic effect of cyclosporine in patients needs to be explored. The treatment with immunosuppressive agents can be timed for the stages in the circadian or other rhythms in the immune system either to achieve maximal immunosuppression with a minimal dose of the agent or to minimize immunosuppression if other effects of the agents are desired.

Further exploration of the time structure of the immune system will provide the background for numerous chronotherapeutic applications to treatment with growth factors, cytokines, and their agonists and antagonists. Immunoenhancement as well as immunosuppression can gain from chronotherapeutic consideration in dosing times (Halberg and Halberg, 1980; Knapp et al., 1980; Liu et al., 1986).

AUTHOR'S CONCLUSIONS

The following conclusions may be drawn from this review:

• The neuroendocrine and immune system form a complex web of interactions and controls at all levels of integration. Most of the variables encountered are not stationary but show rhythms in multiple frequencies (circadian, circaseptan, circannual, and others).

• Some of the rhythms affecting the immune system are genetically fixed (endogenous), but in certain frequencies (e.g., circadian) the rhythm may be adjusted in its timing by periodic environmental factors (synchronizers, entraining agents, "zeitgeber"), such as light-darkness, activity-rest pattern, temperature, and for some parameters in human subjects less than in experimental animals, the time of food uptake.

• Rhythmic changes in the functional stage of cell and organ systems are predictable in their timing if (1) the rhythm is known to be synchronized by a rhythmic environmental factor (e.g., light-darkness, activity-rest), (2) if the rhythm can be monitored directly (e.g., the response of lymphocytes to mitogens), or (3) if the rhythm has a fixed phase relation to a variable that can be studied as time reference or so-called marker rhythm (e.g., sleep-wakefulness pattern, body temperature, activity, salivary solutes, circulating leukocytes).

• Environmental factors, as they are encountered in daily life and especially in the military climate, can transiently alter (mask) the expression of rhythms (e.g., plasma catecholamines or cortisol) without necessarily changing the underlying rhythmic mechanisms.

• Factors that affect neuroendocrine rhythms also affect immune functions (e.g., sleep and sleep deprivation; physical exercise, moderate or exhaustive; phase shifts; or other rhythm disturbances, including shift work).

• The rhythmic variations in immune-related parameters must be taken into account in any studies and testing procedures. For some of these parameters, the amplitude of these rhythms may be quite large. Experimental designs in animal as well as in human studies can take advantage of the relative predictability of rhythmic variations and detect these rhythm alterations (e.g., a phase shift). Failure to do so may lead to misleading results.

• Rhythms in immune-related functions may determine differences in the primary immune response and in the response to antigenic challenge depending on the stage of the rhythm in which the exposure occurs.

• Rhythms in immune-related functions can lead to time-dependent differences in the response to vaccination. In the circadian range, a stronger immune response was noted in diurnally active subjects after vaccination in the afternoon (hepatitis B vaccine) or in subjects vaccinated at noon or during the afternoon (influenza vaccine). In the latter study this temporal difference in vaccination effect was observed for some antigens, but not for others. The clearance of the antigen (viral particles) and the metabolic response showed differences in extent and duration as a function of the time of vaccination (Venezuelan equine encephalitis attenuated viral vaccine), with more pronounced changes in subjects vaccinated at 20:00 as compared with 08:00 .

The local response to vaccination and/or revaccination was most pronounced after antigen exposure in the afternoon. However, the observed changes were quantitative, and all subjects in these studies did achieve immunity irrespective of the circadian time of vaccination. Nevertheless, some investigators suggest that the timing of vaccination may have some importance in subjects with poor antibody formation.

• Rhythmic infradian (most frequently circaseptan) response patterns are found during tissue regeneration, the regeneration of organs of the immune system after immunosuppression, and in the development of humoral- and cell-mediated immunity after introduction of an antigen. Similar reaction patterns can be triggered by metabolic loads. It is not known if exposure to prolonged stress as experienced in the military climate leads to the manifestation of rhythmic reaction patterns.

• Allograft rejection is characterized by rhythmicity of its clinical manifestations, with circadian and circaseptan periods observed. The relative predictability of these rhythmically occurring events may allow preventive treatment at the time when needed and no treatment or decreased dosage at times when rejection reactions are unlikely, thus decreasing undesirable side effects and cost. The feasibility of such an approach has been shown in animal experiments.

• Timing of administration according to circadian or infradian rhythm stages can be of help in treatment with growth factors and cytokines, or with their agonists or antagonists, and in treatment with immunosuppressive or chemotherapeutic agents in which immunosuppression is an undesirable side effect. Timing of treatment according to the stages of a sensitivity or resistance cycle may attain optimal effects with a minimal dose of an agent and/or the desired effects with minimal toxicity (e.g., cancer chemotherapy). These possibilities have been widely explored in animal experiments and recently have also been applied to clinical medicine where they are expected to gain much wider use in the near future.

• In disorders of the immune system (e.g., AIDS), changes in the rhythmic variations of some of its components may be of importance and may precede the clinical manifestations of the disease.

REFERENCES

Abo, T., T. Kawate, K. Itoh, and K. Kumagai. 1981. Studies on the bioperiodicity of the immune response. I. Circadian rhythms of human T-, B-, and K-cell traffic in the peripheral blood. J. Immunol. 126:1360–1363.

Alevizatos, A.C., R.W. McKinney, and R.D. Feigin. 1967. Live attenuated equine encephalomyelitis virus vaccine. I. Clinical response of man to immunization. Am. J. Trop. Med. Hyg. 16:762–768.

Angeli, A., G. Gatti, M.L. Sartori, and R.G. Masora. 1992. Chronobiological aspects of the neuroendocrine immune network. Regulation of human natural killer (NK) cells as a model. Chronobiologia 19:93–110.

Araneo, B.A., M.L.I. Woods, and R.A. Daynes. 1993. Reversal of the immunosenescent phenotype by dehydroepiandrosterone: Hormone treatment provides an adjuvant effect on the immunization of aged mice with recombinant hepatitis B surface antigen. J. Infect. Dis. 167:830–840.

Arendt, J. 1994. The pineal. Pp. 348–362. In Biologic Rhythms in Clinical and Laboratory Medicine, Y. Touitou and E. Haus, editors. 2nd ed. Heidelberg: Springer-Verlag.

Arvidson, N.G., B. Gudbjornson, L. Elfman, and A.C. Ryden. 1994. Circadian rhythm of serum interleukin 6 in rheumatoid arthritis. Ann. Rheum. Dis. 53(8):521–524.

Auernhammer, C.J., and C.J. Strasburger. 1995. Effects of growth hormone and insulin-like growth factor I on the immune system. Eur. J. Endocrinol. 133:635–645.

Auzeby, A., A. Bogdan, Z. Krosi, and Y. Touitou. 1988. Time dependence of urinary neopterin, a marker of cellular immune activity. Clin. Chem. 34:1866–1867.

Badwe, R.A., W.M. Gregory, M.A. Chaudary, and M.A. Richards. 1991. Timing of surgery during the menstrual cycle and survival of the premenopausal woman with operable breast cancer. Lancet 337:1261–1264.

Banchereau, J. 1991. Interleukin-4. Pp. 119–149 in The Cytokine Handbook, A. Thomson, ed. London: Academic Press.

Barnes, P.J. 1984a. Autonomic control of the airways in nocturnal asthma. Pp. 69–73 in Nocturnal Asthma, P.J. Barnes and J. Levy, eds. Oxford: Oxford University Press.

Barnes, P.J. 1984b. Nocturnal asthma: Mechanisms and treatment. Br. Med. J. 288:1397–1398.

Barton, B.E., and J.V. Jackson. 1993. Protective role of interleukin-6 in the lipopolysaccharide-galactosamine septic shock model. Infect. Immun. 61:1496–1499.

Bayle, J.E., M. Guellati, F. Ibos, and J. Roux. 1991. *Brucella abortus* antigen stimulates the pituitary-adrenal axis through the extrapituitary B-lymphoid system. Prog. Neuroendocrinol. Immunol. 4:99–105.

Bellido, T., G. Girasole, G. Passeri, X.P. Yu, H. Mocharla, R.L. Jilka, A. Notides, and S.C. Manolagas. 1993. Demonstration of estrogen and vitamin D receptors in bone marrow-derived stromal cells: Upregulation of the estrogen receptor by 1,25-dihydroxyvitamin D3. Endocrinology 133:553–562.

Benatar, S.R. 1986. Fatal asthma. N. Engl. J. Med. 314:423–429.

Beneviste, E.N. 1992. Cytokines: Influence on glial cell gene expression and function. Pp. 106–153 in Neuroimmunoendocrinology: Chemical Immunology, 2d ed., J.E. Blalock, ed. Basel: Karger.

Berczi, I., F.D. Baragar, I.M. Chalmers, E.C. Keystone, E. Nagy, and R.J. Warrington. 1993. Hormones in self tolerance and autoimmunity: A role in the pathogenesis of rheumatoid arthritis. Autoimmunity 16:45–56.

Bernton, E., M.S. Meltzer, and J.W. Holaday. 1988. Suppression of macrophage activation and T-lymphocyte function in hypoprolactinemic mice. Science 239:401–404.

Besedovsky, H.O., and A. del Rey. 1992. Immune-neuroendocrine circuits: Integrative role of cytokines [Review]. Front Neuroendocrinology. 13(1) 61–94.

Besedovsky, H.O., and A. del Rey. 1996. Immune-neuro-endocrine interactions: Facts and hypothesis. Endocr. Rev. 17:64–102.

Bixby, E.K., F. Levi, R. Haus, F. Halberg, and W. Hrushesky. 1982. Circadian aspects of murine nephrotoxicity of cisdiamminedichloroplatinum (II). Pp. 339–347 in Toward Chronopharmacology, R. Takahashi, ed. Oxford, New York: Pergamon Press.

Bjarnason, G.A., and W.J.M. Hrushesky. 1994. Cancer chronotherapy. Pp. 241–263 in Circadian Cancer Therapy, W.J.M. Hrushesky, ed. Boca Raton, Fla.: CRC Press.

Blalock, J.E. 1989a. A molecular basis for bidirectional communication between the immune and neuroendocrine systems. Physiol. Rev. 69:1–32.

Blalock, J.E. 1989b. A production of peptide hormones and neurotransmitters by the immune system. Pp. 1–19 in Neuroimmunoendocrinology: Chemical Immunology, 2d ed., J.E. Blalock, ed. Basel: Karger.

Blalock, J.E. 1994. The immune system: Our sixth sense. Immunologist 1994:8–15.

Bourin, P., F. Levi, I. Mansour, C. Doinel, and M. Joussemet. 1990. Circadian rhythm of interleukin-1 (IL-1) in serum of healthy men. Ann. Rev. Chronopharmacol. 7:201–204.

Bourin, P., I. Mansour, F. Levi, J.M. Villette, R. Roue, J. Fiet, P. Rouger, and C. Doinel. 1989. Perturbations precoces des rhythmes circadiens des lymphocytes T et B au cours de l'immunodeficience humaine (VIH). CR Acad. Sci. (Paris) 308:431–436.

Bratescu, A., and M. Teodorescu. 1981. Circannual variations in the B-cell/T-cell ratio in normal human peripheral blood. J. Allergy Clin. Immunol. 68:273–280.

Breedveld, F. 1994. Tenidap: A novel cytokine-modulating antirheumatic drug for the treatment of rheumatoid-arthritis. Scand. J. Rheumatol. 100:31–44.

Breus, T.K., F.I. Komarov, M.M. Musin, I.V. Naborov, and S.I. Rapoport. 1989. Heliogeophysical factors and their influence on cyclical processes in biosphere. Itogi Nauki i Techniki: Medicinskaya Geografica 18:138–142.

Britton, S., and G.H. Moller. 1968. Regulation of antibody synthesis against *Escherichia coli* endotoxin. I. Suppressive effects of endogenously produced and passively transferred antibodies. J. Immunol. 100:1326–1334.

Brock, M.A. 1983. Seasonal rhythmicity in lymphocyte blastogenesis persists in a constant environment. J. Immunol. 130:2586–2588.

Brock, M.A. 1987. Age-related changes in circannual rhythms of lymphocyte blastogenic response in mice. Am. J. Physiol. 252:R299–R305.

Brock, M.A. 1991. Chronobiology of aging. J. Am. Geriatr. Soc. 39:74–91.

Brown, R., G. Pang, A.J. Husband, and M.C. King. 1989. A suppression of immunity to influenza virus infection in the respiratory tract following sleep deprivation. Regul. Immunol. 2:321–325.

Calderon, R.A., and D.B. Thomas. 1980. *In vivo* cyclic change in B-lymphocyte susceptibility to T-cell control. Nature (Lond.) 285:662–664.

Cannon, J.G., and C.A. Dinarello. 1985. Increased plasma interleukin-1 activity in women after ovulation. Science 227:1247–1249.

Canon, C., F. Levi, Y. Touitou, J. Sulon, E. Demey-Ponsart, A. Reinberg, and G. Mathe. 1986. Variations circadienne et saisonniere du rapport inducteur: Suppresseur (OKT4 + OKT8+) dans la sang veineux de l'homme adulte sain. C.R. Acad. Sci. III 302:519–524.

Carandente, F., and F. Halberg. 1976. Chronobiologic view of shift-work and ulcers. Pp. 273–283 in NIOSH Research Symposium, Shift-Work and Health, Cincinnati, P.G. Rentos and R.D. Shepard, eds. Cincinnati: National Institute for Occupational Safety and Health.

Carr, D.J.J. 1991. The role of endogenous opioids and their receptors in the immune system. Soc. Exp. Biol. Med. 198:710–720.

Carr, D.J.J. 1992. Neuroendocrine peptide receptors on cells of the immune system. Pp. 49–83 in Neuroimmunoendocrinology: Chemical Immunology, 2d ed., J.E. Blalock, ed. Basel: Karger.

Clark, R., J. Strasser, S. McCabe, K. Robbins, and P. Jardieu. 1993. Insulin-like growth factor-1 stimulation of lymphopoiesis. J. Clin. Invest. 92:540–548.

Clarke, B.L., and K.L. Bost. 1989. Differential expression of functional adrenocorticotropic hormone receptors by subpopulations of lymphocytes. J. Immunol. 143:464–469.

Clevenger, C.V., D.H. Russell, P.M. Appasamy, and M.B. Prystowsky. 1990. Regulation of interleukin-2 driven T-lymphocyte proliferation by prolactin. Proc. Natl. Acad. Sci. USA 87:6460–6464.

Cornélissen, G., T.K. Breus, C. Bingham, R. Zaslavskaya, M. Varshitsky, B. Mirsky, M. Teibloom, B. Tarquini, E. Bakken, and F. Halberg. 1993. Beyond circadian chronorisk: Worldwide circaseptan-circasemiseptan patterns of myocardial infarctions, other vascular events, and emergencies. Chronobiologia 20:87–115.

Cove-Smith, J.R., P. Kabler, R. Pownall, and M.S. Knapp. 1978. Circadian variation in an immune response in man. Br. Med. J. 2(6132):253–254.

Covelli, V., F. Massari, C. Fallarca, I. Munno, F. Jirrilo, S. Savastano, A. Tommaselli, and G. Lombardi. 1992. Interleukin-1β and β-endorphin circadian rhythms are inversely related in normal and stress-altered sleep. Int. J. Neurosci. 63:299–305.

Cricchio, I., G. Arcara, G. Abbate, and M.F. Cannonito. 1978. Aspetti cronobiologia delle immunoglobuline sieriche. Folia Allergol. Immunol. Clin. 24:470.

Cricchio, I., G. Aracara, G. Abbate, T. Ferrar, R. Tarantino, and S. Romano. 1979. Circadian rhythms of serum immunoglobulins in patients affected with allergic rhinitis, atopic asthma and chronic urticaria. Pp. 55–63 in Recent Advances in the Chronobiology of Allergy and Immunology, M.H. Smolensky, A. Reinberg, and J.P. McGovern, eds. Oxford: Pergamon Press.

Da Silva, J.A., and G.M. Hall. 1992. The effect of gender and sex hormones on outcome in rheumatoid arthritis. Clin. Rheumatol. 6:196–219.

Damle, N.K., and S. Gupta. 1982. Autologous mixed lymphocyte reaction in man. III. Regulation of autologous MLR by theophylline-resistant and sensitive human T-lymphocyte subpopulations. Scand. J. Immunol. 15:493–499.

Daniel, L., G. Souweine, J.C. Monier, and S. Saez. 1983. Specific estrogen binding sites in human lymphoid cells and thymic cells. Esteroid Biochem. 18:559–563.

Daynes, R.A., and B.A. Araneo. 1992. Prevention and reversal of some age-associated changes in immunologic responses by supplemental dehydroepiandrosterone sulfate therapy. Aging Immunol. Infect. Dis. 3:135–154.

Daynes, R.A., B.A. Araneo, J. Hennebold, E. Enioutina, and H.M. Hong. 1995. Steroids as regulators of the mammalian immune response. J. Invest. Dermatol. 105:14S–19S.

Del Prete, G., E. Maggi, and S. Romagnani. 1994. Human Th1 and Th2 cells: Functional properties, mechanisms of regulation and role in disease. Lab. Invest. 70:299–307.

DeLeonardis, V., and M.L. Brandi. 1984. Total IgE serum levels: A chronobiologic approach. Pp. 395–398 in Chronobiology 1982–1983, E. Haus and H.F. Kabat, eds. Basel: Karger.

Depres-Brummer, P., F. Levi, M. Palma, A. Beliard, P. Lebon, S. Marion, C. Jasmin, and J. Misset. 1991. A phase I trial of 21-day continuous venous infusion of α-interferon at circadian rhythm modulated rate in cancer patients. J. Immunother. 10:440–447.

DeSarro, G.B., Y. Masuda, C. Ascioti, M.G. Audino, and G. Nistico. 1990. Behavioral and ECoG spectrum changes induced by intracerebral infusion of interferons and interleukin-2 in rats are antagonized by naloxone. Neuropharmacology 29:167–179.

Dethlefsen, U., and R. Repges. 1985. Ein neues Therapieprinzip bei nachtlichem Asthma. Med. Klin. 80:40–47.

DeVecchi, A., F. Halberg, R.B. Sothern, A. Cantaluppi, and C. Ponticelli. 1981. Circaseptan rhythmic aspects of rejection in treated patients with kidney transplant. Pp. 339–353 in Chronopharmacology and Chemotherapeutics, C.A. Walker, C.M. Winget, and K.F.A. Soliman, eds. Tallahassee, FL: A and M University Foundation.

DeVries, K., J.T. Goei, H. Booy-Noord, and N.G.M. Orie. 1962. Changes during 24 hours in the lung function and histamine hyperreactivity of the bronchial tree in asthmatic and bronchitic patients. Int. Arch. Allerg. 20:93–101.

Dixon-Northern, A.L., S.M. Rutter, and C.M. Peterson. 1994. Cyclic changes in the concentration of peripheral blood immune cells during the normal menstrual cycle. Proc. Soc. Exp. Biol. Med. 207:81–88.

Edmunds, L.N.J. 1994. Cellular and molecular aspects of circadian oscillators: Models and mechanisms for biological timekeeping. Pp. 35–54 in Biologic Rhythms in Clinical and Laboratory Medicine, 2d ed., Y. Touitou and E. Haus, eds. Heidelberg: Springer-Verlag.

Eichler, F., and R. Keiling. 1988. Variations in the percentages of lymphocyte subtypes during the menstrual cycle in women. Biomed. Pharmacother. 42:285–288.

Everson, C.A. 1993. Sustained sleep deprivation impairs host defense. Am. J. Physiol. 265:R1148–R1154.

Fabris, N., E. Mocchegiani, and M. Provinciali. 1995. Pituitary-thyroid axis and immune system: A reciprocal neuroendocrine-immune interaction. Horm. Res. 43:29–38.

Feigin, R.D., R.F. Jaeger, R.W. McKinney, and A.C. Alevizatos. 1967a. Live, attenuated Venezuelan equine encephalomyelitis virus vaccine. II. Whole-blood amino-acid and fluorescent-antibody studies following immunization. Am. J. Trop. Med. Hyg. 16:769–777.

Feigin, R.D., A.S. Klainer, and W.R. Beisel. 1967b. Circadian periodicity of whole-blood amino acids in adult men. Nature 215:512–514.

Feldman, J.F. 1985. Genetic and physiological analysis of a clock gene in *Neurospora crassa*. Pp. 238–245 in Temporal Order, L. Rensing and N.I. Jaeger, eds. Berlin, Heidelberg, and New York: Springer.

Fernandes, G. 1994. Chronobiology of immune functions: Cellular and humoral aspects. Pp. 493–503 in Biologic Rhythms in Clinical and Laboratory Medicine, Y. Touitou and E. Haus, eds. Heidelberg: Springer-Verlag.

Fernandes, G., F. Halberg, and R.A. Good. 1980. Circadian dependent chronoimmunological responses of T-, B-, and natural killer cells. Allergology 3:164–170.

Fernandes, G., F. Halberg, E. Yunis, and R.A. Good. 1976. Circadian rhythmic plaque-forming cell response of spleens from mice immunized by SRBC. J. Immunol. 117:962–966.

Fernandes, G., E.J. Yunis, and F. Halberg. 1977. Circadian aspect of immune response in the mouse. Pp. 233–249 in Chronobiology in Allergy and Immunology, J.P. McGovern, M.H. Smolensky, and A. Reinberg, eds. Springfield, Ill.: Charles C Thomas.

Fernandes, G., E.J. Yunis, W. Nelson, and F. Halberg. 1974. Differences in immune response of mice to sheep red blood cells as a function of circadian phase. Pp. 329–338 in Chronobiology. Proceedings of the International Society for the Study of Biological Rhythms, L.E. Scheving, F. Halberg, and J.E. Pauly, eds. Stuttgart and Tokyo: Thime/Igaku Shoin.

Finocchiaro, L.E., E. Nahmod, and J.M. Launay. 1991. Melatonin biosynthesis and metabolism in peripheral blood mononuclear leukocytes. Biochem. J. 280:727–732.

Finocchiaro, L.M.E., E.S. Arzt, S. Fernandez-Castelo, M. Criscuolo, S. Finkielman, and V.E. Nahmod. 1988. Serotonin and melatonin synthesis in peripheral blood mononuclear cells: Stimulation by interferon-γ as part of an immunomodulatory pathway. J. Interferon Res. 1988:705–716.

Fletscher, B. 1993. Zirkadiane Variation der Antikorperbildung nach Hepatitis-B-Impfung. Deutsch. Med. Wschr 118:999.

Fox, D.A. 1995a. Biological therapies: A novel approach to the treatment of autoimmune disease. Am. J. Med. 99:82–88.

Fox, H.S. 1995b. Sex steroids and the immune system [Review]. CIBA Foundation Symposium. 191:203–211.

Fox, H.S., B.L. Bond, and T.G. Parslow. 1991. Estrogen regulates the INF-γ promoter. J. Immunol. 146:4362–4367.

Fuller, R. and H. Snoddy. 1968. Feeding schedule alteration of daily rhythm in tyrosine α-ketoglutaride transaminase in rat liver. Science 159:738.

Gala, R.R., and E.M. Shevach. 1993. Identification by analytical flow cytometry of prolactin receptors on immunocompetent cell population in the mouse. Endocrinology 133:1617–1623.

Gala, R.R., and E.M. Shevach. 1994. Evidence for the release of a prolactin-like substance by mouse lymphocytes and macrophages. Proc. Soc. Exp. Biol. Med. 205:12–19.

Gamaleya, N.F., E.D. Silisko, and A.P. Cherny. 1988. Preservation of circadian rhythms by human leukocytes *in vitro*. Byull. Eksper. Biol. Med. 106:598–600.

Garg, M., and S. Bondada. 1993. Reversal of age-associated decline in immune response to pnu-immune vaccine by supplementation with the steroid hormone dehydroepiandrosterone. Infect. Immun. 61:2238–2241.

Gatti, G., R. Cavallo, M.L. Sartori, R. Carignola, R. Masera, D. Delponte, A. Salvadori, and A. Angeli. 1988. Circadian variations of interferon-induced enhancement of human natural killer (NK) cell activity. Cancer Detect. 12:431–438.

Gatti, G., R. Cavallo, M.L. Sartori, D. Delponte, R.G. Masera, A. Salvadori, R. Carignola, and A. Angeli. 1987. Inhibition by cortisol of human natural killer (NK) cell activity. Steroid. Biochem. 26:49–58.

Gatti, G., R. Cavallo, M.I. Sartori, C. Marinone, and A. Angeli. 1986. Cortisol at physiological concentrations and prostaglandin E2 are additive inhibitors of human nature killer cell activity. Immunopharmacology 11:119–128.

Gatti, G., R.G. Masera, R. Carignola, M.L. Sartori, E. Margro, and A. Angeli. 1990. Circadian-single-dependent enhancement of human natural killer cell activity by melatonin. J. Immunol. Res. 2:108–116.

Gaultier, C., G. DeMontis, A. Reinberg, and Y. Motohashi. 1987. Circadian rhythm of serum total immunoglobulin E (IgE) in asthmatic children. Biomed. Pharmacother. 41:186–188.

Gibinski, K., A. Nowak, J. Rybicka, and K. Czarnecka. 1979. An endoscopic study on the natural history of gastroduodenal ulcer disease. Mater. Med. Pol. 11:265–269.

Gibson, L.F., D. Piktel, and K.S. Landreth. 1993. Insulin-like growth factor-I potentiates expansion of interleukin-7-dependent pro-B-cells. Blood 82:3005–3011.

Gilblett, E.R., J.E. Anderson, F. Cohen, B. Pollara, and H.J. Meuwissen. 1972. Adenosine deaminase deficiency in two patients with severely impaired cellular immunity. Lancet II:1067–1069.

Goetz, F., J. Bishop, F. Halberg, R. Sothern, R. Brunning, B. Senske, B. Greenberg, D. Minors, P. Stoney, I.D. Smith, G.D. Rosen, D. Cressey, E. Haus, and M. Apfelbaum. 1976. Timing of single daily meal influences relations among human circadian rhythms in urinary cyclic AMP and hemic glucagon, insulin, and iron. Experientia (Basel) 32:1081–1084.

Graf, M.V., and A.J. Kastin. 1984. Delta-sleep-inducing peptide (DSIP): A review. Neurosci. Biobehav. Rev. 8:83–93.

Grossman, Z., R. Asofsky, and C. Delisi. 1980. The dynamics of antibody secreting cell production, regulation of growth, and oscillations in the response to T-independent antigens. J. Theor. Biol. 84:49–92.

Gudewill, S., T. Pollmacher, H. Vedder, W. Schreuber, K. Fassbender, and F. Holsboer. 1992. Nocturnal plasma levels of cytokines in healthy men. Eur. Arch. Psych. Clin. Neurosci. 242:53–56.

Haen, E., I. Langenmayer, A. Pangerl, B. Liebl, and J. Remien. 1988. Circannual variation in the expression of β2 adrenoceptors on human peripheral mononuclear leukocytes (MNLs). Klin. Wschr. 66:579–582.

Halberg, E., and F. Halberg. 1980. Chronobiologic study design in everyday life, clinic, and laboratory. Chronobiologia 7:95–120.

Halberg, F. 1974. From iatrotoxicosis and iatrosepsis towards chronotherapy. Pp. 1–34 in Chronobiologic Aspects of Endocrinology, J. Aschoff, F. Ceresa, and F. Halberg, eds. Stuttgart: Schattaner-Verlag.

Halberg, F., and C. Hamburger. 1964. 17-ketosteroids and volume of human urine. Weekly and other changes with low frequency. Minn. Med. 47:916–925.

Halberg, F., and A.N. Stephens. 1959. Susceptibility to ouabain and physiologic circadian periodicity. Proc. Minn. Acad. Sci. 27:139–143.

Halberg, F., C.P. Barnum, R. Silber, and J.J. Bittner. 1958. 24-hour rhythms at several levels of integration in mice on different lighting regimens. Proc. Soc. Exp. Biol. Med. 97:897–900.

Halberg, F., D. Duffert, and H. Von Mayersbach. 1977. Circadian rhythm in serum immunoglobulins of clinically healthy young men [abstract]. Chronobiologia 4:114.

Halberg, F., E. Haus, and G. Cornélissen. 1995. From biologic rhythms to chronomes relevant for nutrition. Pp. 361–372 in Not Eating Enough, Overcoming

Underconsumption of Military Operational Rations, B.M. Marriott, ed. Committee on Military Nutrition Research, Food and Nutrition Board, Institute of Medicine. Washington, D.C.: National Academy Press.

Halberg, F., E.A. Johnson, B.W. Brown, and J.J. Bittner. 1960. Susceptibility rhythm to *E. coli* endotoxin and bioassay. Proc. Soc. Exp. Biol. Med. 103:142–144.

Halberg, J., E. Halberg, W. Runge, J. Wicks, L. Cadotte, E. Yunis, G. Katinas, O. Stutman, and F. Halberg. 1974. Transplant chronobiology. Pp. 320–328 in Chronobiology. Proceedings of the International Society for the Study of Biological Rhythms, L.E. Scheving, F. Halberg, and J.E. Pauly, eds. Stuttgart and Tokyo: Thieme/Igaku Shoin.

Hansson, I., R. Holmdahl, and R. Mattsson. 1992. The pineal hormone melatonin exaggerates development of collagen-induced arthritis in mice. J. Neuroimmunol. 39:23–30.

Hartmann, D.P., J.W. Holday, and E.W. Bernton. 1989. Inhibition of lymphocyte proliferation by antibodies to prolactin. FASEB J. 3:2194–2202.

Hasty, L.A., J.D. Lambris, B.A. Lessey, K. Pruksananonda, and C.R. Lyttle. 1994. Hormonal regulation of complement and receptors throughout the menstrual cycle. Am. J. Obstet. Gynecol. 170:168–175.

Hattori, N., A. Shimatsu, M. Sugita, S. Kumagai, and H. Imura. 1990. Immunoreactive growth hormone (GH) secretion by human lymphocytes: Augmented release by exogenous GH. Biochem. Biophys. Res. Commun. 168:396–401.

Haus, E. 1959. Endokrines system und Blut. Pp. 181–286 in Handbuch der gesamten Hämatologie, L. Heilmeyer and A. Hittmair, eds. Munich: Urban und Schwarzenberg.

Haus, E. 1994. Chronobiology of circulating blood cells and platelets. Pp. 504–526 in Biologic Rhythms in Clinical and Laboratory Medicine, 2d ed., Y. Touitou and E. Haus, eds. Heidelberg: Springer Verlag.

Haus, E. 1996. Biologic rhythms in hematology. Path. Biol. 44(6):618–630.

Haus, E., and F. Halberg. 1978. Cronofarmacologia della neoplasia con speciale riferimento alla leucemia. Pp. 29–85 in Farmacologia Clinica e Terapia, A. Bertelli, ed.Turin: Edizioni.

Haus, E., and Y. Touitou. 1994a. Chronobiology in laboratory medicine. Pp. 673–708 in Biologic Rhythms in Clinical and Laboratory Medicine, 2d ed., Y. Touitou and E. Haus, eds. Heidelberg: Springer-Verlag.

Haus, E., and Y. Touitou. 1994b. Principles of clinical chronobiology. Pp. 6–34 in Biologic Rhythms in Clinical and Laboratory Medicine, 2d ed., Y. Touitou and E. Haus, eds. Heidelberg: Springer-Verlag.

Haus, E., L. Dumitriu, G.Y. Nicolau, D.J. Lakatua, H. Berg, E. Petrescu, L. Sackett-Lundeen, and R. Reilly. 1995. Time relation of circadian rhythms in plasma dehydroepiandrosterone and dehydroepiandrosterone-sulfate to ACTH, cortisol, and 11-desoxycortisol-#107 [abstract]. Biol. Rhythm Res. 26:(4)399.

Haus, E., F. Halberg, J.F.W. Juhl, and D.J. Lakatua. 1974a. Chronopharmacology in animals. Chronobiologia 1:122–156.

Haus, E., F. Halberg, M.K. Loken, and Y.S. Kim. 1974b. Circadian rhythmometry of mammalian radiosensitivity. Pp. 435–474 in Space Radiation Biology, C.A. Tobias and P. Todd, eds. New York: American Institute of Biological Science Academic Press.

Haus, E., F. Halberg, L.E. Scheving, J.E. Pauly, S. Cardoso, J.F.W. Kuhl, R.B. Sothern, R.N. Shiotsuka, and D.S. Hwang. 1972. Increased tolerance of leukemic mice to arabinosyl cytosine with schedule adjusted to circadian system. Science 177:80–82.

Haus, E., D.J. Lakatua, F. Halberg, E. Halberg, G. Cornélissen, L. Sackett, H. Berg, T. Kawasaki, M. Ueno, K. Uezono, M. Matsouka, and T. Omae. 1980.

Chronobiological studies of plasma prolactin in women in Kyushu, Japan, and Minnesota, U.S.A. J. Clin. Endocrinol. Metab. 51:632–640.

Haus, E., D.J. Lakatua, L. Sackett-Lundeen, and J. Swoyer. 1984. Chronobiology in laboratory medicine. Pp. 13–82 in Clinical Aspects of Chronobiology, W.J. Rietveld, ed. The Netherlands: Meducation Service Hoechst.

Haus, E., D.J. Lakatua, L. Sackett-Lundeen and M. White. 1984. Circannual variation of intestinal cell proliferation in BDF male mice on three lighting regimens. Chronobiol. Int. 1:185–194.

Haus, E., D.J. Lakatua, J. Swoyer, and L. Sackett-Lundeen. 1983. Chronobiology in hematology and immunology. Am. J. Anatomy 168:467–517.

Haus, E., G.Y. Nicolau, D.J. Lakatua, and L. Sackett-Lundeen. 1988. Reference values for chronopharmacology. Chronopharmacology 4:333–424.

Haus, M., L. Sackett-Lundeen, D. Lakatua, and E. Haus. 1984. Circannual variation of ^{3}H-thymidine uptake in DNA of lymphatic organs irrespective of relative length of light and dark span [abstract]. J. Minn. Acad. Sci. 49(2):19.

Hayashi, O.K., and M. Kikuchi. 1982. The effects of the light-dark cycle on humoral and cell-mediated immune responses of mice. Chronobiologia 9:291–300.

Hedner, L., and G. Bynke. 1985. Endogenous iridocyclitis relieved during treatment with Bromocriptine. Am. J. Ophthal. 100:618–619.

Heifets, M., G.F. Cooney, L.M. Shaw, and G. Lebetti. 1995. Diurnal variation of cyclosporine clearance in stable renal transplant recipients receiving continuous infusion. Transplantation 60:1615–1617.

Herberman R.B., and D.H. Callewaert, eds. 1985. Mechanisms of Cytotoxicity by NK Cells. Orlando, Fla.: Academic Press.

Hetzel, M.R., T.J.H. Clark, and M.A. Branthwaite. 1977. Asthma: Analysis of sudden deaths and ventilatory arrest in hospital. Br. Med. J. 1:808–811.

Hiestand, P.C., P. Mekler, R. Nordmann, A. Grieder, and C. Permmongkol. 1986. Prolactin as a modulator of lymphocyte responsiveness provides a possible mechanism of action for cyclosporine. Proc. Natl. Acad. Sci. USA 83:2599–2603.

Homo-Delarche, F. 1984. Glucocorticoid receptors and steroid sensitivity in normal and neoplastic human lymphoid tissue: A review. Cancer Res. 44:431–437.

Homo-Delarche, F., F. Fitzpatrick, N. Christeff, E.A. Nunez, J.F. Bach, and M. Dardenne. 1991. Sex steroids, glucocorticoids, stress, and autoimmunity. J. Steroid Biochem. Mol. 40:619–637.

Hooghe, R., M. Delhase, P. Vergani, A. Malur, and E.L. Hooghe-Peters. 1993. Growth hormone and prolactin are paracrine growth and differentiation factors in the haemopoietic system. Immunol. Today 14:212–214.

Hoopes, P.C., and C.E. McCall. 1977. The effect of cobra venom factor (CVF) on activation of the complement cascade on leukocyte circadian variation in the rat. Experientia 33:224–226.

Hrushesky, W.J.M., ed. 1994. Circadian Cancer Therapy. Boca Raton, Fla.: CRC Press.

Hrushesky, W.J.M., and W.J. März. 1994. Chronochemotherapy of malignant tumors: Temporal aspects of antineoplastic drug toxicity. Pp. 611–634 in Biologic Rhythms in Clinical and Laboratory Medicine, 2d ed., Y. Touitou and E. Haus, eds. Heidelberg: Springer-Verlag.

Huber, C., J.R. Batchelor, D. Fuchs, A. Hauser, A. Lang, D. Niederwieser, G. Reitnegger, P. Swetly, J. Troppmair, and H. Wachter. 1984. Immune response associated production of neopterin. Release from macrophages primarily under control of interferon-γ. J. Exp. Med. 160:310–316.

Hübner, K. 1967. Kompensatorische Hypertrophie, Wachstum und Regeneration der Rattenniere. Ergebn Allg. Path. Path. Anat. 48:1–80.

Hughes, E.C., R.L. Johnson, and C.W. Whitaker. 1977. Circadian rhythmic aspects of secretory immunoglobulin A. Pp. 216–232 in Chronobiology in Allergy and Immunology, J.P. McGovern, M.H. Smolensky, and A. Reinberg, eds. Springfield, Ill.: Charles C Thomas.

Husband, A.J. 1993. Role of central nervous system and behavior in the immune response. Vaccine 11:805–816.

Indiveri, F., I. Pierri, S. Rogna, A. Poggi, P. Montaldo, R. Romano, A. Pende, A. Morgano, A. Barabino, and S. Ferrone. 1985. Circadian variations of autologous mixed lymphocyte reactions and endogenous cortisol. J. Immunol. Meth. 82:17–24.

Isenberg, D.A., A.J. Guisp, W.J.W. Morrow, D. Newham, and M.L. Snaith. 1981. Variations in circulating immune complex levels with diet, exercise, and sleep: A comparison between normal controls and patients with systemic lupus erythematosis. Ann. Rheum. Dis. 40:466–469.

Johnson, H.M., M.O. Downs, and C.H. Pontzer. 1992. Neuroendocrine peptide hormone regulation of immunity [Review]. Chemical Immunology 52:49–83.

Johnson, H.M., E.M. Smith, B.A. Torres, and J.E. Blalock. 1982. Neuroendocrine hormone regulation of in vitro antibody production. Proc. Natl. Acad. Sci. USA 79:4171–4174.

Jouvet, M. 1984. Neuromediateurs et facteurs hypnogenes. Rev. Neurol. 140:389–400.

Katila, H., K. Cantell, B. Appelberg, and R. Rimon. 1993. Is there a seasonal variation in the interferon-producing capacity of healthy subjects? J. Interferon Res. 13:233–234.

Kelso, A., and A. Munck. 1984. Glucocorticoid inhibition of lymphokine secretion by alloreactive T-lymphocyte clones. J. Immunol. 133:784–791.

Kern, J.A., R.J. Lamb, J.C. Reed, R.P. Daniele, and P.C. Nowell. 1988. Dexamethasone inhibition of interleukin-1β production by human monocytes. Postranscriptional Mechanisms. J. Clin. Invest. 81:237–244.

Kim, Y., M. Pallansch, F. Carandente, G. Reissmann, E. Halberg, and F. Halberg. 1980. Circadian and circannual aspects of the complement cascade—new and old results, differing in specificity? Chronobiologia 7:189–204.

Kimata, H., and A. Yoshida. 1994. Differential effect of growth hormone and insulin-like growth factor-I, insulin-like growth factor-II, and insulin on Ig production and growth in human plasma cells. Blood 83:1569–1574.

Kishida, T., M. Kita, M. Yamaji, E. Kaneta, and T. Teramatsu. 1987. Interferon-producing capacity in patients with liver diseases, diabetes mellitus, chronic diseases, and malignant diseases. Pp. 435–441 in The Biology of the Interferon System 1986, K. Cantel and H. Schellekens, eds. Dordrecht: Martinus Nijhoff Publishers.

Knapp, M.S., N.P. Byron, R. Pownall, and P. Mayor. 1980. Time of day of taking immunosuppressive agents after renal transplantation. Br. Med. J. 281:1382–1385.

Knapp, M.S., R. Pownall, and J.R. Cove-Smith. 1981. Circadian variations in cell-mediated immunity and in the timing of human allograft rejection. Pp. 329–338 in Chronopharmacology and Chronotherapeutics, C.A. Walker, C.M. Winget, and K.F.A. Soliman, eds. Tallahassee, Fla.: A&M University Foundation.

Konopka, R.J. 1979. Genetic dissection of the Drosophila circadian system. Fed. Proc. 38:2602–2605.

Kopp, W.C., J.T. Holmlund, and W.J. Urba. 1994. Immunologic monitoring and clinical trials of biological response modifiers. Cancer Chemother. Biol. Response Modif. 15:226–286.

Koren, S., and W.R. Fleischmann. 1993. Circadian variations in myelosuppressive activity of interferon-α in mice: Identification of an optimal treatment time associated with reduced myelosuppressive activity. Exp. Hematol. 21:552–559.

Kort, W.J., and J.M. Weijma. 1982. Effect of chronic light-dark shift stress on the immune response of the rat. Physiol. Behav. 29:1083–1087.

Krueger, J.M. 1990. Somnogenic activity of immune response modifiers. Trends Pharmacol. Sci. 11(3):122–126.

Krueger, J.M., C.A. Dinarello, and L. Chedid. 1983. Promotion of slow wave sleep (SWS) by a purified Interleukin-1(IL-1) preparation [abstract]. Fed. Proc. 42:356.

Krueger, J.M., J.R. Pappenheimer, and M.L. Karnovsky. 1982. The composition of sleep-promoting factor isolated from human urine. J. Biol. Chem. 25:1664–1669.

Krueger, J.M., E.J. Walter, C.A. Dinarello, S.M. Wolff, and L. Chedid. 1984. Sleep-promoting effects of endogenous pyrogen (Interleukin-1). Am. J. Physiol. 246:R994–R999.

Kruger, T.E., L.R. Smith, D.V. Harbour, and J.E. Blalock. 1989. Thyrotropin: An endogenous regulator of the in vitro immune response. J. Immunol. 142:744–747.

Kunkel, G., and L. Jusuf. 1984. Theoretical and practical aspects of circadian rhythm for theophylline therapy. Pp. 149–155 in New Perspectives in Theophylline Therapy, M. Turner-Warwick and J. Levy, eds. London: Royal Society of Medicine.

Lakatua, D.J. 1994. Molecular and genetic aspects of chronobiology. Pp. 65–77 in Biologic Rhythms in Clinical and Laboratory Medicine, 2d ed., Y. Touitou and E. Haus, eds. Heidelberg: Springer-Verlag.

Lakatua, D.J., E. Haus, K. Labrosse, C. Veit, and L. Sackett-Lundeen. 1986. Circadian rhythm in mammary cytoplasmic estrogen receptor content of Balb/C female mice with and without pituitary isografts. Chronobiol. Int. 3(4):213–219.

Lakatua, D.J., M. White, L.L. Sackett-Lundeen, and E. Haus. 1983. Change in phase relations of circadian rhythms in cell proliferation induced by time-limited feeding in Balb/C x D8A/2F1 mice bearing a transplantable Harding-Passey tumor. Cancer Res. 43:4068–4072.

Landreth, K.S., R. Narayanan, and K. Dorshkind. 1992. Insulin-like growth factor I regulates pro-B-cell differentiation. Blood 80:1207–1212.

Langlois, P.H., M.H. Smolensky, W.P. Glezen, and W.A. Keitel. 1995. Diurnal variation in responses to influenza vaccine. Chronobiol. Int. 12:28–36.

Lavie, P., and B. Weller. 1989. Timing of naps: Effects on post-nap sleepiness levels. EEG Clin. Neurophysiol. 72:218–224.

Lee, C., P. Vaishali, T. Itsukaichi, B. Kiho, and I. Edery. 1996. Resetting the Drosophila clock by photic regulation of PER and a PER-TIM complex. Science 271:1740–1744.

Lee, R.E., M.H. Smolensky, C.S. Leach, and J.P. McGovern. 1977. Circadian rhythms in the cutaneous reactivity to histamine and selected antigens, including phase relationship to urinary cortisol excretion. Ann. Allergy 38(4):231–236.

Lemmer, B., ed. 1989. Chronopharmacology, Cellular, and Biochemical Interactions. New York: Marcel Dekker.

Lemmer, B., U. Schwulera, A. Thrun, and R. Lissner. 1992. Circadian rhythm of soluble interleukin-2 receptor in healthy individuals. Eur. Cytokine Netw. 3:335–336.

Levi, F. 1994. Chronotherapy of cancer: Biological basis and clinical application. Pathol. Biol. (Paris) 42:338–341.

Levi, F. 1996a. Chronotherapy for gastrointestinal cancers. Curr. Opin. Oncol. 8:334–341.

Levi, F. 1996b. Chronopharmacologie et chronothérapie des cancers. Path. Biol. 44:631–644.

Levi, F. 1997. Chronopharmacology of Anticancer Agents. Pp. 299-332 in Physiology and Pharmacology of Biologic Rhythms. Handbook of Experimental Pharmacology. Volume 125, P.H. Redfern and B. Lemmer, eds. Heidelberg: Springer-Verlag.

Levi, F., and F. Halberg. 1982. Circaseptan (about 7 day) bioperiodicity—spontaneous and reactive—and the search for pacemakers. Ric. Clin. Lab. 12:323–370.

Levi, F., I. Blazsek, and A. Ferle-Vidovic. 1988a. Circadian and seasonal rhythms in murine bone marrow colony-forming cells affect tolerance for the anti-cancer agent 4-0-tetrahydropyranyl adriamycin (THP). Exp. Hematol. 16:696–701.

Levi, F., N.A. Boughattas, and I. Blazsek. 1986. Comparative murine chronotoxicity of anticancer agents and related mechanisms. Ann. Rev. Chronopharmacol. 4:283–331.

Levi, F., C. Canon, J.P. Blum, M. Mechkouri, A. Reinberg, and G. Mathe. 1985. Circadian and/or circahemidian rhythms in nine lymphocyte-related variables from peripheral blood of healthy subjects. J. Immunol. 134:217–222.

Levi, F., C. Canon, M. Dipalma, I. Florentin, and J.L. Misset. 1991. When should the immune clock be reset? From circadian pharmacodynamics to temporally optimized drug delivery. Ann. N.Y. Acad. Sci. 618:312–329.

Levi, F., C. Canon, Y. Touitou, A. Reinberg, and G. Mathe. 1988b. Seasonal modulation of the circadian time structure of circulating T- and natural killer lymphocyte subsets from healthy subjects. J. Clin. Invest. 81:407–413.

Levi, F.A., R. Zidani, J.M. Vannetzel, B. Perpoint, C. Focan, R. Faggiuolo, P. Chollet, C. Garufi, M. Itzhaki, and L. Dogliotti. 1994. Chronomodulated versus fixed-infusion-rate delivery of ambulatory chemotherapy with oxaliplatin, fluorouracil, and folinic acid (leucovorin) in patients with colorectal cancer metastases: a randomized multi-institutional trial. J. Natl. Cancer Inst. 86(21):1608–1617.

Lipa, B.J., P.A. Sturrock, and E. Rogot. 1976. Search for correlation between geomagnetic disturbances and mortality. Nature 259:302–304.

Lissoni, P., S. Barni, C. Archili, G. Cattaneo, F. Rovelli, A. Conti, G.J.M. Maestroni, and G. Tancini. 1990. Endocrine effects of a 24-hour intravenous infusion of interleukin-2 in the immunotherapy of cancer. Anticancer Res. 10:753–758.

Lissoni, P., S. Barni, G. Tancini, A. Ardizzoia, G. Ricci, R. Aldeghi, F. Brivio, E. Tisi, R. Rescaldani, G. Quadro, and G.J.M. Maestroni. 1994. A randomized study with subcutaneous low dose interleukin-2 alone vs. interleukin-2 plus the pineal neurohormone melatonin in advanced solid neoplasms other than renal cancer and melanoma. Br. J. Cancer 69:196–199.

Lissoni, P. S. Barni, G. Tancini, A. Ardizzoia, F. Rovelli, M. Cazzaniga, F. Brivio, A. Piperno, R. Aldeghi, D. Fossati, D. Characiejus, L. Kothari, A. Conti, and G.J.M. Maestroni. 1993. Immunotherapy with subcutaneous low dose interleukin-2 and the pineal indole melatonin as a new effective therapy in advanced cancers of the digestive tract. Br. J. Cancer 67:1404–1407.

Lissoni, P., S. Barni, G. Tancini, E. Maini, F. Piglia, G.J.M. Maestroni, and A. Lewinski 1995. Immunoendocrine therapy with low-dose subcutaneous interleukin-2 plus melatonin of locally advanced or metastatic endocrine tumors. Oncology 52:163–166.

Liu, T., M. Cavallini, F. Halberg, G. Cornélissen, J. Field, and D.E.R. Sutherland. 1986. More of the need for circadian, circaseptan, and circannual optimization of cyclosporine therapy. Experientia 42:20–22.

Lu, M.C., M.H. Smolensky, B. Hsi, and J.P. McGovern. 1979. Seasonal changes in immunoglobulin and complement levels in atopic and non-atopic persons. Pp. 261–272 in Recent Advances in the Chronobiology of Allergy and Immunology, M.H. Smolensky, A. Reinberg, and J.P. McGovern, eds. Oxford: Pergamon Press.

Lundeen, W., G.Y. Nicolau, D.J. Lakatua, L. Sackett-Lundeen, E. Petrescu, and E. Haus. 1990. Circadian periodicity of performance in athletic students. Progr. Clin. Biol. Res. 341B:337–343.

Mackiewicz, A., A. Kof, and P.B. Sehgal, eds. 1995. Interleukin-6-type cytokines. New York: New York Academy of Science. Pp. 1–522.

Maestroni, G.J.M. 1993. The immunoneuroendocrine role of melatonin. J. Pineal Res. 14:1–10. 1995. T-helper-2 lymphocytes as a peripheral target of melatonin. J. Pineal Res. 18:84–89.

Maestroni, G.J.M., and A. Conti. 1993. Melatonin in relation with the immune system. Pp. 229–311 in Melatonin: Biosynthesis, Physiological Effects, and Clinical Applications, Y. Hing-Su and R.J. Reiter, eds. Boca Raton, Fla.: CRC Press.

Maestroni, G.J.M., and W. Pierpaoli. 1981. Pharmacological control of the hormonally mediated immune-response. Pp. 405–425 in Psychoneuroimmunology, R. Ader, ed. New York: Academic Press.

Maestroni, G.J.M., A. Conti, and W. Pierpaoli. 1986. Role of the pineal gland in immunity. Circadian synthesis and release of melatonin modulates the antibody response and antagonizes the immunosuppressive effect of corticosterone. J. Neuroimmunol. 13:19–30.

Maestroni, G.J.M., A. Conti, and W. Pierpaoli. 1987a. The pineal gland and the circadian opiatergic immunoregulatory role of melatonin. Ann. N.Y. Acad. Sci. 496:67–77.

Maestroni, G.J.M., A. Conti, and W. Pierpaoli. 1987b. Role of the pineal gland in immunity. II. Melatonin enhances the antibody response via an opiatergic mechanism. Clin. Exp. Immunol. 68:384–391.

Maestroni, G.J.M., A. Conti, and W. Pierpaoli. 1988. Pineal melatonin: Its fundamental immunoregulatory role in aging and cancer. Ann. N.Y. Acad. Sci. 521:140–148.

Maini, R.N., M. Elliott, F.M. Brennan, R.O. Williams, and M. Feldmann. 1994. Targeting TNF-α for the therapy of rheumatoid arthritis. Clin. Exp. Rheumatol. 12(11):S63–S66.

Many, A., and R.S. Schwartz. 1971. Periodicity during recovery of the immune response after cyclophosphamide treatment. Blood 37:692–695.

Martini, E., J.Y. Muller, C. Doinel, C. Gastal, H. Roquin, L. Douay, and C. Salmon. 1988a. Disappearance of CD4 lymphocyte circadian cycles in HIV-infected patients: Early even during asymptomatic infection. AIDS 2:133–134.

Martini, E., J.Y. Muller, C. Gastal, C. Doinel, M.C. Meyohas, H. Roquin, J. Frottier, and C. Salmon. 1988b. Early anomalies of CD4 and CD20 lymphocyte cycles in human immunodeficiency virus. Presse Med. 17:2167–2168.

Masek, K., and O. Kadlec. 1983. Sleep factor, muramyl peptides, and the serotoninergic system [letter]. Lancet 2(8336):1277.

Mattson, R., I. Hannsson, and R. Holmdah. 1994. Pineal gland in autoimmunity: Melatonin-dependent exaggeration of collagen-induced arthritis in mice. Autoimmunity 17:83–86.

Menzio, P., B. Morra, A. Sartoris, R. Molino, M. Bussi, and G. Cortesina. 1980. Nasal secretory IgA circadian rhythm: A single-dose suppression. Ann. Otol. 89:173–175.

Mercola, K.E., M.J. Cline, and D.W. Golde. 1981. Growth hormone stimulation of normal and leukemic human T-lymphocyte proliferation in vitro. Blood 58:337–340.

Milos, P., D. Morse, and J.W. Hastings. 1990. Circadian control over synthesis of many Gonyaulax proteins is at a translational level. Naturwissenschaften 77:87–89.

Moldofsky, H. 1994. Central nervous system and peripheral immune functions and the sleep-wake system. J. Psychiatr. Neurosci. 19(5):368–374.

Moldofsky, H., F.A. Lue, J.R. Davidson, J. Jephthah-Ochola, K. Carayanniotis, and R. Gorczynski. 1989. The effect of 64 hours of wakefulness on immune functions and plasma cortisol in humans. Pp. 185–187 in Sleep '88, J. Horne, ed. New York: Gustav Fischer Verlag.

Moldofsky, H., F.A. Lue, J. Eisen, E. Keyston, and R.M. Gorczynski. 1986. The relationship of interleukin-1 and immune functions to sleep in humans. Psychosom. Med. 48:309–318.

Morley, A., E.A. King-Smith, and F.J. Stohlman. 1970. The oscillatory nature of hemopoiesis. Pp. 3–14 in Symposium on Hemopoietic Cellular Proliferation, F. Stohlman Jr., ed. New York: Grune and Stratton.

Mormont, M.C., R. von Roemeling, R.B. Sothern, J.S. Berestka, T.R. Langevin, M. Wick, and W.J.M. Hrushesky. 1988. Circadian rhythm and seasonal dependence in the toxicologic response of mice to epirubicin. Invest. New Drugs 6:273–283.

Morrey, M.K., J.A. McLachlan, Serkin C.D., and O. Bakouche. 1994. Activation of human monocytes by the pineal hormone melatonin. J. Immunol. 153:2671–2680.

Morse, D., P.M. Milos, E. Roux, and J.W. Hastings. 1989. Circadian regulation of bioluminescence in Gonyaulax involves translational control. Proc. Natl. Acad. Sci. USA 86:172–176.

Mortin, R., and G. Courchay. 1994. Pregnenolone and dehydroepiandrosterone as precursors of native 7-hydroxylated metabolites which increase the immune response in mice. J. Steroid Biochem. Mol. Biol. 50:91–100.

Mukaida, N., G.L. Gussella, T. Kasahara, Y. Ko, C.O. Zachariae, T. Kawai, and K. Matsushima. 1993. Molecular analysis of the inhibition of interleukin-8 production by dexamethasone in a human fibrosarcoma cell line. Immunology 75:674–679.

Murphy, W.J., H. Rui, and D.L. Longo. 1995. Effects of growth hormone and prolactin immune development and function. Life Sci. 57:1–14.

Myers, M.P., K. Wager-Smith, A. Rothenfluh-Hilfiker, and M.W. Young. 1996. Light-induced degradation of TIMELESS and entrainment of the Drosophila circadian clock. Science 271:1736–1740.

Nagy, E., I. Berczi, G.E. Wren, S.L. Asa, and K. Kovacs. 1983. Immunomodulation by bromocriptine. Immunopharmacology 6:231–243.

Naitoh, Y., J. Fukata, T. Tominaga, Y. Nakai, S. Tamai, K. Mori, and H. Imura. 1988. Interleukin-6 stimulates the secretion of adrenocorticotrophic hormone in conscious, freely moving rats. Biochem. Biophys. Res. Commun. 155:1459–1463.

Nakano, Y., T. Miura, I. Hara, H. Aono, N. Miyano, and K. Miyajima. 1982. The effect of shift work on cellular immune function. J. Hum. Ergol. 11(suppl.):131–137.

Nechaev, A., F. Halberg, A. Mittelman, and G.L. Tritsch. 1977. Circannual variation in human erythrocyte adenosine aminohydrolase. Chronobiologia 4:191–198.

Nelson, W., L. Scheving, and F. Halberg. 1975. Circadian rhythms in mice fed a single daily "meal" at different stages of LD 12:12 lighting regimen. J. Nutr. 105:171–184.

Nelson, W., Y.L. Tong, J.K. Lee, and F. Halberg. 1979. Methods for cosinor rhythmometry. Chronobiologia 6:305–323.

Nicolau, G.Y., and E. Haus. 1994. Chronobiology of the hypothalamic-pituitary-thyroid axis. Pp. 330–347 in Biologic Rhythms in Clinical and Laboratory Medicine, 2d ed., Y. Touitou and E. Haus, eds. Heidelberg: Springer-Verlag.

Nicolau, G.Y., D.J. Lakatua, L. Sackett-Lundeen, and E. Haus. 1984. Circadian and circannual rhythms of hormonal variables in elderly men and women. Chronobiol. Int. 1:301–319.

Nye, L., T.G. Merret, J. Landon, and R.J. White. 1975. A detailed investigation of circulating IgE levels in a normal population. Clin. Allergy 5(1):13–24.

O'Dorisio, M.S., C.L. Wood, and T.M. O'Dorisio. 1984. Vasoactive intestinal peptide and neuropeptide modulation of the immune response. J. Immunol. 135:792S–796S.

Ohlman, S., A. Lindholm, H. Hagglund, J. Sawe, and B.D. Kahan. 1993. On the intraindividual variability and chronobiology of cyclosporine pharmacokinetics in renal transplantation. Eur. J. Clin. Pharmacol. 44:265–269.

Olsen, N.J., and W.J. Kovacs. 1996. Steroids and immunity. Endocr. Rev. 17:369–384.

Opp, M.R., H. Kapas, and L.A. Toth. 1992. Cytokine involvement in the regulation of sleep. Proc Soc Exp Biol Med. 201:16–27.

Opstad, P.K. 1991. Alterations in the morning plasma levels of hormones and the endocrine responses to bicycle exercise during prolonged strain. The significance of energy and sleep deprivation. Acta Endocrinol. (Cophenh.) 125:14–22.

Opstad, P.K. 1992. Androgenic hormones during prolonged physical stress, sleep, and energy deficiency. J. Clin. Endocrinol. Metab. 74:1176–1183.

Opstad, P.K. 1994. Circadian rhythm of hormones is extinguished during prolonged physical stress, sleep, and energy deficiency in young men. Eur. J. Endocrinol. 131:56–66.

Palestine, A.G., C.G. Muellenberg-Coulombre, M.K. Kim, M.C. Gelato, and R.B. Nussenblatt. 1987. Bromocriptine and low dose cyclosporine in the treatment of experimental autoimmune uveitis in the rat. J. Clin. Invest. 79:1078–1081.

Palmblad, J., K. Cantell, H. Strander, J. Froberg, C.G. Karlsson, L. Levi, M. Granstom, and P. Unger. 1976. Stressor exposure and immunological response in man: Interferon-producing capacity and phagocytosis. J. Psychosom. Res. 20:193–199.

Palmblad, J., B. Petrini, J. Wasserman, and T. Akerstedt. 1979. Lymphocyte and granulocyte reactions during sleep deprivation. Psychosom. Med. 41:273–278.

Pangerl, A., J. Remien, and E. Haen. 1986. The number of β-adrenoceptor sites on intact human lymphocytes depends on time of day, on season, and on sex. Ann. Rev. Chronopharmacol. 3:331–334.

Pappenheimer, J.R. 1983. Induction of sleep by muramyl peptides. J. Physiol. 335:1–2.

Pati, A.K., I. Florentin, V. Chung, M. DeSousa, F. Levi, and G. Mathe. 1987. Circannual rhythm in natural killer activity and mitogen responsiveness of murine splenocytes. Cell. Immunol. 108:227–234.

Peleg, L., M.N. Nesbitt, and I.E. Ashkenazi. 1989. Strain dependent response of circadian rhythms during exposure to continuous illumination. Life Sci. 44:893–900.

Petrovsky, N., P. McNair, and L.C. Harrison. 1994. Circadian rhythmicity of interferon-γ production in antigen-stimulated whole blood. Chronobiologia 21:293–300.

Pöllman, L., and B. Pöllman. 1988. Variations of the efficiency of hepatitis B vaccination. Annual Rev. Chronopharmacol. 5:45–48.

Portaluppi, F., P. Cortelli, P. Avoni, and L. Vergnani. 1994. Progressive disruption of the circadian rhythm of melatonin in fatal familial insomnia. J. Clin. Endocrinol. Metab. 78(5):1075–1078.

Pownall, R., and M.S. Knapp. 1980. Immune responses have rhythms. Are they important? Immunol. Today 1:7–10.

Pownall, R., P.A. Kabler, and M.S. Knapp. 1979. The time of day of antigen encounter influences the magnitude of the immune response. Clin. Exp. Immunol. 36:347–354.

Provinciali, M., G. DiStefano, and N. Fabris. 1992. Improvement in the proliferative capacity and natural killer cell activity of murine spleen lymphocytes by thyrotropin. J. Immunopharmacol. 14:865–870.

Raine, C.S., V. Traugott, and S.H. Stone. 1978. Suppression of chronic allergic encephalomyelitis: Relevance to multiple sclerosis. Science 201:445–448.

Rankin, E.C., E.H. Choy, D. Kassimos, and G.H. Kingsley. 1995. The therapeutic effects of an engineered human anti-tumor necrosis factor-α antibody (CDP571) in rheumatoid arthritis. Br. J. Rheumatol. 34(4):334–342.

Ratté, J., F. Halberg, and J.F.W. Kuhl. 1973. Circadian variation in the rejection of rat kidney allografts. Surgery 73:102–108.

Reinberg, A. 1967. The hours of changing responsiveness or susceptibility. Perspect. Biol. Med. 11:111–128.

Reinberg, A. 1989. Chronopharmacology of corticosteroids and ACTH. Pp. 137–167 in Chronopharmacology, Cellular, and Biochemical Interactions, B. Lemmer, ed. New York: Marcel Dekker.

Reinberg, A., and E. Sidi. 1966. Circadian changes in the inhibitory effects of an antihistaminic drug in man. J. Invest. Dermatol. 46:415–419.

Reinberg, A., and M.H. Smolensky. 1994. Night and Shift Work and Transmeridian and Space Flights. Pp. 243-255 in Biologic Rhythms in Clinical and Laboratory Medicine, 2d ed., Y. Touitou and E. Haus, eds. Heidelberg: Springer-Verlag.

Reinberg, A., P. Gervais, M. Morin, and C. Abulker. 1971. Human circadian rhythm in threshold of the bronchial response to acetylcholine. C.R. Acad. Sci. Hebd. Seances Acad. Sci. D. 272:1879–1881.

Reinberg, A., J. Ghata, and E. Sidi. 1963. Nocturnal asthma attacks: Their relationship to the circadian adrenal cycle. J. Allerg. 34:323–330.

Reinberg A., G. Labreque, and M.H. Smolensky, eds. 1991. Chronobiologie et Chronotherapeutique. Heme Optimale d'Administration des Medicamcuts. Paris: Flamarion-Medecine-Sciences.

Reinberg, A., E. Schuller, J. Clench, and M.H. Smolensky. 1979. Circadian and circannual rhythms of leukocytes, proteins, and immunoglobulins. Pp. 251–259 in Recent Advances in the Chronobiology of Allergy and Immunology, M.H. Smolensky, A. Reinberg, and J.P. McGovern, eds. Oxford: Pergamon Press.

Reinberg, A., E. Sidi, and J. Ghata. 1965. Circadian reactivity rhythms of human skin to histamine or allergen and the adrenal cycle. J. Allerg. 36:273–283.

Reinberg, A., M.H. Smolensky, G.E. D'Alonzo, and J.P. McGovern. 1988a. Chronobiology and asthma. III. Timing corticotherapy to biological rhythms to optimize treatment goals. J. Asthma 25:219–248.

Reinberg, A., Y. Touitou, M. Botbol, P. Gervais, D. Chaouat, F. Levi, and A. Bicakova-Rocher. 1988b. Oral morning dosing of corticosteroids in long term treated cortico-dependent asthmatics: Increased tolerance and preservation of the adrenocortical function. Ann. Rev. Chronopharmacol. 5:209–212.

Reinberg, A., Y. Touitou, A. Restoin, C. Migraine, F. Levi, and H. Montagner. 1985. The genetic background of circadian and ultradian rhythm patterns of 17-hydroxycorticosteroids: A cross twin study. J. Endocrinol. 105:247–253.

Rensing L. 1997. Genetics and molecular biology of circadian clocks. Pp. 55–77 in Physiology and Pharmacology of Biologic Rhythms. Handbook of Experimental Pharmacology, Volume 125, P.H. Redfern and B. Lemmer, eds. Heidelberg: Springer-Verlag.

Richtsmeier, W.S. 1985. Interferon. Present and future prospects. CRC Crit. Rev. Clin. Lab. Sci. 20:57–93.

Ritchie, A.W.S., I. Oswald, H.S. Micklem, J.E. Boyd, R.A. Elton, E. Jazwinska, and K. James. 1983. Circadian variation of lymphocyte subpopulations: A study with monoclonal antibodies. Br. Med. J. 286:1773–1775.

Rivard, G.E., C. Infante-Rivard, M.F. Dresse, J.M. Leclerc, and J. Champagne. 1993. Circadian time-dependent response of childhood lymphoblastic leukemia to chemotherapy: A long-term follow-up study of survival. Chronbiol. Int. 10:201–204.

Rivier, C., and S. Rivest. 1993. Mechanisms mediating the effects of cytokines on neuroendocrine functions in the rat. Ciba Found. Symp. 172:204–220.

Romball, C.G., and W.O. Weigle. 1973. A cyclical appearance of antibody producing cells after a single injection of serum protein antigen. J. Exp. Med. 138:1426–1442.

Romball, C.G., and W.O. Weigle. 1976. Modulation of regulatory mechanisms operative in the cyclical production of antibody. J. Exp. Med. 143:497–510.

Rosenblatt, L.S., M. Shifrine, N.W. Hetherington, T. Paglierioni, and M.R. Mackenzie. 1982. A circannual rhythm in rubella antibody titers. J. Interdiscipl. Cycle Res. 13:81–88.

Russell, D.H., K.T. Mills, F.J. Talamantes, and H.A. Bern. 1988. Neonatal administration of prolactin antiserum alters the development pattern of T- and B-lymphocytes in the thymus and spleen in Balb/C female mice. Proc. Natl. Acad. Sci. USA 85:7404–7407.

Russo, M.F. 1992. Macrophages and the glucocorticoids. J. Neuroimmunol. 40:281–286.

Sabate, I., J.M. Grino, A.M. Castelao, B. Arranz, C. Gonzalez, E. Guillin, C. Diaz, J. Huguet, and S. Gracia. 1990. Diurnal variations of cyclosporine and metabolites in renal transplant patients. Transplant. Proc. 22:1700–1701.

Scheving, L.E., E. Burns, J.E. Pauly, S. Tsai, and F. Halberg. 1976. Meal scheduling, cellular rhythms, and the chronotherapy of cancer [abstract]. Chronobiologia 3:80.

Scheving, L.E., E.L. Kanabrocki, F. Halberg, and J.E. Pauly. 1977. Circadian variations in total and electrophoretically fractioned serum proteins of presumably healthy man. Pp. 204–214 in Chronobiology in Allergy and Immunology, J.P. McGovern, M.H. Smolensky, and A. Reinberg, eds. Springfield, Ill.: Charles C Thomas.

Scheving, L.E., J.E. Pauly, and T. Tsai. 1968. Circadian fluctuation in plasma proteins of the rat. Am. J. Physiol. 215:1096–1101.

Schuurs, A.H., and H.A. Verheul. 1990. Effects of gender and sex steroids on the immune system. J. Steroid Biochem. 25:157–172.

Schwab, R., C.A. Waiters, and M.E. Weksler. 1989. Host defense mechanisms and aging. Semin. Oncol. 16:20–27.

Schweiger, H.G., R. Hartwig, and M. Schweigher. 1986. Cellular aspects of circadian rhythms. J. Cell Sci. 4(suppl.):181–200.

Senie, R.T., P.P. Rosen, P. Rhodes, and M.L. Lesser. 1991. Timing of breast cancer excision during the menstrual cycle influences duration of disease-free survival. Ann. Intern. Med. 115:337–342.

Sensi, S., E. Haus, G.Y. Nicolau, F. Halberg, D.J. Lakatua, A. DelPonte, and M.T. Guagnano. 1984. Circannual variation of insulin secretion in clinically healthy subjects in Italy, Romania, and the U.S.A. Riv. Ital. Biol. Med. 4:1–8.

Shahal, B., F.A. Lue, C.G. Jiang, A. MacLean, and H. Moldofsky. 1992. Circadian and sleep-wake related changes in immune functions. J. Sleep Res. 1(suppl.):210.

Sharp, G.W.G. 1960. Reversal of diurnal leukocyte variations in man. J. Endocrinol. 21:107–114.

Shaw, L.M., B. Kaplan, and D. Kaufman. 1996. Toxic effects of immunosuppressive drugs: Mechanisms and strategies of controlling them. Clin. Chem. 42:1316–1321.

Shephard, R.J., S. Rhind, and P.N. Shek. 1995. The impact of exercise on the immune system: NK cells, interleukins-1 and -2, and related responses. Exerc. Sport Sci. Rev. 23:215–241.

Shifrine, M., A. Garsd, and L.S. Rosenblatt. 1982a. Seasonal variation in immunity of humans. J. Interdiscipl. Cycle Res. 12:157–165.

Shifrine, M., L.S. Rosenblatt, N. Taylor, N.W. Hetherington, F.J. Mathews, and F.D. Wilson. 1982b. Seasonal variations in lectin-induced lymphocyte transformation in Beagle dogs. J. Interdiscipl. Cycle Res. 13:151–156.

Shifrine, M., N. Taylor, L.S. Rosenblatt, and F. Wilson. 1980. Seasonal variation in cell-mediated immunity of clinically normal dogs. Exp. Hematol. 8:318–326.

Shoham, S., D. Davenne, A. B. Cady, C.A. Dinarello, and J.M. Krueger. 1987. Recombinant tumor necrosis factor and interleukin-1 enhance slow wave sleep. Am. J. Physiol. 253:R142–R149.

Sitar, J. 1991. Correlation of some parameters of solar wind and sudden cardiovascular deaths. Cas Lek Cesk. 130:44–47.

Slozina, N.M., and G.D. Golovachev. 1986. The frequency of sister chromatin exchanges in human lymphocytes determined at different times within 24 hours. Citologia 28:127–129.

Smith, E.M. 1992. Hormonal activities of cytokines. Chem. Immunol. 52:154–169.

Smith, E.M., W.J. Meyer, and J.E. Blalock. 1982. Virus-induced increases in corticosterone in hypophysectomized mice: A possible lymphoid adrenal axis. Science 218:1311–1313.

Smith, E.M., A.C. Morrill, W.J.I. Meyer, and J.E. Blalock. 1986. Corticotropin-releasing factor induction of lymphocyte-derived immunoreactive ACTH and endorphins. Nature 321:881–882.

Smolensky, M.H., and G.E.D. D'Alonzo. 1994. Nocturnal asthma: mechanisms and chronotherapy. Pp. 453–469 in Biologic Rhythms in Clinical and Laboratory Medicine, 2d ed., Y. Touitou and E. Haus, eds. New York: Springer-Verlag.

Smolensky, M.H., and G.E.D. D'Alonzo. 1997. Progress in the chronotherapy of nocturnal asthma. Pp. 205-250 in Physiology and Pharmacology of Biologic Rhthyms. Handbook of Experimental Pharmacology, Volume 125, P.H. Redfern and B. Lemmer, eds. Heidelberg: Springer-Verlag.

Smolensky, M.H., P.J. Barnes, A. Reinberg, and J.P. McGovern. 1986a. Chronobiology and asthma. I. Day-night differences in bronchial patency and dyspnea and circadian rhythm dependencies. J. Asthma 23:321–343.

Smolensky, M.H., G.E. D'Alonzo, G. Kunkel, and P.J. Barnes. 1987. Circadian rhythm-adapted theophylline chronotherapy for nocturnal asthma. Chronobiol. Int. 4:301–466.

Smolensky, M.H., A. Reinberg, and J.T. Queng. 1981. The chronobiology and chronopharmacology of allergy. Ann. Allergy 47:237–252.

Smolensky, M.H., P.H. Scott, P.J. Barnes, and J.H.G. Jonkman. 1986b. The chronopharmacology and chronotherapy of asthma. Ann. Rev. Chronopharmacol. 2:229–273.

Soiffer, R.J., C. Murray, C. Shapiro, H. Collins, S. Chartier, S. Lazo, and J. Ritz. 1996. Expansion and manipulation of natural killer cells in patients with metastatic cancer by low-dose continuous infusion and intermittent bolus administration of interleukin-2. Clin. Cancer Res. 2:493–499.

Song, J.G., S. Nakano, S. Ohdo, and N. Ogawa. 1993. Chronotoxicity and chronopharmacokinetics of methotrexate in mice: Modification of feeding schedule. Japan J. Pharmacol. 62:373–378.

Sothern, R.B., B. Roitman-Johnson, E.L. Kanabrocki, J.G. Yager, M.M. Roodell, J.A. Weatherbee, M.R. Young, B.M. Nemchausky, and L.E. Scheving. 1995. Circadian characteristics of circulating interleukin-6 in men. J. Allergy Clin. Immunol. 95:1029–1035.

Souba, W.W. 1994. Cytokine control of nutrition and metabolism in critical illness. Curr. Probl. Surg. 31(7):577–652.

Spangelo, B.L., and W.C. Gorospe. 1995. Role of the cytokines in the neuroendocrine immune system axis. Front. Neuroendocrinol. 16:1–22.

Stimpfling, J.H., and A. Richardson. 1967. Periodic variations of the hemagglutinin response in mice following immunization against sheep red blood cells and alloantigens. Transplantation 5:1496–1503.

Stimson, W.H. 1988. Oestrogen and human T-lymphocytes: Presence of specific receptors in the T-suppressor cytotoxic subset. Scand. J. Immunol. 28:345–350.

Suteanu, S., E. Haus, L. Dumitriu, G.Y. Nicolau, E. Petrescu, H. Berg, L. Sackett-Lundeen, I. Ionescu, R. Reilly. 1995. Circadian rhythm of pro- and anti-inflammatory factors in patients with rheumatoid arthritis-#226 [abstract]. Biological Rhythm Research 26:(4)446.

Swoyer, J., P. Irvine, L. Sackett-Lundeen, L. Conlin, D.J. Lakatua, and E. Haus. 1989. Circadian hematologic time structure in the elderly. Chronobiol. Int. 6:131–137.

Swoyer, J., F. Rhame, W. Hrushesky, L. Sackett-Lundeen, R. Sothern, H. Gale, and E. Haus. 1990. Circadian rhythm alterations in HIV-infected patients. Pp. 437–449 in Chronobiology: Its Role in Clinical Medicine, General Biology, and Agriculture, Proceedings of the XIX International Conference of the International Society for Chronobiology, Bethesda, Md., June 20–24, 1989. New York: Wiley-Liss, Inc.

Swoyer, J., L.L. Sackett, E. Haus, D.J. Lakatua, and L. Taddeini. 1975. Circadian lymphocytic rhythms in clinically healthy subjects and in patients with hematologic malignancies [abstract]. Pp. 62-63 in International Congress on Rhythmic Functions in Biological System, Vienna: Egerman.

Tarquini, B. 1980. Physiopathology of peptic ulcer: A new view. Rass. di Medicina Sperimentale 27(5):279.

Tavadia, H.B., K.A. Fleming, P.D. Hume, and H.W. Simpson. 1975. Circadian rhythmicity of human plasma cortisol and PHA-induced lymphocyte transformation. Clin. Exp. Immunol. 22:190–193.

Tobler, I., A.A. Borbely, M. Schwyzer, and A. Fontana. 1984. Interleukin-1 derived from astrocytes enhances slow wave activity in sleep EEG of rat. Eur. J. Pharmacol. 104:191–192.

Touitou, Y., A. Carayon, A. Reinberg, A. Bogdan, and H. Beck. 1983. Differences in the seasonal rhythmicity of plasma prolactin in elderly subjects. Detection in women but not in men. J. Endocrinol. 96:65-71.

Touitou, Y., and E. Haus. 1994. Aging of the human endocrine and neuroendocrine time structure. Ann. N.Y. Acad. Sci. 719:378–397.

Tritsch, G.L., A. Nechaev, and A. Mittelman. 1975. Adenosine aminohydrolase as an indicator of lymphocyte-mediated cytolysis: Possible role of cyclic adenosine monophosphate. Clin. Chem. 21:984.

Turner-Warwick, M. 1988. Epidemiology of nocturnal asthma. Am. J. Med. 85(suppl. 1B):6–8.

Uezono, K., L. Sackett-Lundeen, T. Kawasaki, T. Omae, and E. Haus. 1987. Circaseptan rhythm in sodium and potassium excretion in salt sensitive and salt resistant Dahl rats. Pp. 297–307 in Advances in Chronobiology, Part A, J.E. Pauly and L.E. Scheving, eds. New York: Alan R. Liss, Inc.

Valtora, A., A. Moretta, R. Maccario, M. Bozzola, and F. Severi. 1991. Influence of growth hormone-releasing hormone (GHRH) on phytohemagglutinin-induced lymphocyte activation: comparison of two synthetic forms. Thymus 18:51–59.

Van Cauter, E., and F.W. Turek. 1995. Endocrine and other biologic rhythms. Pp. 2487–2548 in Endocrinology, Degroot, L.J. ed. Philadelphia: W.B. Saunders Company.

Varma, S., P. Sabharwal, J.F. Sheridan, and W.B. Malarkey. 1993. Growth hormone secretion by human peripheral blood mononuclear cells detected by an enzyme-linked immunoplaque assay. J. Clin. Endocrinol. Metab. 76:49–53.

Venkataramanan, R., S. Yang, G.J. Burckard, R.J. Ptachcinski, D.H. Van Thiel, and T.E. Starzl. 1986. Diurnal variation in cyclosporine pharmacokinetics. Ther. Drug Monit. 8:380–381.

Walker, A.M. 1994. Phosphorylated and non-phosphorylated prolactin isoforms. Endocrinol. Metab. 5:195–200.

Weigent, D.A., and J.E. Blalock. 1995. Associations between the neuroendocrine and immune systems. J. Leukocyte Biol. 58:137–150.

Weigle, W.O. 1975. Cyclic production of antibody as a regulatory mechanism in the immune response. Adv. Immunol. 21:87–111.

Wendling, D., E. Racadot, and J. Wijdeness. 1993. Treatment of severe rheumatoid arthritis by anti-interleukin-6 monoclonal antibody. J. Rheumatol. 20(2):259–262.

Westaway, J., C.M. Atkinson, T. Davies, S.A. Petersen, and M.P. Wailoo. 1995. Urinary excretion of cortisol after immunization. Arch. Dis. Child. 72:432–434.

Wilder, R.L. 1995. Neuroendocrine-immune system interactions and autoimmunity. Ann. Rev. Immunol. 13:307–338.

Williams, R.M., L.J. Kraus, D.P. Dubey, E.J. Yunis, and F. Halberg. 1979. Circadian bioperiodicity in natural killer cell activity of human blood [abstract]. Chronobiologia 6:172.

Winget, C.M., M.R.I. Soliman, D.C. Holley, and J.S. Meylor. 1994. Chronobiology of Physical Performance and Sports Medicine. Pp. 230–242 in Biologic Rhythms in Clinical and Laboratory Medicine, 2d ed., Y. Touitou and E. Haus, eds. Heidelberg: Springer-Verlag.

Withyachumnarnkul, B., K.O. Nonaka, C. Santana, A.M. Attia, and R.J. Reiter. 1990. Interferon-γ modulates melatonin production in rat pineal gland in organ culture. J. Interferon Res. 10:403–411.

Wood, P.A., and W.J.M. Hrushesky. 1994. Chronopharmacodynamics of hematopoietic growth factors and antitumor cytokines. Pp. 185–207 in Circadian Cancer Therapy, W.J.M. Hrushesky, ed. Boca Raton, Fla.: CRC Press.

Yehuda, S., B. Shredny, and Y. Kalechman. 1987. Effects of DSIP, 5-HTP, and serotonin on the lymphokine system: A preliminary study. Int. J. Neurosci. 33:185–187.

Young, M.R.I., J.P. Matthews, E.L. Kanabrocki, R.B. Sothern, B. Roitman-Johnson, and L.E. Scheving. 1995. Circadian rhythmometry of serum interleukin-2, interleukin-10, tumor necrosis factor-α, and granulocyte-macrophage colony stimulating factor in men. Chronobiol. Int. 12:19–27.

Young, M.W., ed. 1993. Molecular Genetics of Biological Rhythms. New York: Dekker.

Young, M.W., F.R. Jackson, H.S. Shin, and T.A. Bargiello. 1985. A biological clock in Drosophila. Cold Spring Harbor Symp. Quant. Biol. 50:865–875.

Zabel, P., H. Horst, C. Kreiber, and M. Schlaak. 1990. Circadian rhythm of interleukin-1 production of monocytes and the influence of endogenous and exogenous glucocorticoids in man. Klin Wochenschr. 68:1217–1221.

Zabel, P., K. Linnemann, and M. Schlaak. 1993. Circadian rhythm in cytokines. Immun. Infekt. 20:38–40.

Zimmer, J., A.S. Khalifa, and J.J. Lightbody. 1975. Decreased lymphocyte adenosine deaminase activity in acute lymphocytic leukemic children and their parents. Cancer 35(1):68–70.

Nutrition and Immune Function, 1999
Pp. 497–507. Washington, D.C.
National Academy Press

21

Conclusions: Militarily Important Issues Identified in this Report

William R. Beisel[1]

INTRODUCTION

The workshop held on May 20–21, 1996, and this report provide a broad review of current concepts about nutritional immunology. The task of this chapter is to summarize militarily important issues about a complex subject. LTC Karl E. Friedl's chapter introduces Army concerns that multistressor components of rigorous military training induced weight loss, impairments in immunological indices, and at times, an increased incidence of infectious illnesses (see Chapter 4 in this volume). Because higher energy intakes appeared to preserve immune functions, even in the presence of multiple other military stresses, the Committee on Military Nutrition Research (CMNR) was asked to consider five complex questions:

[1] William R. Beisel, Department of Molecular Microbiology and Immunology, The Johns Hopkins School of Hygiene and Public Health, Baltimore, MD. *Mailing addresses*: 8210 Ridgelea Court, Frederick, MD 21702 *or* 2108 Harlans Run, Naples, FL 34105.

1. What methods for assessment of immune function are most appropriate in military nutrition laboratory research, and what methods are most appropriate for field research?

2. What are the significant military hazards or operational settings most likely to compromise immune function in soldiers?

3. The proinflammatory cytokines have been proposed to decrease lean body mass, mediate thermoregulatory mechanisms, and increase resistance to infectious disease by reducing metabolic activity in a way that is similar to the reduction seen in malnutrition and other catabolic conditions. Interventions to sustain immune function can alter the actions, nutritional costs, and potential changes in the levels of proinflammatory cytokines. What are the benefits and risks to soldiers of such interventions?

4. What are the important safety and regulatory considerations in the testing and use of nutrients or dietary supplements to sustain immune function under field conditions?

5. Are there areas of investigation for the military nutrition research program that are likely to be fruitful in the sustainment of immune function in stressful conditions? Specifically, is there likely to be enough value added to justify adding to operational rations or including an additional component?

GENERAL CONCEPTS

Ranjit Kumar Chandra, for decades a world leader and prolific writer in the field of nutritional immunology, discusses the role of malnutrition in diminishing resistance against infectious diseases and in creating dysfunctions in cell-mediated immunity, in humoral and secretory antibody production, in phagocyte function, in cytokine production, and in complement system effectiveness (see Chapter 7 in this volume).

These effects can be termed generalized or single-nutrient malnutrition, *nutritionally acquired immune dysfunction syndromes*, or NAIDS. NAIDS, in combination with various forms of infectious diseases, are the major cause of human mortality, leading to the deaths of over 20,000 children (largely in underdeveloped nations) each day (along with deaths of countless elderly individuals) and in modern medical centers, deaths of patients with severe medical illnesses and surgical interventions.

Chandra emphasizes the practical applications of nutritional supplementation in both preventive and therapeutic situations. The committee's task will be to translate Chandra's immunological data into meaningful recommendations concerning optimal nutritional support for healthy, well-conditioned, young adults who face the multiple, complex stresses associated with military operations in training situations as well as in operational missions that may include combat.

The chapters by Jeffrey L. Rossio and Seymour Reichlin (see Chapters 8 and Chapter 18, respectively, in this volume) also have broad, general importance. Rossio begins with an overview of the cytokine system; note that almost every speaker at this workshop mentioned cytokines and their importance in nutritional immunology. Rossio brings the general topic of cytokines up-to-date in a chapter that extends and amplifies Lyle L. Moldawer's discussion of cytokine assay methods in an earlier CMNR report (Moldawer, 1997). Rossio defines five types of cytokine activities, and he reviews the complex interactions among cytokines. In discussing their highly intracoordinated controls, Rossio emphasizes the propensity for cytokines to overlap in their multiple activities and to regulate each other. The systems of checks and balances that maintain hormonal homeostasis are minuscule in comparison with the checks and balances that regulate the synthesis and cellular effects of various cytokines.

Cytokine actions on cells can be influenced by the production of cytokine receptors, the release of such receptors into plasma, and the inhibitory proteins that block the cell wall receptors. At the same time, cellular production of individual cytokines can be reduced by other inhibitory cytokines, by hormones, or by other biologically active molecules. Rossio suggests that an unusual profile of serum cytokines (and related molecules) might signify a departure from homeostasis. This concept bears further thought and research.

Rossio warns that scientists have viewed cytokines with individualized perspectives and that his perceptions are as an immunologist. However, from the perspectives of this report, the nutritional role of proinflammatory cytokines that this author's U.S. Army Medical Research Institute of Infectious Diseases (USAMRIID) team discovered a full quarter century ago must be emphasized (Pekarek and Beisel, 1971; Wannemacher et al., 1972). The newly discovered agents were called "leukocytic endogenous mediators," or LEMs, and it was a struggle for many years to gain the LEMs the recognition they deserved. LEMs were never accepted as hormones, although as Reichlin points out, they met all the definitions of hormones. Eventually, the words *interleukin* and *cytokine* were introduced. With new and acceptable immunological names, and the advances in biotechnology that allowed the production of sizable amounts of individual cytokines, the field experienced logarithmic growth. In any event, the immunological benefits and functions of the cytokines often have large nutritional costs for the host. Cytokine-induced "acute phase reactions" are accompanied by cytokine-induced malnutrition.

Rossio points out that cytokine responses might be used as surrogate markers of nutritional adequacy. In this regard, almost every essential nutrient is involved in the production of cytokines and/or in the diverse cellular activities they stimulate.

Reichlin discusses the neuroendocrine consequences of systemic inflammation (see Chapter 18 in this volume). Echoing the presentations of both Leonard P. Kapcala (see Chapter 19 in this volume) and Rossio, Reichlin also emphasizes the primary role of the flood of polypeptide cytokines that are released into the circulation by lymphocytes, monocytes, macrophages, and endothelial cells. These pluripotent mediators induce the relatively stereotyped pathophysiological responses termed the *acute phase reaction*, which is characterized by fever; nutrient catabolism; changes in protein, carbohydrate, and lipid metabolism; and profound changes in hepatic functions and in all components of the endocrine system. Reichlin also points out that associated sickness behaviors during infection can proceed to cognitive deficits, delirium, stupor, and coma if the infection becomes severe.

Proinflammatory cytokines activate the hypothalamic-pituitary-adrenal axis and stimulate a release of growth hormone and prolactin. At the same time, they inhibit pituitary stimulation of both thyroidal and hypothalamic-gonadal functions. As Reichlin points out, certain of these cytokines, such as interleukin (IL)-1 and tumor necrosis factor (TNF), can transduce the endothelia of the blood-brain barrier to exert central nervous system (CNS) effects. Cytokines may also be produced within the CNS.

MILITARILY USEFUL METHODS TO EVALUATE IMMUNOLOGICAL FUNCTIONS

Susanna Cunningham-Rundles discusses measures needed to evaluate human immune functions (see Chapter 9 in this volume). She emphasizes tests of cell-mediated immunity, humoral immunity, cytokine expression, and phagocyte function. She also emphasizes the need to determine the body content of key nutrients, focusing on those that significantly affect immune functions (protein, energy, most vitamins especially A, C, B_6, B_{12}, and folic acid; and trace elements including Fe, Zn, Cu, and Se).

Tim R. Kramer follows up his previous comments before this committee (IOM, 1993; 1997) by discussing methods using whole blood samples collected during field studies to assess cell-mediated immunity and to study the production of cytokines and the cellular release of cytokine receptors (see Chapter 10 in this volume). Such large-scale testing is a military necessity.

As demonstrated by these two presentations and the discussions that followed at the May 1996 workshop, methodological concerns and data interpretation are highly important issues in all studies of nutritional immunology.

HEALTH STATUS, STRESS, AND IMMUNE FUNCTION

David C. Nieman describes the effects of both acute and long-term exercise on natural killer (NK) cells, neutrophils, and macrophage/monocytes, and the somewhat lesser effects on T- and B-lymphocytes (see Chapter 17 in this volume). Nieman cites evidence that neutrophil function is suppressed by strenuous physical training, and this may increase the risk for upper respiratory tract infections (URIs). In contrast, a limited number of studies suggest that URI incidence may be reduced in those who engage in moderate level exercise. A recent paper by Peters et al. (1993) showed that vitamin C supplements could reduce the incidence of post-race URIs in ultramarathon runners.

Kapcala (see Chapter 19 in this volume) amplifies the views of Rossio and Reichlin (see Chapters 8 and 18 in this volume, respectively) by emphasizing the important bidirectional communication and interactions between the immune and neuroendocrine systems. Mediators for these interactions include cytokines, hormones, and neurotransmitters, with responding cells exhibiting the appropriate surface receptors. Stimulation of the hypothalamic-pituitary-adrenal axis by proinflammatory cytokines is of particular importance during inflammatory stresses. Kapcala points out the importance of the array of checks and balances provided by this bidirectionally interactive system, which he demonstrates clearly by studies in laboratory rats.

Kapcala's rat model demonstrates the potential benefits of cytokine release as well as the disastrous consequences of cytokine excesses. Benefits and detriments of cytokine activities are certainly seen during infections in human patients, but the role of glucocorticoids is often exaggerated in rodent models as compared with human disease. A full understanding of cytokine benefits and possible detriments is needed for an optimal management of battlefield casualties and infections seen in military personnel.

Although the CMNR has heard presentations on biological rhythms by speakers at earlier meetings, none were as clearly presented or as specifically focused toward nutritional concerns as the chapter by Erhard Haus (see Chapter 20 in this volume). The data shown by Haus clearly indicate the daily rhythmic changes in circulating lymphocyte numbers and in their subsets, as well as in their propensity to produce or respond to various cytokines. These cytokines also undergo circadian changes in concentration. The same seems to be true for certain soluble cytokine receptors and cytokine antagonists.

Lymphocyte activities and functions, including responses to antigens and antibody production, also exhibit circadian rhythms, a fact of potential military importance. Can responses to military vaccines be improved by administering them at just the right time of day? The same question can be asked about the deleterious effects of infections, or toxemias, if contracted at various times of day.

Abrupt changes in daily living and eating patterns, and in degrees of emotional and physical stress, are characteristic of military operations, as are intercontinental flights. It has long been recognized that military operations may disrupt circadian rhythms. However, relatively little is known about possible immunological rhythms having weekly, monthly, or yearly periodicity. In theory, such long-term rhythms would be less likely to have military relevance. Lymphocyte rhythms and their relationships to other body rhythms may be dramatically altered by the presence of chronic diseases, such as AIDS, or by changes in endocrine rhythms known to occur in acute febrile infections. One might ask if immunological rhythms are also altered by military or by various forms of military stress.

Stephen Morse's discusses emerging infections, nutritional status, and immunity in Appendix A of this volume. As Morse notes, this was an appropriate topic to be presented in the USAMRIID building, the country's finest laboratory for studying newly emerged, highly dangerous infectious microorganisms. Morse points out that environmental and social changes, as well as antibiotic resistance will accelerate the "microbial traffic" that gives animal pathogens the potential chance to infect new host populations, including human beings.

Morse also emphasizes that malnutrition could have added or synergistic effects on these other factors. He points out the propensities for immunosuppression caused by malnutrition to allow pathogens to spread more rapidly through immunocompromised populations, especially those with high population densities. In making his point, Morse cites the collaborative research of Melinda A. Beck and Orville A. Levander, research which showed that an avirulent strain of Coxsackievirus underwent rapid genomic evolution to become virulent when the infection was initiated in selenium-deficient mice.

Pål Wiik (see Chapter 6 in this volume) describes immunological studies in Norwegian Rangers during 7-d training courses that included 90 percent starvation, sleep deprivation, and a variety of other severe military stresses. Although infections were not observed, these Rangers exhibited a two- to threefold increase in blood granulocytes and monocytes and a 30 to 40 percent reduction in B- and T-lymphocytes and in eosinophil numbers. Concentrations of serum immunoglobulins also decreased, and variable responses were detected in cytokine measurements.

Wiik's data confirm and extend observations made in U.S. Rangers, as reviewed in several earlier reports of the CMNR (IOM, 1992, 1993). It must be assumed that the immunological dysfunctions, which develop quickly during Ranger-type military training, will also develop during military combat scenarios. With their longer training exercises, U.S. Army Rangers did experience outbreaks of infectious diseases. It is a historical fact that during major, long-term wars, more casualties are caused by naturally occurring infections than by hostile enemy actions.

The CMNR report must ask and try to differentiate, if possible, the relevance of dietary diminutions during combat and severe military training operations, in contrast to the relevance of numerous other types of stress that might lead to immunological dysfunctions in the military forces.

Is it possible that extraordinary efforts to maintain an adequate dietary intake of energy and essential nutrients during combat situations might prevent these stress-associated immunological dysfunctions? In short, can dietary measures, or supplements, provide as much protection against infectious illness as can the long-term military strategy of using immunizations to provide protection against selected infectious diseases? Wiik's chapter certainly raises some interesting questions.

NEW RESEARCH DIRECTIONS

CMNR member Douglas W. Wilmore changes the direction of the chapters by discussing the potential nutrient needs for a single amino acid, glutamine, during periods of military stress (see Chapter 11 in this volume). As Wilmore points out, glutamine is of great importance in diverse biochemical reactions. It is a major substrate for gluconeogenesis, and a major fuel for lymphocytes and macrophages. The functional capacity of the immune system is related to the availability of glutamine in a dose-dependent manner.

Although not an essential amino acid under ordinary circumstances, glutamine's consumption in cells increases beyond its rates of synthesis during periods of malnutrition, injury, or infection. This creates a "relative" deficiency state in which glutamine supplementation is beneficial, as confirmed by clinical studies. Wilmore suggests that glutamine supplements may also be of value for military personnel exposed to radiation or chemical injury or to bacterial pathogens. He postulates that glutamine supplementation might benefit the performance of healthy soldiers by supporting muscle protein synthesis and glycogen stores and by stimulating the production of growth hormone as well as bicarbonate.

LTC Ronald L. Shippee (see Chapter 19 in this volume) follows on this same theme with data from recent studies in military personnel exposed to severe stresses, including dietary deprivation. Micronutrient intervention studies, which included glutamine and selected antioxidant vitamins and minerals, demonstrated the potential military significance of such supplements.

Laura C. Rall and Simin Nikbin Meydani (see Chapter 13 in this volume) amplify the points raised by LTC Shippee about the relationship of antioxidants to the immune system. They call attention to the importance of oxidant-antioxidant balance in maintaining integrity and functionality of membrane lipids, cellular proteins, and nucleic acids. A balanced need for antioxidants also contributes to the control of signal transduction and gene expression in immune cells. Meydani's data show the immunological value of antioxidant supplements in aged individuals and in laboratory animals exposed to the oxidative stress of environmental pollutants. These comments about the broad protective roles of antioxidant vitamins also relates to the immunological value of glutamine supplements and the importance of glutamine in the synthesis of glutathione, one of the major intracellular antioxidants, as pointed out by Wilmore.

The data presented by Wilmore, Shippee and Meydani at the May 1996 workshop regarding glutamine and antioxidant supplements will receive careful evaluation by this committee. It will also need to evaluate the possible needs for arginine supplements. Arginine is the sole source of nitric oxide (NO) (Stamler et al., 1992). NO is thought to have bactericidal powers as effective as those of the better-known free oxygen radicals. The synthesis of NO is stimulated by proinflammatory cytokines, and gives rise to an excretion of nitrate (Wishnok et al., 1996

Single nutrients were also discussed by the last four speakers. The research studies of Richard D. Semba (see Chapter 12 in this volume) have contributed to a renewed interest in vitamin A during the past decade, in terms of its immunological and anti-infection value in malnourished children. Vitamin A undoubtedly provides considerable support for immune system functions. Programs for vitamin A supplementation are now reducing childhood morbidity and mortality throughout the world.

The CMNR must consider these data in terms of military needs. Military diets provide quite adequately for normal vitamin requirements. Healthy service personnel should therefore possess adequate stores of vitamin A in their bodies. It has been presumed that stores of vitamin A were sufficient to see soldiers through relatively short periods of severe military stress, even if those stresses include semistarvation. However, it must now be asked whether these stresses generate an increased degradation of vitamin A and other essential single nutrients. The military must also find out if the urinary excretion of vitamin A increases during military stress situations, as it does during infectious illnesses. The committee must also look into the unsettled question of whether beta-carotene possesses immunostimulatory properties that are absent in vitamin A.

After reviewing the roles of zinc and copper in supporting the immune system, Beck describes her own studies of selenium deficiency in mice, work done in collaboration with Levander (see Chapter 16 in this volume). These scientists demonstrated changes in the infecting Coxsackievirus B3 genome in the presence of selenium deficiency in the mouse host. A genetic mutation involving six nucleotide changes caused the avirulent virus to become virulent. These surprising findings are of great biological significance, for, as pointed out earlier by Morse (see Appendix A in this volume), effects of malnutrition in the host could possibly allow newly virulent microorganisms to emerge as a threat to humans.

Several pertinent questions must now be asked. Is there any evidence of selenium deficiency in the military's well-nourished troops? Could selenium deficiency emerge as a problem as a result of military stress, including that of partial starvation? Moreover, would selenium supplements provide any benefits, including those ascribed to its antioxidant properties? Selenium supplements are reportedly widely used in Europe, with little, if any, apparent evidence of toxicity.

Similar questions can be asked about possible copper deficiency. Is it present in U.S. troops? Could it occur during stress or semistarvation?

Of greater concern is the possible zinc deficiency in military personnel. Although zinc is sequestered during cytokine-induced acute phase reactions, there is normally no pool of stored zinc in the body. Furthermore, losses of zinc from the body appear to parallel losses of nitrogen during infections. The question arises, are losses of body zinc commonplace during military stresses that do not include infection? Nonetheless, there are concerns about zinc supplements, based on evidence that even slightly increased intakes of zinc might have immunosuppressive effects.

Darshan S. Kelley discusses interactions between essential polyunsaturated fatty acids (PUFAs) and the immune system (see Chapter 14 in this volume). He points out that lipid excesses as well as deficiencies can have immunosuppressive effects and that proper dietary balances between n-3 and n-6 PUFA are also important. The composition of cell wall lipids can be altered in animals and in humans, by dietary changes involving n-3 versus n-6 PUFA intakes.

More information is needed about the practical immunological importance of changes in cell wall lipids, as introduced by dietary manipulations. A diet high in n-3 PUFA can cause the cytokine-stimulated production of eicosanoids to shift to less-potent 5-series leukotrines and 3-series prostaglandins. The committee must ask if such dietary manipulations might have military relevance.

As an example, data have been obtained from horses fed supplements of n-3 PUFA containing linseed oil in an effort to induce the formation of eicosanoid mediators that might help resist endotoxin challenge. The concept worked fine when cells from n-3 PUFA-fed horses were tested *in vitro* against endotoxin (Morris et al., 1989), but in contrast, the donor horses supplemented by linseed oil retained their full, characteristically dangerous *in vivo* hypersensitivity to endotoxin (Henry et al., 1991). Although the composition of eicosanoid-generating cell wall PUFA can be altered by the manipulation of human diets, it is not yet known if such changes will affect the outcome of infectious illnesses.

Gerald T. Keusch rounds out the discussions on essential nutrients with a presentation on iron metabolism, microbial virulence, and host defense mechanisms (see Chapter 15 in this volume). Keusch points out that the normal state of iron nutrition in humans is one of significant physiological limitations in the availability of free iron. Iron is required by various microorganisms to support growth and replication. The possibility that an excess of iron (as related to the binding capacity of iron-transport proteins) could increase the severity of infectious illnesses has been an unsettled point for decades. Keusch's chapter, in agreement with newly published data (Gordeur et al., 1992; van Hensbroek et al., 1995), shows that the question is still unsettled, especially in regard to malaria. Oral iron therapy can be given safely to malarial patients who are receiving appropriate antimalarial drugs (van Hensbroek et al., 1995). At the same time, use of iron chelation therapy can hasten recovery from severe cerebral malaria. The military has poured much time, effort, and money into malaria research, including a 40-y screening program involving over 250,000 possible drugs, plus major vaccine development efforts (Wyler, 1992); thus, the potential contribution of iron is of considerable interest.

Iron nutrition is clearly a prominent concern, especially in female military personnel, whose physical performance is impaired in the presence of iron deficiency anemia. This committee has recently made formal recommendations concerning military problems of iron nutrition. As was summarized in a recent report from the CMNR (IOM, 1995b), 56 percent of women recruits enter basic training with low iron stores as assessed by serum ferritin, and 84 percent have low stores at the end of basic training. As a result, the CMNR recommended that women with reduced iron stores should not be enlisted until this problem has been corrected (IOM, 1995b). The prevalence of iron deficiency among men in the military is low. Nevertheless, because combat and even training can result in injuries causing blood loss, the role of iron deficiency in reducing immune function is of potential importance for men as well. Also, military personnel often are exposed to less than sanitary conditions and infectious organisms. Thus, the periodic monitoring of iron status is important for men and especially for women.

SUMMARY

As the workshop and resulting report elaborate so clearly, a variety of nutritional deficiencies can initiate clinically apparent forms of NAIDS. These clinical forms of NAIDS result from deficiencies of protein, energy, vitamins A and C, zinc, and iron. An isolated deficiency of many other essential nutrients can induce NAIDS in experimental animals, and some nutrients—such as the B-group vitamins, vitamins D and E, copper, selenium, essential fatty acids, and amino acids such as glutamine and arginine—may be of value in providing additional dietary support for the human immune system.

Even short-term dietary restrictions during stressful military training operations can induce laboratory evidence of NAIDS while longer periods of military stress can also predispose soldiers to the development of infectious illnesses. It remains unclear if derangements in immunological indices observed during strenuous military exercises are due solely to dietary deprivation, to other military stresses, or to some combination of both.

Much additional research is needed to generate a full understanding of the genesis of NAIDS and its practical importance in military operations.

An array of difficult questions have been posed to the CMNR. Data presented at this workshop will assist the committee in formulating answers to the questions posed and in developing recommendations for future research and operational practices. Finally, the words of Hippocrates may still hold much truth, "Let your food be your medicine, and your medicine be your food."

REFERENCES

Gordeur, V., P. Thuma, G. Brittenham, C. McLaren, D. Parry, A. Backenstose, G. Biema, R. Msiska, L. Holmes, E. McKinley, L. Vargas, R. Gilkeson, and A.A. Poltera. 1992. Effect of iron chelation therapy on recovery from deep coma in children with cerebral malaria. N. Engl. J. Med. 327:1473–1477.

Henry, M.M., J.N. Moore, and J.K. Fisher. 1991. Influence of an omega-3 fatty acid-enriched ration on *in vivo* responses of horses to endotoxin. Am. J. Vet. Res. 52:523–527.

IOM (Institute of Medicine). 1992. A Nutritional Assessment of U.S. Army Ranger Training Class 11/91 [brief report]. A brief report of the Committee on Military Nutrition Research, Food and Nutrition Board. March 23. Washington, D.C.

IOM (Institute of Medicine). 1993b. Review of the Results of Nutritional Intervention, U.S. Army Ranger Training Class 11/92 (Ranger II), B.M. Marriott, ed. A report of the Committee on Military Nutrition Research, Food and Nutrition Board. Washington, D.C.: National Academy Press.

IOM (Institute of Medicine). 1995b. A Review of Issues Related to Iron Status of Women During U.S. Army Basic Combat Training [letter report]. Committee on Military Nutrition Research, Food and Nutrition Board. December 19. Washington, D.C.

IOM (Institute of Medicine). 1997. Emerging Technologies for Nutrition Research, Potential for Assessing Military Performance Capability, S.J. Carlson-Newberry and R.B. Costello, eds. A report of the Committee on Military Nutrition Research, Food and Nutrition Board, Institute of Medicine. Washington, D.C.: National Academy Press.

Moldawer, L.L. 1997. The validity of blood and urinary cytokine measurements for detecting the presence of inflammation. Pp. 417–430 in Emerging Technologies for Nutrition Research: Potential for Assessing Military Performance Capability, S.J. Carlson-Newberry and R.B. Costello, eds. Committee on Military Nutrition Research, Food and Nutrition Board, Institute of Medicine. Washington, D.C.: National Academy Press.

Morris, D.M., M.M. Henry, J.N. Moore, and K. Fisher. 1989. Effect of dietary linoleid acid on indotoxin-induced thromboxane and prostacyclin production by equine peritoneal macrophages. Circ. Shock 29:311–318.

Pekarek, R.S., and W.R. Beisel. 1971. Characterization of the endogenousmediator(s) of serum zinc and iron depression during infection and other stresses. Proc. Soc. Exp. Biol. Med. 138:728–732.

Peters, E.M., J.M. Goetzsche, B. Gobbelaar, and T.D. Noakes. 1993. Vitamin C supplementation reduces the incidence of postrace symptoms of upper-respiratory-tract infection in ultramarathon runners. Am. J. Clin. Nutr. 57:170–174.

Stamler, J.S., D.J. Singel, and J. Loscalzo. 1992. Biochemistry of nitric oxide and its redox-activated form. Science 258:1898–1902.

van Hensbroek, M.B., S. Morris-Jones, S. Meisner, S. Jaffar, L. Bayo, R. Dackour, C. Phillips, and B.M. Greenwood. 1995. Iron, but not folic acid, combined with effective antimalarial therapy promotes phaematological recovery in African children after acute falciparum malaria. Trans. Soc. Trop. Med. Hyg. 89:672–676.

Wannemacher Jr., R.W., H.L. DuPont, R.S. Pekarek, M.C. Powanda, A. Schwartz, R.B. Hornick, and W.R. Beisel. 1972. An endogenous mediator of depression of amino acids and trace metals during typhoid fever. J. Infect. Dis. 126:77–86.

Wishnok, J.S., J.A. Glogowski, S.R. Tannenbaum S.R. 1996. Quantitation of nitrate, nitrite, and nitrosating agents. Methods Enzymol. 268:130–141.

Wyler, D.J. 1992. Bark, weeds, and iron chelators—drugs for malaria. N. Engl. J. Med. 327:1519–1521.

APPENDIXES

Nutrition and Immune Function, 1999
Pp. 511–525. Washington, D.C.
National Academy Press

A

Overview of the Immune System and Other Host Defense Mechanisms

William R. Beisel[1]

Immunity, if defined broadly, encompasses all mechanisms and responses used by the body to defend itself against foreign substances, microorganisms, toxins, and noncompatible living cells. Such immunity may be conferred by the immune system itself, or by the protective role of other generalized host defensive mechanisms. Every aspect of immunity and host defense is dependent upon a proper supply and balance of nutrients (Chandra, 1988; Cunningham-Rundles, 1993; Forse, 1994; Gershwin et al., 1985; Watson, 1984).

The generalized primary forms of host defense are termed "innate," "inborn," or "nonspecific" immunity (Abbas et al., 1995; Brostoff et al., 1991). These initial defensive mechanisms guard the body by contributing protective responses that are effective against a diverse variety of threats. Nonspecific defensive mechanisms may be active or passive in nature (Beisel, 1991). Although nonspecific immunity does not require participation of the immune system per se, it may trigger secondary immune system actions.

[1] William R. Beisel, Department of Molecular Microbiology and Immunology, The Johns Hopkins School of Hygiene and Public Health, Baltimore, MD. *Mailing addresses*: 8298 Waterside Court, Frederick, MD 21701 *or* 21701 Harlans Run, Naples, FL 33942.

The second, or subsequent, form of host defense is termed "adaptive," "acquired," or "antigen-specific" immunity. This form of protection is delivered by the immune system itself, with its complex and highly interactive network of lymphocyte species and their products. The immune system is characterized by antigen specificity and antigen-related memory. Beginning at birth and continuing throughout life, the immune system's immunological repertoire expands as a myriad of new and different antigens are encountered.

GENERALIZED (NONSPECIFIC) HOST DEFENSES

Nonspecific host defenses are provided by both passive and active mechanisms. These mechanisms are involved in defining host susceptibility or resistance to infection, trauma, or other disease threats, and they may be drastically impaired by diverse forms of malnutrition.

Passive Defensive Measures

Passive defenses include anatomical barriers and pathways (skin and mucous membranes, fascial planes, body spaces, tubular structures); exogenous body secretions (mucin, saliva, bronchial fluids, gastric HCl, properdin, opsonins, lysozyme, etc.); physicochemical environments within normal tissues; normal ciliary activity; normal physiological factors (age, sex, race, circadian rhythms); normal microbiological flora in various locations; and even occupational and environmental factors.

Passive defenses can be compromised by malnutrition, injury or trauma, fatigue, specific illnesses (for example, diabetes, leukemia, Hodgkin's disease, alcoholism), prescribed or addictive drugs (for example, corticosteroids, antimetabolites, antimicrobials, hallucinogens, crack cocaine), and medically implanted foreign bodies (for example, vascular prostheses, catheters, drains).

Active Nonspecific Defenses

Nonspecific active defensive measures include a diverse variety of physiological responses (for example, elevated body temperatures tachycardia, vomiting and diarrhea, pituitary–adrenal activation), phagocytic cell activation, creation of inflammatory reactions, formation of nitric oxide from arginine, and a stereotyped pattern of acute-phase reactions (including fever, myalgias, arthralgias, headache and somnolence, anorexia, and a markedly altered pattern of protein synthesis and breakdown in liver and muscle, respectively). In contrast to the synthesis of antigen-specific antibodies by the immune system, nonspecific active humoral defense mechanisms include the production of cytokines, hormones, acute-phase plasma proteins, and sometimes the activation of protein components of the complement, kinin, and coagulation systems.

However, it is important to point out that not all of these components may come into play in any one inflammatory or nonantigen-specific response.

Cytokines

Cytokines are small peptides that function as intercellular signals and mediators. Cytokines are produced by many different types of cells throughout the body. Most cytokines have a diverse variety of actions, depending on the cells they stimulate. Cytokines involved in immune function include interleukins, interferons, colony stimulating factors, and a variety of other closely related mediators. In addition to their multiplicity of actions, cytokines tend to have great redundancy, with overlapping actions being common. Moreover, certain cytokines can stimulate the synthesis and release of other cytokines.

In their role as active participants in nonspecific immunity, a group of "proinflammatory cytokines" (that is, interleukin-1 [IL-1], IL-6, IL-8, tumor necrosis factor [TNF], and interferon-gamma [INF-γ]) initiate acute-phase reactions, launch immune system activities, trigger central nervous system (CNS) responses, and stimulate the release (or suppression) of hormones. Proinflammatory cytokines also participate in inflammatory reactions. Interferons have both antiviral and immunological properties. INF-γ (produced by lymphocytes) also participates in inflammatory and acute-phase processes. Yet another category of cytokines, colony stimulating factors, whose main functions are as hematopoietic factors, may also play a role in inflammation in select responses (Aggarwal and Puri, 1995).

Although new information about the cytokines is still being generated, the fundamental importance of their diverse functions is now fully recognized. As an example of cytokine biology, when macrophages or monocytes are activated (by microorganisms, antigen–antibody complexes, toxins, chemicals, etc.), they quickly respond by producing IL-1, TNF, and other cytokines. These cytokines travel via the blood or interstitial fluid between cells to interact with specific receptor proteins located on the walls of many different target cells throughout the body. The union of a cytokine with its specific cellular receptor leads to the activation of phospholipase enzymes within the target cell wall and the subsequent release into the cell of arachidonic acid (from n-6 polyunsaturated fatty acids [PUFAs] in the plasma membrane), or eicosapentaenoic acid (from n-3 PUFA).

Then, depending on the enzymes (cyclooxygenases or lipoxygenases) contained within a target cell, the arachidonic and eicosapentaenoic acids (EPAs) are converted into eicosanoids (for example, prostaglandins, leukotrienes, thromboxanes, lipoxins) of different potencies. These eicosanoid messenger–effector molecules, in turn, initiate target cell-specific responses (some of which can be blocked by glucocorticoids, aspirin, or ibuprofen) (Beisel, 1995).

Although these cytokine-induced responses are generally protective in nature, an excess production and/or activity of cytokines can be harmful. In fact, an excess of proinflammatory cytokines can lead to hypotensive shock, multiorgan failure, and death. The body possesses an elaborate system of checks and balances to control the production and activity of individual cytokines, a system far more complicated than those that regulate endocrine functions.

The effects of cytokines can be inhibited by a number of different mechanisms. Cytokines with inhibitory actions can block the synthesis and release of other cytokines. In addition, target cells release cytokine receptors into the plasma, and these soluble free receptors can intercept and inactivate the cytokine before it reaches the target cell. Blocking proteins can obstruct cell wall receptors so that cytokines cannot exert their cellular effects. Finally, hormones such as the glucocorticoids can inhibit the intracellular effects of certain cytokines.

Every aspect of cytokine biology requires proper nutrition. A full range of essential nutrients is required to (1) permit the replication of cytokine-producing cells; (2) allow the activation of these cells and the subsequent synthesis and release of cytokines into plasma; (3) allow target cells to synthesize receptor proteins and cytokine-related enzymes; (4) provide a full spectrum of cell wall PUFAs and permit their multistep conversion into eicosanoids; (5) enable target cells to respond appropriately to specific eicosanoid stimuli; and (6) allow the simultaneous development of mechanisms used for controlling excess cytokine activity (Beisel, 1995; Cunningham-Rundles, 1993; Jeng et al., 1995; see Jeffrey Rossio, Chapter 8).

Acute-Phase Reactions

Acute-phase reactions constitute an interrelated group of physiologic and metabolic changes that occur in response to generalized acute infectious illnesses, trauma, severe inflammatory processes, tissue injury, and other medical and surgical diseases (Beisel, 1995; Cunningham-Rundles, 1993; Forse, 1994). Acute-phase reactions are initiated by proinflammatory cytokines and generally have an acute onset.

Acute-phase reactions include fever, generalized malaise, somnolence, anorexia, arthralgia or myalgia, skeletal muscle proteolysis, endocrine system participation, water and salt retention, and cachexia accompanied by negative body balances of nitrogen, phosphate, magnesium, and zinc (Beisel, 1991). Acute-phase reactions are accompanied by a stimulated production of white blood cells and by immune system activation, and are characterized metabolically by a transient intolerance to glucose, hypertriglyceridemia, the sequestration of iron and zinc, and a diminished production of hemoglobin. Numerous other metabolic responses include a massive reprioritization of hepatocyte functions that involves the synthesis of acute-phase reactant glycoproteins, hepatic enzymes, and metallothioneins, concomitant with a depressed production of plasma albumin (Beisel, 1991).

Acute-phase proteins are synthesized within hours; they include C-reactive protein (CRP), haptoglobin, ceruloplasmin, orosomucoid, α_1-antitrypsin, serum amyloid A protein, fibrinogen, and others.

Proinflammatory cytokines, especially IL-1 and TNF, trigger all of these physiological and cellular events. Cytokine actions within the CNS trigger the onset of fever (by causing the release of prostaglandins within the temperature-regulating center), anorexia, somnolence, and the release (or suppression) of hormones produced in the CNS and pituitary gland.

Inflammatory Reactions

Localized inflammatory reactions serve to control and confine infectious microorganisms, to attract cells and their products to localized areas of injury, and to initiate the healing process. Inflammatory reactions involve many pathophysiological processes and cell types.

Inflammatory reactions are characterized by heat and redness, swelling, and pain. Despite these noxious symptoms, inflammatory reactions serve to localize a disease process and prevent it from becoming generalized.

Inflammatory reactions initially include dilation of local blood vessels, vascular congestion, and the binding of white blood cells to the endothelium. At the same time, immunoglobulin G (IgG) molecules become attached to mast cells and basophils, activating them to release histamine and other inflammation-producing complement activation aids in this process. Polymorphonuclear (PMN) leukocytes, monocytes, and other cells penetrate blood vessel endothelium to enter the area of inflammation; this penetration is abetted by the release of chemoattractants.

These initial inflammatory reactions are accompanied by extensive cellular activation that may include the following: the release of prostaglandins, defensins, cathepsins, and thromboxanes from phagocytes; release of lysozyme from macrophages or monocytes; release of histamine from basophils; release of cationic and basic proteins by eosinophils; deposition of fibrin; binding of iron to PMN-synthesized lactoferrin; microbicidal killing; and destruction of many participating cells with localized release of their contents, including enzymes and free oxygen radicals.

The healing process involves the proliferation of fibroblasts, the synthesis of collagen and glucosaminoglycans, phagocytic removal of inflammatory debris, and eventual disappearance of vascular congestion and edema.

The Complement System

As one of the principal mediators of the inflammatory reaction, the complement system participates in both adaptive and cell-mediated immunological responses. It assists in phagocytosis, chemotaxis, cellular activation, the respiratory burst of phagocytes, anaphylaxis, increased capillary permeability, and damage to microorganism surfaces (Abbas et al., 1994; Brostoff et al., 1991) (see Figure A-1). It is a highly adaptive system of profound importance, but its activity can be curtailed by malnutrition.

The complement system consists of a group of 17 plasma proteins that, when the system is activated, are cleaved and/or linked in a sequential manner (termed the complement cascade). Induction of the cascade by antibodies produces the "classic activation pathway," and initiation by endotoxins or microbial antigens produces the "alternate activation pathway."

In the classic complement activation pathway, aggregated antigen–antibody complexes bind to C1 (first complement component), converting it to a protease enzyme that activates C4 and C2, in turn, to produce fragments C4b and C2a. These fragments then form a complex that activates C3.

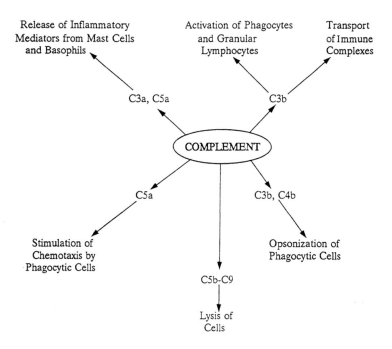

FIGURE A-1 Actions of complement fragments. After complement component C3 is activated via either the classic or the alternate pathway, C3 cleavage fragments have a variety of actions, as shown. C3b is also the starting point for the lytic pathway, which involves complement components C5–C9, to initiate cellular lysis. Lytic pathway fragments also help stimulate chemotaxis.

In the alternate pathway, the presence of microbial cell wall lipopolysaccharides activates plasma proteins, including properdin, to trigger the cleavage of C3 to C3b.

Each complement pathway leads to the activation of C3, which in turn is cleaved into the biologically active molecules C3a (anaphylatoxin) and C3b. The effector molecule C3b is the starting point of the lytic pathway, which proceeds via the participation of C5, C6, C7, C8, and C9. Lytic components can stimulate chemotaxis or produce lesions in cell membranes.

ANTIGEN-SPECIFIC HOST DEFENSES

Assisting the nonspecific defenses of the host, the immune system provides additional defensive measures by focusing on and reacting to the highly specific molecular structures of antigens (unique molecular components of microorganisms, food, tissues, inert substances, chemicals, etc.).

The immune system is divided into two major branches that provide (1) antigen-specific cell-mediated immunity (CMI) and (2) humoral immunity (see Figure A-2). CMI is controlled by the thymus gland and provided by T-lymphocytes and natural killer (NK) cells. Humoral immunity is generated by B-lymphocytes. When stimulated appropriately by an antigen plus IL-2 and other cytokines, B-cells undergo clonal expansion and/or are converted into plasma cells, the cellular factories that produce antigen-specific antibodies. The ability of the immune system to recognize and respond to foreign antigens has five cardinal features (Abbas et al., 1995):

1. *specificity*, the ability of lymphocytes to recognize determinant configurations, known as epitopes, on antigenic molecules;

2. *diversity*, the huge number ($>10^9$) of distinct antigenic determinants recognizable in the human lymphocyte repertoire;

3. *memory*, the primary and secondary recognition of a specific antigen by lymphocytes: after the first lymphocytic identification of a new foreign antigen, clonal proliferation occurs, memory cells eventually survive as programmed lymphocytes that will respond to that same antigenic determinant for the indefinite future;

4. *self-limitation*, the waning of an immune response after initial interactions with (and generally, elimination of) a foreign antigen; and

5. *discrimination of self from nonself*, the ability of lymphocytes to distinguish foreign antigens from the self-antigens contained in body tissues. Abnormalities in the maintenance of "self-tolerance" lead to autoimmune diseases.

Immune responses occur in three distinct phases: *cognitive, activation*, and *effector* (Abbas et al., 1995). (1) In the initial *cognitive phase*, foreign antigens

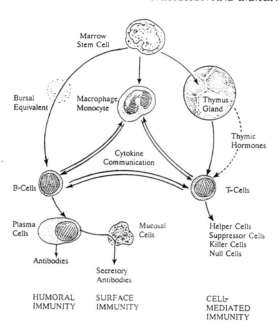

FIGURE A-2 Overview of the immune system. Lymphocytes, derived initially from marrow stem cells, comprise the humoral or cell-mediated arms of the immune system. Humoral immunity is provided by B-cells, which are influenced in mammals by an unidentified equivalent of the bursa of chickens. When stimulated by an appropriate antigen, B-cells undergo clonal expansion and transformation into antibody-producing plasma cells. IgA molecules are joined by J and "secretory" pieces produced by mucosal and epithelial cells, and the resultant IgA dimers are then secreted to generate surface immunity. Cell-mediated immunity is provided by T-cells that originate in the thymus gland and remain thereafter under the influence of circulating thymic hormones. B- and T-cells also are stimulated (or inhibited) by a complex network of cytokines (released by macrophages/monocytes and a variety of other body cells, including the lymphocytes themselves), which provide cell-to-cell communications. T-cells also assist antigen-presenting cells in the cell-to-cell delivery of processed antigen to B-cells.

become bound to specific receptors on the cell wall of mature lymphocytes. B-lymphocytes express specific antibodies on their surfaces that can bind soluble foreign proteins, polysaccharides, or lipids, while T-lymphocytes express receptors that recognize only short peptide sequences on foreign antigens (including those located on the surfaces of other cells). (2) In the *activation phase*, lymphocytes that have recognized a foreign antigen proliferate, leading to the creation of lymphocyte clones. This involves both of the major arms, or branches, of the immune system. In the *humoral arm* (see Figure A-2), humoral immunity is generated by B-cells, which, when stimulated by an antigen plus IL-2 and other cytokines, differentiate into antibody-secreting plasma cells. Simultaneously, in the CMI arm of the immune system, antigen-stimulated T-cells (Figure A-2) differentiate from null cells to helper or suppressor cells or into killer cells. The CMI arm is controlled by the thymus gland and its zinc-containing hormones. The CMI serves to support the *humoral arm* of the immune system, recruit other defensive cells, and kill any cell recognized as foreign. Responding T- and B-lymphocytes eventually migrate to sites of antigen administration or antigen penetration into body tissues. (3) In the third, *effector phase*, newly secreted antibodies serve to eliminate the foreign antigen and also to activate the complement cascade, stimulate the degranulation of mast cells, and initiate the release of mediators from other cells. Activated T-cells secrete cytokines that enhance the functions of B-cells and phagocytes and stimulate nonspecific inflammatory responses.

The immune system performs its unique functions in two anatomically distinct but interrelated loci. A systemic component generates both CMI and humoral responses whenever it is penetrated by a foreign antigen. A second and separate (but cofunctioning) surface component of the immune system recognizes foreign antigens on body surfaces (including the respiratory and intestinal mucosa) and produces antibodies for secretion in tears and in mucosal, dermal, and intestinal fluids.

Other functioning aspects of the immune system can generate inappropriate or exaggerated tissue-damaging responses. Hypersensitivity or allergic reactions, or autoimmunity, result in damaging long-term immune responses as the body makes antibodies against its own tissues.

Cell-Mediated Immunity

CMI protects the specific, genetically determined tissue type of the body (host) from anything foreign. Through CMI, the body recognizes and defends against infusions of incompatible blood cells or transplanted tissues. Constant surveillance by NK-cells is maintained to detect any body cells that may undergo malignant mutations and, if possible, destroy them (Abbas et al., 1995; Bostoff et al., 1991). NK-lymphocytes arise from "previously uncommitted or null" cells and can, with the help of IL-2, lyse individual bloodborne tumor stem cells without prior sensitization or major histocompatibility complex (MHC). NK-cells also function in graft-versus-host reactions and have been implicated in antibacterial and antiviral defense mechanisms.

Antibody responses to T-cell-dependent antigens require direct physical contact (regulated by genetically determined MHC proteins and adhesion molecules on cell surfaces) between T-helper cells, antigen-presenting cells, and B-cells, and the activation of B-cells to produce appropriate antibodies. CMI includes the lymphocytic secretion of and response to a variety of cytokines. CMI also is involved in eliciting delayed hypersensitivity reactions, that is, reactions that result 24–48 h after contact with an antigen to which the body has been exposed previously.

CMI, particularly T-cell number and function, is a major target of malnutrition. Generalized protein-energy malnutrition (PEM) may cause severe atrophy of lymphoid tissues, especially in their T-cell areas. Deficiencies of other nutrients, including vitamins A and B_6 and the minerals iron, zinc, copper, and selenium, also can produce CMI dysfunction. Zinc is of special concern because, in addition to its role in nucleic acid synthesis and the activity of many metalloenzymes, it is a component of the thymic hormones and is essential for their functions. Severe generalized malnutrition also causes the disappearance of clinical allergies and hypersensitivities (Chandra, 1988; Cunningham-Rundles, 1993; Forse, 1994; Gershwin et al., 1985; Watson, 1984).

T-Cells

T-cells are long-lived lymphocytes that circulate continually throughout the body, periodically returning (homing) to the site of their individual origins. At all locations, T-cell activities are influenced by the thymus gland through the effects of its thymic hormones.

T-cells have diverse functions and activities, many of which are triggered when a native T-cell is first stimulated by a new foreign antigen. These functional responses develop in three distinct phases: (1) the cognitive phase, (2) the activation phase, and (3) the effector phase (see Figure A-3).

Many different subsets of T-cells exist. Each T-cell subset has unique (but sometimes overlapping) actions and can be identified by specific cluster of differentiation (CD) antigens (glycoproteins localized on their exterior cell membranes). Subsets include CD4+ T-helper cells, CD8+ T-suppressor cells, and killer cells. T-cells may recognize both specific antigens presenting on membranes of body cells and antigen fragments associated with MHC proteins on these membranes.

CD4+ T-cells recognize antigen fragments associated with Class II MHC molecules in *antigen-presenting cells* (APCs). APCs engulf (endocytose) and process antigens and link recognizable antigenic fragments to the Class II MHC molecules on their surfaces, which stimulates initiating or helping activities.

When CD4+ cells recognize complexes of antigen and Class II (MHC) molecules on the surface of a macrophage, they activate the macrophage, stimulating it to destroy engulfed organisms. However, if the complexes are on the surface of a B-lymphocyte, the CD4+ cells release cytokines, including IL-2, that lead to B-cell activation, clonal expansion, and antibody production.

CD8+ T-cells recognize antigen fragments associated with Class I MHC molecules on cell surfaces. Cells infected by a virus may exhibit viral peptide antigens linked to surface Class I molecules. CD8+ T-cells thus can recognize and destroy virally infected cells.

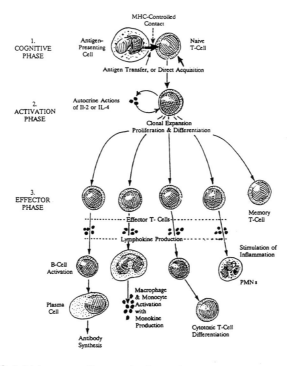

FIGURE A-3 Initial contact of a new foreign antigen with a naive T-cell initiates the cognitive phase. This is immediately followed by the release of lymphokines (IL-2 and/or IL-4) that function as autocrines to stimulate growth, proliferation, and differentiation of the newly stimulated T-cell during the activation phase to produce clones of effector and memory T-cells. Effector T-cells have many functions, including the triggering of antibody production by B-cells, activation of monocytes and macrophages, the stimulation of inflammatory reactions, and further differentiation into cytotoxic T-cells.

Humoral Immunity

Humoral immunity involves the production of antibodies against specific antigens. Like CMI, humoral immunity has both a systemic component (which produces serum antibodies IgG, IgM, and IgA) and a surface component (which produces secretory IgA).

B-Cells

B-cells are primarily responsible for humoral immunity. They recognize both intact, "whole," extracellular antigens and processed antigens delivered by antigen-presenting cells. B-cells receive help from CD4+ T-helper cells and stimulatory cytokines. During B-cell interactions with antigen-presenting cells, the role of MHC molecules is essential. There are many genetically determined

MHC haplotypes that vary in their efficiency, resulting in differences in the quantity and quality of subsequent immune responses.

Following the presentation of an antigen to a naive B-cell, the B-cell undergoes clonal expansion to produce daughter cells that will respond to the same antigen whenever it is encountered in the future. Antigen-activated B-cells, stimulated further by IL-2 and other cytokines, mature into plasma cells, the major antibody-producing cells.

Antibodies

Antibodies are bifunctional (immunoglobulin) molecules created to interact with specific antigens. The primary molecular structure of antibodies consists of four peptides (chains) connected by sulfhydryl bonds and arranged in the shape of a Y. Two heavy chains form the Y, and two light chains are attached to the arms of the Y. These arms are termed the Fab (fragment-antibody) regions, and they serve to interact with (bind to) specific intact antigens, either free or on the surface of a microorganism or cell. The stem of the Y is termed the Fc region, and it interacts with receptors on lymphocytes and other cells, or directly with complement.

There are several types of antibodies (immunoglobulins): IgG, IgM, IgA, secretory IgA, IgD, and IgE. A brief description of these immunoglobulins is provided in the glossary (Appendix B).

After the first exposure of a B-cell to a new foreign antigen, systemic antibody production focuses predominantly on IgM, with relatively little IgG produced. Subsequent exposures to the same antigen result in predominant production of IgG (Figure A-4). In contrast, the formation of a secretory antibody by the mucosal immune system involves the initial production of IgA molecules, the joining of two IgAs by a small protein J (joiner) peptide, and actual secretion of the IgA dimer by epithelial or mucosal cells, which add another secretory fragment or peptide to the process.

Antibodies have a variety of distinct functions such as the direct neutralization of circulating antigens and the formation of immune complexes with circulating antigens. After creation of an immune complex in plasma, the Fc regions of the antibody can act as adapters that cross-link the antigen–antibody complex to Fc receptors on the surface of host phagocytic cells (that is, macrophages and PMN leukocytes) that express Fc receptors. This linkage then can lead to the cellular uptake and destruction of the antigen–antibody complex:

• *Recognition and sensitization of "foreign" cell targets or parasites for attack by cytotoxic killer cells that possess Fc receptors.* This is called antibody-dependent cell-mediated cytotoxicity and is used by eosinophils and large, granular lymphocytes.

• *Participation in inflammatory reactions.* IgG antibodies can bind to and sensitize mast cells and basophils via their Fc receptors. This binding activates the cells to release inflammation-producing mediators, such as histamine, that contribute to the local inflammatory reaction.

• *Activation of complement.* This is followed by the release of proinflammatory mediators.

The effects of malnutrition on humoral immunity are far less pronounced than on CMI. Atrophy of B-cell areas of lymphoid tissues is relatively small, and preexisting antibodies continue to be produced. In fact, a slightly paradoxical increase in plasma antibody concentrations is a common finding in children with severe PEM. Antibody responses to new antigens, such as those in vaccines, can generally be detected, although the titers and activities of such new antibodies may be reduced.

Hypersensitivity (or Allergic) Reactions

When immune responses are inappropriate or exaggerated and lead to tissue damage, the terms "hypersensitivity" or "allergy" are used. These responses occur only in certain individuals, as a result of second (or numerous)

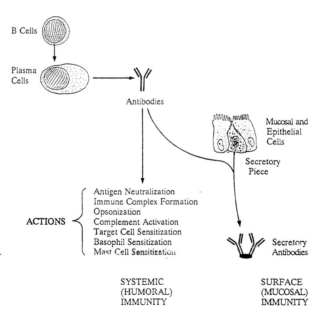

FIGURE A-4 Antibody actions. Plasma antibodies have a multiplicity of actions that provide the interior of the body with systemic humoral immunity. Plasma IgA molecules are joined by J- and "secretory" pieces produced by mucosal and epithelial cells, and the resultant IgA dimers are then secreted to generate surface (mucosal and epithelial) immunity.

contacts with a particular antigen (antigens that produce these reactions are generally termed allergens). Hypersensitivity responses can occur in a variety of distinct but sometimes overlapping types, as listed below.

- *Type I* reactions are immediate reactions that result from the interaction of an allergen with IgE-sensitized mast cells and basophils. Histamine and other mediators are released, causing acute responses in the skin (weal and flare reactions, urticaria), eyes, nose, bronchial tree, and so forth. These reactions are commonly called allergies. If of extreme, immediate, life-threatening severity, they are termed anaphylactic responses.
- *Type II* reactions are cytolytic or cytotoxic reactions triggered by the interaction of IgG or IgM with antigens on the surface of specific cells or tissues. These reactions lead to tissue destruction, as seen in autoimmune diseases; the rejection of transplanted foreign tissue; or skin diseases such as pemphigus.
- *Type III* reactions are immune complex reactions that are also triggered by IgG or IgM and are caused by the interaction of soluble antigen–antibody complexes with complement. If these complexes are deposited within certain tissues, they can cause localized damage. In the kidney, they induce glomerulonephritis, and in the skin, diseases such as erythema multiforme and erythema induratum. Interaction with fungal antigens causes farmer's lung disease. Skin testing with the inciting allergen produces Arthus reactions of 5- to 24-h duration.
- *Type IV* reactions are delayed-type dermal hypersensitivity reactions to the intracutaneous injection of tuberculin or other antigens. If positive, these modified inflammatory responses progress slowly and peak in 24 to 48 h. In deeper tissues, these reactions induce granulomatous responses that are characteristic of tuberculosis.

Severe malnutrition, by resulting in immunological dysfunction, can cause both hypersensitivity and allergic reactions to disappear.

REFERENCES

Abbas, A.K., A.H. Lichtman, and J.S. Pober, eds. 1994. Cellular and Molecular Immunology, 2nd ed. Philadelphia: W.B. Saunders Co.

Abbas, A.K., V.L. Perez, L. Van Parijs, and R.C. Wong. 1995. Differentiation and tolerance of CD4+ T lymphocytes. Ciba Found. Symp. 195:7–13.

Aggarwal, B.B., and R.K. Puri, eds. 1995. Human Cytokines: Their Role in Disease and Therapy. Cambridge, MA: Blackwell Science.

Anderson, A.O. 1997. New technologies for producing systemic and mucosal immunity by oral immunization: Immunoprophylaxis in Meals, Ready-to-Eat. Pp. 451–500 in Emerging Technologies for Nutrition Research: Potential for Assessing Military Performance Capability, S.J. Carlson-Newberry and R.B. Costello, eds. Committee on Military Nutrition Research, Food and Nutrition Board, Institute of Medicine. Washington, D.C.: National Academy Press.

Beisel, W.B. 1991. Nutrition and infection. Pp. 507–542 in Nutritional Biochemistry and Metabolism, 2nd ed., M.C. Linder, ed. New York: Elsevier.

Beisel, W.R. 1995. Herman Award Lecture, 1995: Infection-induced malnutrition—From cholera to cytokines. Am. J. Clin. Nutr. 62:813–819.

Brostoff, J., G.K. Scadding, D. Male, and I.M. Roitt, eds. 1991. Clinical Immunology. London: Gower Medical Publishing.

Chandra, R.K., ed. 1988. Nutrition and Immunology. New York: Alan R. Liss, Inc.

Cunningham-Rundles, S., ed. 1993. Nutritional Modulation of the Immune Response. New York: Marcel Decker, Inc.

Forse, R.A., ed. 1994. Diet, Nutrition, and Immunity. Boca Raton, Fla.: CRC Press.

Gershwin, M.E., R.S. Beach, and L.S. Hurley, eds. 1985. Nutrition and Immunology. Orlando, Fla.: Academic Press.

Jeng, K-C.G., C-S. Yang, W-Y. Siu, Y-S. Tsai, W-J. Liao, and J-S. Kuo. 1996. Supplementation with vitamins C and E enhances cytokine production by peripheral blood mononuclear cells in healthy adults. Am. J. Clin. Nutr. 64:960–965.

Watson, R.R., ed. 1984. Nutrition, Disease Resistance, and Immune Function. New York: Marcel Decker, Inc.

Nutrition and Immune Function, 1999
Pp. 527–536. Washington, D.C.
National Academy Press

B

Glossary of Immunological Terms

William R. Beisel[1]

Activation phase. The second phase of the immune response in that lymphocytes which recognize and bind a foreign antigen undergo initial proliferation to become cloned memory cells and to amplify the protective response. B-cells then differentiate into clones of antibody-producing plasma cells.

Allergen. Any substance capable of inducing an allergic reaction.

Allergy. A clinically manifest hypersensitivity state to a specific allergen or antigen causing a range of harmful immunologic reactions, (e.g., hay fever, asthma, food intolerance, skin rash).

Anaphylactic reaction. Sudden generalized allergic reactions of life-threatening severity.

---

[1] William R. Beisel, Department of Molecular Microbiology and Immunology, The Johns Hopkins School of Hygiene and Public Health, Baltimore, MD. *Mailing addresses*: 8298 Waterside Court, Frederick, MD 21701 *or* 21701 Harlans Run, Naples, FL 33942.

Anaphylatoxin. A fragment (also known as C3a) of complement C3 that causes cellular release of histamine.

Antibody. An immunoglobulin protein produced by the immune system, designed to bind to a specific single antigen. Antibodies neutralize foreign antigens; form immune complexes; activate complement; sensitize target cells, mast cells, and basophiles; and initiate opsonization.

Antigen. Any substance (or molecule) capable of inducing a specific immune response. Antigens include a wide variety of plant and microorganism components or toxins.

α_1–**antitrypsin.** An acute-phase reactant plasma glycoprotein.

Arthus reactions. Dermal skin test reactions (characteristic of Type III hypersensitivities), that occur during a 4–12 h interval.

Autoimmune disease. Any disease caused by the immune system's erroneous and destructive actions on the body's own tissues, such as thyroiditis, myocarditis, glomerulonephritis, and lupus erythematosus.

Basophil. A white blood cell (WBC) with granules that can be stained by basic dyes. Basophils participate in inflammatory processes and in allergic and hypersensitivity reactions by releasing histamine.

B-cells (or B-lymphocytes). Thymus-independent, bursa-equivalent lymphocytes produced by bone marrow to populate all lymphoid organs and tissues. They are capable of producing antibodies and maturing into plasma cells. B-cells express antibody on their surfaces that can respond to foreign protein, polysaccharide, and lipid antigens in soluble form.

Cathepsin. A proteinase enzyme released by polymorphonuclear leukocytes during inflammation.

Cell-mediated immunity. Antigen-specific and nonspecific immunity provided by the direct localized cellular activity of T-lymphocytes and natural killer cells. Specific cells include T–helper cells (Th) and T–cytotoxic cells (Tc); nonspecific cells include macrophages, neutrophils, eosinophils, and NK-cells.

CD4+ cells. Helper T-cells recognized by the presence of cluster of differentiation antigen 4 on their exterior cell surfaces.

CD8+ cells. Suppressor T-cells recognized by the presence of cluster of differentiation antigen 8 on their exterior cell surfaces.

Chemotaxis. The purposeful movement of phagocytes toward invading bacteria, cell debris, or foreign particles.

Cognitive phase. The phase of the immune response in which foreign antigens are bound to specific receptors on mature lymphocytes.

Colony Stimulating Factors. Cytokines that stimulate the generation of additional white blood cells. These have been produced by biotechnology and are available for therapeutic or investigative use.

    GCSF. Granulocyte colony stimulating factor

    GMCSF. Granulocyte macrophage colony stimulating factor

    MCSF. Monocyte colony stimulating factor

Complement system. A group of plasma proteins that interact to form complement, an important mediator of inflammation. Active complement fragments play important roles in both nonspecific and cell-mediated immunity. (See Appendix A for details concerning this complex system.)

Concanavalin A (ConA). A plant lectin with mitogenic effects on T-cells.

C-reactive protein. An acute-phase reactive glycoprotein widely used as a clinical indicator of acute-phase reactions.

Cytokines. Small peptide molecules released by a variety of cells. Acting in the nature of hormones, apocrines, and/or paracrines, they allow intercellular communication and stimulate a diverse variety of responses by target cells. Cytokines include, but are not limited to, interleukins, interferons, and colony stimulating factors.

Defensins. Basic polymorphonuclear leukocyte proteins released during inflammation that kill bacteria by damaging their cell walls.

Delayed hypersensitivity. An exaggerated immune response that is delayed for a day or more. It is mediated by the response of T-cells to a foreign antigen or allergen.

Discrimination of self from nonself. A remarkable feature of the immune system that enables it to distinguish between foreign antigens and self-antigens. Tolerance to self-antigens is acquired by individual lymphocytes. If the tolerance process becomes defective, autoimmune diseases may develop.

Diversity. Immune system diversity constitutes the entire, extremely large number of different antigens that can be recognized. See Lymphocyte repertoire.

Effector phase. The third phase of the immune response in which multifaceted mechanisms become focused on the elimination of the foreign antigen. Antibodies bind to the antigen to enhance its elimination by phagocytes, to activate the complement cascade, to stimulate mast-cell degranulation, and to assist in the inflammatory reaction. Cytokines are released to enhance the immunological reaction, recruit phagocytic cells, and induce generalized acute-phase reactions.

Eicosanoids. Small lipid molecules derived from polyunsaturated fatty acids (contained in cellular plasma membranes) that initiate a diverse variety of cellular and physiological activities. Eicosanoids include families of prostaglandins, thromboxanes, leukotrines, and so forth.

Enzyme-linked immunosorbent assay (ELISA). A sensitive method for serodiagnosis of specific infectious diseases; an in vitro competitive binding in which an enzyme and its substrate, rather than a radioactive substance, serve as the indicator system.

Eosinophil. A white blood cell with granules that can be stained by eosin dyes. Eosinophils participate in allergic and hypersensitivity reactions.

Epitopes (or determinants). The precise molecular configurations of an antigen that can be recognized by an individual lymphocyte.

Fab (antibody fragment) parts. The two arms of Y-shaped antibody molecules that bind to a specific antigen.

Fc (crystalline fragment) part. The bottom leg of Y-shaped antibody molecules that can bind to complement or various WBCs.

Haplotypes. *See* Major histocompatibility complex.

Haptoglobin. A plasma glycoprotein, also an acute-phase reactant, that functions to bind and inactivate (detoxify) free hemoglobin.

Helper cell. A CD4+ T-lymphocyte that helps initiate and stimulate the production of immunoglobulins by B-cells or plasma cells. Also provides help to Tc-cells.

Histamine. A small amine compound, $C_5H_9N_3$, released by mast cells during allergic reactions, which causes dilation of blood vessels, bronchoconstriction, itching, and other symptoms.

Humoral immunity. Antigen-specific immunity mediated by B- and plasma-cell production of circulating or secretory immunoglobulins.

Hypersensitivity reaction. An allergic response to an allergen or antigen.

Immediate hypersensitivity. Exaggerated immune response to a foreign allergen or antigen induced largely by the release of histamine and occurring within minutes.

Immune responses. The humoral and cell-mediated responses of the immune system to antigens. These responses occur in three distinct phases (cognitive, activation, and effector phases) and exhibit five cardinal properties, or features (specificity, diversity, memory, self-limitation, and discrimination of self from nonself).

Immunity. High protective resistance to a disease threat that is produced by the immune system or by some other nonspecific protective mechanism.

Immunoglobulin. An antibody of one of several types (IgA, IgD, IgE, IgG, IgM).

    IgA. A mature polymeric immunoglobulin secreted in response to antigens on mucosal and epithelial surfaces, and the precursor of secretory IgA, possessing the primary four-chain structure typical of IgG. Its normal concentration is 3 mg/mL serum.

    IgD. An immunoglobulin intrinsic to the surface of B-cells that, when contacted by a specific homologous antigen, initiates B-cell proliferation (cloning), differentiation, and antibody production. Normal IgD concentration in serum is 0.03 mg/mL.

    IgE. An antibody that can sensitize mast cells and basophils during allergic reactions, causing them to release histamine and other inflammatory mediators. Normal IgE concentration is 0.0001 mg/mL serum.

    IgG. The mature antibody of the humoral immune response, possessing the primary molecular structure described above. Normal IgG concentration in serum is 12 mg/mL.

IgM. The initial antibody produced during a humoral immune response. IgM is a large polymer consisting of five of the primary Y-shaped antibody structures connected by a J-chain. Normal IgM concentration in serum is 1 mg/mL.

Secretory IgA. An IgA dimer (two IgAs connected by a J-piece) to which a secretory piece has been added by an epithelial cell prior to IgA secretion into a body fluid such as tears, milk, or saliva. Although the serum concentration of IgA is lower that of IgG, far more IgA is actually produced each day because it is constantly being secreted into body fluids.

Interferon. Cytokine that interferes with the propagation of viruses and fills other immunological roles. INF-α is produced by phagocytic leukocytes, INF-β by fibroblasts, and INF-γ by lymphocytes.

Interleukin. Cytokine that permits communication among white blood cells and other tissues. Interleukins include the following:

IL-1 (endogenous pyrogen, leukocytic endogenous mediator, lymphocyte activating substance). A proinflammatory cytokine with scores of reported activities, including the generation of fever, skeletal muscle proteolysis, and metabolic wasting. IL-1 also enhances the proliferation of T-helper and B-cells.

IL-2 (T-cell growth factor). A lymphokine derived from helper cells, predominantly responsible for T-cell proliferation, the generation of lymphokine activated killer (LAK) cells, and the activation of B-cells.

IL-3 (multicolony stimulating factor). A cytokine derived from monocytes, fibroblasts, and endothelial cells that increases the production of monocytes.

IL-4 (B-cell differentiating factor, T-cell growth factor-2). A lymphokine that stimulates both T- and B-cells.

IL-5 (B-cell growth factor-2, eosinophil-differentiating factor). A lymphokine that activates B-cells and eosinophils.

IL-6 (B-cell stimulatory factor-2, interferon-β2). A proinflammatory cytokine with many diverse actions, including stimulation of hepatocellular responses during the acute-phase reaction.

IL-7 (lymphopoietin I, pre-B-cell growth factor). A cytokine that stimulates proliferation of both B- and T-cells.

IL-8 (neutrophil-activating peptide, neutrophil chemotactic [or chemoattractant] factor). A proinflammatory cytokine produced by numerous cell types that also causes chemotaxis of polymorphonuclear leukocytes.

IL-9 (P40, mast-cell growth-enhancing factor, T-cell growth factor-3). A lymphokine that stimulates growth and proliferation of T-cells and mast cells.

IL-10 (cytokine synthesis inhibitory factor). A cytokine produced by various cells that inhibits T-cell production of INF-γ and the synthesis of monokines by macrophage or monocytes.

IL-11 (adipogenesis inhibitory factor). A cytokine produced by marrow stromal cells that stimulates the hepatic synthesis of acute-phase glycoproteins.

IL-12 (NK-cell stimulating factor, cytotoxic lymphocyte maturation factor). A cytokine that induces INF-γ gene expression in lymphocytes.

IL-13 (P600). A lymphokine that inhibits the synthesis of proinflammatory cytokines by monocytes and other cells.

IL-14 (high molecular weight B-cell growth factor). A lymphokine that stimulates B-cell proliferation while inhibiting antibody production.

IL-15 (no prior common name). A lymphokine that stimulates T-cell proliferation and NK-cell activation.

Lymphocyte repertoire. The more than 10^9 distinct antigenic determinants (epitopes) that can be recognized by antigen-specific clones of human lymphocytes.

Lymphokine. A cytokine secreted by a lymphocyte.

Lysozyme. An enzyme present in tears and body secretions and fluids that helps in the destruction of bacterial cell walls.

Macrophages. Large mononuclear tissue phagocytes that secrete cytokines when activated and interact with T-cells in processing and presenting antigens to B-cells. They are termed monocytes when bloodborne.

Major histocompatibility complex haplotypes. Genetically controlled proteins on cell surfaces that indicate its specific tissue type. The cellular HLA (human leukocyte antigen) locus is expressed by at least four blocks of genes. A correct arrangement and recognition of MHC surface proteins is necessary for direct cell-to-cell contact between antigen-presenting cells and lymphocytes and for the identification of nonforeign body cells. Two classes of MHC molecules exist, each containing two polymorphic polypeptide chains that traverse the cell membranes of body cells. Molecular transcription rates of both MHC classes are influenced by cytokines, thus providing an important amplification mechanism for T-cell responses. Both classes were originally recognized for their role in triggering rejection of transplanted tissues, but their larger roles in forming complexes with diverse kinds of foreign protein antigens is now known.

Class I MHC molecules are expressed on virtually all nucleated body cells. MHC molecules of both types possess peptide-binding, Ig-like, transmembrane, and cytoplasmic regions. The peptide-binding regions of both types are the principal determinants of the specificities and affinities of peptide antigens that can be bound, wherever the Ig-like regions appear to be important for noncovalent interactions between the two molecular chains. Antigens associated with Class I MHC molecules are recognized by CD8+ T-suppressor lymphocytes.

Class II MHC molecules are expressed primarily on cells involved in the presentation of foreign antigens (i.e., lymphocytes, macrophages, dendritic cells, endothelial cells, etc.). In contrast to Class I molecules, Class II molecules show differences in cell expression and cytokine responsiveness among these cell types. Class II-associated molecules are recognized by CD4+ T-helper cells.

Memory. The exquisite recall exhibited by the immune system that enables it to mount a more vigorous and effective response whenever it is restimulated by a specific foreign antigen.

Memory cells. Lymphocytes that have previously responded to a specific antigenic stimulus. They survive for exceedingly long periods and can respond rapidly to the same antigen.

Monocyte. A large white blood cell with a single nucleus, with phagocytic, cytokine-producing, and antigen-processing capabilities. Tissue forms are called macrophages.

Monokine. A cytokine secreted by a monocyte or macrophage.

Neopterin. A small protein produced by monocyte–macrophages (often in combination with IL-6 and other proinflammatory cytokines) that has immunosuppressive properties.

Neutrophil. The most numerous of the white blood cells (also called polymorphonuclear leukocytes). The principal cellular participant in inflammatory reactions, neutrophils act by engulfing and destroying microbial invaders, cell debris, and particulate matter.

Nitric oxide. A multifunctional molecule derived from arginine that has microbicidal and parasiticidal properties.

NK (natural killer) cells. Specialized T-cells with the continuous task of identifying and eliminating cells recognized as being foreign or nonself. Large, granular NK-lymphocytes can mediate antibody-dependent cellular cytotoxity as well as lysing target cells (tumor cells and modified host cells.

Nonspecific immunity. Resistance against disease threats produced by diverse physiological mechanisms that do not require the recognition of or response to specific antigens.

Null cells. Lymphocytes lacking the surface CD markers of the principal lymphocyte subsets.

Opsonins. Constituents of serum that bind to antigens, making invading microorganism more susceptible to the destructive action of phagocytes.

Opsinization. The process of altering bacterial walls to increase susceptibility to phagocytosis.

Orosomucoid. An acute-phase reactant plasma glycoprotein, α1-acid glycoprotein.

Oxidative burst. Sudden uptake and utilization of oxygen by phagocytic cells (neutrophils, monocytes, macrophages) whenever they engulf a bacterium or other foreign particle. *See* Respiratory burst.

Phagocyte. A blood cell that ingests and destroys foreign particles, bacteria, and cell debris.

Phagocytosis. The process of engulfing particles, bacteria, and cell debris.

Phytohemagglutinin (PHA). A plant mitogen that stimulates T-lymphocytes.

Plasma cells. Antibody-producing cells that have matured from antigen-stimulated B-cells.

Pleiotropy. Ability to exert multiple effects.

Polymorphonuclear leukocyte (also termed PMN or poly). See Neutrophil.

Proinflammatory cytokines. Cytokines that are especially linked to the production of inflammatory processes and acute-phase responses. They include IL-1, IL-6, IL-8, TNF, and INF-γ.

Properdin. A nonimmune gamma-globulin that can be activated to a convertase enzyme, which in turn causes activation of the alternative pathway of the complement system.

Respiratory burst. A sudden increase in cellular respiration that occurs when phagocytes become activated. This process generates free oxygen radicals with microbicidal properties.

Self-limitation. The waning over time of immune responses to antigenic stimulation.

Siderophores. Iron-binding proteins secreted by bacteria that gather the iron needed for bacterial growth. Siderophores compete with mammalian iron-binding proteins for the iron they carry.

Specificity. Property of the immune system that enables it to recognize and respond to each of the myriads of foreign, molecularly unique antigens encountered throughout an individual's lifetime.

Suppressor cell. A CD8+ T-lymphocyte that helps control (suppress) an excess production of specific immunoglobulins.

T-cells (or T-lymphocytes). Thymus gland-dependent lymphocytes responsible for the development and maintenance of cell-mediated immunity. T-cells recognize only short peptide sequences on intracellular protein antigens expressed on cell surface membranes; T-cells may exert a helper, suppressor, or effector function.

Thymosin. A zinc-containing hormone produced by stromal cells of the thymus gland that abets the actions of T-cells throughout the body.

Tumor necrosis factor (cachexin, lymphotoxin). Cytokine with action closely similar to IL-1. In addition, TNF stimulates cytotoxicity by PMN and eosinophils and inhibits the activity of lipoprotein lipase.

Urticaria. Itchy dermal wheals caused by type I hypersensitivity reactions.

Nutrition and Immune Function, 1999
Pp. 537–542. Washington, D.C.
National Academy Press

C

Overview of Immune Assessment Tests

BASIC TESTS OF IMMUNE STATUS

The Agency for Toxic Substances and Disease Registry (ATSDR) basic panel of immune function tests consists of a group of assessments that are performed with serum and several that are performed on whole blood. Assays of serum include the following:

- C-reactive protein (CRP), a marker of acute-phase reactions and a sensitive indicator of tissue damage from a variety of causes;
  - immunoglobulins (Ig) G and M, indicators of humoral immune status;
  - IgA, an indicator of mucosal humoral immunity;
  - antinuclear antibody, an indicator of autoantibodies; and
  - total protein, used to correct the concentration of immunoglobulins for concentration of blood proteins.

537

Whole blood measures include the following:

- a complete blood count with a five-part differential to determine total white cells, total lymphocytes, and total eosinophils; and
- number of CD4+ lymphocytes and the CD4+:CD8+ ratio, by lymphocyte phenotyping. CD4+ lymphocytes are helper–inducer T-lymphocytes, whereas CD8+ cells are suppressor or cytotoxic T-cells. A decrease in CD4+ and a CD4+:CD8+ ratio of less than 1.5 is correlated with immune impairment and increased susceptibility to infection (Bloom et al., 1992). Although lymphocyte phenotyping with a complete panel of major phenotypes is recommended by the ATSDR as the most predictive test for immunotoxicity in animals (Luster et al., 1992, 1993) and can be performed with small samples of whole blood (making the tests amenable to field studies), these tests are not able to evaluate functional status. Lymphocyte subpopulations vary over time and between individuals. In addition, peripheral immune cells and compartments, although easy to sample, may not reflect immune function in the lymphoid tissues where the most significant changes in lymphocyte subpopulations are likely to occur, and samples drawn from peripheral pools may be more reflective of one part of the immune system than the other (humoral versus systemic) (see Susanna Cunningham-Rundles, see Chapter 9). Monoclonal antibodies (Mabs) that identify cell-surface markers associated with T-cell activation (such as CD25, the interleukin-2 (IL-2) receptor) are now becoming available and may alleviate some of the problems mentioned.

Focused Tests of Immune (Deficiency) Function

For individuals whose basic test results provide evidence of immune deficiency, a panel of more specific tests may be performed.

Tests of Serum

Secondary humoral response (IgM and IgG responses to an antigen to which the subject has been exposed previously) can be assessed in samples of serum drawn before and after immunization with the recall antigen, making this a suitable technique for use in the field (Straight et al., 1994). Factors that must be considered include the timing of blood sampling (to take into account variations in immune function resulting from biological rhythms [see Erhard Haus, Chapter 20]) and the background ("before") antibody titer expected. An additional consideration is the great degree of variability observed in response to immunization, including a fairly high percentage of nonresponders.

Antibody response to primary immunization with a novel antigen may be measured as an alternative. This test requires identification of an antigen to which the subject has not been exposed previously (see Cunningham-Rundles, Chapter 9).

A specific antibody response can also be assessed by measuring the titer of isohemagglutinins, the antibodies to blood type A or B antigens present in everyone except those with type AB blood (Straight et al., 1994).

Complement assays (CH50 is the most common) can detect deficiencies in components of the complement system, which can manifest as recurrent infections with normal concentrations of plasma IgG (Straight et al, 1994).

ADVANCED IMMUNE FUNCTION ASSESSMENTS

Advanced immune function assessments are performed in whole blood or in cultures of cells isolated from blood. Granulocyte nitroblue tetrazolium dye reduction provides an assessment of granulocyte function but should be replaced eventually by lymphocyte phenotyping.

Studies of lymphocyte proliferation or function are in vitro assays of the ability of plant mitogens, lymphokines, recall antigens, or allogeneic cells to stimulate lymphocyte blastogenesis and proliferation. The use of a recall antigen permits the evaluation of immunologic memory as well as proliferation (Straight et al., 1994). Measurable indicators of proliferation include [^{3}H]thymidine incorporation into DNA (see Tim R. Kramer, Chapter 10), expression of cell-surface activation antigens such as CD25, release of cytokines, and shedding of soluble receptors for the cytokine IL-2 (Straight et al., 1994). Functional assays such as measurement of IL-2 release (via enzyme-linked immunosorbent assay [ELISA]) and IL-2 receptor expression (CD25) in cell culture supernatants may be a more physiological as well as reliable index of T-helper 1 (Th1) cell proliferation and would obviate the need for radioisotopes. The measure of Th1 proliferation in this way has been shown to be associated with stress levels and with the frequency of upper respiratory infections (URIs), although there is disagreement regarding the use of cytokine release as an index of proliferation.

A number of factors must be considered with regard to tests of lymphocyte stimulation by mitogens. One factor is that not all plant lectin mitogens are specific for T-cells; some have B-cell stimulatory properties as well. Also, mitogens are polyclonal activators that bypass the early events in lymphocyte stimulation. Thus, they may not produce the same response as a defined antigen. Plant lectins are not often encountered in vivo by the immune systems of most people (Shephard et al., 1994). Thus, any inferences regarding the type of cell responding must be made with caution, particularly since it may not be possible to account for differential changes in various subpopulations of cells due to illness or other stressors.

In addition to tests on serum and whole blood, ATSDR includes delayed hypersensitivity skin testing in its second tier of assays. Using a panel of four to five antigens such as mumps and diphtheria, this test measures functional T-cell-mediated immunity. However, the test is difficult to perform in large population-based studies, in part because it requires two visits (48 h apart) to the clinic.

Assays of Circulating Cytokines and Soluble Receptors

A large number of cytokines, including at least 18 identifiable interleukins and 3 interferons, have been characterized thus far. All can be measured by immunoassay, and many can also be measured by bioassay.

Many methodological issues must be considered in planning a strategy for the assessment of cytokines, their receptors, and inhibitors. A prime factor, which will not be discussed here, is the cost of individual assays. A second factor, or group of factors, of considerable importance for field studies is the proper means of sample collection, storage, and shipping; this is discussed below. A third and somewhat related factor is the inaccuracy that may be introduced by the assay of the plasma or serum rather than the supernatant of cultured lymphocytes. In his dicussion of on the use of whole blood cultures to measure lymphocyte proliferation, Kramer (Chapter 10) described attempts of his laboratory to identify cytokines whose production in response to phytohemagglutinin (PHA)-stimulation not only paralleled [³H]thymidine incorporation but also would be measurable in blood samples. Currently, such a parallel substance would obviate the need to use tritiated thymidine and would permit actual analyses to be performed in the field. Kramer and coworkers compared the parameters of [³H]thymidine incorporation to those of immunoassayable production and release of the soluble receptor for IL-2 (sIL-2r), as well as tumor necrosis factor α (TNF-α), interferon-γ (IFN-γ) and IL-10, in supernatants from whole blood. When the coefficients of variation (CVs) were compared between whole blood and isolated cell supernatants for measurements of TNF, sIL-2r, IFN-γ, and IL-10, the CVs for TNF and sIL-2r compared well with that for [³H]thymidine, but those for IFN-γ and IL-10 did not; Kramer indicated that this was an area of ongoing investigation. Two possible explanations for the results were offered by J.G. Cannon (Pennsylvania State University, University Park, personal communication, 1996), who emphasized the need to correlate cytokine production by whole blood with that of isolated blood cells. In a study by his group (Nerad et al., 1992), it was observed that when whole blood cultures were stimulated by lectins, IL-1β production compared favorably with that in standard peripheral blood mononuclear cell (PBMC) cultures. In contrast, because neutrophils in blood synthesize large numbers of TNF receptors as well as TNF itself, there was a reduction in measurable TNF compared with that in standard cultures. Cannon also mentioned that commercial assays, developed for measurement of cytokines in cell culture supernatants, can be unpredictable in measuring factors in samples that contain serum or plasma.

Cannon et al. (1993) reviewed the factors that must be considered in the measurement of circulating cytokines. With respect to the samples themselves, they pointed out that differences in plasma and serum affect assays in ways that must be tested; that white blood cells (WBCs) collected in blood samples are, themselves, a source of cytokines; and that contaminants on some types of assay tubes are capable of stimulating the ex vivo synthesis of cytokines by these WBCs.

Assays of circulating cytokines are affected by three types of cytokine-binding proteins and by cytokine antagonists found in plasma (Cannon et al., 1993). The binding proteins include immunoglobulins, α_2-macroglobulin, and soluble receptors. All three types of proteins are affected by changes in physiological status, not necessarily in parallel with changes in the cytokines themselves. In addition, although most soluble receptors inhibit the effects of the cytokines that bind to them, the soluble receptor for IL-6 actually increases the activity of the cytokine. Cytokine antagonists inhibit the effects of cytokines by competing with them for binding to receptors.

The assessment of cytokine values in urine, where circulating receptors are less prevalent, is suggested by Virella et al. (1997) and Moldawer (1997). These authors caution, however, that the effect of hydration status (diuresis) must be corrected for by the concurrent assessment of urinary creatinine or a similar substance. Another potential problem is that urinary concentrations of the cytokine of interest may be too low to detect changes (G. Sonnenfeld, University of Kentucky, Louisville, personal communication, 1997).

Other considerations in the assay of cytokines include the low sensitivity of most immunoassays. Concentrations of cytokines in blood and urine are often near the lower limit of detection for many assays in current use. Although bioassays are much more sensitive, they are far less specific. Antibody-based assays, such as ELISA, detect the presence of the epitope to which the antibody is directed, which may or may not assess biological activity. In addition, combinations of cytokines can cause synergistic effects. Thus, it is necessary to perform numerous assays with the specific types of samples and assay of interest, including many types of controls and standards.

An additional problem with cytokine assays is that the correlation between circulating levels of cytokines or their membrane receptors and functional immune status is still not well characterized (G. Sonnenfeld, University of Kentucky, Louisville, personal communication, 1997). This problem is compounded by the possible lack of relevance of circulating levels of cytokines compared to those in the lymphoid tissues of origin or other cytokine-producing cells. According to Cannon and coworkers (1993), factors that affect the measurement of cytokines also affect their biological activity in vivo. Thus, for example, the measurement of a cytokine without measurement of its antagonist gives a false picture of the role of the cytokine in a physiological process or disease state. Binding proteins can influence the half-life of cytokines as well as their distribution to other tissue compartments and their association with cell-surface receptors. In addition, because some cytokines remain primarily cell associated, they may never be detected in plasma, or their presence in plasma may not be meaningful. Finally, cytokines rarely act alone, but instead function in synergy with or opposition to others. Thus, it is important, but not always possible, to know how the concentration of one cytokine relates to that of others.

Nevertheless, Sonnenberg and coworkers include assays of IL-4, IL-6, IL-12, TNF-α and β, and IFN-γ in PBMC supernatants of shuttle astronauts (G. Sonnenfeld, University of Kentucky, Louisville, personal communication, 1997). The influence of exercise on IL-1 and IL-2 and on IL-2 receptors has been reviewed by Shephard and coworkers (1995).

Natural Killer Cell Activity

Natural killer cytolytic activity is assessed by measuring the in vivo release of radiolabeled chromium from target cells, usually a human myeloid tumor cell line.

REFERENCES

Bloom, B.R., R.L. Modlin, and P. Salgame. 1992. Stigma variations: observations on suppressor T cells and leprosy. Annu. Rev. Immunol. 10:453–88.

Cannon, J.G, J.L. Nerad, D.D. Poutsiaka, C.A. Dinarello. 1993. Measuring circulating cytokines. J. Appl. Physiol. 75(4):1897–902.

Luster, M.I., C. Portier, D.G. Pait, G.J. Rosenthal, D.R. Germolec, E. Corsini, B.L. Blaylock, P. Pollock, Y. Kouchi, and W. Craig. 1993. Risk assessment in immunotoxicology. II. Relationships between immune and host resistance tests. Fundam. Appl. Toxicol. 21(1):71–82.

Luster, M.I., C. Portier, D.G. Pait, K.L. White Jr., C. Gennings, A.E. Munson, G.J. Rosenthal. 1992. Risk assessment in immunotoxicology. I. Sensitivity and predictability of immune tests. Fundam. Appl. Toxicol. 18(2):200–210.

Moldawer, L.L. 1997. The validity of blood and urinary cytokine measurements for detecting the presence of inflammation. Pp. 417–430 in Emerging Technologies for Nutrition Research: Potential for Assessing Military Performance Capability, S.J. Carlson-Newberry and R.B. Costello, eds. Committee on Military Nutrition Research, Food and Nutrition Board. Washington, D.C.: National Academy Press.

Nerad, J.L., J.K. Griffiths, J.W. Van der Meer, S. Endres, D.D. Poutsiaka, G.T. Keusch, M. Bennish, M.A. Salam, C.A. Dinarello, and J.G. Cannon. 1992. Interleukin-1 beta (IL-1 beta), IL-1 receptor antagonist, and TNF alpha production in whole blood. J. Leukoc. Biol. 52(6):687–692.

Shephard, R.J., S. Rhind, and P.N. Shek. 1994a. Exercise and the immune system. Natural killer cells, interleukins and related responses. Sports Med. 18(5):340–69.

Shephard, R.J., and P.N. Shek. 1995. Exercise, aging and immune function. Int. J. Sports Med. 16(1):1–6 .

Straight, J.M., H.M. Kipen, R.F. Vogt, and R.W. Amler. 1994. Immune Function Test Batteries for Use in Environmental Health Studies. U.S. Department of Health and Human Services, Public Health Service. Publication Number: PB94-204328.

Virella, G., C. Enockson, and M. La Via. 1997. New approaches to the study of abnormal immune function. Pp. 431–450 in Emerging Technologies for Nutrition Research: Potential for Assessing Military Performance Capability, S.J. Carlson-Newberry and R.B. Costello, eds. Committee on Military Nutrition Research, Food and Nutrition Board. Washington, D.C.: National Academy Press.

Nutrition and Immune Function, 1999
Pp. 543–551. Washington, D.C.
National Academy Press

D

Emerging Infections, Nutritional Status, and Immunity

Presentation by Stephen S. Morse,
Edited by William R. Beisel

Seldom-recognized infections are likely to be encountered by U.S. troops who are deployed in unusual places (Morse, 1997). This problem has long been under investigation by the military, and as Susanna Cunningham-Rundles has said so very eloquently (see Chapter 9), one should expect the unexpected. Some of the lessons already obtained by studying the pathogenesis of newly emerged infections have been fruitful. However, there may also be some contradictory lessons to be gained from these studies.

Popularly speaking, emerging infections are the ones that suddenly appear in the news, such as the Ebola outbreak in Africa or, more recently, the Ebola–Reston virus, which appeared in monkeys in Reston, Virginia, and more recently in Alice, Texas. The most important emerging infection, which contributes to the realization that surprises will always occur, is the HIV (human immunodeficiency virus) infection that leads to AIDS. Like other emerging infections, AIDS was unknown to humans prior to the early 1980s. At that time, the major causes of death among men aged 25 to 44 years, a prime age group, did not include infectious disease death. Rather, the predominant causes of death were injuries, automobile accidents, and so on. This cohort of men was similar to those in the military—soldiers who were preparing to fight. In the last decade, AIDS has shown a remarkably steep slope of increase and is now the leading cause of death among men of prime age. In this case, expecting the unexpected is not only necessary, but also something that must be prepared for.

Emerging infections are more formally defined as infections that appear suddenly in a population or that rapidly increase in prevalence or in some new geographic range. Many of these conditions will be faced by troops deployed to distant places, which is why the military has a long-standing interest in emerging infections.

During the Korean War, almost 4,000 U.S. and UN troops acquired a viral disease called Korean hemorrhagic fever. The virus was not identified until the mid-1970s, and it is now known as *Hantavirus*, after a river in Korea near where it was first isolated. Almost 400 troops died, many more were incapacitated, and military demoralization occurred. Thus, emerging infections certainly can affect military operations, in addition to having a civilian impact. Soldiers serve as sentinels, intentionally or unintentionally, for emerging infections.

Viral emergence or, in general terms, infectious disease emergence is a process that involves two steps. The first step is introduction. Where do these apparently mysterious viruses or other agents come from, and how are they introduced into the human population? This has long been the most mysterious step.

Pathogen dissemination is the second step. Many infections are introduced into the human population, but most fail to make the leap to wide dissemination. Infections that are geographically localized cause problems for troops and others who are deployed in those areas, but they do not necessarily lead to a worldwide pandemic. Influenza does on occasion, and AIDS certainly has.

A number of factors can be associated with the emergence of a new infection (IOM, 1992a; Morse, 1997). These factors promote either the introduction or the dissemination step, and sometimes they influence both steps. Introduction factors include ecological changes, which involve the changing relationship between humans and their environment. They typically involve land-use changes or people interposing themselves into formerly sequestered natural environments. The result is increased human contact with a natural host. For example, a rodent species carries an infection that is natural to the wild host, but not to humans. As a result of increased rodent–human contact, an apparently new zoonotic infection can be introduced into the human population and disease may occur.

Other factors leading to the introduction of disease include land-use changes, such as clearing the land for agriculture, which may precipitate the introduction of a new infection.

Human demographics and behavior also play a very important role. The role of human behavior is illustrated by the dissemination of HIV and AIDS. Isolated infections can be introduced from a zoonotic source in an isolated geographic setting; then, the infection becomes disseminated as people move from rural areas into cities. Such movement is occurring with increasing frequency throughout the world. The United Nations estimates that, by the year 2025, two-thirds of the world's population will live in cities. Probably a dozen cities have populations of 8 million or more, and this trend will continue, largely for economic reasons related to demographic upheavals or war. In the case of HIV, this trend transposed once localized viruses to a larger population. The population in these burgeoning Third World cities such as Bangkok, Mexico City, Cairo, and Lagos, Nigeria (all larger than New York City), is often at high density, which facilitates the spread of potentially transmissible viruses. Malnutrition is also common in these high-density areas. Soldiers who are deployed in such areas—as they have been in Haiti, Panama, and Somalia—will be at risk of disease.

International travel and commerce include the rapid movement of people and goods around the world, which can allow previously isolated pathogens that have made the leap from the country into the city to disseminate even further. Such movement may be aided by advances in technology and industry such that biological products contaminating a single batch of a product become introduced to a larger final product. For example, hemolytic uremic syndrome is caused by a particular strain of *E. scherichia coli* that makes a toxin that contaminates hamburger. In high-density settings in which cattle are kept, the bacteria are largely disseminated by way of a small number of cattle who pick up the infection and transmit it to others. This scenario has also happened with bovine spongiform encephalopathy (BSE). Changes in rendering processes in England allowed the feeding of cattle with contaminated material very likely from sheep, although the transmission path has not been definitely identified. The oil shortage may also have influenced the transmission of BSE, in that portions of the rendering process were modified. Thus, technology and industry often create high-density settings in which biological products contaminated by an agent can flourish and spread.

A highly important factor in the spread of infection involves microbial adaptation and change, sometimes resulting in antibiotic-resistant organisms. Virus evolution is not usually the engine of a new disease, simply because so many viruses exist in various zoonotic species.

Reemerging diseases are also an important factor. These are infections that have reappeared in places where they were thought to be eliminated. Diphtheria, for example, is now making a massive reappearance in the former Soviet Union. Reemerging diseases are usually an indication of a breakdown in public health measures, such as sanitation, immunization, and all of the nineteenth-century control measures that were so effective in reducing infectious diseases in the past.

It is important to ask where and in what manner future infections might emerge, including pathogenetic mechanisms and the extent of human susceptibility during nutritional deficiency states. Where do these infections come from? The answer is from nature. In most cases, ecological changes underlie these events. They often involve previously sequestered natural hosts—in many cases, though not always, a rodent. There is a great biodiversity of rodents throughout the world carrying their own infections, and sometimes they come in contact with humans under suitable conditions. For example, hantaviruses, named after the prototype Hantaan, the virus of Korean hemorrhagic fever, is a virus carried by a common field mouse *Apodemis aggrarious*. This mouse flourishes in rice fields, as well as in somewhat more pristine environments occupied by military troops. As rice planting increases throughout Asia, the incidence of Korean hemorrhagic fever in Korea and China also increases, probably 100,000 to 200,000 cases occur per year. This particular rodent consumes rice in the fields prior to harvest. With their rice harvest, humans may also accidentally reap a virus that is left behind from the urine of infected mice. After the urine dries, the virus becomes airborne. Humans can then inhale this virus and become infected.

Historically, *Hantavirus* has been considered exotic. Although it was known to be in North America, none was associated with disease until the famous outbreak of *Hantavirus* pulmonary syndrome (HPS), as it is now called, in the Four-Corners region of the southwestern United States in 1993. The setting in which it occurred was not a jungle and not one where a new and unknown disease would be expected. The rodent that transmitted the virus is *Peromyscus meniculatas*, the common deer mouse, which is commonly found over most of North America. In fact, it appears to be the natural host of the virus that causes HPS. Probably the virus has been widespread in the United States and in North America, since there are related viruses now known in South America. It is now well-documented by ecologists in the area that a temporary change in the climate resulted in a rodent population explosion and an increase in rodent–human contact.

Various human activities may also provide opportunities for larger numbers of people to come in contact with diseases and spread them--for example, international travel. Troop movements follow the same pattern. This phenomenon underscores the need to be prepared, both diagnostically and in terms of surveillance.

Comparatively little is known about the role of nutrition in many of these infections, even for some that are quite familiar. Regarding pathogenesis and the effect of nutritional interventions on the pathogenesis of many of these infections, very little is known, aside from the truism that "malnutrition is bad."

One of the most common of the emerging infections in the world is dengue hemorrhagic fever (Bhamarapravati, 1989; Fan et al., 1989; Halstead, 1989; Krishnamurti and Alving, 1989; LeDuc, 1989; Rosen, 1989), a severe manifestation of dengue infection in children. Dengue is a common, tropical, mosquito-borne infection that most people living in the tropics eventually experience. The more severe forms of infection lead to something not unlike septic shock, and one assumes there is an underlying mechanism. Interest has focused on cytokines in recent years, but few details have been elucidated. The pathogenesis of dengue hemorrhagic fever is probably similar to the pathogenesis of other hemorrhagic fevers and perhaps similar to the pathogenesis of septic shock. Scott Halstead working in Thailand some years ago noted clinically that he rarely saw dengue hemorrhagic fever in undernourished children. It was only the better-nourished children who seemed to mount this particular response. In 1993, an epidemiological study in Thailand confirmed this observation (Thisyakorn and Nimmannitya, 1993). The children studied were ages 3 to 15, and it was relatively uncommon, compared with the entire population, to see dengue hemorrhagic fever in those who were malnourished. Because little is understood about the pathogenesis of dengue hemorrhagic fever, one wonders about the effect of nutritional intervention on the release of cytokines.

Indeed, comparatively little is known in vivo about the effects of nutrition or malnutrition on the cytokines. Indeed, this may be a double-edged sword. Why do children seem to be most susceptible to dengue hemorrhagic fever, and why are those who become clinically ill better nourished rather than malnourished? The answer is not known.

However, the dangers of poor nutrition are clear and palpable. Measles in Africa, for example, appeared in unusual manifestations, causing immunosuppressive disease with much more severe manifestations than normally expected. Although the pathogenesis is not known, a widespread suspicion suggests that malnutrition may have altered the presentation of disease. Indeed, when working in places with high operational, environmental, and nutritional stresses, unusual manifestations can be expected—even of well-known infections—and we may be fooled by them.

Finally, relatively little is known about the many factors affecting resistance to viral infection in humans. The macrophage is an important target for many of the infections that might be classified as emerging, including HIV and many of those causing hemorrhagic fevers. Macrophages are also important cells for releasing TNF (tumor necrosis factor) and IL-1 (interleukin-1), which may be important as a pathogenic mechanism.

Finally, the role of the immune system itself in the evolution of viruses is still unknown. One expects, for example, that immunosuppression might lead to viral variation and mutation. However, in some situations, the opposite may be true. The immune response itself may help to drive variation. In contrast, there are remarkable and unexpected effects of even micronutrient malnutrition on viral evolution.

Melinda Beck's work (see Chapter 16) with mice deficient in selenium or vitamin E illustrates this viral evolution—the appearance in these animals of a variant that was virulent for them and also for healthy animals. In other words, a malnourished mouse who gets this infection is a danger to itself, but also to the others next to it who now become infected. This work came out of a clinical observation of humans in China where a similar disease was seen in areas of low selenium.

To understand, in sum, there are many more questions than answers, and it is important to look at biological outcomes and the relationship between nutritional factors and pathogenesis. These factors can be defined, and they can be studied. Attention to cytokines is an important research task.

Certainly, military troops deployed in distant, hazardous locations and experiencing a diverse variety of stresses will always face these potential problems of emerging infections. This threat argues for the systematic study of potential infections in a combined research program that would also make intervention studies possible.

REFERENCES

Bhamarapravati, N. 1989. Hemostatic defects in dengue hemorrhagic fever. Rev. Infect. Dis. 11(suppl. 4):S826–S829.

Fan, W.F., S.R. Yu, and T.M. Cosgriff. 1989. The reemergence of dengue in China. Rev. Infect. Dis. 11(suppl. 4):S847–S853.

Halstead, S.B. 1989. Antibody, macrophages, dengue virus infection, shock, and hemorrhage: A pathogenetic cascade. Rev. Infect. Dis. 11(suppl. 4):S830–S839.

IOM (Institute of Medicine). 1992a. Emerging Infections: Microbial Threats to Health in the United States, J. Lederberg, R.E. Shope, and S.C. Oaks Jr., eds. Committee on Emerging Microbial Threats Health, Division of Health Sciences Policy, Division of International Health. Washington, D.C.: National Academy Press.

Krishnamurti, C., and B. Alving. 1989. Effect of dengue virus on procoagulant and fibrinolytic activities of monocytes. Rev. Infect. Dis. 11(suppl. 4):S843–S846.

LeDuc, J.W. 1989. Epidemiology of hemorrhagic fever viruses. Rev. Infect. Dis. 11(suppl. 4):S730–S735.

Morse, S.S. 1997. The public health threat of emerging viral diseases. J. Nutr. 127(5 suppl.):951S–957S.

Rosen, L. 1989. Disease exacerbation caused by sequential dengue infections: Myth or reality? Rev. Infect. Dis. 11(suppl. 4):S840–842.

Thisyakorn, U., and S. Nimmannitya. 1993. Nutritional status of children with dengue hemorrhagic fever. Clin. Infect. Dis. 16(2):295–297.

DISCUSSION

G. RICHARD JANSEN: Your talk reminded me so much of a book that Renee Dubose wrote like 40 or 50 years ago called *The Mirage of Health*. Essentially what he was saying is that we cannot keep up with it because there is always going to be something new coming along.

STEPHEN MORSE: Yes. There is a great biodiversity of microbes out there that have been evolving far longer than we have. They have evolved all sorts of strategies for better evolution. I am afraid that Dubose was right.

The good news though is that these factors can be studied, they can be identified, and I think we can better understand the complex interactions of these multifactorial interactions.

There are a lot of surprises out there. Certainly, Melinda Beck's work is a surprise and opens up a lot of questions about how some of the things like nutrients could in fact shape evolution in ways that we had not originally expected. I think that it is an exciting time to be studying this. Perhaps we have more of an advantage. We are more vulnerable, but we also have more advantages for studying these factors than were available in Dubose's time.

WILLIAM BEISEL: Talking about the possible disease effects in healthy children for dengue hemorrhagic fever earlier, Dr. Chandra showed a picture. The third man in that picture was Dr. Nevin Scrimshaw, and he introduced the concept of synergism and antagonism. I went through all of his quoted papers, and antagonism was about 50/50 in virus diseases with synergism. Microbiologists cannot grow viruses unless their cultured cells have a beautifully balanced nutritional status. So this is a possible reason as to why the healthy children developed the dengue hemorrhagic fever symptoms. They were better nourished. They could maybe grow more viruses in the body than the malnourished kids.

STEPHEN MORSE: That is entirely possible. It would also be ironic, of course, if their nutritional status made children less able to mount an effective immune response and, therefore, in some sense, less able to make some of the mediators that caused the immunopathology that was really the problem.

JOHANNA DWYER: Just a quick question. Richard Mung, from Harvard, says it is a big, bad world out there, but also that part of the problem lies in ourselves, that we use paradigms that are outdated and so forth. Can you suggest any that might be helpful to the committee in its deliberations?

STEPHEN MORSE: In terms of ecological paradigms, or infectious disease paradigms, or nutrition paradigms?

JOHANNA DWYER: Both infectious disease, which I think is what he deals with, and nutritional.

STEPHEN MORSE: This is certainly a subject that one could speculate about for hours. First of all, we know relatively little about the biodiversity of organisms that we might potentially be exposed to, and we know relatively little about how we would respond to them. For example, at this point, we cannot look at a sequence of any given virus and say what effect it is going to cause in a human being. I find that not surprising. But I think that we are in a position where soon we may be able to change that. For example, Ebola–Reston is arguably less virulent than Ebola–Zaire in humans. There is some natural evidence from the monkey handlers and others who became infected. It appears to be less virulent, and yet it is fairly closely related to known virulent strains.

The *Hantavirus* pulmonary syndrome, caused by *Hantavirus* Muerto Canyon, is fairly closely related to other hantaviruses that are not associated with human disease. Smallpox and vaccinia are another pair. One is not very virulent for humans by most measures. In fact, we used it as a vaccine, and one is highly virulent.

One of the underlying problems is our lack of pathogenesis models. We know so little about dengue because we have no pathogenesis model. If we had better pathogenesis models, nutrition could also be studied, and the factors isolated in those models could be further tested through interventional studies.

Now, on sort of the broad global scale, I would argue that the military is one of a number of components that is well positioned to be doing infectious disease surveillance and providing those data both to themselves and, when available, to others. Military operations may occur anywhere in the world. When troops are sent somewhere, they become effectively sentinels. So this requires watchfulness. We have long argued—every expert group like the Institute of Medicine Committee on Emerging Microbial Threats to Health—for the importance of surveillance, but we are not there yet. The World Health Organization, for example, is beginning to formulate effective plans for global surveillance, but it is going to take years to do that.

JOHN VANDERVEEN: One of the comments we are hearing occasionally now—not only that we are concerned about public health being a major cause for disease spread, but also there is some suggestion that perhaps we made some of our environment too clean, in that we are ridding ourselves of beneficial organisms that may cut down on the possibility of the spread of more harmful organisms. What is your opinion on that?

STEPHEN MORSE: We know relatively little. It is an interesting question. I cannot speak with authority on it. The impression I have is that we know relatively little about that. On sort of a macroscale, if I can get to just something a little bit larger, namely the rodents, we know that many of these outbreaks that have occurred in natural settings are very likely to be the result of an ecological change, some sort of agricultural change that favored a particular rodent. The result was that that rodent, which was best adapted to that environment, outcompeted the others who were holding it in check.

It is interesting that we know relatively little about beneficial effects and about what maintains these balances in nature at the detailed level of being able to model and predict them.

Nutrition and Immune Function, 1999
Pp. 553–558. Washington, D.C.
National Academy Press

E

Workshop Agenda

**NUTRITION AND IMMUNE FUNCTION:
STRATEGIES FOR SUSTAINMENT IN THE FIELD**

A Workshop Sponsored by

Committee on Military Nutrition Research

U.S. Army Medical Research Institute of Infectious Diseases
Fort Detrick, Maryland

Monday, May 20, 1996

I   WELCOMES AND INTRODUCTION TO THE TOPIC

8:00 a.m.–8:15 a.m.   Welcome and Introductions
                           Robert O. Nesheim
                           Chair, Committee on Military Nutrition Research

8:15 a.m.–8:30 a.m.   Welcome on Behalf of the U.S. Army Medical
                           Research and Materiel Command
                           Frederick W. Hegge
                           USAMRMC, Fort Detrick, Maryland

8:30 a.m.–9:00 a.m.   Why Is the Army Interested in Nutrition and
                           Immune Function?
                           LTC Karl E. Friedl
                           USAMRMC, Fort Detrick, Maryland

9:00 a.m.–9:10 a.m.   Discussion

9:10 a.m.–9:40 a.m.   Overview: What Do We Know About Nutrition
                           and Immune Function?
                           Ranjit K. Chandra
                           Janeway   Child   Health   Centre,   St.   John's,
                           Newfoundland, Canada

9:40 a.m.–9:50 a.m.   Discussion

9:50 a.m.–10:10 a.m.   Coffee Break

II   ISSUES OF METHODS AND ASSESSMENT

10:10 a.m.–10:40 a.m.   Issues   and   Assessment   of   Human   Immune
                           Function
                           Susanna Cunningham-Rundles
                           New York Hospital–Cornell University Medical
                           Center, New York

10:40 a.m.–10:50 a.m.   Discussion

10:50 a.m.–11:20 a.m.	Use of Whole Blood Cultures in Measurement of Cellular Immune Functions in Field Studies *Tim R. Kramer* USDA Agricultural Research Service, Beltsville, Maryland
11:20 a.m.–11:30 a.m.	Discussion
11:30 a.m.–12:00 p.m.	Part II Discussion
12:00 p.m.–1:00 p.m.	Lunch

III   HEALTH STATUS, STRESS, AND IMMUNE FUNCTION

1:00 p.m.–1:30 p.m.	Exercise, Infection, and Immunity: Practical Applications *David C. Nieman* Appalachian State University, Boone, North Carolina
1:30 p.m.–1:40 p.m.	Discussion
1:40 p.m.–2:10 p.m.	Inflammatory Stress and the Immune System *Leonard P. Kapcala* University of Maryland School of Medicine, Baltimore
2:10 p.m.–2:20 p.m.	Discussion
2:20 p.m.–2:50 p.m.	Biologic Rhythms in the Immune System and Nutrition *Erhard Haus* University of Minnesota and St. Paul–Ramsey Medical Center, Minnesota
2:50 p.m.–3:00 p.m.	Discussion
3:00 p.m.–3:20 p.m.	Coffee Break

3:20 p.m.–3:50 p.m.	Emerging Infections, Nutritional Status, and Immunity *Stephen S. Morse* The Rockefeller University, New York
3:50 p.m.–4:00 p.m.	Discussion
4:00 p.m.–4:30 p.m.	Part III Discussion
4:30 p.m.–4:45 p.m.	Concluding Remarks *Robert O. Nesheim*
Dinner Address:	Immune Function Studies During the Ranger Training Course of the Norwegian Military Academy *Pål Wiik* Norwegian Defence Research Establishment

Tuesday, May 21, 1996

8:00 a.m.–8:15 a.m.	Opening Remarks *Robert O. Nesheim*

IV NEW RESEARCH DIRECTIONS IN NUTRITION AND IMMUNE SYSTEM INTERACTIONS

8:15 a.m.–8:45 a.m.	The Cytokine System *Jeffrey Rossio* National Cancer Institute–Frederick Cancer Research and Development Center, Frederick, Maryland
8:45 a.m.–8:55 a.m.	Discussion
8:55 a.m.–9:25 a.m.	Neuroendocrine Consequences of Systemic Inflammation *Seymour Reichlin* University of Arizona–Arizona Health Sciences Center, Tucson
9:25 a.m.–9:35 a.m.	Discussion

9:35 a.m.–10:05 a.m.	Amino Acids: Glutamine *Douglas W. Wilmore* Brigham and Women's Hospital, Boston, Massachusetts
10:05 a.m.–10:15 a.m.	Discussion
10:15 a.m.–10:35 a.m.	Coffee Break
10:35 a.m.–11:05 a.m.	Physiological and Immunological Impact of U.S. Army Special Operations Training: A Model for the Assessment of Nutritional Intervention Effects on Temporary Immunosuppression *LTC Ronald L. Shippee* USARIEM, Natick, Massachusetts
11:05 a.m.–11:15 a.m.	Discussion
11:15 a.m.–11:45 a.m.	Antioxidants and Immune Response *Simin Nikbin Meydani* USDA Human Nutrition Research Center for Aging at Tufts, Boston, Massachusetts
11:45 a.m.–11:55 a.m.	Discussion
11:55 a.m.–12:05 p.m.	Vitamin A and Immune Function *Richard D. Semba* The Johns Hopkins University Hospital, The Wilmer Ophthalmological Institute, Baltimore, Maryland
12:05 p.m.–12:15 p.m.	Discussion
12:15 p.m.–1:00 p.m.	Lunch
1:00 p.m.–1:30 p.m.	Trace Minerals, Immune Function, and Viral Evolution *Melinda A. Beck* Child Development Center, University of North Carolina at Chapel Hill
1:30 p.m.–1:40 p.m.	Discussion

1:40 p.m.–2:10 p.m.	Dietary Fatty Acids and Immune Functions *Darshan S. Kelley* USDA Western Human Nutrition Research Center, Presidio of San Francisco, California
2:10 p.m.–2:20 p.m.	Discussion
2:20 p.m.–2:50 p.m.	Iron Metabolism, Microbial Virulence, and Host Defenses *Gerald T. Keusch* Tufts University School of Medicine, Boston, Massachusetts
2:50 p.m.–3:00 p.m.	Discussion
3:00 p.m.–3:30 p.m.	Part IV Discussion
3:30 p.m.–3:50 p.m.	Coffee Break

V   CONCLUSIONS

3:50 p.m.–4:20 p.m.	Conclusions: Militarily Important Issues Identified at This Workshop *William R. Beisel* The Johns Hopkins University School of Hygiene and Public Health, Baltimore, Maryland
4:20 p.m.–4:50 p.m.	Final Discussion
4:50 p.m.–5:00 p.m.	Closing Remarks *Robert O. Nesheim*

Nutrition and Immune Function, 1999
Pp. 559–574. Washington, D.C.
National Academy Press

F

Biographical Sketches

COMMITTEE ON MILITARY NUTRITION RESEARCH

ROBERT O. NESHEIM (*Chair, through June 30, 1998*) was vice president of research and development and later of science and technology for the Quaker Oats Company; he retired in 1983. Before his retirement in 1992, he was vice president of science and technology and president of the Advanced Health Care Division of Avadyne, Inc. During World War II, he served as captain in the U.S. Army. Dr. Nesheim has served on the Institute of Medicine's (IOM's) Food and Nutrition Board (FNB), currently chairing the Committee on Military Nutrition Research and formerly chairing the Committee on Food Consumption Patterns and serving as a member of several other committees. He also was active in the Biosciences Information Service (as board chairman), American Medical Association, American Institute of Nutrition, Institute of Food Technologists, and *Food Reviews International* editorial board. Dr. Nesheim's academic services included professor and head of the Department of Animal Science at the University of Illinois, Urbana. He is a fellow of the American Institute of Nutrition and American Association for the Advancement of Science and a member of several professional organizations. Dr. Nesheim holds a B.S. in agriculture, an M.S. in animal science, and a Ph.D. in nutrition and animal science from the University of Illinois.

JOHN E. VANDERVEEN (*Chair*) is the retired director of the Food and Drug Administration's (FDA) Office of Plant and Dairy Foods and Beverages in Washington, D.C. His previous position at the FDA was director of the Division of Nutrition, at the Center for Food Safety and Applied Nutrition. He also served in various capacities at the U.S. Air Force (USAF) School of Aerospace Medicine at Brooks Air Force Base, Texas. He has received accolades for service from the FDA and the USAF. Dr. Vanderveen is a member of the American Society for Clinical Nutrition, American Institute of Nutrition, Aerospace Medical Association, American Dairy Science Association, Institute of Food Technologists, and American Chemical Society. In the past, he was the treasurer of the American Society of Clinical Nutrition and a member of the Institute of Food Technology, National Academy of Sciences Advisory Committee. Dr. Vanderveen holds a B.S. in agriculture from Rutgers University, New Jersey, and a Ph.D. in chemistry from the University of New Hampshire.

LAWRENCE E. ARMSTRONG is an associate professor of exercise science at the University of Connecticut. He has joint appointments in the Department of Physiology and Neurobiology and the Department of Nutritional Sciences. Dr. Armstrong received his Ph.D. in human bioenergetics–exercise physiology from Ball State University. His research interests include thermoregulation, fluid electrolyte balance, energy metabolism, exercise physiology, and the human heat illnesses. He previously served as a research physiologist at the U.S. Army Research Institute of Environmental Medicine. He is a fellow of the American College of Sports Medicine and a member of the Federation of American Societies for Experimental Biology and the Aerospace Medical Association.

WILLIAM R. BEISEL is adjunct professor in the Department of Molecular Microbiology and Immunology at The Johns Hopkins University School of Hygiene and Public Health. He held several positions at the U.S. Army Medical Research Institute of Infectious Diseases at Fort Detrick, Maryland, including in turn, chief of the Physical Sciences Division, scientific advisor, and deputy for science. He then became special assistant for biotechnology to the Surgeon General. After serving in the U.S. military during the Korean War, Dr. Beisel was the chief of medicine at the U.S. Army Hospital in Fort Leonard Wood, Missouri, before becoming the chief of the Department of Metabolism at the Walter Reed Army Hospital. He was awarded a Commendation Ribbon, Bronze Star for the Korean War, Hoff Gold Medal at the Walter Reed Army Institute of Research, B. L. Cohen Award of the American Society for Microbiology, the Robert Herman Award from the American Association for Clinical Nutrition, and Department of Army Decoration for Exceptional Civilian Service. He was named a diplomate of the American Board of Internal Medicine and a fellow of the American College of Physicians. In addition to his many professional memberships, Dr. Beisel is a *Clinical Nutrition* contributing editor and *Journal of Nutritional Immunology* associate editor. He received his A.B. from Muhlenberg College in Allentown, Pennsylvania, and M.D. from the Indiana University School of Medicine.

GAIL E. BUTTERFIELD is director of nutrition research, Palo Alto Veterans Affairs Health Care System in California. Concurrently, she is lecturer in the Department of Medicine, Stanford University Medical School; visiting assistant professor in the Program of Human Biology, Stanford University; and director of nutrition in the Program in Sports Medicine, Stanford University Medical School. Her previous academic appointments were at the University of California, Berkeley. Dr. Butterfield belongs to the American Institute of Nutrition, American Society for Clinical Nutrition, American Dietetic Association, and American Physiological Society. As a fellow of the American College of Sports Medicine, she serves as chair of the Pronouncements Committee and was recently elected vice president; she also was president and executive director of the Southwest Chapter of this organization. She is a member of the Respiratory and Applied Physiology Study Section of the NIH (National Institutes of Health) and is on the editorial boards of the following journals: *Medicine and Science in Sports and Exercise, Health and Fitness Journal of the American College of Sports Medicine, Canadian Journal of Clinical Sports Medicine,* and *International Journal of Sports Nutrition.* Dr. Butterfield earned her A.B. in biological sciences, M.A. in anatomy, and M.S. and Ph.D. in nutrition from the University of California, Berkeley, and she is a registered dietitian. Her current research interests include nutrition in exercise, effect of growth factors on protein metabolism in the elderly, and metabolic fuel use in women exposed to high altitude.

WANDA L. CHENOWETH (*from September 18, 1996*) is professor in the Department of Food Science and Human Nutrition at Michigan State University. Previously, she held positions as teaching associate at the University of Iowa and University of California, Berkeley. Other work experience includes positions as research dietitian and head clinical dietitian at the University of Iowa Hospitals and research dietitian at Mayo Clinic. She is a member of the American Society for Nutritional Sciences, American Dietetic Association, and Institute of Food Technology. She serves as a reviewer for several journals, including the *Journal of the American Dietetic Association, American Journal of Clinical Nutrition,* and *Journal of Nutrition,* and is a member of the associate editorial board of *Plant Foods for Human Nutrition.* She has served on a technical review committee for the Diet, Nutrition, and Cancer Program of the National Cancer Institute and as a site evaluator, Commission on Evaluation of Dietetic Education of the American Dietetic Association. Her research interests are in the area of mineral bioavailability and clinical nutrition. Dr. Chenoweth completed a B.S. in dietetics at the University of Iowa, dietetic internship and M.S. in nutrition at the University of Iowa, and Ph.D. in nutrition at the University of California, Berkeley.

JOHN D. FERNSTROM is professor of psychiatry, pharmacology, and behavioral neuroscience at the University of Pittsburgh School of Medicine and director, Basic Neuroendocrinology Program at the Western Psychiatric Institute and Clinic. He received his S.B. in biology and his Ph.D. in nutritional biochemistry from the Massachusetts Institute of Technology (MIT). He was a postdoctoral fellow in neuroendocrinology at the Roche Institute for Molecular Biology in Nutley, New Jersey. Before coming to the University of Pittsburgh, Dr. Fernstrom was an assistant and then associate professor in the Department of Nutrition and Food Science at MIT. He has served on numerous governmental advisory committees. He presently is a member of the National Advisory Council of the Monell Chemical Senses Center, chair of the Neurosciences Section of the American Society for Nutritional Sciences (ASNS), and a member of the ASNS Council. He is a member of numerous professional societies, including the American Institute of Nutrition, American Society for Clinical Nutrition, American Physiological Society, American Society for Pharmacology and Experimental Therapeutics, American Society for Neurochemistry, Society for Neuroscience, and Endocrine Society. Among other awards, Dr. Fernstrom received the Mead-Johnson Award of the American Institute of Nutrition, a Research Scientist Award from the National Institute of Mental Health, a Wellcome Visiting Professorship in the Basic Medical Sciences, and an Alfred P. Sloan Fellowship in Neurochemistry. His current major research interest concerns the influence of the diet and drugs on the synthesis of neurotransmitters in the central and peripheral nervous systems.

G. RICHARD JANSEN (*through August 31, 1997*) is professor emeritus in the Department of Food Science and Human Nutrition at Colorado State University, where he was head of the department from 1969 to 1990. He was a research fellow at the Merck Institute for Therapeutic Research and senior research biochemist in the Electrochemical Department at E. I. DuPont de Nemours. Prior to his stint in private industry, he served in the U.S. Air Force. Dr. Jansen is a past member of the U.S. Department of Agriculture (USDA) Human Nutrition Board of Scientific Counselors and the *Journal of Nutrition*, *Nutrition Reports International*, and *Plant Foods for Human Nutrition* editorial boards. His research interests deal with protein-energy relationships during lactation and new foods for developing countries based on low-cost extrusion cooking. He received the Babcock–Hart Award of the Institute of Food

Technologists and a Certificate of Merit from the USDA's Office of International Cooperation and Development for his work on low-cost extrusion cooking, and he is a fellow of the IFT. He is a member of the American Society for Nutritional Sciences, Institute of Food Technologists, and American Society for Biochemistry and Molecular Biology among others. Dr. Jansen holds a B.A. in chemistry and Ph.D. in biochemistry from Cornell University in Ithaca, New York.

ROBIN B. KANAREK is professor of psychology and of nutrition at Tufts University in Medford, Massachusetts, where she also is the chair of psychology. Her prior experience includes Research Fellow, Division of Endocrinology, University of California–Los Angeles (UCLA) School of Medicine and research fellow in Nutrition at Harvard University. In addition to reviewing for several journals, including *Science, Brain Research Bulletin, Journal of Nutrition, American Journal of Clinical Nutrition*, and *Annals of Internal Medicine*, she is an editorial board member of *Physiology and Behavior* and the *Tufts Diet and Nutrition Newsletter* and is a past editor-in-chief of *Nutrition and Behavior*. Dr. Kanarek has served on ad hoc review committees for the National Science Foundation, NIH, and USDA Nutrition Research, as well as the Member Program Committee of the Eastern Psychological Association. She is a fellow of the American College of Nutrition, and her other professional memberships include the American Institute of Nutrition, New York Academy of Sciences, Society for the Study of Ingestive Behavior, and Society for Neurosciences. Dr. Kanarek received a B.A. in biology from Antioch College in Yellow Springs, Ohio, and M.S. and Ph.D. in psychology from Rutgers University in New Brunswick, New Jersey.

ORVILLE A. LEVANDER is research leader for the USDA Nutrient Requirements and Functions Laboratory in Beltsville, Maryland. He was research chemist at the USDA's Human Nutrition Research Center, resident fellow in biochemistry at Columbia University's College of Physicians and Surgeons, and research associate at Harvard University's School of Public Health. Dr. Levander served on the FNB's Committee on the Recommended Dietary Allowances. He also served on panels of the National Research Council's (NRC's) Committee on Animal Nutrition and Committee on the Biological Effects of Environmental Pollutants. He was a member of the U.S. National Committee for the International Union of Nutrition Sciences and temporary advisor to the World Health Organization's Environmental Health Criteria Document on Selenium. Dr. Levander was awarded the Osborne and Mendel Award by the American Institute of Nutrition. His society memberships include the American Institute of Nutrition, American Chemical Society, and American Society for Clinical Nutrition. Dr. Levander received his B.A. from Cornell University and his M.S. and Ph.D. in biochemistry from the University of Wisconsin–Madison.

GILBERT A. LEVEILLE (*through December 31, 1996*) recently retired as vice president for research and technical services at the Nabisco Foods Group in East Hanover, New Jersey. His other industry experience was as the director of nutrition and health science for the General Foods Corporation. He was chair and professor of food science and human nutrition at Michigan State University, professor of nutritional biochemistry at the University of Illinois–Urbana, and a biochemist at the U.S. Army Medical Research and Nutrition Laboratory in Colorado. Dr. Leveille was a member of the Committee on International Nutrition, a joint FNB–Board on International Health project. He won a research award from the Poultry Science Association, the Mead Johnson Research Award from the American Institute of Nutrition, the Distinguished Faculty Award from Michigan State University, and the Carl R. Fellers Award from the Institute of Food Technologists. He is a member of the American Association for the Advancement of Science, American Institute of Nutrition (past president), American Society for Clinical Nutrition, American Chemical Society, Institute of Food Technologists (past president), and Sigma Xi. Dr. Leveille received his B.V.A. from the University of Massachusetts and M.S. and Ph.D. in nutrition and biochemistry from Rutgers University, New Jersey.

ESTHER STERNBERG is chief of the Section on Neuroendocrine Immunology and Behavior, and associate branch chief of the Clinical Neuroendocrinology Branch of the National Institute of Mental Health Intramural Research Program at NIH. Dr. Sternberg received her M.D. degree and trained in rheumatology at McGill University, Montreal, Canada. She did postdoctoral training at Washington University, Barnes Hospital, St. Louis, Missouri, in the Division of Allergy and Immunology. She was subsequently a Howard Hughes Associate and instructor in medicine at Washington University and Barnes Hospital before joining NIH. Dr. Sternberg is internationally recognized for her ground-breaking discoveries in the area of central nervous system–immune system interactions. She has received the Arthritis Foundation William R. Felts Award for Excellence in Rheumatology Research Publications, has been awarded the Public Health Service Superior Service Award, and has been elected to the American Society for Clinical Investigation in recognition of this work. Dr. Sternberg is also internationally recognized as a foremost authority on the l-tryptophan eosinophilia myalgia syndrome (L-TRP-EMS). She was the first to describe this syndrome in relation to a similar drug l-5-hydroxytryptophan, and published this landmark article in the *New England Journal of Medicine* in 1980.

DOUGLAS W. WILMORE, the Frank Sawyer Professor of Surgery at Harvard Medical School, is a senior staff scientist and surgeon at Brigham and Women's Hospital, Boston, Massachusetts. Concurrently, he is also a consultant for the Dana-Farber Cancer Center, Children's Hospital Medical Center, the Beth Israel/Deaconess Hospital, Wrentham State School, and Youville Hospital and Rehabilitation Center. Dr. Wilmore's main interests are related to metabolic and nutritional means to support critically ill patients and enhance recovery. His basic research has been applied to patients with thermal and accidental injury, with infectious complications, and multiple organ failure. He worked with the team that developed the current method of intravenous nutrition used for patients throughout the world. This technique has been improved in Dr. Wilmore's laboratory; new amino acid solutions have been developed utilizing the amino acid glutamine, and anabolic factors such as growth hormone have been incorporated in to this new feeding program with dramatic therapeutic results. Dr. Wilmore serves on the advisory board of the Tufts Pediatric Trauma Center, international editorial committee of the *Chinese Nutritional Sciences Journal* of the Chinese Academy of Medical Sciences, and editorial boards of *Annals of Surgery* and *Journal of the American College of Surgeons*. He is senior editor of *Scientific American Surgery*, the surgical text published by the American College of Surgeons that serves as the basis for the care of general surgical patients. He also has published more than 300 scientific papers and 4 books. Among his professional memberships, Dr. Wilmore includes the American College of Surgeons, American Surgical Association, American Medical Association, Society of University Surgeons, and American Society for Enteral and Parenteral Nutrition. He holds a B.A. and honorary Ph.D. from Washburn University of Topeka, M.D. from the University of Kansas School of Medicine in Kansas City, and honorary M.S. from Harvard University.

JOHANNA T. DWYER (*FNB Liaison*) is the director of the Frances Stern Nutrition Center at New England Medical Center and professor in the Departments of Medicine and of Community Health at the Tufts Medical School and School of Nutrition Science and Policy in Boston. She is also senior scientist at the Jean Mayer–USDA Human Nutrition Research Center on Aging at Tufts. Dr. Dwyer is the author or coauthor of more than 120 research articles and 200 review articles published in scientific journals. Her work centers on life-cycle-related concerns such as the prevention of diet-related disease in children and adolescents and the maximization of quality of life and health in the elderly. She also has a long-standing interest in vegetarian and other alternative life-styles.

Dr. Dwyer is a past president of the American Institute of Nutrition, past secretary of the American Society for Clinical Nutrition, and past president and current fellow of the Society for Nutrition Education. She served on the Program Development Board of the American Public Health Association from 1989 to 1992 and is a member of the FNB, the Technical Advisory Committee of the Nutrition Screening Initiative, and the Board of Directors of the American Institute of Wine and Food. As a Robert Wood Johnson Health Policy Fellow (1980–1981), she served on the personal staffs of Senators Richard Lugar (R-Indiana) and Barbara Mikulski (D-Maryland).

Dr. Dwyer has received numerous honors and awards for her work in the field of nutrition, including the 1996 W.O. Atwater Award of the USDA and J. Harvey Wiley Award from the Society for Nutrition Education. She gave the Lenna Frances Cooper Lecture at the annual meeting of the American Dietetic Association in 1990. Dr. Dwyer is currently editor of *Nutrition Today*, on the editorial board of *Family Economics* and *Nutrition Review* and the advisory board of *Clinics in Applied Nutrition*, and is a contributing editor for *Nutrition Reviews*, as well as a reviewer for the *Journal of the American Dietetic Association, American Journal of Clinical Nutrition*, and *American Journal of Public Health*. She received her D.Sc. and M.Sc. from the Harvard School of Public Health and an M.S. from the University of Wisconsin, and completed her undergraduate degree with distinction from Cornell University.

REBECCA B. COSTELLO (*Project Director, through May 1998*) was project director for the Committee on Military Nutrition Research (CMNR) and Committee on Body Composition, Nutrition, and Health of Military Women (BCNH). Prior to joining the FNB staff, she served as research associate and program director for the Risk Factor Reduction Center, a referral center for the detection, modification, and prevention of cardiovascular disease through dietary and/or drug interventions at the Washington Adventist Hospital in Takoma Park, Maryland. She received her B.S. and M.S. in biology from the American University, Washington, D.C., and a Ph.D. in clinical nutrition from the University of Maryland at College Park. She has active membership in the American Institute of Nutrition, American College of Nutrition, American Dietetic Association, and American Heart Association Council on Epidemiology. Dr. Costello's areas of research interest include mineral nutrition, dietary intake methodology, and chronic disease epidemiology.

MARY I. POOS (*Project Director*) joined the IOM's Food and Nutrition Board in November 1997. She has been a project director for the National Academy of Sciences since 1990. Prior to officially joining the FNB staff, she served as a project director for the NRC's Board on Agriculture for more than seven years, two of which were spent on loan to the FNB. Her work with the FNB includes senior staff officer for the IOM report *The Program of Research for Military Nursing*, and study director for the reports *A Review of the Department of Defense's Program for Breast Cancer Research* and *Vitamin C Fortification of Food Aid Commodities*. Currently, she also serves as study director to the Subcommittee on Interpretation and Uses of Dietary Reference Intakes, and directs the planning activities in Global Food and Nutrition. While working with the Board on Agriculture, Dr. Poos was responsible for the Committee on Animal Nutrition and directed the production of seven reports in the *Nutrient Requirements of Domestic Animals* series, including a letter report to the commissioner of the FDA concerning the importance of selenium in animal nutrition. Prior to joining the National Academy of Sciences she was consultant/owner of Nutrition Consulting Services of Greenfield, Massachusetts; assistant professor in the Department of Veterinary and Animal Sciences at the University of Massachusetts, Amherst, and adjunct assistant professor in the Department of Animal Sciences, University of Vermont. She received her B.S. in biology from Virginia Polytechnic Institute and State University, and a Ph.D. in animal sciences (nutrition/biochemistry) from the University of Kentucky, and completed a postdoctoral fellowship in the Department of Animal Sciences Area of Excellence Program at the University of Nebraska. Dr. Poos's areas of research interest include protein and nitrogen metabolism and nutrition–reproduction interactions.

SYDNE J. CARLSON-NEWBERRY (*Program Officer*) is program officer for the CMNR and BCNH. Prior to joining the FNB staff, she served as project director for the Women's Health Project and adjunct assistant professor in the Department of Family Medicine, Wright State University School of Medicine; as a behavioral health educator for a hospital-based weight management program in Dayton, Ohio; and as a research associate at the Ohio State University Biotechnology Center. She received her B.A. from Brandeis University and her Ph.D. in nutritional biochemistry and metabolism from MIT and completed an NIH postdoctoral fellowship in the Departments of Biochemistry and Molecular Genetics at Ohio State. Dr. Carlson-Newberry's areas of research interest include eating disorders and diabetes management.

AUTHORS

MELINDA A. BECK is an assistant professor of pediatrics and a fellow at the Frank Porter Graham Child Development Center at the University of North Carolina at Chapel Hill. She has a Ph.D. in medical microbiology and immunology from Ohio State University, Columbus; an M.S. in biological sciences from California Polytechnic State University, San Luis Obispo; and a B.A. in zoology from the University of California, Berkeley. Her work focuses on the influences of antioxidant nutrients on viral pathogenesis.

RANJIT KUMAR CHANDRA is research professor and director of immunology, Memorial University of Newfoundland, St. John's, Newfoundland, Canada. He is also an adjunct professor at John Hopkins University School of Hygiene, New York Medical College, and the University of Napoli. He is the founding editor-in-chief of the monthly peer-reviewed journal *Nutrition Research*. Dr. Chandra has served on several advisory committees of the World Health Organization, International Union of Nutritional Sciences, Health Canada and the NIH. He was President of the 16th International Congress of Nutrition held in Montreal in 1997. Previously, Dr. Chandra served as visiting professor of nutritional immunology and associate program director of the Clinical Research Centre, MIT, and lecturer in pediatrics at Harvard Medical School. He was an assistant professor of pediatrics at the All-India Institute of Medical Sciences, New Delhi. Dr. Chandra is a member of 21 scientific societies and has received six honorary doctoral degrees. Dr. Chandra received an MBBS degree from Punjab University and an M.D. from the All-India Institute of Medical Sciences. Dr. Chandra is an officer of the Order of Canada.

SUSANNA CUNNINGHAM-RUNDLES is associate professor of immunology and vice chair for academic affairs in the Department of Pediatrics of Cornell University Medical College in New York City where she directs the Immunology Research Laboratory. She also is director of the Immunology Core Laboratory for the Clinical Research Nutrition Unit, an NIH-funded consortium among Cornell University, Memorial Sloan Kettering Cancer Center, and the Rockefeller University. She is chair of the Immunology Working Group for the Hemophilia Growth and Development Study Group, a national group of investigators studying hemophilia. Dr. Cunningham-Rundles is currently the chair of the Scientific Advisory Panel, National Institute of Child Health and Human Development: Adolescent Medicine HIV/AIDS Research Network, and recently completed a 2-year term as chair of the Microbial Immunology Review Group Study Section, AIDS and Related Diseases, ARR-1. She is a member of the Pediatric Advisory Committee of the Pediatric AIDS Foundation and the Scientific Advisory Committee of the American Foundation for AIDS Research. She is a fellow of the American Institute of Nutrition and American Academy of Microbiology and is currently serving a 2-year term as divisional group representative for the American Society for Microbiology. Dr. Cunningham-Rundles received her Ph.D. in biochemical genetics from New York University and postdoctoral training in immunobiology and immunogenetics at Memorial Sloan Kettering Cancer Center.

KARL E. FRIEDL is deputy director of the Army Operational Medicine Research Program at the U.S. Amy Medical Research and Materiel Command (USAMRMC), Fort Detrick, Maryland. Prior to this assignment, he was an Army Research Physiologist in the Occupational Physiology Division at the U.S. Army Research Institute of Environmental Medicine (USARIEM), where he specialized in the physical and biochemical limits of prolonged, intensive military training. Previously, LTC Friedl worked in the Department of Clinical Investigation at Madigan Army Medical Center in Tacoma, Washington, performing studies in endocrine physiology. He received his Ph.D. in physiology in 1984 from the Institute of Environmental Stress at the University of California, Santa Barbara.

ERHARD HAUS is a professor in the Department of Laboratory Medicine and Pathology of the University of Minnesota and chairman of the Department of Pathology of Health Partners and Regions Hospital in St. Paul, Minnesota. Dr. Haus is president of the American Association of Medical Chronobiology and Chronotherapeutics (AAMCC), honorary member of the Romanian Academy of Medical Sciences, member of the Endocrine Society, honorary member of the Romanian Society of Endocrinology, member of American Association for Cancer Research, the American Association of Clinical Pathologists, and several other professional organizations. Dr. Haus is involved in the study of the human time structure and the application of temporal parameters, diagnosis and treatment in human medicine. Dr. Haus has edited two books on medical chronobiology and published extensively on related topics.

LEONARD P. KAPCALA graduated from the University of Scranton with a B.S. in biology in 1970 and from the University of Pittsburgh School of Medicine in 1974 with his M.D. Subsequently, he received training in internal medicine at Case Western Reserve University School of Medicine and clinical and research training in endocrinology at the Tufts New England Medical Center. His first faculty position as assistant professor was at Case Western Reserve University School of Medicine. He is presently an associate professor of medicine and physiology at the University of Maryland School of Medicine in Baltimore. Dr. Kapcala is also a member of the university's Center for Studies in Reproduction and the Graduate School faculty. His neuroendocrinological research focus has been on the regulatory relationships of stress neuropeptides (corticotropin-releasing hormone, β-endorphin, adrenocorticotropin) in brain. More recently, his research has focused on several aspects of immune–neuroendocrine interactions including (1) the protective role of the hypothalamic–pituitary–adrenal axis against inflammatory stress, (2) immune-cytokine regulation of stress neuropeptides in brain, and (3) immune-cytokine regulation of cytokine gene expression in brain. Dr. Kapcala's basic research has been funded continuously since 1985 by federal grants from the NIH and the Veterans Administration. He is the author of more than 90 peer-reviewed publications, abstracts, and chapters. He is the founding coordinator of the Baltimore–Washington Stress Society and the Maryland Endocrine Society and hold memberships in the Society for Neuroscience and the Endocrine Society.

DARSHAN KELLEY is a research chemist at the Western Human Nutrition Research Center (WHNRC), San Francisco, CA. Dr. Kelley previously served as a research leader at the WHNRC, and research assistant professor at the West Virginia University. Dr. Kelley is a member of the American Society for Biochemistry and Molecular Biology, the American Institute of Nutrition, the American Diabetic Association, and the International Immunology Group.

Dr. Kelley received a B.Sc. in Agriculture and M.Sc. in Biochemistry from Punjab Agricultural University, and a Ph.D. in Biochemistry from Oklahoma University.

GERALD T. KEUSCH is professor of medicine at Tufts University School of Medicine, chief of the Division of Geographic Medicine and Infectious Diseases at the New England Medical School, and a faculty associate at Harvard Institute for International Development. His research interests include defining the role of nutrition in the host immune response and the interactions of malnutrition and infection, and he is currently chair of the U.S. component of the Nutrition and Metabolism Panel for the U.S.–Japan Cooperative Medical Sciences Program. Dr. Keusch previously served on the FNB's Committee on International Nutrition Programs, and he is a former member and chair of its Subcommittee on the Interaction of Nutrition and Infection. Dr. Keusch is a member of the American Association for the Advancement of Science and a fellow of the Infectious Diseases Society of America, as well as many other professional societies. He obtained his A.B. in art history from Columbia College and an M.D. from Harvard Medical School.

TIM R. KRAMER is a research biologist at the USDA Agricultural Research Service (ARS), Beltsville Human Nutrition Research Center in Maryland. He received his Ph.D. in medical sciences with emphasis in pathology and immunology in 1973 and M.S. in medical microbiology and immunology in 1970 from the University of Oklahoma Health Sciences Center, Oklahoma City. He spent 1973–1976 as a research fellow at the Sloan Kettering Institute for Cancer Research, New York City, and 1976–1979 as an assistant professor in pathology at Saint Louis University School of Medicine, during which he spent 2 years at the Anemia and Malnutrition Research Center in Chiang Mai, Thailand. In 1979, he joined the USDA–ARS as a research microbiologist at the Grand Forks Human Nutrition Research Center, North Dakota, followed by transfer to his current position in 1988. He currently serves as the editor-in-chief of the *Journal of Nutritional Immunology*.

SIMIN NIKBIN MEYDANI is professor of nutrition and immunology at Tufts University and chief of the Nutritional Immunology Laboratory at the Jean Mayer USDA Human Nutrition Research Center on Aging at Tufts University, where she directs studies related to the impact of nutritional factors on the immune response of the elderly. Her research interests focus on the effect of nutrients on immune responses of the young and the aged, with emphasis on the role of arachidonic acid metabolites, the molecular mechanisms, and clinical implications of antioxidant and prooxidant nutrient-induced changes in the aging immune response. She is the recipient of several awards, including the 1998 Lederle Award in Nutrition Research, Tufts University Outstanding Faculty Award for 1996, 1994 HERMES Vitamin Research Award, 1993

Nutritional Immunology Group Award, Denham Harman Lecture Award of the American College for the Advancement in Medicine, Alborz Institute Award, and Pahlavi Royal Gold Medal. Dr. Meydani is a member of the American Association of Immunologists, the American Institute of Nutrition, the American College of Nutrition, the American Aging Association, the Gerontological Society of America, the International Nutritional Immunology Group, and numerous other professional scientific societies. She has served on the editorial boards of the *Journal of Nutritional Immunology*, *Nutrition Research*, and *Journal of Nutrition*.

DAVID C. NIEMAN graduated from Loma Linda University in 1984 with the doctor of public health degree. Prior to this time, he had taught health and physical education for 8 years at the collegiate level. From 1984 to 1990, he was assistant and associate professor in the School of Public Health, Loma Linda University. He presently is professor of health and exercise science at Appalachian State University in North Carolina. His research focus from 1985 to the present, has been on obesity, sports, nutrition, aging, and exercise immunology, with more than 85 peer-reviewed publications in journals and books. He is also the primary author of three textbooks on sports medicine, physical fitness, and nutrition, and a coauthor on two others. Dr. Nieman sits on the editorial boards of the *International Journal of Sports Nutrition*; *Sports Medicine, Training, and Rehabilitation*; and *Exercise Immunology Annual*. He also serves as president-elect of the International Society of Exercise and Immunology.

LAURA C. RALL is currently assistant professor, foods and nutrition, and the American Dietetic Association Didactic Program Director at the University of Wisconsin–Stevens Point. She received a B.A. in sociology/community health, M.S. in nutrition, and Ph.D. in nutritional sciences from Tufts University. She is a member of the American Dietetic Association and American Society for Nutritional Sciences.

SEYMOUR REICHLIN is research professor of medicine at the University of Arizona College of Medicine, where he conducts research on neuroendocrine immunomodulation. His previous academic appointment was as professor of medicine, chief of the Endocrine Division, and director of the General Research Center at the Tufts–New England Medical Center. Dr. Reichlin has also been professor and chair of the Department of Medical and Pediatric Specialties, University of Connecticut, and professor of medicine and chief of the Endocrine Division at the University of Rochester School of Medicine. He has served on the Council of the National Institute of Kidney, Diabetes, and Digestive Disease and among other organizational activities is a fellow of the American Association for Advancement of Science and of the American Academy of Arts and Science; he has as president of the Endocrine

Society, the Association of Research in Nervous and Mental Diseases, and the Pituitary Society. He received a B.A. in biology from Antioch College, M.D. from Washington University, and Ph.D. in physiology from the University of London.

JEFFREY L. ROSSIO is a senior scientist for SAIC, Inc., at the National Cancer Institute–Frederick Cancer Research & Development Center (NCI-FCRDC) in Frederick, Maryland. He works in the AIDS Vaccine Program, specializing in measurement of human and non–human primate immune responses. From 1984 to 1992, Dr. Rossio was head of Clinical Immunology Services and also directed the Cytokine Testing Laboratories at NCI-FCRDC. He is the incoming chairman (1998) of the Clinical and Diagnostic Immunology Division (Division V) of the American Society of Microbiology. Dr. Rossio is also an associate professor of biology at Hood College in Frederick, Maryland. He is a member of several professional organizations, serves on the editorial board of *Clinical and Diagnostic Immunology*, and has published many research papers and books. Dr. Rossio received his B.S. from the University of Michigan, and his M.S. and Ph.D. degrees in microbiology and immunology from the Ohio State University. He served a postdoctoral fellowship in the Department of Biochemistry and Molecular Biology at the University of Texas Medical Branch, Galveston.

RICHARD D. SEMBA is an assistant professor, Department of Ophthalmology, the Johns Hopkins University School of Medicine in Baltimore, Maryland. He received his B.S. from Yale University in 1978, M.A. and M.D. from Stanford University in 1983, and M.P.H. form the Johns Hopkins University in 1991. He was a resident in ophthalmology at the Wilmer Institute from 1984 to 1987 and has been a faculty member in the School of Medicine at Johns Hopkins University for 10 years. Dr. Semba serves on the editorial board of the *Journal of Nutrition*. He has been active in research on vitamin A deficiency for nearly a decade, and his research interests include the role of vitamin A in immunity and response to infection, and the role of nutrition in the pathogenesis of HIV/AIDS.

RONALD L. SHIPPEE entered active military service in 1970 and completed the Infantry Officer's Basic Course and the U.S. Army Aviation Rotary Wing Course. LTC Shippee then served a combat tour in Vietnam, assigned to an Air Calvary Troop. Shortly after returning from Vietnam, he left active military duty to complete an M.S. and Ph.D. in nutritional biochemistry at the University of Connecticut. After graduate school, he returned to active military service and served as a research biochemist and chief of clinical chemistry at the U.S. Army Institute of Surgical Research, Fort Sam Houston, Texas. From April 1992 to August 1996, LTC Shippee was assigned to USARIEM in Natick, Massachusetts. During this period, LTC Shippee served as the principal investigator on numerous studies designed to determine the interaction of nutritional status and host resistance of soldiers involved in U.S. Army Special Operations Training. He is currently the deputy commander, chief of technical services, U.S. Army Forensic Toxicology Drug Testing Laboratory, Fort George Meade, Maryland.

PÅL WIIK has been a principal scientist at the Norwegian Defence Research Establishment since 1992. He received his M.D. in 1981 and his Ph.D. in 1989 from the University of Oslo. He was awarded a postdoctoral grant from the Norwegian Research Council from 1989 to 1991. At the Norwegian Defence Research Establishment, Dr. Wiik has especially been working with studies of the effects of military stress on the immune system.

Nutrition and Immune Function, 1999
Pp. 575–579. Washington, D.C.
National Academy Press

G

Acronyms and Abbreviations

AA	arachidonic acid
AAs	amino acids
ACH	acetylcholine
ACTH	adrenocorticotrophic hormone
ADH	antidiuretic hormone
ADX	adrenalectomy
AIDS	acquired immunodeficiency syndrome
ALA	α-linolenic acid
APC	antigen-presenting cell
ARC	AIDS-related complex
ARS	Agricultural Research Service
ASNS	American Society for Nutritional Sciences
ATSDR	Agency for Toxic Substances and Disease Registry
AVP	arginine vasopressin

BCG	Bacillus Calmette–Guérin (vaccine)
BCNH	Committee on Body Composition, Nutrition, and Health of Military Women
BCT	basic combat training
BIA	bioelectrical impedance
Bq	becquerel
BSE	bovine spongiform encephalopathy
BW	body weight
CD	cluster of differentiation
CEHR	Center for Environmental Health Research
CHD	coronary heart disease
CMI	cell-mediated immunity
CMNR	Committee on Military Nutrition Research
CNS	central nervous system
ConA	concanavalin A
CORT	corticosterone
CRDA	Cooperative Research and Development Agreement
CRH	corticotropin-releasing hormone
CRP	C-reactive protein
CVB4	coxsackievirus B4
CVO	circumventricular organ
DCM	dilated cardiomyopathy
DDH	delayed dermal hypersensitivity
DGLA	dihomo-gamma-linolenic acid
DHA	docosohexaenoic acid
DHEA	dehydroepiandrosterone
DLW	doubly labeled water
DNA	deoxyribonucleic acid
DNFB	dinitrofluorobenzene
DoD	Department of Defense
DRI	Dietary Reference Intake
DTH	delayed-type hypersensitivity
DWHRP	Defense Women's Health Research Program
DXA	dual-energy x-ray absorptiometry
EFA	essential fatty acid
ELISA	enzyme-linked immunosorbent assay
en%	energy percent
EPA	eicosapentaenoic acid
ESR	erythrocyte sedimentation rate
Fab	fragment-antibody
Fc	
FDA	Food and Drug Administration
FFA	free fatty acid

FFM	fat-free mass
FNB	Food and Nutrition Board
FTX	field training exercises
GABA	gamma-aminobutyric acid
GC	glucocorticoids
GH	growth hormone
GMCSF	granulocyte macrophage colony stimulating factor
GnRH	gonadotropin-releasing hormone
GTP	guanosine triphosphate
HAPE	high-altitude pulmonary edema
HDL	high-density lipoprotein
HDT	Human Dimensions Teams
HIV	human immunodeficiency virus
HLA	human leukocyte antigen
HPAA	hypothalamic–pituitary–adrenal axis
HYPOX	hypophysectomy
icv	intracerebroventricular
Ig	immunoglobulin
IGF-I	insulin-like growth factor-I
IL	interleukin
IL-1ra	interleukin-1 receptor antagonist
IOM	Institute of Medicine
ip	intraperitoneal
IR	immune response
IRE	iron-responsive element
IRE-BP	iron-responsive element-binding protein
iv	intravenous
KD	Keshan disease
LA	linoleic acid
LAK	lymphokine-activated killer (cell)
LDL	low-density lipoprotein
LH	luteinizing hormone
LLRP	Long-Life Ration Packet
LPS	lipopolysaccharide
LTB$_4$	leukotriene-B$_4$
L-TRP-EMS	l-tryptophan eosinophilia myalgia syndrome
Mabs	monoclonal antibodies
MDA	malondialdehyde
MFA	monounsaturated fatty acid
MHC	major histocompatibility complex
MIT	Massachusetts Institute of Technology
MN-CS	multiple nutrients for cellular synthesis
MN-PS	multiple nutrients for protein synthesis

MND	Military Nutrition Division (currently Military Nutrition and Biochemistry Division)
MOA	Memorandum of Agreement
MR	mitogenic responsiveness
MRDA	Military Recommended Dietary Allowance
MRDR	modified relative dose response (test)
MRE	Meal, Ready-to-Eat
MUFA	monounsaturated fatty acid
NAD	nicotinamide–adenine dinucleotide
NAIDS	nutritionally acquired immune dysfunction syndromes
NATO	North Atlantic Treaty Organization
NBT	nitroblue tetrazolium
NCI-FCRDC	National Cancer Institute–Frederick Cancer Research & Development Center
NIH	National Institutes of Health
NRC	National Research Council
NK	natural killer (cell)
OLVT	organum vasculosum of lamina terminalis
PBMC	peripheral blood mononuclear cell
PEM	protein-energy malnutrition
PGE_2	prostaglandin E_2
PHA	phytohemagglutinin
PHA-T	phytohemagglutinin-stimulated T-cell proliferation
PMN	polymorphonuclear neutrophil
PPD	purified protein derivative (skin test)
PSS	pituitary stalk section
PUFA	polyunsaturated fatty acid
PVFS	postviral fatigue syndrome
PVN	paraventricular nuclear
RA	rheumatoid arthritis
RDA	Recommended Dietary Allowance
RE	retinol equivalent
REM	rapid eye movement
RfD	reference dose
RGR-I	first U.S. Army Ranger training course
RGR-II	second U.S. Army Ranger training course
ROS	reactive oxygen species
RTB	U.S. Army Ranger Training Brigade
RT-PCR	reverse transcriptase–polymerase chain reaction
SAA	serum amyloid antecedent

SCID	severe combined–immunodeficient
SFA	saturated fatty acid
SFAS	Special Forces Assessment and Selection
SIADH	syndrome of inappropriate ADH secretion
sIL-2r	soluble receptor for IL-2
SOZ	serum opsonized zymosan
SRBC	sheep red blood cell
SSCOM	Soldier System Command
T_3	triiodothyronine
T_4	thyroxine
TBG	thyroid-binding globulin
TDEE	total daily energy expenditure
TE	tocopherol equivalent
TfR	transferrin receptor
Th1	T-helper 1 (cell)
TNF	tumor necrosis factor
TPN	total parenteral nutrition
TRH	thyrotropin-releasing hormone
TSH	thyroid-stimulating hormone
UCLA	University of California–Los Angeles
URI	upper respiratory infection
URTI	upper respiratory tract infection
USAF	U.S. Air Force
USAMRIID	U.S. Army Medical Research Institute of Infectious Diseases
USAMRMC	U.S. Army Medical Research and Materiel Command
USARIEM	U.S. Army Research Institute of Environmental Medicine
USDA	U.S. Department of Agriculture
VIP	vasoactive intestinal polypeptide
VP	vasopressin
WBC	white blood cell
WHO	World Health Organization
WRAIR	Walter Reed Army Institute of Research

Nutrition and Immune Function, 1999
Pp. 581–656. Washington, D.C.
National Academy Press

H

Nutrition and Immune Function: A Selected Bibliography

Abbas, A.K., A.H. Lichtman, and J.S. Prober, eds. 1991. Cellular and Molecular Immunology. Philadelphia, Pa.: W.B. Saunders Co.

Abbas, A.K., A.H. Lichtman, and J.S. Pober, eds. 1994. Cellular and Molecular Immunology, 2nd ed. Philadelphia, Pa.: W.B. Saunders Co.

Abbas, A.K., V.L. Perez, L. Van Parijs, and R.C. Wong. 1995. Differentiation and tolerance of CD4+ T lymphocytes. Ciba Found. Symp. 195:7–13.

Abe, F., H. Inaba, T. Katoh, and M. Hotachi. 1990 Effects of iron and desferrioxamine on *Rhizopus* infection. Mycopathologia 110:87–91.

Abo, T., T. Kawate, K. Itoh, and K. Kumagai. 1981. Studies on the bioperiodicity of the imune response. I. Circadian rhythms of human T-, B-, and K-cell traffic in the peripheral blood. J. Immunol. 126: 1360–1363.

Ader, R., and N. Cohen. 1993. Psychoneuroimmunology: Conditioning and stress. Ann. Rev. Psychol. 44:53–85.

Aggarwal, B.B., and R.K. Puri, eds. 1995. Human Cytokines: Their Role in Disease and Therapy. Cambridge, Mass.: Blackwell Science.

Ahmed, F., D.B. Jones, and A.A. Jackson. 1990. The interaction of vitamin A deficiency and rotavirus infection in the mouse. Br. J. Nutr. 63:363–373.

Akana, S.F., C.S. Cascio, J. Shinsako, and M.F. Dallman. 1985. Corticosterone: Narrow range required for normal body and thymus weight and ACTH. Am. J. Physiol. 249:R527–R532.

Akbar, A.N., P.A. Fitzgerald-Bacarsly, M. deSousa, P.J. Giardina, M.W. Hilgartner, and R.W. Grady. 1986. Decreased natural killer activity in thalassemia major: A possible consequence of iron overload. J. Immunol. 136:1635–1640.

Aldred, A.R., and G. Schreiber. 1993. The negative acute phase proteins. Pp. 21–37 in Acute Phase Proteins: Molecular Biology, Biochemistry, and Clinical Applications, A. Mackiewicz, I. Kushner, and H. Bauman, eds. Boca Raton, Fla.: CRC Press.

Alevizatos, A.C., R.W. McKinney, and R.D. Feigin. 1967. Live attenuated equine encephalomyelitis virus vaccine. I. Clinical response of man to immunization. Am. J. Trop. Med. Hyg. 16:762–768.

Alexander, J.W. 1993. Immunoenhancement via enteral nutrition. Arch. Surg. 128(11):1242–1245.

Almond, J., and J. Pattison. 1997. Human BSE. Nature 389:437–438.

Alvarez, J.O., E. Salazar-Lindo, J. Kohatsu, P. Miranda, and C.B. Stephensen. 1995. Urinary excretion of retinol in children with acute diarrhea. Am. J. Clin. Nutr. 61:1273–1276.

Andelman, M.B., and B.R. Sered. 1966. Utilization of dietary iron by term infants: A study of 1,048 infants from a low socioeconomic population. Am. J. Dis. Child. 111:45–55.

Anderson, A.O. 1997. New Technologies for Producing Systemic and Mucosal Immunity by Oral Immunization: Immunoprophylaxis in Meals, Ready-to-Eat. Pp. 451–500 in Emerging Technologies for Nutrition Research, Potential for Assessing Military Performance Capability, S.J. Carlson-Newberry and R.B. Costello, eds. A report of the Committee on Military Nutrition Research, Food and Nutrition Board, Institute of Medicine. Washington, D.C.: National Academy Press.

Anderson, R., R. Oosthuizen, R. Maritz, A. Heron, and A. J. VanRensburg. 1980. The effects of increasing weekly doses of ascorbate on certain cellular and humoral immune function in volunteers. Am. J. Clin. Nutr. 33:71–76.

Andreis, P.G., G. Neri, A.S. Belloni, M. Giuseppina, A. Kasprzak, and L.G.G. Nussdorfer. 1991. Interleukin-1β enhances corticosterone secretion by acting directly on the rat adrenal gland. Endocrinology 129:53–57.

Angeli, A., G. Gatti, M.L. Sartori, and R.G. Masora. 1992. Chronobiological aspects of the neuroendocrine immune network. Regulation of human natural killer (NK) cells as a model. Chronobiologia 19:93–110.

AR (Army Regulation) 40-25. 1985. See U.S. Departments of the Army, the Navy, and the Air Force, 1985.

Araneo, B.A., M.L.I. Woods, and R.A. Daynes. 1993. Reversal of the immunosenescent phenotype by dehydroepiandrosterone: Hormone treatment provides an adjuvant effect on the immunization of aged mice with recombinant hepatitis B surface antigen. J. Infect. Dis. 167:830–840.

Archibald, F. 1983. Lactobacillus plantarum, an organism not requiring iron. FEMS Microbiol. Lett. 19:29–32.

Ardawi, M.S.M., and E.A. Newsholme. 1983. Glutamine metabolism in lymphocytes of the rat. Biochem. J. 212:835–842.

Ardawi, M.S.M., and E.A. Newsholme. 1985. Fuel utilization in colonocytes of the rat. Biochem. J. 231:713–719.

Arem, R., G.J. Wiener, S.G. Kaplan, H.S. Kim, S. Reichlin, and M.M. Kaplan. 1993. Reduced tissue thyroid hormone levels in fatal illness. Metab. Clin. Exp. 42:1102–1108.

Arendt, J. 1994. The pineal. Pp. 348–362. In Biologic Rhythms in Clinical and Laboratory Medicine, Y. Touitou and E. Haus, editors. 2nd ed. Heidelberg: Springer-Verlag.

Armstrong, R.B., G.L. Warren, and J.A. Warren. 1991. Mechanisms of exercise-induced muscle fibre injury. Sports Med. 12:184–207.

Arthur, J.R., and G.J. Beckett. 1994. Roles of selenium in type I iodothyronine 5'-deiodinase and in thyroid hormone and iodine metabolism. Pp. 93–115 in Selenium in Biology and Human Health, R.F. Burk, ed. New York: Springer-Verlag.

Arvidson, N.G., B. Gudbjornson, L. Elfman, and A.C. Ryden. 1994. Circadian rhythm of serum interleukin 6 in rheumatoid arthritis. Ann. Rheumat. Dis. 53(8):521–524.

Auernhammer, C.J., and C.J. Strasburger. 1995. Effects of growth hormone and insulin-like growth factor I on the immune system. Eur. J. Endocrinol. 133:635–645.

Autenrieth, I.B., E. Bohn, J.H. Ewald, and J. Heesemann. 1995. Deferoxamine B but not deferoxamine G1 inhibits cytokine production in murine bone marrow macrophages. J. Infect. Dis. 172:490–496.

Autenrieth, I.B., R. Reissbrodt, E. Saken, R. Berner, U. Vogel, W. Rabsch, and J. Heesemann. 1994. Desferrioxamine-promoted virulence of *Yersinia enterocolitica* in mice depends on both desferrioxamine type and mouse strain. J. Infect. Dis. 169:562–567.

Auzeby, A., A. Bogdan, Z. Krosi, and Y. Touitou. 1988. Time dependence of urinary neopterin, a marker of cellular immune activity. Clin. Chem. 34:1866–1867.

Badalamenti, S., F. Salerno, E. Lorenzano, G. Paone, G. Como, S. Finnazzi, A.C. Sacchetta, A. Rimola, G. Graziani, D. Galmarini, and C. Ponticelli. 1995. Renal effects of dietary fish oil supplementation with fish oil in cyclosporine-treated liver transplant recipients. Hepatology 22:1695–1701.

Badwe, R.A., W.M. Gregory, M.A. Chaudary, and M.A. Richards. 1991. Timing of surgery during the menstrual cycle and survival of the premenopausal woman with operable breast cancer. Lancet 337:1261–1264.

Baetjer, A.M. 1932. The effect of muscular fatigue upon resistance. Physiol. Rev. 12:453–468.

Bai, J., S. Wu, K. Ge, X. Deng, and C. Su. 1980. The combined effect of selenium deficiency and viral infection on the myocardium of mice. Acta Acad. Med. Sci. Sin. 2:29–31.

Baj, Z., J. Kantorski, E. Majewska, K. Zeman, L. Pokoca, E. Fornalczyk, H. Tchorzewski, Z.Sulowska, and R. Lewicki. 1994. Immunological status of competitive cyclists before and after the training season. Int. J. Sports Med. 15:319–324.

Bala, S., M.L. Failla and J.K. Lunney. 1991. Alterations in splenic lymphoid cell subsets and activation antigens in copper-deficient rats. J. Nutr. 121(5):745–73.

Ballart, I.J., M.E. Estevez, L. Sen, R.A. Diez, J. Giuntoli, S.A. de Miani, and J. Penalver. 1986. Progressive dysfunction of monocytes associated with iron overload and age in patients with thalassemia major. Blood 67:105–109.

Ballmer, P.E. and H.B. Staehlin. 1994. Beta carotene, vitamin E, and lung cancer. N. Engl. J. Med. 330(15):1029–1035.

Ban, E., F. Haour, and R. Lenstra. 1992. Brain interleukin-1 gene expression induced by peripheral lipopolysaccharide administration. Cytokine 4:48–54.

Banchereau, J. 1991. Interleukin-4. Pp. 119–149 in The Cytokine Handbook, A. Thomson, ed. London: Academic Press.

Bandtlow, C.E., M. Meyer, D. Lindholm, M. Spranger, R. Heumann, and H. Thoenen. 1990. Regional and cellular codistribution of interleukin-1β and nerve growth factor mRNA in the adult rat brain: Possible relationship to the regulation of nerve growth factor synthesis. J. Cell Biol. 111:1701–1711.

Banks, W.A., L. Ortiz, S.R. Plotkin, and A.J. Kastin. 1991. Human interleukin (IL)-1 (IL-1α) and murine IL-1β are transported from blood to brain in the mouse by a shared saturable mechanism. J. Pharm. Exp. Ther. 259:988–996.

Barbanel, G., S. Gaillet, M. Mekaouche, L. Givalois, G. Ixtart, P. Siaud, A. Szafarczyk, F. Malaral, and I. Assenmacher. 1993. Complex catecholaminergic modulation of the stimulatory effect of interleukin-1β on the corticotropic axis. Brain Res. 626:31–36.

Barber, A.E., S.M. Coyle, M.A. Marano, E. Fischer, S.E. Calvano, Y. Fong, L.L. Moldawer, and S.F. Lowry. 1993. Glucocorticoid therapy alters hormonal and cytokine responses to endotoxin in man. J. Immunol. 150:1999–2006.

Barbul, A., D.A. Sisto, H.L. Wasserkrug, and G. Efron. 1981. Arginine stimulates lymphocyte immune response in healthy human beings. Surgery 90(2):244–251.

Barger, L.K., J.E. Greenleaf, F. Baldini, and D. Huff. 1995. Effects of space missions on the human immune system: A meta-analysis. Sports Med. Train. Rehabil. 5:293–310.

Barnes, P.F., L. Shuzhuang, J.S. Abrams, E. Wang, M. Yamamura, and R.L. Modlin. 1993. Cytokine production at the site of disease in human tuberculosis. Infect. Immun. 61(8):3482–3489.

Barnes, P.J. 1984a. Autonomic control of the airways in nocturnal asthma. Pp. 69–73 in Nocturnal Asthma, P.J. Barnes and J. Levy, eds. Oxford: Oxford University Press.

Barnes, P.J. 1984b. Nocturnal asthma: Mechanisms and treatment. Br. Med. J. 288:1397–1398.

Barone, J., J.R. Herbert, and M.M. Reddy. 1989. Dietary fat and natural-killer-cell activity. Am. J. Clin. Nutr. 50(4):861–867.

Barret-Connor, E. 1971. Bacterial infection and sickle-cell anaemia. An analysis of 250 infections in 166 patients and a review of the literature. Medicine 50:97–112.

Barrett S., and V. Herbert. 1994. The Vitamin Pushers. How the "Health Food" Industry Is Selling America a Bill of Goods. Amherst, N.Y.: Prometheus Books.

Barry, D.M.J., and A.W. Reeve. 1973. Iron injections and serious gram negative infection in Polynesian newborn. N. Zeal. J. Med. 78:376.

Barry, D.M.J., and A.W. Reeve. 1977. Increased incidence of gram-negative neonatal sepsis with intramuscular iron administration. Pediatrics 60:908–912.

Barton, B.E., and J.V. Jackson. 1993. Protective role of interleukin-6 in the lipopolysaccharide-galactosamine septic shock model. Infect. Immun. 61:1496–1499.

Baslund, B., K. Lyngberg, V. Andersen, J. Halkjaer-Kristensen, M. Hansen, M. Klokker, and B.K. Pedersen. 1993. Effect of 8 weeks of bicycle training on the immune system of patients with rheumatoid arthritis. J. Appl. Physiol. 75:1691–1695.

Basta, S.S., Soekirman, A. Karyadi, and N.S. Scrimshaw. 1979. Iron-deficiency anaemia and the productivity of adult males in Indonesia. Am. J. Clin. Nutr. 32:916–925.

Bateman, A., A. Singh, R. Kral, and S. Solomon. 1989. The immune-hypothalamic-pituitary-adrenal axis. Endocr. Rev. 10:92–112.

Baurenfreund, J.C. 1980. The safest use of vitamin A. International Vitamin A Consultative Group. Washington, D.C.: The Nutrition Foundation.

Bayle, J.E., M. Guellati, F. Ibos, and J. Roux. 1991. Brucella abortus antigen stimulates the pituitary-adrenal axis through the extrapituitary B-lymphoid system. Prog. Neuroendocrinol. Immunol. 4:99–105.

Beard, J. 1993. Iron dependent pathologies. Pp. 99–111 in Iron Deficiency Anemia, Recommended Guidelines for the Prevention, Detection, and Management Among U.S. Children and Women of Childbearing Age, R. Earl and C.E. Woteki, eds. A report of the Committee on the Prevention, Detection, and Management of Iron Deficiency Anemia Among U.S. Children and Women of Childbearing Age, Food and Nutrition Board, Institute of Medicine. Washington, D.C.: National Academy Press.

Beaton, G.H. 1996. Basic biology and biology of interventions: A synthesis view. In Beyond Nutritional Recommendations: Implementing Science for Healthier Populations, C. Garza, J.D. Haas, J-P. Habicht, and D.L. Pelletier, eds. Proceedings from the 14th Annual Bristol-Myers Squibb/Mead Johnson Nutrition Research Symposium, June 5–7, 1995. Ithaca, N.Y.: Cornell University.

Beaton, G.H., R. Martorell, K.J. Aronson, B. Edmonston, G. McCabe, A.C. Ross, and B. Harvey. 1993. Effectiveness of vitamin A supplementation in the control of young child morbidity and mortality in developing countries. State-of-the-Art Series Nutrition Policy Discussion Paper No. 13. Geneva: Administrative Committee on Coordination/Subcommittee on Nutrition of the United Nations.

Beck, M.A., and O.A. Levander. 1997. Effects of nutritional antioxidants and other dietary constituents on coxsackievirus-induced myocarditis. In The Coxsackie B viruses, S. Tracy and N. M. Chapman, and B.W.J. Mahy, eds. Berlin; New York: Springer.

Beck, M.A., B.R. Blakly, and D.L. Hamilton. 1987. The effect of copper deficiency on the immune response in mice. Drug Nutr. Interact. 5:103–111.

Beck, M.A., P.C. Kolbeck, L.H. Rohr, Q. Shi, V.C. Morris, and O.A. Levander. 1994a. Benign human enterovirus becomes virulent in selenium-deficient mice. J. Med. Virol. 43:166–170.

Beck, M.A., P.C. Kolbeck, L.H. Rohr, Q. Shi, V.C. Morris, and O.A. Levander. 1994b. Vitamin E deficiency intensifies the myocardial injury of coxsackievirus B3 infection of mice. J. Nutr. 124:345–358.

Beck, M.A., P.C. Kolbeck, Q. Shi, L.H. Rohr, V.C. Morris, and O.A. Levander. 1994c. Increased virulence of a human enterovirus (coxsackievirus B3) in selenium-deficient mice. J. Infect. Dis. 170:351–357.

Beck, M.A., Q. Shi, V.C. Morris, and O.A. Levander. 1995. Rapid genomic evolutuion of a non-virulent Coxsackievirus B3 in selenium-deficient mice results in selection of identical virulent isolates. Nature Medicine 1(5):433–436.

Beck, M.A., Q. Shi, V.C. Morris, and O.A. Levander. 1996. From avirulent to virulent: Vitamin E deficiency in mice drives rapid genomic evolution of a CVB3 virus [abstract]. FASEB J. 10(3):A191.

Beckman, K.B., and B.N. Ames. 1997. Oxidative decay of DNA. J. Biol. Chem. 272:19633–19636.

Beisel, W.R. 1977. Symposium on impact of infection on nutritional status of the host. Am. J. Clin. Nutr. 30:1203–1371, 1439–1566.

Beisel, W.R. 1982. Single nutrients and immunity. Am. J. Clin. Nutr. 35 (suppl.):415–468.

Beisel, W.R. 1991. Nutrition and infection. Pp. 507–542 in Nutritional Biochemistry and Metabolism, 2nd ed., M.C. Linder, ed. New York: Elsevier.

Beisel, W.R. 1992 Metabolic responses of the host to infections. Pp. 1–13 in Textbook of Pediatric Infectious Diseases, 3d ed., R.D. Feigin and J.D. Cherry, eds. Philadelphia: W.B. Saunders Co.

Beisel, W.R. 1995. Herman Award Lecture, 1995: Infection-induced malnutrition—From cholera to cytokines. Am. J. Clin. Nutr. 62:813–819.

Beisel, W.R., and P.Z. Sobocinski. 1980. Metabolic Aspects of Fever. Pp. 39–48 in Fever, J.M. Lipton, ed. New York: Raven Press.

Beisel, W.R., and J.M. Talbot, eds. 1985. Research Opportunities on Immunocompetence in Space. Report of the Life Science Research Office, FASEB. Prepared for the Life Science Division, Office of Space Science and Applications, NASA, Washington, D.C. Bethesda, Md.: Life Science Research Office, FASEB.

Beisel, W.R., W.D. Sawyer, E.D. Ryll, and D. Crozier. 1967. Metabolic effects of intracellular infections in man. Ann. Int. Med. 67:744–779.

Beisel, W.R., K.A. Woeber, P.J. Bartelloni, and S.H. Ingbar. 1968. Groeth hormone response during sandfly fever. J. Clin. Endocrinol. Metab. 28(8):1220–1223.

Bellido, T., G. Girasole, G. Passeri, X.P. Yu, H. Mocharla, R.L. Jilka, A. Notides, and S.C. Manolagas. 1993. Demonstration of estrogen and vitamin D receptors in bone marrow-derived stromal cells: Upregulation of the estrogen receptor by 1,25-dihydroxyvitamin D3. Endocrinology 133:553–562.

Benatar, S.R. 1986. Fatal asthma. N. Engl. J. Med. 314:423–429.

Bendich, A. 1992. Safety issues regarding the use of vitamin supplements. Ann. N.Y. Acad. Sci. 669:300–310.

Bendich, A., and R.K. Chandra, ed. 1990. Micronutrients and immune functions. New York, N.Y.: New York Academy of Sciences.

Beneviste, E.N. 1992. Cytokines: Influence on glial cell gene expression and function. Pp. 106–153 in Neuroimmunoendocrinology: Chemical Immunology, 2d ed., J.E. Blalock, ed. Basel: Karger.

Bentham, J., J. Rodriguez-Arnao, and R.J. Ross. 1993. Acquired growth hormone resistance in patients with hypercatabolism. Horm. Res. 40:87–91.

Berczi, I., F.D. Baragar, I.M. Chalmers, E.C. Keystone, E. Nagy, and R.J. Warrington. 1993. Hormones in self tolerance and autoimmunity: A role in the pathogenesis of rheumatoid arthritis. Autoimmunity 16:45–56.

Bernstein, A.L., and L.S. Lobitz. 1988. A clinical and electro-physiologic study of the treatment of painful diabetic neuropathies with pyridoxine. Pp. 415–423 in Clinical and Physiological Applications and Vitamin B-6, J.E. Leklem and R.E. Reynolds. New York: Alan R. Liss.

Bernton, E., H. Bryant, J. Holaday, and J. Dave. 1992. Prolactin and prolactin secretagogues reverse immunosuppression in mice treated with cysteamine, glucocorticoid, or cyclosporin-A. Brain Behav. Immunol. 6:394–408.

Bernton, E., R. Galloway, and D. Hoover. 1994. Immune function II: Monocyte and granulocyte function. Chapter 10 in Nutritional and Immunological Assessment of Ranger Students with Increased Caloric Intake. Technical Report T95-5. Natick, Mass.: U.S. Army Research Institute of Environmental Medicine.

Bernton, E., D. Hoover, R. Galloway, and K. Popp. 1995. Adaptation to chronic stress in military trainees. Adrenal androgens, testosterone, glucocorticoids, IGF-I, and immune function. Ann. N.Y. Acad. Sci. 774:217–231.

Bernton, E., M.S. Meltzer, and J.W. Holaday. 1988. Suppression of macrophage activation and T-lymphocyte function in hypoprolactinemic mice. Science 239:401–404.

Berry, E.M., J. Hirsch, J. Most, D.J. McNamara, and S. Cunningham-Rundles. 1987. Dietary fat, plasma lipoproteins, and immune functions in middle-aged American men. Nutr. Cancer 9:129–142.

Berry, M.J., and P.R. Larsen. 1992. The role of selenium in thyroid hormone action. Endocr. Rev. 13:207–219.

Berthoux, F.C., C. Guerin, and G. Burgard. 1992. One-year randomized controlled trial with omega-3 fatty acid-fish oil in clinical renal transplant. Transplant. Proc. 24:2578–2582.

Bertini, R., M. Bianchi, and P. Ghezzi. 1988. Adrenalectomy sensitizes mice to the lethal effects of interleukin 1 and tumor necrosis factor. J. Exp. Med. 167:1708–1712.

Besedovsky, H.O., and A. del Rey. 1992. Immune-neuroendocrine circuits: Integrative role of cytokines [Review]. Front Neuroendocrinology. 13(1) 61–94.

Besedovsky, H.O., and A. del Rey. 1996. Immune–neuroendocrine interactions: Facts and hypotheses. Endocr. Rev. 17(1):64–102.

Bessey, P.Q., J.M. Watters, T.T. Aoki, and D.W. Wilmore. 1984. Combined hormonal infusion simulates the metabolic response to injury. Ann. Surg. 200:264–281.

Bhamarapravati, N. 1989. Hemostatic defects in dengue hemorrhagic fever. Rev. Infect. Dis. 11(suppl. 4):S826–S829.

Bistrian, B.R., G.L. Blackburn, N.S. Scrimshaw, J.P. Flatt. 1975. Cellular immunity in semistarved states in hospitalized adults. Am. J. Clin. Nutr. 28:1148–1155.

Bixby, E.K., F. Levi, R. Haus, F. Halberg, and W. Hrushesky. 1982. Circadian aspects of murine nephrotoxicity of cisdiamminedichloroplatinum (II). Pp. 339–347 in Toward Chronopharmacology, R. Takahashi, ed. Oxford, New York: Pergamon Press.

Bjarnason, G.A., and W.J.M. Hrushesky. 1994. Cancer chronotherapy. Pp. 241–263 in Circadian Cancer Therapy, W.J.M. Hrushesky, ed. Boca Raton, Fla.: CRC Press.

Bjerve, K.S., S. Fischer, F. Wammer, and T. England. 1989. α-linolenic acid and long-chain omega-3 fatty acid supplementation in three patients with omega-3 fatty acid deficiency. Am. J. Clin. Nutr. 49:290–300.

Black, M.M., R.E. Zachrau, and R.H. Ashikari. 1988. Skin window reactivity to autologous breast cancer: An index of prognostically significant cell-mediated immunity. Cancer 62:72–83.

Black, P.H., L.J. Kunz, and M.N. Swartz. 1960. Salmonellosis—A review of some usual aspects. N. Engl. J. Med. 262:811–817, 921–927.

Blackfan, K.D., and S.B. Wolbach. 1933. Vitamin A deficiency in infants. A clinical and pathological study. J. Pediatr. 3:679–706.

Blake, P.A., M.H. Merson, R.E. Weaver, D.G. Hollis, and P.C. Heublein. 1979. Disease caused by a marine Vibrio: Clinical characteristics and epidemiology. N. Engl. J. Med. 300:1–5.

Blakley, B.R., and D.L. Hamilton. 1987. The effect of copper deficiency on the immune response in mice. Drug Nutr. Interact. 5:103–111.

Blalock, J.E. 1989a. A molecular basis for bidirectional communication between the immune and neuroendocrine systems. Physiol. Rev. 69:1–32.

Blalock, J.E. 1989b. A production of peptide hormones and neurotransmitters by the immune system. Pp. 1–19 in Neuroimmunoendocrinology: Chemical Immunology, 2d ed., J.E. Blalock, ed. Basel: Karger.

Blalock, J.E. 1994. The immune system: Our sixth sense. Immunologist 1994:8–15.

Blazar, B.A., M.L. Rodrick, J.B. O'Mahoney, J.J. Wood, P.Q. Bessey, D.W. Wilmore, and J.A. Mannick. 1986. Suppression of natural killer-cell function in humans following thermal and traumatic injury. J. Clin. Immunol. 6:26–36.

Blei, F., and D.R. Puder. 1993. Yersinia enterocolitica bacteremia in a chronically transfused patient with sickle-cell anemia. Case report and review of the literature. Am. J. Pediatr. Hematol. Oncol. 15:430–434.

Bliese, P., and K. Wright. 1995. Stress in Today's Army: Human Dimension Research Team Findings. Information Briefing to Secretary of the Army. May 22. Washington, D.C.

Block, G. 1992. Vitamin C status and cancer: Epidemiologic evidence of reduced risk. Ann. N.Y. Acad. Sci. 669:280–292.

Bloemena, E., M.T.L. Roos, J.L.A.M. Van Heijst, J.M.J.J. Vossen, and P.T.A. Schellekens. 1989. Whole-blood lymphocyte cultures. J. Immunol. Meth. 122:161–167.

Bloom, B.R., R.L. Modlin, and P. Salgame. 1992. Stigma variations: observations on suppressor T cells and leprosy. Annu. Rev. Immunol. 10:453–88.

Blot,W.J., J.Y. Li, P.R. Taylor, W. Guo, S. Dawsey, G.Q. Wang, C.S. Yang, S.F. Zheng, M. Gail, G.Y. Li, Y. Yu, B. Liu, J. Tangrea, Y. Sun, F. Liu, J.F. Fraumeni, Jr., Y.H. Zhang, and B. Li. 1993. Nutrition intervention trials in Linxian, China: Supplementation with specific vitamin/mineral combinations, cancer incidence, and disease specific mortality in the general population. J. Natl. Cancer Inst. 85(18):1483–1491.

Bluthe, R.M., V. Walter, P. Parnet, S. Laye, J. Lestage, D. Verrier, S. Poole, B.E. Stenning, K.W. Kelley, and R. Dantzer. 1994. Lipopolysaccharide induces sickness behavior in rats by a vagal mediated mechanism. C.R. Acad. Sci. Paris, Sciences de la via/Life sciences. 317:499–503.

Bocchieri, M.H., M.A. Talle, L.M. Maltese, I.R. Ragucci, C-C. Hwang, and G. Goldstein. 1995. Whole blood culture for measuring mitogen induced T cell proliferation provides superior correlations with disease state and T cell phenotype in asymptomatic HIV-infected subjects. J. Immunol. Meth. 181:233–243.

Boelen, A., M.C. Platvoet-Ter Schiphorst, O. Bakker, and W.M. Wiersinga. 1995. The role of cytokines in the lipopolysaccharide-induced sick euthyroid syndrome in mice. J. Endocrinol. 146:475–483.

Boelen, A., M.C. Platvoet-Ter Schiphorst, and W.M. Wiersinga. 1993. Association between serum interleukin-6 and serum 3,5,3'-triiodothyronine in nonthyroidal illness. J. Clin. Endocrinol. Metab. 77:1695–1699.

Bogden, J.D., J.M. Oleske, M.A. Lavenhar, E.M. Munves, P.W. Kemp, K.S. Bruening, K.J. Holding, T.N. Denny, M.A. Guarino, L.M. Krieger, and B.K. Holland. 1988. Zinc and immunocompetence in elderly people: Effects of zinc supplementation for 3 months. Am. J. Clin. Nutr. 48:655–663.

Booher, L.E., E.C. Callison, and E.M. Hewston. 1939. An experimental determination of the minimum vitamin A requirements of normal adults. J. Nutr. 17:317–331.

Borelli, M.I. F.E. Estivariz, and J.J. Gagliardino. 1996. Evidence for the paracrine action of islet-derived corticotrophin-like peptides on the regulation of insulin release. Metabolism. 45(5):565–570.

Bothwell, T.H. 1995. Overview and mechanisms of iron regulation. Nutr. Rev. 53:237–245.

Bourin, P., F. Levi, I. Mansour, C. Doinel, and M. Joussemet. 1990. Circadian rhythm of interleukin-1 (IL-1) in serum of healthy men. Ann. Rev. Chronopharmacol. 7:201–204.

Bourin, P., I. Mansour, F. Levi, J.M. Villette, R. Roue, J. Fiet, P. Rouger, and C. Doinel. 1989. Perturbations precoces des rhythmes circadiens des lymphocytes T et B au cours de l'immunodeficience humaine (VIH). CR Acad. Sci. (Paris) 308:431–436.

Bourne, P.G., R.M. Rose, and J.W. Mason. 1967. Urinary 17-OHCS levels. Data on seven helicopter ambulance medics in combat. Arch. Gen. Psychiatry 17:104–110.

Bower, R.H., F.B. Cerra, B. Bershadsky, J.J. Licari, D.B. Hoyt, G.L. Jensen, C.T. Van Buren, M.M. Rothkopf, J.M. Daly and B.R. Adelsberg. 1995. Early enteral administration of a formula (Impact) supplemented with arginine, nucleotides, and fish oil in intensive care unit patients: results of a multicenter, prospective, randomized, clinical trial. Crit. Care Med. 23(3):436–449.

Bøyum, A. 1977. Separation of lymphocytes, lymphocyte subgroups and monocytes: A review. Lymphology 10:71–76.

Bøyum A., P. Wiik, E. Gustavson, O.P. Veiby, J. Reseland, A.H. Haugen, and P.K. Opstad. 1996. The effect of strenuous exercise, calorie deficiency and sleep deprivation on white blood cells, plasma immunoglobulins and cytokines. Scand. J. Immunol. 43:228–235.

Brady, L.S., A.B. Lynn, M. Herkenham, and Z. Gottesfeld. 1994. Systemic interleukin-1 induces early and late patterns of c-fos mRNA expression in brain. J. Neurosci. 14:4951–4964.

Bratescu, A., and M. Teodorescu. 1981. Circannual variations in the B-cell/T-cell ratio in normal human peripheral blood. J. Allergy Clin. Immunol. 68:273–280.

Bray, R.M., L.A. Kroutil, S.C. Wheeless, M.E. Marsden, S.L. Bailey, J.A. Fairbank, and T.C. Harford. 1995. Health behavior and health promotion. Department of Defense Survey of Health-Related Behaviors among Military Personnel. Report No. RTI/6019/06-FR. Research Triangle Park, N.C.: Research Triangle Institute.

Breder, C.D., C.A. Dinarello, and C.B. Saper. 1988. Interleukin-1 immunoreactive innervation of the human hypothalamus. Science 240:321–324.

Breder, C.D., C. Hazuka, T. Ghayur, C. Klug, M. Huginin, K.Yasuda, M. Teng, and C.B. Saper. 1994. Regional induction of TNF-α expression in the mouse brain after systemic lipopolysaccharide administration. Proc. Nat. Acad. Sci. USA 91:11393–11397.

Breedveld, F. 1994. Tenidap: A novel cytokine-modulating antirheumatic drug for the treatment of rheumatoid-arthritis. Scand. J. Rheumatol. 100:31–44.

Breman, J.G., G. van der Groen, C.J. Peters, and D.L. Heymann. 1997. International colloquium on Ebola virus research: summary report. J. Infect. Dis. 176(4):1058–1063.

Brenner, I.K.M., P.N. Shek, and R.J. Shephard. 1995. Heat exposure and immune function: Potential contribution to the exercise response. Exerc. Immunol. Rev. 1:49–80.

Brenner, S., and L.J. Roberts. 1943. Effects of vitamin A depletion in young adults. Arch. Intern. Med. 71:474–482.

Brent, G.A., and J.M. Hershman. 1986. Thyroxine therapy in patients with severe nonthyroidal illnesses and low serum thyroxine concentration. J. Clin. Endocrinol. Metab. 63:1–8.

Breus, T.K., F.I. Komarov, M.M. Musin, I.V. Naborov, and S.I. Rapoport. 1989. Heliogeophysical factors and their influence on cyclical processes in biosphere. Itogi Nauki i Techniki: Medicinskaya Geografica 18:138–142.

Briggs, J.D., C.A. Kennedy, and A. Goldberg. 1963. Urinary white cell excretion after iron–sorbitol–citric acid. Br. Med. J. ii:352–354.

Britton, J.R., I.D. Pavord, K.A. Richards, A.J. Knox, A.F. Wisniewski, S.A. Lewis, A.E. Tattersfield, and S.T. Weiss. 1995. Dietary antioxidant vitamin intake and lung function in the general population. Am. J. Respir. Crit. Care Med. 151:1383–1387.

Britton, S., and G.H. Moller. 1968. Regulation of antibody synthesis against *Escherichia coli* endotoxin. I. Suppressive effects of endogenously produced and passively transferred antibodies. J. Immunol. 100:1326–1334.

Brock, J.H., and M.C. Rankin. 1981. Transferrin binding and iron uptake by mouse lymph-node cells during transformation in response to concanavalin A. Immunology 43:393–398.

Brock, M.A. 1983. Seasonal rhythmicity in lymphocyte blastogenesis persists in a constant environment. J. Immunol. 130:2586–2588.

Brock, M.A. 1987. Age-related changes in circannual rhythms of lymphocyte blastogenic response in mice. Am. J. Physiol. 252:R299–R305.

Brock, M.A. 1991. Chronobiology of aging. J. Am. Geriatr. Soc. 39:74–91.

Brostoff, J., G.K. Scadding, D. Male, and I.M. Roitt, eds. 1991. Clinical Immunology. London: Gower Medical Publishing.

Brown, K.H., A. Gaffar, and S.M. Alamgir. 1979. Xerophthalmia, protein-caloric malnutrition, and infections in children. J. Pediatr. 95:651–656.

Brown, L.S., R.Y. Phillips, C.L. Brown, D. Knowlan, L. Castle, and J. Moyer. 1994. HIV/AIDS policies and sports: The National Football League. Med. Sci. Sports Exerc. 26:403–407.

Brown, R., G. Pang, A.J. Husband, and M.C. King. 1989. A suppression of immunity to influenza virus infection in the respiratory tract following sleep deprivation. Regul. Immunol. 2:321–325.

Brubacher, G.B., and H. Weiser. 1985. The vitamin A activity of β carotene. J. Vit. Nutr. Res. 55:5–15.

Buchanan, W.M. 1971. Shock in Bantu siderosis. Am. J. Clin. Pathol. 55:401–406.

Buck, J., G. Ritter, L. Dannecker, V. Katta, S.L. Cohen, B.T. Chait, and U. Hämmerling. 1990. Retinol is essential for growth of activated human B-cells. J. Exp. Med. 171:1613–1624.

Bullen, J.J., and E. Griffiths, eds. 1987. Iron and Infection. London: John Wiley & Sons.

Bullen, J.J., C.G. Ward, and S.N. Wallis. 1978. Virulence and the role of iron in *Pseudomonas aeruginosa* infection. Infect. Immun. 10:443–450.

Burch, R.E., R.V. Williams, H.K.J. Hahn, M.M. Jetton, and J.F. Sullivan. 1975. Serum and tissue enzyme activity and trace element content in response to zinc deficiency in the pig. Clin. Chem. 21:568–577.

Burk, R.F. 1997. Selenium-dependent gluthathione peroxidases. In Comprehensive Toxicology, vol. 3, Biotransformation, F.P. Guengerich, ed. Oxford: Pergamon.

Burney, P. 1995. The origins of obstructive airways disease: A role for diet? Am. J. Respir. Crit. Care Med. 151:1292–1293.

Burrought, M., C. Cabellos, S. Prasad, and E. Tuomanen. 1992. Bacterial components and the pathophysiology of injury to the blood–brain barrier: Does cell wall add to the effects of endotoxin in gram-negative meningitis? J. Infect. Dis. 165 (suppl. 1):S82–S85.

Butler, L.D., N.K. Layman, P.E. Riedl, R.L. Cain, and J. Shellhaas. 1989. Neuroendocrine regulation of in vivo cytokine production and effects: I. In vivo regulatory networks involving the neuroendocrine system, interleukin-1 and tumor necrosis factor-α. J. Neuroimmunol. 24:143–153.

Byers, T., and N. Guerrero. 1995. Epidemiologic evidence for vitamin C and vitamin E in cancer prevention. Am. J. Clin. Nutr. 62:1385S–1392S.

Cacioppo, J.T., G.G. Berntson, W.B. Malarkey, J.K. Kiecolt-Glaser, J.F. Sheridan, K.M. Poehlmann, M.H. Burleson, J.M. Ernst, L.C. Hawkley, and R. Glaser. 1998. Autonomic, neuroendocrine, and immune responses to psychological stress: the reactivity hypothesis. Ann. NY Acad. Sci. 840:664–673.

Calabrese, L.H., and A. LaPerriere. 1993. Human immunodeficiency virus infection, exercise and athletics. Sports Med. 15:6–13.

Calder, P.C. 1997. n-3 polyunsaturated fatty acids and cytokine production in health and disease. Ann. Nutr. Metab. 41:203-34.

Calder, P.C. 1998. Dietary fatty acids and the immune system. Nutr. Rev. 56:S70–83.

Calderon, R.A., and D.B. Thomas. 1980. *In vivo* cyclic change in B-lymphocyte susceptibility to T-cell control. Nature (Lond.) 285:662–664.

Callard, R., and A.J.H. Gearing. 1994. The Cytokine Facts Book. London: Academic Press.

Callewaert, D.M., V.K. Moudgil, G. Radcliff, and R. Waite. 1991. Hormone specific regulation of natural killer cells by cortisol: Direct inactivation of the cytotoxic function of cloned human NK cells without an effect on cellular proliferation. FEBS Lett. 285:108 015–110.

Calvano, S.E., J.D. Albert, A. Legaspi, B.C. Organ, K.J. Tracey, S.F. Lowry, G.T. Shires, and A.C. Antonacci. 1987. Comparison of numerical and phenotypic leukocyte changes during constant hydrocortisone infusion in normal humans with those in thermally injured patients. Surg. Gynecol. Obstet. 164:509–520.

Camilli, A., D. Beattie, and J.J. Mekalanos. 1994. Use of genetic recombination as a reporter of gene expression. Proc. Natl. Acad. Sci. USA 91:2634–2638.

Cannon, J.G. 1993. Exercise and resistance to infection. J. Appl. Physiol. 74:973–981.

Cannon, J.G., and C.A. Dinarello. 1985. Increased plasma interleukin-1 activity in women after ovulation. Science 227:1247–1249.

Cannon, J.G., S.N. Meydani, R.A. Fielding, M.A. Fiatarone, M. Meydani, M. Farhangmehr, S.F. Orencole, J.B. Blumberg, and W.J. Evans. 1991. The acute-phase response in exercise. II. Associations between vitamin E, cytokines and muscle proteolysis. Am. J. Physiol. 260:R1235–R1240.

Cannon, J.G, J.L. Nerad, D.D. Poutsiaka, C.A. Dinarello. 1993. Measuring circulating cytokines. J. Appl. Physiol. 75(4):1897–902.

Cannon, J.G., S.F. Orencole, R.A. Fielding, M. Meydani, S.N. Meydani, M.A. Fiatarone, J.B. Blumberg, and W.J. Evans. 1990. Acute phase response in exercise: Interaction of age and vitamin E on neutrophils and muscle enzyme release. Am. J. Physiol. 259:R1214–R1219.

Canon, C., F. Levi, Y. Touitou, J. Sulon, E. Demey-Ponsart, A. Reinberg, and G. Mathe. 1986. Variations circadienne et saisonniere du rapport inducteur: Suppresseur (OKT4 + OKT8+) dans la sang veineux de l'homme adulte sain. C.R. Acad. Sci. III 302:519–524.

Cantinieaux, B., C. Hariga, A. Ferster, E. de Maerterlaerre, M. Toppet, and P. Fondu. 1987. Neutrophil dysfunctions in thalassemia major: The role of iron overload. Eur. J. Haematol. 389:28–34.

Cantorna, M.T., F.E. Nashold, T.Y. Chun, and C.E. Hayes. 1996. Vitamin A downregulation of IGN-γ synthesis in cloned mouse Th1 lymphocytes depends upon the CD28 costimulatory pathway. J. Immunol. 156:2674–2679.

Carandente, F., and F. Halberg. 1976. Chronobiologic view of shift-work and ulcers. Pp. 273–283 in NIOSH Research Symposium, Shift-Work and Health, Cincinnati, P.G. Rentos and R.D. Shepard, eds. Cincinnati: National Institute for Occupational Safety and Health.

Caravalho, J., Jr. 1992. Knee protection during Ranger school. Mil. Med. 157:A3.

Carniel, E., D. Mazigh, and H.H. Mollaret. 1987. Expression of iron-regulated proteins in *Yersinia* species and their relation to virulence. Infect. Immun. 55:277–280.

Carniel, E., O. Mercereau-Puijalon, and S. Bonnefoy. 1989. The gene coding for the 190,000-dalton iron-regulated protein of *Yersinia* species is present only in the highly pathogenic strains. Infect. Immun. 57:1211–1217.

Carr, A., D.A. Cooper, and R. Penny. 1991. Allergic manifestations of human immunodeficiency (HIV) infection. J. Clin. Immunol. 11:55–64.

Carr, D.J.J. 1991. The role of endogenous opioids and their receptors in the immune system. Soc. Exp. Biol. Med. 198:710–720.

Carr, D.J.J. 1992. Neuroendocrine peptide receptors on cells of the immune system. Pp. 49–83 in Neuroimmunoendocrinology: Chemical Immunology, 2d ed., J.E. Blalock, ed. Basel: Karger.

Casciari, J.J., H. Sato, S.K. Durum, J. Fiege, and J.N. Weinstein. 1996. Reference databases of cytokine structure and function. Cancer Chemother. Biol. Response Modif. 16:315–346.

Castell, L.M., J.R. Poortmans, and E.A. Newsholme. 1996. Does glutamine have a role in reducing infections in athletes? Eur. J. Appl. Physiol. 73:488–490.

Caughey, G.E., E. Montzioris, R.A. Gibson, L.G. Cleland, and M.J. James. 1996. The effect on human tumor necrosis factor α and interleukin-1β production of diets enriched in n-3 fatty acids from vegetable oil or from fish oil. Am. J. Clin. Nutr. 63:116–122.

CDC (Centers for Disease Control and Prevention). 1998. Recommendations to Prevent and Control Iron Deficiency in the United States. MMWR 47(RR-3):1–36.

Celada, A., V. Herreros, P. Pugin, and M. Rudolf. 1979. Reduced leukocyte alkaline phosphatase activity and decreased NBT reduction test in induced iron deficiency. Br. J. Haematol. 43:457–463.

Chandra, R.K. 1972. Immunocompetence in undernutrition. J. Pediatr. 81:1194–1200.

Chandra, R.K. 1973. Reduced bactericidal capacity of polymorphs in iron deficiency. Arch. Dis. Child. 48:864–866.

Chandra, R.K. 1975. Impaired immunocompetence associated with iron deficiency. J. Pediatr. 86:899–902.

Chandra, R.K. 1982. Excessive intake of zinc impairs immune response. J. Am. Med. Assoc. 252:1443–1446.

Chandra, R.K. 1984. Excessive intake of zinc impairs immune responses. J. Am. Med. Assoc. 252:1443–1446.

Chandra, R.K., ed. 1988. Nutrition and Immunology. New York: Alan R. Liss, Inc.

Chandra, R.K. 1991. 1990 McCollum award lecture. Nutrition and immunity: Lessons from the past and new insights into the future. Am. J. Clin. Nutr. 53:1087–1101.

Chandra, R.K. 1992a. Effect of vitamin and trace-element supplementation on immune responses and infection in elderly subjects. Lancet 340:1124–1127.

Chandra, R.K. 1992b. Experience of an old traveller and recent observations. Pp. 9–43 in The First INIG Award Lecture: Nutrition and Immunology. St. John's, Newfoundland: ARTS Biomedical Publishers and Distributors.

Chandra, R.K. 1993. Nutrition and the immune system. Proc. Nutr. Soc. (England) 52(1):77–84.

Chandra, R.K. 1996. Nutrition, immunity and infection: From basic knowledge of dietary manipulation of immune responses to practical application of ameliorating suffering and improving survival. Proc. Natl. Acad. Sci. USA 93:14304–14307.

Chandra, S., and R.K. Chandra. 1986. Nutrition, immune response, and outcome. Prog. Food Nutr. Sci. 10:1–7.

Chandra, R.K., and S. Kumari. 1994. Nutrition and immunity: an overview. J. Nutr. 124(8 Suppl):1433S–1435S.

Chandra, R.K., and P.M. Newberne. 1977. Nutrition, Immunity, and Infection: Mechanisms of Interactions. New York: Plenum.

Chandra, R.K., and A.K. Saraya. 1975. Impaired immuno-competence associated with iron deficiency. J. Pediatr. 86:899–901.

Chandra, R.K., M. Baker, S. Whang, and B. Au. 1991. Effect of two feeding formulas on immune responses and mortality in mice challenged with Listeria monocytogenes. Immunol. Lett. 27:45–48.

Chandra, R.K., S. Whang, and B. Au. 1992. Enriched feeding formula and immune responses and outcome after Listeria monocytogenes challenge in mice. Nutrition 8:426–429.

Chang, S.L., T. Ren, and J.E. Zadina. 1993. Interleukin-1 activation of fos proto-oncogene protein in the rat hypothalamus. Brain Res. 617:123–130.

Chart, H., and E. Griffiths. 1985. The availability of iron and the growth of Vibrio vulnificus in sera from patients with haemochromatosis. FEMS Microbiol. Lett. 26:227–231.

Chart, H., P. Stevenson, and E. Griffiths. 1988. Iron-regulated outer-membrane proteins of Escherichia coli strains associated with enteric or extraintestinal diseases of man and animals. J. Gen. Microbiol. 134:1549–1559.

Chaudiere, J., E.C. Wilhelmsen, and A.L. Tappel. 1984. Mechanism of selenium-glutathione peroxidase and its inhibition by mercaptocarboxylic acids and other mercaptans. J. Biol. Chem. 259:1043–1050.

Chikanza, I.C., P. Petrou, G. Kingsley, G. Chrousos, and G.S. Panayi. 1992. Defective hypothalamic response to immune and inflammatory stimuli in patients with rheumatoid arthritis. Arthritis Rheum. 35:1281–1288.

Chow, L.H., K.W. Beisel, and B.M. McManus. 1992. Enteroviral infection of mice with severe combined immunodeficieny. Evidence for direct viral pathogenesis of myocardial injury. Lab. Invest. 66:24–31.

Chowdhury, B.A., and R.K. Chandra. 1987. Biological and health implications of toxic heavy metal and essential trace element interactions. Prog. Food Nutr. Sci. 11:55–113.

Christadoss, P., N. Talal, J. Lindstrom, and G. Fernandes. 1984. Suppression of cellular and humoral immunity to T-dependent antigens by calorie restriction. Cell Immunol. 88:1–8.

Christian, P., K.P. West Jr., S.K. Khatry, J. Katz, R.J. Stoltzfus, and R.P. Pokhrel. 1996. Epidemiology of night blindness during pregnancy in rural Nepal. P. 8 in Abstracts of the XVII International Vitamin A Consultative Group Meeting, Guatemala City, Guatemala, March.

Chrousos, G.P. 1995. The hypothalamic–pituitary–adrenal axis and immune-mediated inflammation. New Engl. J. Med. 332:1351–1362.

Cioffi, W.G., D.C. Gore, L.W. Rue III, G. Carrougher, H.P. Guler, W.F. McManus, and B.A. Pruitt Jr. 1994. Insulin-like growth factor-1 lowers protein oxidation in patients with thermal injury. Ann. Surg. 220:310–316.

Clark, R., J. Strasser, S. McCabe, K. Robbins, and P. Jardieu. 1993. Insulin-like growth factor-1 stimulation of lymphopoiesis. J. Clin. Invest. 92:540–548.

Clarke, B.L., and K.L. Bost. 1989. Differential expression of functional adrenocorticotropic hormone receptors by subpopulations of lymphocytes. J. Immunol. 143:464–469.

Clevenger, C.V., D.H. Russell, P.M. Appasamy, and M.B. Prystowsky. 1990. Regulation of interleukin-2 driven T-lymphocyte proliferation by prolactin. Proc. Natl. Acad. Sci. USA 87:6460–6464.

Coceani, F., J. Lees, and C.A. Dinarello. 1988. Occurrence of interleukin-1 in cerebrospinal fluid of the conscious cat. Brain Res. 446:245–250.

Cohen, J.J. 1994. Cells involved in host defense: The new immunology. J. Nutr. Immunol. 2(4):73–86.

Cohen, S., D.A. Tyrrell, and A.P. Smith. 1991. Psychological stress and susceptibility to the common cold. N. Engl. J. Med. 325:606–612.

Coligan, J.E., A.M. Kruisbeek, D.H. Margulies, E.M. Shevach, and W. Strober, eds. 1994. Current Protocols in Immunology. New York: John Wiley & Sons.

Consolazio C.F., H.L. Johnson, R.A. Nelson, R. Dowdy, H.J. Krzywicki, T.A. Daws, L.K. Lowry, P.P. Warling, W.K. Calhoun, B.W. Schwenneker, and J.E. Canham. 1979. The relationship of diet to the performance of the combat soldier. Minimal calorie intake during combat patrols in a hot humid environment (Panama). Technical Report No. 76. Presidio of San Francisco, Calif.: Letterman Army Institute of Research.

Consolazio, C.F., L.O. Matoush, R.A. Nelson, R.S. Harding, and J.E. Canham. 1966. Nutritional survey: Ranger Department, Fort Benning, Georgia. Laboratory Report No. 291. Denver, Colo.: U.S. Army Medical Research and Nutrition Laboratory, Fitzimons General Hospital.

Cooper, A.L., L. Gibbons, M.A., Horan, R.A. Little, and N.J. Rothwell. 1993. Effect of dietary fish oil supplementation on fever and cytokine production in human volunteers. Clin. Nutr. 12:321–328.

Cornélissen, G., T.K. Breus, C. Bingham, R. Zaslavskaya, M. Varshitsky, B. Mirsky, M. Teibloom, B. Tarquini, E. Bakken, and F. Halberg. 1993. Beyond circadian chronorisk: Worldwide circaseptan-circasemiseptan patterns of myocardial infarctions, other vascular events, and emergencies. Chronobiologia 20:87–115.

Cove-Smith, J.R., P. Kabler, R. Pownall, and M.S. Knapp. 1978. Circadian variation in an immune response in man. Br. Med. J. 2(6132):253–254.

Covelli, V., F. Massari, C. Fallarca, I. Munno, F. Jirrilo, S. Savastano, A. Tommaselli, and G. Lombardi. 1992. Interleukin-1β and β-endorphin circadian rhythms are inversely related in normal and stress-altered sleep. Int. J. Neurosci. 63:299–305.

Cricchio, I., G. Arcara, G. Abbate, and M.F. Cannonito. 1978. Aspetti cronobiologia delle immunoglobuline sieriche. Folia Allergol. Immunol. Clin. 24:470.

Cricchio, I., G. Aracara, G. Abbate, T. Ferrar, R. Tarantino, and S. Romano. 1979. Circadian rhythms of serum immunoglobulins in patients affected with allergic rhinitis, atopic asthma and chronic urticaria. Pp. 55–63 in Recent Advances in the

Chronobiology of Allergy and Immunology, M.H. Smolensky, A. Reinberg, and J.P. McGovern, eds. Oxford: Pergamon Press.

Crofford, L.J., S.R. Pillemer, K.T. Kalogeras, J.M. Cash, D. Michelson, M.A. Kling, E.M. Sternberg, P.W. Gold, G.P. Chrousos, and R.L. Wilder. 1994. Hypothalamic-pituitary–adrenal axis perturbations in patients with fibromyalgia. Arthritis Rheum. 37:1583–1592.

Crofford, L.J., J.I. Rader, M.C. Dalakas, R.H. Hill Jr., S.W. Page, L.L. Needham, L.S. Brady, M.P. Heyes, R.L. Wilder, P.W. Gold, et al. 1990. L-tryptophan implicated in human eosinophilia-myalgia syndrome causes fascitis and perimyositis in the Lewis rat. J. Clin. Invest. 86:1757–1763.

Croteau, W., S.L. Whittemore, M.J. Schneider, and D.L. St. Germain. 1995. Cloning and expression of a cDNA for a mammalian type III iodothyronine deiodinase. J. Biol. Chem. 270:16569–16575.

Cunningham, E.T., and E. DeSouza. 1994. Interleukin 1 receptors in the brain and endocrine tissues. Immunol. Today 14:161–176.

Cunningham-Rundles, S., ed. 1993. Nutritional Modulation of the Immune Response. New York: Marcel Decker, Inc.

Cunningham-Rundles, S. 1994. Malnutrition and gut immune function. Curr. Opin. Gastroenterol. 10:664–670.

Cunningham-Rundles, S., and J.S. Cervia. 1996. "Malnutrition and host defense" in nutrition. Pp. 295–307 in Pediatrics: Basic Science and Clinical Application, 2d ed., W.A. Walker and J.B. Watkins, eds. Basel: Marcel Dekker.

Cunningham-Rundles, S., R.S. Bockman, A. Lin, P.V. Giardina, M.W. Hilgartner, D. Caldwell-Brown, and D.M. Carter. 1990a. Physiological and pharmacological effects of zinc on immune response. Ann. N.Y. Acad. Sci. 587:113–122.

Cunningham-Rundles, S., C. Chen, J.B. Bussel, C. Blankenship, M.B. Veber, D. Sanders-Laufer, T. Hinds, J.S. Cervia, and P. Edelson. 1993. Human immune development: Implications for congenital HIV infections. Ann. N.Y. Acad. Sci. 693:20–34.

Cunningham-Rundles, S., R.R. Yeger-Arbitman, R. Nachman, S.A. Kaul, and M. Fotino. 1990b. New variant of MHC class II deficiency with interleukin-2 abnormality. Clin. Immunol. Immunopathol. 56:116–123.

Cupps, T.R., and A.S. Fauci. 1982. Corticosteroid-mediated immunoregulation in man. Immunol. Rev. 65:133–155.

Da Silva, J.A., and G.M. Hall. 1992. The effect of gender and sex hormones on outcome in rheumatoid arthritis. Clin. Rheumatol. 6:196–219.

Daly, A.L., L.A. Velazquez, S.F. Bradley, and C.A. Kauffman. 1989. Mucormycosis: Association with deferoxamine therapy. Am. J. Med. 87:468–471.

Damle, N.K., and S. Gupta. 1982. Autologous mixed lymphocyte reaction in man. III. Regulation of autologous MLR by theophylline-resistant and sensitive human T-lymphocyte subpopulations. Scand. J. Immunol. 15:493–499.

Damsdaran, M., A.N. Naidu, and K.V.R. Sarma. 1979. Anemia and morbidity in rural preschool children. Indian J. Med. Res. 69:448–456.

Daniel, L., G. Souweine, J.C. Monier, and S. Saez. 1983. Specific estrogen binding sites in human lymphoid cells and thymic cells. Esteroid Biochem. 18:559–563.

Daniels, W.L., D.S. Sharp, J.E. Wright, J.A. Vogel, G. Friman, W.R. Beisel, and J.J. Knapik. 1985. Effects of virus infection on physical performance in man. Milit. Med. 150:8–14.

Dantzer, R., R.M. Bluthe, J.L. Bret-Dibat, S. Laye, R. Parnet, J. Lestage, D. Verrier, S. Poole, B. E. Stenning, and K.W. Kelley. 1994. The neuroimmune basis of sickness behavior [abstract]. P. 41 in Proceedings of the 25th Congress of the International Society for Psychoneuroendocrinology.

Davies, K.J., and A.L. Goldberg. 1987. Proteins damaged by oxygen radicals are rapidly degraded in extracts of red blood cells. J. Biol. Chem. 262:8227–8231.

Davies, K.J.A., L. Packer, and G.A. Brooks. 1982. Free radicals and tissue damage produced by exercise. Biochem. Biophys. Res. Commun. 107:1198–1205.

Davis, G.K., and W. Mertz. 1987. Copper. Pp. 301–364 in Trace Elements in Human and Animal Nutrition, W. Mertz, ed. San Diego: Academic Press.

Davis, J.M., J.D. Albert, K.J. Tracy, S.E. Calvano, S.F. Lowry, G.T. Shires, and R.W. Yurt. 1991. Increased neutrophil mobilization and decreased chemotaxis during cortisol and epinephrine infusions. J. Trauma 31:725–731.

Davis, M.A., W.T. Johnson, M. Briske-Anderson, and T.R. Kramer. 1987. Lymphoid cell functions during copper deficiency. Nutr. Res. 7:211–222.

Daynes, R.A., and B.A. Araneo. 1992. Prevention and reversal of some age-associated changes in immunologic responses by supplemental dehydroepiandrosterone sulfate therapy. Aging Immunol. Infect. Dis. 3:135–154.

Daynes, R.A., B.A. Araneo, J. Hennebold, E. Enioutina, and H.M. Hong. 1995. Steroids as regulators of the mammalian immune response. J. Invest. Dermatol. 105:14S–19S.

De Groote, D., P.F. Zangerle, Y. Gevaert, M.F. Fassotte, Y. Beguin, F. Noizat-Pirenne, J. Pirenne, R. Gathy, M. Lopez, I. Dehart, D. Igot, M. Baudrihaye, D. Delacroix, and P. Franchimont. 1992. Direct stimulation of cytokines (IL-1J, TNF-I, IL-6, IL-2, IFN-K and GM-CSF) in whole blood. I. Comparison with isolated PBMC stimulation. Cytokine 4:239–248.

de Pee, S., C.E. West, Muhilal, D. Karyadi, and J.G. Hautvast. 1995. Lack of improvement in vitamin A status with increased consumption of dark-green leafy vegetables. Lancet 346:75–81.

Dealler, S., and R.W. Lacey. 1990. Beef and bovine spongiform encephalopathy: the risk persists. Nutr. Health. 7(3)117–133.

DeForge, L.E., and D.G. Remick. 1991. Kinetics of TNF, IL-6, and IL-8 gene expression in LPS-stimulated human whole blood. Biochem. Biophys. Res. Commun. 174:18–24.

Deitch, E.A. 1990. Intestinal permeability is increased in burn patients shortly after injury. Surgery 107:411–416.

Deitch, E.A., J. Wintertron, M.A. Li, and R. Berg. 1989. The gut is a portal of entry for bacteremia. Ann. Surg. 205:681–690.

Del Prete, G., E. Maggi, and S. Romagnani. 1994. Human Th1 and Th2 cells: Functional properties, mechanisms of regulation and role in disease. Lab. Invest. 70:299–307.

DeLeonardis, V., and M.L. Brandi. 1984. Total IgE serum levels: A chronobiologic approach. Pp. 395–398 in Chronobiology 1982–1983, E. Haus and H.F. Kabat, eds. Basel: Karger.

Demitrack, M.A. 1994. Chronic fatigue syndrome a disease of the hypothalamic–pituitary–adrenal axis? Ann. Med. 26:1–5.

Denham, S., and I.J. Rowland. 1992. Inhibition of the reactive proliferation of lymphocytes by activated macrophages: The role of nitric oxide. Clin. Exp. Immunol. 87:157–162.

Depres-Brummer, P., F. Levi, M. Palma, A. Beliard, P. Lebon, S. Marion, C. Jasmin, and J. Misset. 1991. A phase I trial of 21-day continuous venous infusion of α-interferon at circadian rhythm modulated rate in cancer patients. J. Immunother. 10:440–447.

DeRijk, R., D. Michelson, B. Karp, J. Petrides, E. Galliven, P. Deuster, G. Paciotti, P.W. Gold, and E.M. Sternberg. 1997. Exercise and circadian rhythm-induced variations in plasma cortisol differentially regulate interleukin-1 β (IL-1 β), Il-6, and tumor necrosis factor-α (TNF α) production in humans: High sensitivity of TNF α and resistance of IL-6. J. Clin. Endocrinol. Metab. 82(7):2182–2191.

DeRijk, R.H., J. Petrides, P. Deuster, P.W. Gold, and E.M. Sternberg. 1996. Changes in corticosteroid sensitivity of peripheral blood lymphocytes after strenuous exercise in humans. J. Clin. Endocrinol. Metab. 81(1):228–235.

DeRijk, R., N. Van Rooijen, F.J.H. Tilders, H.O. Besedovsky, A. Del Rey, and F. Berkenbosch. 1991. Selective depletion of macrophages prevents pituitary–adrenal activation in response to subpyrogenic, but not to pyrogenic, doses of bacterial endotoxin in rats. Endocrinology 129:330–338.

DeSarro, G.B., Y. Masuda, C. Ascioti, M.G. Audino, and G. Nistico. 1990. Behavioral and ECoG spectrum changes induced by intracerebral infusion of interferons and interleukin-2 in rats are antagonized by naloxone. Neuropharmacology 29:167–179.

Desch, C.E., N.L. Kovach, W. Present, C. Broyles, and J.M. Harlan. 1989. Production of human tumor necrosis factor from whole blood ex vivo. Lymphokine Res. 8:141–146.

DeSouza, E.B. 1993. Corticotropin-releasing factor and interleukin-1 receptors in the brain-endocrine–immune axis. Ann. N.Y. Acad. Sci. 697:9–27.

Dethlefsen, U., and R. Repges. 1985. Ein neues Therapieprinzip bei nachtlichem Asthma. Med. Klin. 80:40–47.

DeVecchi, A., F. Halberg, R.B. Sothern, A. Cantaluppi, and C. Ponticelli. 1981. Circaseptan rhythmic aspects of rejection in treated patients with kidney transplant. Pp. 339–353 in Chronopharmacology and Chemotherapeutics, C.A. Walker, C.M. Winget, K.F.A. Soliman, eds.Tallahasse, FL: Aand M University Foundation.

DeVries, K., J.T. Goei, H. Booy-Noord, and N.G.M. Orie. 1962. Changes during 24 hours in the lung function and histamine hyperreactivity of the bronchial tree in asthmatic and bronchitic patients. Int. Arch. Allerg. 20:93–101.

Dhabhar, F.S., A.H. Miller, B.S. McEwen, and R.L. Spencer. 1995. Effects of stress on immune cell distribution. Dynamics and hormonal mechanisms. J. Immunol. 154:5511–5527.

Dhur, A., P. Galan, and S. Hercberg. 1989. Iron status, immune capacity, and resistance to infections. Comp. Biochem. Physiol. 94A:11–19.

Dhur, A., P. Galan, and S. Hercberg. 1990. Relationship between selenium, immunity, and resistance against infection. Comp. Biochem. Physiol. 96C:271–280.

Dillard, C.J., R.E. Litov, W.M. Savin, E.E. Dumelin, and A.L. Tappel. 1978. Effects of exercise, vitamin E, and ozone on pulmonary function and lipid peroxidation. J. Appl. Physiol. 45:927–932.

Dinarello, C.A. 1992. The biology of interleukin-1. Mol. Biol. Immunol. 51:1–32.

Dinarello, C.A. 1994. The biological properties of interleukin-1. Euro. Cytokine Netw. 5:517–531.

Dinarello, C.A., and S.M. Wolff. 1993. The role of interleukin-1 in disease. N. Engl. J. Med. 328:106–113.

Dinarello, C.A., T. Ikejima, S.J.C. Warner, S.F. Orencole, and G. Lonnemann. 1987. Interleukin-1 induces interleukin-1. I. Induction of circulating interleukin-1 in rabbits in vivo and in human mononuclear cells in vitro. J. Immunol. 139:1902–1910.

Dinges, D.F., S.D. Douglas, S. Hamarman, L. Zaugg, and S. Kapoor. 1995. Sleep deprivation and human immune function. Adv. Neuroimmunol. 5:97–110.

Dinges, D.F., S.D. Douglas, L. Zaugg, D.E. Campbell, J.M. McMann, W.G. Whitehouse, E.C. Orne, S.C. Kapoor, E. Icaza, and M.T. Orne. 1994. Leukocytosis and natural killer cell function parallel neurobehavioral fatigue induced by 64 hours of sleep deprivation. J. Clin. Invest. 93:1930–1939.

Dishman, R.K., J.M. Warren, S.D. Youngstedt, H. Yoo, B.N. Bunnell, E.H. Mougey, J.L. Meyerhoff, L. Jaso-Friedmann, and D.L. Evans. 1995. Activity-wheel running attenuates suppression of natural killer cell activity after footshock. J. Appl. Physiol. 78:1547–1554.

Dixon-Northern, A.L., S.M. Rutter, and C.M. Peterson. 1994. Cyclic changes in the concentration of peripheral blood immune cells during the normal menstrual cycle. Proc. Soc. Exp. Biol. Med. 207:81–88.

DoD (Department of Defense). 1983. DoD Coordination on Food, Agriculture, Forestry, Nutrition, and Other Designated Research with the U.S. Department of Agriculture. Directive 3210.4. July 5, 1983. Washington, D.C.

Dong, Q., F. Hawker, D. McWilliam, M. Bangah, H. Bureger, and D.J. Handelsman. 1992. Circulating immunoreactive inhibin and testosterone levels in men with critical illness. Clin. Endocrinol. 36:399–404.

Donnerer, J., R. Amann, G. Skofitsch, and F. Lembeck. 1992. Substance P afferents regulate ACTH-corticosterone release. Ann. N.Y. Acad. Sci. 632:296–303.

Dresser, D.W. 1968. Adjuvanticity of vitamin A. Nature 217:527–529.

Dreyfuss, D., F. Leviel, M. Paillard, J. Rahmani, and I. Coste. 1988. Acute infectious pneumonia is accompanied by a latent vasopressin-dependent impairment of renal water excretion. Am. Rev. Resp. Dis. 138:583–585.

Driessen, C., K. Hirv, H. Kirchner, and L. Rink. 1995. Zinc regulates cytokine induction by superantigens and lipopolysaccharide. Immunology 84:272–277.

Duitsman, P.K., L.R. Cook, S.A. Tanumihardjo, and J.A. Olson. 1995. Vitamin A inadequacy in socioeconomically disadvantaged pregnant Iowan women as assessed by the modified relative dose response (MRDR) test. Nutr. Res. 15:1263–1276.

Dulchavsky, S.A., S.M. Ksenzenko, A.A. Saba, and L.N. Diebel. 1995. Triiodothyronine (T3) supplementation maintains surfactant biochemical integrity during sepsis. J. Trauma 39:53–57.

Dunn, A.J. 1992. The role of interleukin-1 and tumor necrosis factor-α in the neurochemical and neuroendocrine responses to endotoxin. Brain Res. Bull. 29:807–812.

Dunn, A.J., and H.E. Chuluyan. 1992. The role of cyclo-oxygenase and lipoxygenase in the interleukin-1-induced activation of HPA axis. Life Sci. 51:219–225.

Dwyer, J., C. Wood, J. McNamara, A. Williams, W. Andiman, L. Rink, T. O'Connor, and H. Pearson. 1987. Abnormalities in the immune system of children with β-thalassemia. Clin. Exp. Immunol. 63:621–629.

Eagle, H., V.L. Oyama, M. Levy, C.L. Horton, and R. Fleischman. 1956. The growth response of mammalian cells in tissue culture to L-glutamine and L-glutamic acid. J. Biol. Chem. 218:607–616.

Ebisui, O., J. Fukata, N. Murakami, H. Kobayashi, H. Segawa, S. Muro, I. Hanaoka, Y. Naito, Y. Masui, Y. Ohmmoto, H. Imura, and K. Nakao. 1994. Effects of IL-1 receptor antagonist and antiserum to TNF-α on LPS-induced plasma ACTH and corticosterone rise in rats. Am. J. Physiol. 29:E986–E992.

Edmunds, L.N.J. 1994. Cellular and molecular aspects of circadian oscillators: Models and mechanisms for biological timekeeping Pp. 35–54 in Biologic Rhythms in Clinical and Laboratory Medicine, 2d ed., Y. Touitou and E. Haus, eds. Heidelberg: Springer-Verlag.

Ehrenfried, J.A., J. Chen, J. Li, and B.M. Evers. 1995. Glutamine-mediated regulation of heat shock protein expression in intestinal cells. Surgery 118:352–357.

Eichler, F., and R. Keiling. 1988. Variations in the percentages of lymphocyte subtypes during the menstrual cycle in women. Biomed. Pharmacother. 42:285–288.

Elenkov, I.J., K. Kovacs, J. Kiss, L. Bertok, and E. S. Vizi. 1992. Lipopolysaccharide is able to bypass corticotrophin-releasing factor in affecting plasma ACTH and corticosterone levels: Evidence from rats with lesions of the paraventricular nucleus. J. Endocrinol. 133:231–236.

Ellaurie, M., S.L. Yost, and D.L. Rosenstreich. 1991. A simplified human whole blood assay for measurement of dust mite-specific gamma interferon production in vitro. Ann. Allergy 66:143–147.

Elliott, S.J., and W.P. Schilling. 1992. Oxidant stress alters Na^+ pump and $Na^+K^+Cl^-$ cotransporter activities in vascular endothelial cells. Am. J. Physiol. 263:H96–H102.

Elsässer-Beile, U., S. von Kleist, A. Lindenthal, R. Birken, H. Gallati, and J.S. Mönting. 1993. Cytokine production in whole blood cell cultures of patients undergoing therapy with biological response modifiers or 5-fluorouracil. Cancer Immunol. Immunother. 37:169–174.

Elsayed, N.M., Y.Y. Tyurina, V.A. Tyurin, E.V. Menshikova, E.R. Kisin, and V.E. Kagan. 1996. Antioxidant depletion, lipid peroxidation, and impairment of calcium transport induced by air-blast overpressure in rat lungs. Exp. Lung Res. 22:179–200.

Endres, S., R. Ghorbani, V.E. Kelley, K. Georgilis, G. Lonnemann, J.W.M. van der Meer, J.G. Cannon, T.S. Rogers, M.S. Klempner, P.C. Weber, E.J. Schaefer, S.M. Wolff, and C.A. Dinarello. 1989. The effect of dietary supplementation with n-3 polyunsaturated fatty acids on the synthesis of interleukin-1 and tumor necrosis factor by mononuclear cells. N. Engl. J. Med. 320:265–271.

Endres, S., S.N. Meydani, R. Ghorbani, R. Schindler, and C.A. Dinarello. 1993. Dietary supplementation with n-3 fatty acids suppresses interleukin-2 production and mononuclear cell proliferation. J. Leukocyte Biol. 54:599–603.

Ericsson, A., K.J. Kovacs, and P.E. Sawchenko. 1994. A functional anatomical analysis of central pathways subserving the effects of interleukin-1 on stress-related neuroendocrine neurons. J. Neurosci. 14:897–913.

Erickson, K.L., N.E. Hubbard, and S.D. Sommers. 1992. Dietary fat and immune function. Pp. 81–104 in Nutrition and Immunology, R.K. Chandra, ed. St. John's, Newfoundland: ARTS Biomedical Publishers.

Eskola J., O. Ruuskanen, E. Soppi, M.K. Viljanen, M. Järvinen, H. Toivonen, and K. Kouvalainen. 1978. Effect of sport stress on lymphocyte transformation and antibody formation. Clin. Exp. Immunol. 32:339–345.

Evans, G.W., C.I. Grace, and C. Han. 1974. The effect of copper and cadmium on ^{65}Zn absorption in zinc-deficient and zinc-supplemented rats. Bioinorg. Chem. 3:115–120.

Evans. M.J., C.J. Kovacs, J.M. Gooya, and J.P. Harrell. 1991. Interleukin-1α protects against the toxicity associated with combined radiation and drug therapy. Int. J. Radiat. Oncol. Biol. Phys. 20:303–306.

Everson, C.A. 1993. Sustained sleep deprivation impairs host defense. Am. J. Physiol. 265:R1148–R1154.

Ewald, J.H., J. Heesemann, H. Rudiger, and I.B. Autenrieth. 1994. Interaction of polymorphonuclear leukocytes with Yersinia enterocolitica: Role of the Yersinia virulence plasmid and modulation by the iron-chelator desferrioxamine. Br. J. Infect. Dis. 170:140–150.

Fabris, N., E. Mocchegiani, and M. Provinciali. 1995. Pituitary-thyroid axis and immune system: A reciprocal neuroendocrine-immune interaction. Horm. Res. 43:29–38.

Failla, M., and S. Bala. 1992. Cellular and biochemical functions of copper in immunity. Pp. 129–142 in Nutrition and Immunology, R.K. Chandra, ed. St. John's, Newfoundland: ARTS Biomedical Publishers.

Failla, M.L., U. Babu, and K.E. Seidel. 1988. Use of immunoresponsiveness to demonstrate that the dietary requirement for copper in young rats is greater with dietary fructose than dietary starch. J. Nutr. 118:487–496.

Fairbrother, B., E.W. Askew, M.Z. Mays, R. Shippee, K.E. Friedl, R.W. Hoyt, M. Kramer, T.R. Kramer, and K. Popp. 1993. Nutritional assessment of soldiers during the special forces assessment and selection course. Study Protocol, May 1993. Natick, Mass.: U.S. Army Research Institute of Environmental Medicine.

Faist, E., C. Shinkel, and S. Zimmer. 1996. Update on the mechanisms of immune suppression of injury and immune modulation. World J. Surg. 20:454–459.

Fakir, M., C. Saison, T. Wong, B. Matta, and J.M. Hardin. 1992. Septicemia due to *Yersinia enterocolitica* in a hemodialyzed, iron-depleted patient receiving omeprazole and oral iron supplementation. Am. J. Kidney Dis. 19:282–284.

Fan, J., X. Gong, J. Wu, Y. Zhang, and R. Xu. 1994. Effect of glucocorticoid receptor (GR) blockade on endotoxemia in rats. Circul. Shock 42:76–82.

Fan, W.F., S.R. Yu, and T.M. Cosgriff. 1989. The reemergence of dengue in China. Rev. Infect. Dis. 11(suppl. 4):S847–S853.

Farber, J.M., and R.L. Levine. 1982. Oxidative modification of the glutamine synthetase of *E. coli* enhances its susceptibility to proteolysis [abstract 3482]. Fed. Proc. 41:865.

Farmer, K., and D.M.O. Becroft. 1976. Administration of parenteral iron to newborn infants [letter]. Arch. Dis. Child. 51:486.

Farrell, P.M., and J.G. Bieri. 1975. Megavitamin E supplementation in man. Am. J. Clin. Nutr. 28:1381–1386.

Feigin, R.D., R.F. Jaeger, R.W. McKinney, and A.C. Alevizatos. 1967a. Live, attenuated Venezuelan equine encephalomyelitis virus vaccine. II. Whole-blood amino-acid and fluorescent-antibody studies following immunization. Am. J. Trop. Med. Hyg. 16:769–777.

Feigin, R.D., A.S. Klainer, and W.R. Beisel. 1967b. Circadian periodicity of whole-blood amino acids in adult men. Nature 215:512–514.

Fernandes, G. 1994. Chronobiology of immune functions: Cellular and humoral aspects. Pp. 493–503 in Biologic Rhythms in Clinical and Laboratory Medicine, Y. Touitou and E. Haus, eds. Berlin: Springer-Verlag.

Fernandes, G., F. Halberg, and R.A. Good. 1980. Circadian dependent chronoimmunological responses of T-, B-, and natural killer cells. Allergology 3:164–170.

Fernandes, G., F. Halberg, E. Yunis, and R.A. Good. 1976. Circadian rhythmic plaque-forming cell response of spleens from mice immunized by SRBC. J. Immunol. 117:962–966.

Fernandes, G., M. Nair, K. Onoe, T. Tanaka, R. Gloyd, and R.A. Good. 1979. Impairment of cell-mediated functions by dietary zinc deficiency in mice. Proc. Natl. Acad. Sci. USA 76:457–461.

Fernandes, G., J.T. Venkatraman, and N. Mohan. 1992. Effect of omega-3 lipids in delaying the growth of human breast cancer cells in nude mice. Pp. 283–296 in Nutrition and Immunology, R.K. Chandra, ed. St. John's, Newfoundland: ARTS Biomedical Publishers.

Fernandes, G., E.J. Yunis, and F. Halberg. 1977. Circadian aspect of immune response in the mouse. Pp. 233–249 in Chronobiology in Allergy and Immunology, J.P. McGovern, M.H. Smolensky, and A. Reinberg, eds. Chicago, Ill.: Charles C Thomas.

Fernandes, G., E.J. Yunis, W. Nelson, and F. Halberg. 1974. Differences in immune response of mice to sheep red blood cells as a function of circadian phase. Pp. 329–338 in Chronobiology. Proceedings of the International Society for the Study of Biological Rhythms, L.E. Scheving, F. Halberg, and J.E. Pauly, eds. Stuttgart and Tokyo: Thime/Igaku Shoin.

Finocchiaro, L.E., E. Nahmod, and J.M. Launay. 1991. Melatonin biosynthesis and metabolism in peripheral blood mononuclear leukocytes. Biochem. J. 280:727–732.

Finocchiaro, L.M.E., E.S. Arzt, S. Fernandez-Castelo, M. Criscuolo, S. Finkielman, and V.E. Nahmod. 1988. Serotonin and melatonin synthesis in peripheral blood mononuclear cells: Stimulation by interferon-γ as part of an immunomodulatory pathway. J. Interferon Res. 1988:705–716.

Fischer, C.P., B.P. Bode, S.F. Abcouwer, G.C. Lukaszewicz, and W.W. Souba. 1995. Hepatic uptake of glutamine and other amino acids during infection and inflammation [editorial]. Shock 3:315–322.

Fisher, Jr., C.J., J.F. Dhainaut, S.M. Opal, J.P. Pribble, R.A. Balk, G.J. Slotman, T.J. Iberti, E.C. Rackow, M.J. Shapiro, R.L. Greenman et al. 1994a. Recombinant human interleukin 1 receptor antagonist in the treatment of patients with sepsis syndrome. Results from a randomized, double-blind, placebo-controlled trial. Phase III rhIL-1ra Sepsis Syndrome Study Group. J. Am. Med. Assoc. 271:1836–1843.

Fisher, Jr., C.J., G.J. Slotman, S.M. Opal, J.P. Pribble, R.C. Bone, G. Emmanuel, D. Ng, D.C. Bloedow, and M.A. Catalano. 1994b. Initial evaluation of human recombinant interleukin-1 receptor antagonist in the treatment of sepsis syndrome: A randomized, open-label, placebo-controlled multicenter trial. The IL-1ra Sepsis Syndrome Study Group. Crit. Care Med. 22:12–21.

Fisher, M., P.H. Levine, B.H. Weiner, M.H. Johnson, E.M. Doyle, P.A. Ellis, J.J. Hoogasian. 1990. Dietary n-3 fatty acid supplementation reduces superoxide production and chemiluminescence in a monocyte-enriched preparation of leukocytes. Am. J. Clin. Nutr. 51(5):804–8.

Fitzgerald, L. 1988. Exercise and the immune system. Immunol. Today 9:337–339.

Flament, J., M. Goldman, Y. Waterlot, E. Dupont, J. Wybran, and J.L. Vanherweghem. 1986. Impairment of phagocyte oxidative metabolism in hemodialysed patients with iron overload. Clin. Nephrol. 25:227–230.

Fleet, J.C. 1995. A new role for lactoferrin: DNA binding and transcription activation. Nutr. Rev. 53:226–227.

Fleshner, M., L.E. Goehler, J. Hermann, J.K. Relton, S.F. Maier, and L.R. Watkins. 1995. Interleukin-1β induced corticosterone elevation and hypothalamic NE depletion is vagally mediated. Brain Res. Bull. 37:605–610.

Fletcher, J., and E. Goldstein. 1970. The effect of parenteral iron preparation on experimental pyelonephritis. Br. J. Exp. Pathol. 51:280–285.

Fletcher, J., J. Mather, M.J. Lewis, and G. Whiting. 1975. Mouth lesions in iron-deficiency anemia: Relationship to Candida albicans in saliva and to impairment of lymphocyte transformation. J. Infect. Dis. 131:44–50.

Fletcher, M.A., N. Klimas, R. Morgan, and G. Gjerset. 1992. Lymphocyte proliferation. Pp. 213–219 in Manual of Clinical Laboratory Immunology, 4th ed., N.R. Rose, E. Conway DeMacario, J.L. Fahey, H. Friedman, and G.M. Penn, eds. Washington, D.C.: American Society for Microbiology.

Fletscher, B. 1993. Zirkadiane Variation der Antikorperbildung nach Hepatitis-B-Impfung. Deutsch. Med. Wschr 118:999.

Forse, R.A., ed. 1994. Diet, Nutrition, and Immunity. Boca Raton, Fla.: CRC Press.

Fox, D.A. 1995a. Biological therapies: A novel approach to the treatment of autoimmune disease. Am. J. Med. 99:82–88.

Fox, H.S. 1995b. Sex steroids and the immune system [Review]. CIBA Foundation Symposium. 191:203–211.

Fox, H.S., B.L. Bond, and T.G. Parslow. 1991. Estrogen regulates the INF-γ promoter. J. Immunol. 146:4362–4367.

Fraker, P.J., P. DePasqual-Jardieu, C.M. Zwick, and R.W. Luecke. 1978. Regeneration of T-cell helper function in zinc-deficient adult mice. Proc. Natl. Acad. Sci. USA 75:5660–5664.

Fraker, P.J., M.E. Gershwin, R.A. Good, and A. Prasad. 1986. Interrelationships between zinc and immune function. Fed. Proc. 45:1474–1479.

Fraker, P.J., L.E. King, B.A. Garry, and C.A. Medina. 1993. The immunopathology of zinc deficiency in humans and rodents. Pp. 267–283 in Human Nutrition—A Comprehensive Treatise, D.M. Klurfeld, ed., vol. 8: Nutrition and Immunology. New York: Plenum Press.

Frei, B., R. Stocker, and B.N. Ames. 1988. Antioxidant defenses and lipid peroxidation in human blood plasma. Proc. Natl. Acad. Sci. USA 85:9748–9752.

Fridovich, I. 1978. The biology of oxygen radicals. Science 201:875–880.

Friedl, K.E. 1997. Variability of fat and lean tissue loss during physical exertion with energy deficit. Pp. 431–450 in Physiology, Stress, and Malnutrition: Functional Correlates, Nutritional Intervention, J. Kinney and H. Tucker, eds. New York: Lippincott-Raven.

Friedl, K.E., L.J. Marchitelli, D.E. Sherman, and R. Tulle. 1990. Nutritional assessment of cadets at the U.S. Military Academy: Part 1. Anthropometric and biochemical measures. Technical Report No. T4-91. Natick, Mass.: U.S. Army Research Institute of Environmental Medicine.

Friedl, K.E, M.Z Mays, and T.R Kramer. 1995a. Acute recovery of physiological and cognitive function in U.S. Army Ranger students in a multistressor field environment. Workshop on the Effect of Prolonged Exhaustive Military Activities on Man—Physiological and Psychological Changes—Possible Means of Rapid Recuperation. NATO AC/243 Panel VIII. April 3–5. Holmenkollen, Oslo, Norway.

Friedl, K.E., K.A. Westphal, and L.J. Marchitelli. 1995b. Reproductive status and menstrual cyclicity of premenopausal women in Army basic combat training (BCT). FASEB J. 9:A292.

Friedman, E.M., and M.R. Irwin. 1995. A role for CRH and the sympathetic nervous system in stress-induced immunosuppression. Ann. N.Y. Acad. Sci. 771:396–418.

Friman, G., N.G. Ilbäck, D.J. Crawford, and H.A. Neufeld. 1991. Metabolic responses to swimming exercise in *Streptococcus pneumoniae* infected rats. Med. Sci. Sports Exerc. 23:415–421.

Friman, G., E. Larsson, and C. Rolf. 1997. Interaction between infection and exercise with special reference to myocarditis and the increased frequency of sudden deaths among young Swedish orienteers 1979–1992. Scand. J. Infect. Dis. Supp. 104:41–49.

Friman, G., J.E. Wright, N.G. Ilbäck, W.R. Beisel, J.D. White, D.S. Sharp, E.L. Stephen, W.L. Daniels, and J.A. Vogel. 1985. Does fever or myalgia indicate reduced physical performance capacity in viral infections? Acta. Med. Scand. 217:353–361.

Fritze, D., and P. Dystant. 1984. Detection of impaired mitogen responses in autologous whole blood of cancer patients using an optimized method of lymphocyte stimulation. Immunol. Lett. 8:243–247.

Fuchs, B.A., and V.M. Sanders. 1994. The role of brain–immune interactions in immunotoxicology. Crit. Rev. Toxicol. 24:151–176.

Fuller, R. and H. Snoddy. 1968. Feeding schedule alteration of daily rhythm in tyrosine α-ketoglutaride transaminase in rat liver. Science 159:738.

Fuster, V., B.J. Gersh, E.R. Giuliani, A.J. Tajik, R.O. Brandenburg, and R.L. Frye. 1981. The natural history of idiopathic dilated cardiomyopathy. Am. J. Cardiol. 47:525–531.

Futran, J., J.D. Kemp, E.H. Field, A. Ora, and R.F. Ashman. 1989. Transferrin receptor synthesis is an early event in B-cell activation. J. Immunol. 143:787–792.

Gabriel, H., L. Schwarz, P. Born, and W. Kindermann. 1992. Differential mobilization of leukocyte and lymphocyte subpopulations into the circulation during endurance exercise. Eur. J. Appl. Physiol. 65:529–534.

Gaillard, R.C. 1994. Neuroendocrine-immune system interactions. Trends in Endocrinology and Metabolism 7:303–309.

Gala, R.R., and E.M. Shevach. 1993. Identification by analytical flow cytometry of prolactin receptors on immunocompetent cell population in the mouse. Endocrinology 133:1617–1623.

Gala, R.R., and E.M. Shevach. 1994. Evidence for the release of a prolactin-like substance by mouse lymphocytes and macrophages. Proc. Soc. Exp. Biol. Med. 205:12–19.

Gallagher, H.J., and J.M. Daly. 1993. Malnutrition, injury, and the host immune response: Nutrient substitution. Curr. Opin. Gen. Surg. 1993:92–104.

Gamaleya, N.F., E.D. Silisko, and A.P. Cherny. 1988. Preservation of circadian rhythms by human leukocytes in vitro. Byull. Eksper. Biol. Med. 106:598–600.

Gao, Y., J.R. He, and L.P. Kapcala. 1996. Interleukin-1β and lipopolysaccharide regulation of interleukin-1β and interleukin-1 type 1 receptor in hypothalamic neurons and glia [abstract 336.3]. Soc. Neurosci. 21.

Gapinski, J.P., J.V. VanRuiswyk, G.R. Henderbert, and G.S. Schectman. 1993. Preventing restenosis with fish oils following coronary angioplasty. Arch. Intern. Med. 153:1595–1601.

Garbe, A., J. Buck, and U. Hämmerling. 1992. Retinoids are important cofactors in T-cell activation. J. Exp. Med. 176:109–117.

Gardner, D.F., M.M. Kaplan, C.A. Stanley, and R.D. Utiger. 1979. Effect of triiodothyronine replacement on the metabolic and pituitary responses to starvation. N. Engl. J. Med. 300:579–584.

Garg, M., and S. Bondada. 1993. Reversal of age-associated decline in immune response to pnu-immune vaccine by supplementation with the steroid hormone dehydroepiandrosterone. Infect. Immun. 61:2238–2241.

Garrey, W.E., and W.R. Bryan. 1935. Variations in white blood cell counts. Physiol. Rev. 15:597–638.

Gatti, G., R. Cavallo, M.L. Sartori, R. Carignola, R. Masera, D. Delponte, A. Salvadori, and A. Angeli. 1988. Circadian variations of interferon-induced enhancement of human natural killer (NK) cell activity. Cancer Detec. 12:431–438.

Gatti, G., R. Cavallo, M.L. Sartori, D. Delponte, R.G. Masera, A. Salvadori, R. Carignola, and A. Angeli. 1987. Inhibition by cortisol of human natural killer (NK) cell activity. Steroid. Biochem. 26:49–58.

Gatti, G., R. Cavallo, M.I. Sartori, C. Marinone, and A. Angeli. 1986. Cortisol at physiological concentrations and prostaglandin E2 are additive inhibitors of human nature killer cell activity. Immunopharmacology 11:119–128.

Gatti, G., R.G. Masera, R. Carignola, M.L. Sartori, E. Margro, and A. Angeli. 1990. Circadian-single-dependent enhancement of human natural killer cell activity by melatonin. J. Immunol. Res. 2:108–116.

Gaultier, C., G. DeMontis, A. Reinberg, and Y. Motohashi. 1987. Circadian rhythm of serum total immunoglobulin E (IgE) in asthmatic children. Biomed. Pharmacother. 41:186–188.

Gauntt, C.J., E.K. Godeny, and C.W. Lutton. 1988. Host factors regulating viral clearance. Path. Immunol. Res. 7:251–265.

Gaykema, R.P.A., I. Dijkstra, and F.J.H. Tilders. 1995. Subdiaphragmatic vagotomy suppresses endotoxin-induced activation of hypothalamic corticotropin-releasing hormone neurons and ACTH secretion. Endocrinology 136:4717–4770.

Ge, K.Y., J. Bai, X.J. Deng, S.Q. Wu, S.Q. Wang, A.N. Xue, and C.Q. Su. 1987. The protective effect of selenium against viral myocarditis in mice. Pp. 761–768 in Selenium in Biology and Medicine, Part B, G.F. Combs, O.A. Levander, J.J. Spallholz, and J.E. Oldfield, eds. New York: Van Nostrand/Reinhold.

Germain, R.N., and D.H. Margulies. 1993. The biochemistry and cell biology of antigen processing and presentation. Ann. Rev. Immunol. 11:403–450.

Gershwin, M.E., R.S. Beach, and L.S. Hurley, eds. 1985. Nutrition and Immunology. Orlando, Fla.: Academic Press.

Ghighineishvili, G.R., V.V. Nicolaeva, A.J. Belousov, P.G. Sirtori, V. Balsamo, A. Miani, R. Franceschini, M. Ripani, M. Crosina, and G. Cosenza. 1992. Correction by physiotherapy of immune disorders in high-grade athletes. Clin. Ter. 140:545–550.

Gibinski, K., A. Nowak, J. Rybicka, and K. Czarnecka. 1979. An endoscopic study on the natural history of gastroduodenal ulcer disease. Mater. Med. Pol. 11:265–269.

Gibson, L.F., D. Piktel, and K.S. Landreth. 1993. Insulin-like growth factor-I potentiates expansion of interleukin-7-dependent pro-B-cells. Blood 82:3005–3011.

Gibson-Berry, K.L., J.C. Whitin, and H.J. Cohen. 1993. Modulation of the respiratory burst in human neutrophils by isoproterenol and dibutyryl cyclic AMP. J. Neuroimmunol. 43:59–68.

Gifford, R., R. Halverson, D. Ritzer, J. Valentine, and L. Newkirk. 1996. Operation Joint Endeavor: Psychological status of the deployed force—June 1996. Summary brief/report, July. Washington, D.C.: Division of Neuropsychiatry, Walter Reed Army Institute of Research.

Gilblett, E.R., J.E. Anderson, F. Cohen, B. Pollara, and H.J. Meuwissen. 1972. Adenosine deaminase deficiency in two patients with severely impaired cellular immunity. Lancet II:1067–1069.

Glaser, R., and J.K. Kiecolt-Glaser, 1997. Chronic stress modulates the virus-specific immune response to latent herpes simplex virus type 1. Ann. Behav. Med. 19:78–82.

Glaser, R., J.K. Kiecolt-Glaser, W.B. Malarkey, and J.F. Sheridan. 1998. The influence of psychological stress on the immune response to vaccines. Ann. NY Acad. Sci. 840:649–655.

Gleeson, M., W.A. McDonald, A.W. Cripps, D.B. Pyne, R.L. Clancy, and P.A. Fricker. 1995. The effect on immunity of long-term intensive training in elite swimmers. Clin. Exp. Immunol. 102:210–216.

Goetz, F., J. Bishop, F. Halberg, R. Sothern, R. Brunning, B. Senske, B. Greenberg, D. Minors, P. Stoney, I.D. Smith, G.D. Rosen, D. Cressey, E. Haus, and M. Apfelbaum. 1976. Timing of single daily meal influences relations among human circadian rhythms in urinary cyclic AMP and hemic glucagon, insulin, and iron. Experientia (Basel) 32:1081–1084.

Goldblatt, H., and M. Benischek. 1927. Vitamin A deficiency and metaplasia. J. Exp. Med. 46:699–707.

Goldenberg, D.L. 1993. Fibromyalgia, chronic fatigue syndrome, and myofascial pain syndrome. Curr. Opin. Rheumatol. 5:199–208.

Golding, S., and S.P. Young. 1995. Iron requirements of human lymphocytes: Relative contributions of intra- and extracellular iron. Scand. J. Immunol. 41:229–236.

Goldsmith, M.F. 1992. World health organization consensus statement. Consultation on AIDS and sports. J. Am. Med. Assoc. 267:1312–1314.

Good, R.A., and E. Lorenz. 1992. Nutrition and cellular immunity. Int. J. Immunopharmacol. 14:361–366.

Good, M.F., L.W. Powell, and J.W. Halliday. 1988. Iron status and cellular immune competence. Blood Rev. 2:43–49.

Goodili, J.J., and J.G. Abuelo. 1987. Mucormycosis—A new risk of deferrioxamine therapy in dialysis patients with aluminum or iron overload? [letter]. N. Engl. J. Med. 317:54.

Goodwin, J.S. 1995. Decreased immunity and increased morbidity in the elderly. Nutr. Rev. 53:S41–S46.

Gorbach, S.L., T.A. Knox, and R. Roubenoff. 1993. Interactions between nutrition and infection with human immunodeficiency virus. Nutr. Rev. 51:226–234.

Gorbunov, N.V., A.N. Osipov, M.A. Sweetland, B.W. Day, N.M. Elsayed, and V.E. Kagan. 1996. NO-redox paradox: Direct oxidation of alpha-tocopherol and alpha-tocopherol-mediated oxidation of ascorbate. Biochem. Biophys. Res. Commun. 27:835–841.

Gordeur, V., P. Thuma, G. Brittenham, C. McLaren, D. Parry, A. Backenstose, G. Biema, R. Msiska, L. Holmes, E. McKinley, L. Vargas, R. Gilkeson, and A.A. Poltera. 1992. Effect of iron chelation therapy on recovery from deep coma in children with cerebral malaria. N. Engl. J. Med. 327:1473–1477.

Gore, D.C., and F. Jahoor. 1994. Glutamine kinetics in burn patients. Arch. Surg. 129:1318–1323.

Grady, R.W., A. Akbar, P.J. Giardina, M.W. Hilgartner, and M. deSousa. 1985. Disproportionate lymphoid cell subsets in thalassemia major: The relative contributions of transfusion and splenectomy. Br. J. Haematol. 72:361–367.

Graf, M.V., and A.J. Kastin. 1984. Delta-sleep-inducing peptide (DSIP): A review. Neurosci. Biobehav. Rev. 8:83–93.

Granowitz, E.V., R. Porat, J.W. Mier, S.F. Orencole, M.V. Callahan, J.G. Cannon, E.A. Lynch, K. Ye, D.D. Poutsiaka, E. Vannier et al. 1993. Hematologic and immunomodulatory effects of an interleukin-1 receptor antagonist coinfusion during low-dose endotoxemia in healthy adults. Blood 82:2985–2990.

Gray, A.B., Y.C. Smart, R.D. Telford, M.J. Weidemann, and T.K. Roberts. 1992. Anaerobic exercise causes transient changes in leukocyte subsets and IL-2R expression. Med. Sci. Sports Exerc. 24:1332–1338.

Green, N.S. 1992. *Yersinia* infections in patients with homozygous β-thalassemia associated with iron overload and its treatment. Pediatric Hematol. Oncol. 9:247–254.

Griep, E.N., J.W. Boersma, and E.R. de Kloet. 1993. Altered reactivity of the hypothalamic–pituitary–adrenal axis in the primary fibromyalgia syndrome. J. Rheumatol. 20:469–474.

Griffin, P.M. and R.V. Tauxe. 1991. The epidemiology of infections caused by *Escherichia coli* O157:H7, other enterohemorrhagic *E. coli*, and the associated hemolytic uremic syndrome. Epidemiol. Rev.

Griffith, R.D., C. Jones, and T.E.A. Palmer. 1997. Six month outcome of critically ill patients given glutamine supplemental parenteral nutrition. Nutrition 13:295–302.

Griffiths, E. 1987. Iron in biological systems. Pp. 1–25 in Iron and Infection, J.J. Bullen and E. Griffiths, eds. London: John Wiley & Sons.

Griffiths, R.D., C. Jones, and T.E. Palmer. 1997. Six month outcome of critically ill patients given glutamine-supplemental parenteral nutrition. Nutrition 13:295–302.

Grimble, R.F. 1994. Malnutrition and immune response. 2. Impact of nutrients on cytokine biology in infection [abstract]. Trans. R. Soc. Trop. Med. Hyg. 88(6):615–619.

Grimble, R.F. 1995. Interactions between nutrients and the immune system. Nutr. Health 10:191–200.

Grosch-Warner, I., H. Grosse-Wilde, C. Bender-Gotze, and K.H. Schafer. 1984. Lymphozytenfunktionen bei kindern mit eisenmangel. Klin. Wochenschr. 62:1091–1093.

Gross, R.L., and P.M. Newberne. 1976. Malnutrition, the thymolymphatic system and immunocompetence. Adv. Exp. Med. Biol. 73:179–187.

Gross, R.L., J.V.O. Reid, P.M. Newberne, B. Burgess, R. Marston, and W. Hift. 1975. Depressed cell-mediated immunity in megaloblastic anemia due to folic acid deficiency. Am. J. Clin. Nutr. 28:225–232.

Grossman, Z., R. Asofsky, and C. Delisi. 1980. The dynamics of antibody secreting cell production, regulation of growth, and oscillations in the response to T-independent antigens. J. Theor. Biol. 84:49–92.

Gruchalla, R.S., and T.J. Sullivan. 1991. Detection of human IgE to sulfamethoxazole by skin testing with sulfamethoxazoyl-poly-l-tyrosine. J. Allergy Clin. Immunol. 88:784–792.

Gu, B.Q. 1983. Pathology of Keshan disease: A comprehensive review. Chinese Med. J. 96:251–261.

Gubler, D.J., and D.W. Trent. 1993. Emergence of epidemic dengue/dengue hemorrhagic fever as a public health problem in the Americas. Infect. Agents Dis. 2:383–393.

Gudewill, S., T. Pollmacher, H. Vedder, W. Schreuber, K. Fassbender, and F. Holsboer. 1992. Nocturnal plasma levels of cytokines in healthy men. Eur. Arch. Psych. Clin. Neurosci. 242:53–56.

Guerinot, M.L. 1994. Microbial iron transport. Ann. Rev. Microbiol. 48:743–772.

Gupta, K.K., P.S. Dhatt, and H. Singh. 1982. Cell-mediated immunity in children with iron-deficiency anemia. Indian J. Pediatr. 49:507–510.

Gwosdow, A.R., N.A. O'Connell, J.A. Spencer, and M.S.A. Kuman. 1992. Interleukin-1-induced corticosterone release occurs by an adrenergic mechanism from rat adrenal gland. Am. J. Physiol. 263:E461–E466.

Hack, V., G. Strobel, J-P. Rau, and H. Weicker. 1992. The effect of maximal exercise on the activity of neutrophil granulocytes in highly trained athletes in a moderate training period. Eur. J. Appl. Physiol. 65:520–524.

Hack, V., G. Strobel, M. Weiss, and H. Weicker. 1994. PMN cell counts and phagocytic activity of highly trained athletes depend on training period. J. Appl. Physiol. 77:1731–1735.

Haen, E., I. Langenmayer, A. Pangerl, B. Liebl, and J. Remien. 1988. Circannual variation in the expression of β2 adrenoceptors on human peripheral mononuclear leukocytes (MNLs). Klin. Wschr. 66:579–582.

Halberg, E., and F. Halberg. 1980. Chronobiologic study design in everyday life, clinic, and laboratory. Chronobiologia 7:95–120.

Halberg, F. 1974. From iatrotoxicosis and iatrosepsis towards chronotherapy. Pp. 1–34 in Chronobiologic Aspects of Endocrinology, J. Aschoff, F. Ceresa, and F. Halberg, eds. Stuttgart: Schattaner-Verlag.

Halberg, F., and C. Hamburger. 1964. 17-ketosteroids and volume of human urine. Weekly and other changes with low frequency. Minn. Med. 47:916–925.

Halberg, F., and A.N. Stephens. 1959. Susceptibility to ouabain and physiologic circadian periodicity. Proc. Minn. Acad. Sci. 27:139–143.

Halberg, F., C.P. Barnum, R. Silber, and J.J. Bittner. 1958. 24-hour rhythms at several levels of integration in mice on different lighting regimens. Proc. Soc. Exp. Biol. Med. 97:897–900.

Halberg, F., D. Duffert, and H. Von Mayersbach. 1977 Circadian rhythm in serum immunoglobulins of clinically healthy young men [abstract]. Chronobiologia 4:114.

Halberg, F., E. Haus, and G. Cornélissen. 1995. From biologic rhythms to chronomes relevant for nutrition. Pp. 361–372 in Not Eating Enough, Overcoming Underconsumption of Military Operational Rations, B.M. Marriott, ed. Committee on Military Nutrition Research, Food and Nutrition Board, Institute of Medicine. Washington, D.C.: National Academy Press.

Halberg, F., E.A. Johnson, B.W. Brown, and J.J. Bittner. 1960. Susceptibility rhythm to E. coli endotoxin and bioassay. Proc. Soc. Exp. Biol. Med. 103:142–144.

Halberg, J., E. Halberg, W. Runge, J. Wicks, L. Cadotte, E. Yunis, G. Katinas, O. Stutman, and F. Halberg. 1974. Transplant chronobiology. Pp. 320–328 in Chronobiology.

Proceedings of the International Society for the Study of Biological Rhythms, L.E. Scheving, F. Halberg, and J.E. Pauly, eds. Stuttgart and Tokyo: Thieme/Igaku Shoin.

Hallberg, L., C. Bengtsson, L. Lapidus, G. Lindstedt, P.A. Lundberg and L. Hulten. 1993. Screening for iron deficiency: an analysis based on bone-marrow examinations and serum ferritin determinations in a population sample of women. Br. J. Haematol. 85(4):787–798.

Halstead, S.B. 1989. Antibody, macrophages, dengue virus infection, shock, and hemorrhage: A pathogenetic cascade. Rev. Infect. Dis. 11(suppl. 4):S830–S839.

Halvorsen, R.R., P.D. Bliese, R.E. Moore, and C.A. Castro . 1995. Psychological well-being and physical health symptoms of soldiers deployed for Operation Uphold Democracy. A summary of human dimensions research in Haiti. Washington, D.C.: Division of Neuropsychiatry, Walter Reed Army Institute of Research.

Hammarqvist, F., J. Wernerman, R. Ali, A. von der Decken, and E. Vinnars. 1989. Addition of glutamine to total parenteral nutrition after elective abdominal surgery spares free glutamine in muscle, counteracts the fall in muscle protein synthesis, and improves nitrogen balance. Ann. Surg. 209:455–461.

Hansson, I., R. Holmdahl, and R. Mattsson. 1992. The pineal hormone melatonin exaggerates development of collagen-induced arthritis in mice. J. Neuroimmunol. 39:23–30.

Harbige, L.S. 1996. Nutrition and immunity with emphasis on infection and autoimmune disease. Nutr. Health 10:285–312.

Harbuz, M.S., and S.L. Lightman. 1992. Stress and the hypothalamo–pituitary–adrenal axis: Acute, chronic, and immunological activation. J. Endocrinol. 134:327–339.

Harbuz, M.S., R.G. Rees, D. Eckland, D.S. Jessop, D. Brewerton, and S.L. Lightman. 1992a. Paradoxical responses of hypothalamic corticotropin-releasing factor (CRF) messenger ribonucleic acid (mRNA) and CRF-41 peptide and adenohypophysial proopiomelanocortin mRNA during chronic inflammatory stress. Endocrinology. 130:1394–1400.

Harbuz, M.S., R.G. Rees, and S.L. Lightman. 1993. HPA axis responses to acute stress and adrenalectomy during adjuvant-induced arthritis in the rat. Am. J. Physiol. 264:R179–R185.

Harbuz, M.S., A. Stephanou, N. Sarlis, and S.L. Lightman. 1992b. The effects of recombinant human interleukin (IL)-1α, IL-1β, or IL-6 on hypothalamo-pituitary-adrenal axis activation. J. Endocrinol. 133:349–355.

Hardy, C.A., J. Quay, S. Livast, and R. Ader. 1990. Altered T-lymphocyte response following aggressive encounters in mice. Physiol. Behav. 47:245–251.

Harford, J.B., and R.D. Klausner. 1990. Coordinate posttranscriptional regulation of ferritin and transferrin receptor expression: The role of regulated RNA–protein interaction. Enzyme 44:28–41.

Harford, J.B., J.L. Casey, D.M. Koeller, and R.D. Klausner. 1990. Structure, function, and regulation of the transferrin receptor: Insights from molecular biology. Pp. 302–334 in Intracellular Trafficking of Proteins, C.J. Steer and J.A. Hanover, eds. Cambridge: Cambridge University Press.

Hartmann, D.P., J.W. Holday, and E.W. Bernton. 1989. Inhibition of lymphocyte proliferation by antibodies to prolactin. FASEB J. 3:2194–2202.

Hasty, L.A., J.D. Lambris, B.A. Lessey, K. Pruksananonda, and C.R. Lyttle. 1994. Hormonal regulation of complement and receptors throughout the menstrual cycle. Am. J. Obstet. Gynecol. 170:168–175.

Hatch, G.E. 1995. Asthma, inhaled oxidant, and dietary antioxidants. Am. J. Clin. Nutr. 61:625S–630S.

Hattori, N., A. Shimatsu, M. Sugita, S. Kumagai, and H. Imura. 1990. Immunoreactive growth hormone (GH) secretion by human lymphocytes: Augmented release by exogenous GH. Biochem. Biophys. Res. Commun. 168:396–401.

Hauger, S.E., and P. Wiik. 1997. Glucocorticoid and ACTH regulation of rat peritoneal phagocyte chemiluminescence and nitric oxide production in culture. Acta Physiol. Scand. 161:93–101.

Haus, E. 1959. Endokrines system und Blut. Pp. 181–286 in Handbuch der gesamten Hämatologie, L. Heilmeyer and A. Hittmair, eds. Munich: Urban und Schwarzenberg.

Haus, E. 1994. Chronobiology of circulating blood cells and platelets. Pp. 504–526 in Biologic Rhythms in Clinical and Laboratory Medicine, 2d ed., Y. Touitou and E. Haus, eds. Heidelberg: Springer Verlag.

Haus, E. 1996. Biologic rhythms in hematology. Path. Biol. 44(6):618–630.

Haus, E., and F. Halberg. 1978. Cronofarmacologia della neoplasia con speciale riferimento alla leucemia. Pp. 29–85 in Farmacologia Clinica e Terapia, A. Bertelli, ed.Turin: Edizioni.

Haus, E., and Y. Touitou. 1994a. Chronobiology in laboratory medicine. Pp. 673–708 in Biologic Rhythms in Clinical and Laboratory Medicine, 2d ed., Y. Touitou and E. Haus, eds. Heidelberg: Springer-Verlag.

Haus, E., and Y. Touitou. 1994b. Principles of clinical chronobiology. Pp. 6–34 in Biologic Rhythms in Clinical and Laboratory Medicine, Y. Touitou and E. Haus, eds. Berlin: Springer-Verlag.

Haus, E., L. Dumitriu, G.Y. Nicolau, D.J. Lakatua, H. Berg, E. Petrescu, L. Sackett-Lundeen, and R. Reilly. 1995. Time relation of circadian rhythms in plasma dehydroepiandrosterone and dehydroepiandrosterone-sulfate to ACTH, cortisol, and 11-desoxycortisol-#107 [abstract]. Biol. Rhythm Res. 26:(4)399.

Haus, E., F. Halberg, J.F.W. Juhl, and D.J. Lakatua. 1974a. Chronopharmacology in animals. Chronobiologia 1:122–156.

Haus, E., F. Halberg, M.K. Loken, and Y.S. Kim. 1974b. Circadian rhythmometry of mammalian radiosensitivity. Pp. 435–474 in Space Radiation Biology, C.A. Tobias and P. Todd, eds. New York: American Institute of Biological Science Academic Press.

Haus, E., F. Halberg, L.E. Scheving, J.E. Pauly, S. Cardoso, J.F.W. Kuhl, R.B. Sothern, R.N. Shiotsuka, and D.S. Hwang. 1972. Increased tolerance of leukemic mice to arabinosyl cytosine with schedule adjusted to circadian system. Science 177:80–82.

Haus, E., D.J. Lakatua, F. Halberg, E. Halberg, G. Cornélissen, L. Sackett, H. Berg, T. Kawasaki, M. Ueno, K. Uezono, M. Matsouka, and T. Omae. 1980. Chronobiological studies of plasma prolactin in women in Kyushu, Japan, and Minnesota, U.S.A. J. Clin. Endocrinol. Metab. 51:632–640.

Haus, E., D.J. Lakatua, L. Sackett-Lundeen, and T Swoyer. 1984. Chronobiology in laboratory medicine. Pp. 13–82 in Clinical Aspects of Chronobiology, W.J. Rietveld, ed. The Netherlands: Meducation Service Hoechst.

Haus, E., D.J. Lakatua, L. Sackett-Lundeen and M. White. 1984. Circannual variation of intestinal cell proliferation in BDF male mice on three lighting regimens. Chronobiol. Int. 1:185–194.

Haus, E., D.J. Lakatua, J. Swoyer, and L. Sackett-Lundeen. 1983. Chronobiology in hematology and immunology. Am. J. of Anatomy 168:467–517.

Haus, E., G.Y. Nicolau, D.J. Lakatua, L. Sackett-Lundeen, E. Petrescu, and J. Swoyer. 1993. Chronobiology in laboratory medicine. Ann. 1st. Super. Sanita. 29(4):581–606.

Haus, M., L. Sackett-Lundeen, D. Lakatua, and E. Haus. 1984. Circannual variation of ^{3}H-thymidine uptake in DNA of lymphatic organs irrespective of relative length of light and dark span [abstract]. J. Minn. Acad. Sci. 49(2):19.

Hayashi, O.K., and M. Kikuchi. 1982. The effects of the light-dark cycle on humoral and cell-mediated immune responses of mice. Chronobiologia 9:291–300.

Haynes, B.F., S.M. Denning, P.T. Le, and K.H. Singer. 1990. Human intrathymic T-cell differentiation. Semin. Immunol. 2:67–77.

He, J.R., Y. Gao, and L.P. Kapcala. 1996. Induction of interleukin-1β gene expression in specific brain sites by peripheral interleukin-1β and lipopolysaccharide [abstract 336.1]. Soc. Neurosci. 21.

Hedner, L., and G. Bynke. 1985. Endogenous iridocyclitis relieved during treatment with Bromocriptine. Am. J. Ophthal. 100:618–619.

Heifets, M., G.F. Cooney, L.M. Shaw, and G. Lebetti. 1995. Diurnal variation of cyclosporine clearance in stable renal transplant recipients receiving continuous infusion. Transplantation 60:1615–1617.

Helms, S.D., J.D. Oliver, and J.C. Travis. 1984. Role of heme compounds and haptoglobin in *Vibrio vulnificus* pathogenicity. Infect. Immun. 45:345–349.

Helyar, L., and A.R. Sherman. 1987. Iron deficiency and interleukin-1 production by rat leukocytes. Am. J. Clin. Nutr. 46:346–352.

Helzlsouer, C.K., R. Jacobs, and S. Morris. 1985. Acute selenium intoxication in the United States. Fed. Proc. 44:1670.

Hemila, H. 1997. Vitamin C intake and susceptibility to the common cold. Br. J. Nutr. 77(1):59–72.

Henkin, R.I., and R.L. Aamodt. 1983. A redefinition of zinc deficiency. Pp. 83–105 in Nutritional Bioavailability of Zinc, G.E. Inglett, ed. Washington, D.C.: American Chemical Society.

Henry, M.M., J.N. Moore, and J.K. Fisher. 1991. Influence of an omega-3 fatty acid-enriched ration on *in vivo* responses of horses to endotoxin. Am. J. Vet. Res. 52:523–527.

Heppner, D.G., A.J. Magill, R.A. Gasser, and C.N. Oster. 1993. The threat of infectious diseases in Somalia. N. Engl. J. Med. 328:1061–1068.

Herberman R.B., and D.H. Callewaert, eds. 1985. Mechanisms of Cytotoxicity by NK Cells. Orlando, Fla.: Academic Press.

Herbert, V. 1979. Ascorbic acid and vitamin B12. JAMA 242(21):2285.

Herbert, V. 1997. Destroying immune homeostasis in normal adults with antioxidant supplements. Am. J. Clin. Nutr. 65(6):1901-1903.

Herbert, V., and T.S. Kasdan. 1994. Alfalfa, vitamin E, and autoimmune disorders. Am. J. Clin. Nutr. 60:639–640.

Herbeth, B., A. Lemoine, B.P. Zhu, and M. Chavance. 1992. Vitamin status, immunity and infections in the elderly. Pp. 225–237 in Nutrition and Immunology, R.K. Chandra, ed. St. John's, Newfoundland: ARTS Biomedical Publishers.

Heresi, G., M. Olivaress, F. Pizarro, M. Cayazo, E. Hertrampf, E. Walter, and A. Stekel. 1985. Effect of iron fortification on infant morbidity [abstract]. XIII International Congress of Nutrition, Brighton, England, p. 129.

Hershko, C. 1992. Iron and infection. Pp. 53–64 in Nutritional Anemias. Nestle Nutrition Workshop Series, vol. 30, S.J. Fomon and S. Zlotkin, eds. New York: Nestec Ltd Vevey Raven Press Ltd.

Hershko, C., and T.E.A. Peto. 1987. Non-transferrin plasma iron. Brit. J. Haematology 66:149–151.

Hershko, C., and T.E.A. Peto. 1988. Deferoxamine inhibition of malaria is independent of host iron status. J. Exp. Med. 168:375–387.

Hershko, C., T.E.A. Peto, and D.J. Weatherall. 1988. Iron and infection. Br. Med. J. 296:660–664.

Herskovitz, A., K.W. Beisel, L.J. Wolfgram, and N.R. Rose. 1985. Coxsackievirus B3 murine myocarditis: Wide pathologic spectrum in genetically defined inbred strains. Human Pathol. 16:671–673.

Hetzel, M.R., T.J.H. Clark, and M.A. Branthwaite. 1977. Asthma: Analysis of sudden deaths and ventilatory arrest in hospital. Br. Med. J. 1:808–811.

Hickson, R.C., L.E. Wegrzyn, D.F. Osborne, and I.E. Karl. 1996. Glutamine interferes with glutamine-induced expression of glutamine synthetase in skeletal muscle. Am. J. Physiol. 270:E912–E917.

Hiestand, P.C., P. Mekler, R. Nordmann, A. Grieder, and C. Permmongkol. 1986. Prolactin as a modulator of lymphocyte responsiveness provides a possible mechanism of action for cyclosporine. Proc. Natl. Acad. Sci. USA 83:2599–2603.

Higgins, G.A., and J.A. Olschowka. 1991. Induction of interleukin-1β mRNA in adult rat brain. Mol. Brain Res. 9:143–148.

Hinshaw, L.B., B.K. Beller-Todd, and L.T. Archer. 1982. Current management of the septic shock patient: Experimental basis for treatment. Circ. Shock 9:543–553.

Hinton, P.S., C.A. Peterson, H.C. Lo, H. Yang, D. McCarthy, and D.M. Ney. 1995. Insulin-like growth factor-I enhances immune response in dexamethasone-treated or surgically stressed rats maintained with total parenteral nutrition. JPEN J. Parenter. Enter. Nutr. 19:444–452.

Hodges, R.E., W.B. Bean, M.A. Ohlson, and R.E. Bleiler. 1962. Factors affecting human antibody response. IV. Pyridoxine deficiency. Am. J. Clin. Nutr. 11:180–186.

Hoffman-Goetz, L., and B.K. Pedersen. 1994. Exercise and the immune system: A model of the stress response? Immunol. Today 8:382–387.

Hollander, D., C.M. Vadheim, E. Brettholz, G.M. Petterson, T. Delahunty, and J.I. Rotter. 1986. Increased intestinal permeability in patients with Crohn's disease and their relatives. Ann. Int. Med. 105:883–885.

Hollingsworth, J.W., and J. Carr. 1973. 3H-uridine incorporation as a T lymphocyte indicator in the rat. Cell Immunol. 8(2):270–279.

Homo-Delarche, F. 1984. Glucocorticoid receptors and steroid sensitivity in normal and neoplastic human lymphoid tissue: A review. Cancer Res. 44:431–437.

Homo-Delarche, F., F. Fitzpatrick, N. Christeff, E.A. Nunez, J.F. Bach, and M. Dardenne. 1991. Sex steroids, glucocorticoids, stress, and autoimmunity. J. Steroid Biochem. Mol. 40:619–637.

Hong, R.W., J.D. Rounds, W.S. Helton, M.K. Robinson, and D.W. Wilmore. 1992. Glutamine preserves liver glutathione after lethal hepatic injury. Ann. Surg. 215:114–119.

Hooghe, R., M. Delhase, P. Vergani, A. Malur, and E.L. Hooghe-Peters. 1993. Growth hormone and prolactin are paracrine growth and differentiation factors in the haemopoietic system. Immunol. Today 14:212–214.

Hoopes, P.C., and C.E. McCall. 1977. The effect of cobra venom factor (CVF) on activation of the complement cascade on leukocyte circadian variation in the rat. Experientia

Hopkins, R.G., and M.L. Failla. 1997. Copper deficiency reduces interleukin-2 (IL-2) production and IL-2 mRNA in human T-lymphocytes. J. Nutr. 127(2):257–262.

Hrushesky, W.J.M., ed. 1994. Circadian Cancer Therapy. Boca Raton, Fla.: CRC Press.

Hrushesky, W.J.M., and W.J. März. 1994. Chronochemotherapy of malignant tumors: Temporal aspects of antineoplastic drug toxicity. Pp. 611–634 in Biologic Rhythms in Clinical and Laboratory Medicine, 2nd ed., Y.Touitou and E.Haus, eds. Heidelberg: Springer-Verlag.

Huber, C., J.R. Batchelor, D. Fuchs, A. Hauser, A. Lang, D. Niederwieser, G. Reitnegger, P. Swetly, J. Troppmair, and H. Wachter. 1984. Immune response associated production of neopterin. Release from macrophages primarily under control of interferon-γ. J. Exp. Med. 160:310–316.

Hübner, K. 1967. Kompensatorische Hypertrophie, Wachstum und Regeneration der Rattenniere. Ergebn Allg. Path. Path. Anat. 48:1–80.

Hughes D.A., A.C. Pinder, Z. Piper, I.T. Johnson, and E.K. Lund. 1996. Fish oil supplementation inhibits the expression of major histocompatibility complex class II molecules and adhesion molecules on human monocytes. Am. J. Clin. Nutr. 63:267–272.

Hughes, E.C., R.L. Johnson, and C.W. Whitaker. 1977. Circadian rhythmic aspects of secretory immunoglobulin A. Pp. 216–232 in Chronobiology in Allergy and Immunology, J.P. McGovern, M.H. Smolensky, and A. Reinberg, eds. Springfield, Ill.: Charles C Thomas.

Huhman, K.L., M.A. Hebert, J.L. Meyerhoff, and B.N. Bunnell. 1991. Plasma cyclic AMP increases in hamsters following exposure to a graded footshock stressor. Psychoneuroendocrinology 16:559–563.

Huhman, K.L., T.O. Moore, E.H. Mougey, and J.L. Meyerhoff. 1992. Hormonal responses to fighting in hamsters: Separation of physical and psychological causes. Physiol. Behav. 51:1083–1086.

Hume, E.M., and H.A. Krebs. 1949. Vitamin A requirements of human adults: An experimental study of vitamin A deprivation in man. Medical Research Council Special Report Series 264. London: Her Majesty's Stationery Office.

Hummell, D.S. 1993. Dietary lipids and immune function. Prog. Food Nutr. Sci. 17:287–329.

Husband, A.J. 1993. Role of central nervous system and behavior in the immune response. Vaccine 11:805–816.

Hussein, M.A., H.A. Hassan, A.A. Abdel-Ghaffar and S. Salem. 1988. Effect of iron supplements on occurrence of diarrhea among children in rural Egypt. Food Nutr. Bull. 10(2):35–49.

Hussein, M.A., M.A. Hassan, S. Salem, N. Scrimshaw, G. Keusch, and E. Pollit. 1985. Field work on the effects of iron supplementation [abstract]. XIII International Congress of Nutrition, Brighton, England, p. 129.

Hussey, G., J. Hughes, S. Potgieter, G. Kessow, J. Burgess, D. Beatty, M. Keraan, and E. Carelse. 1996. Vitamin A status and supplementation and its effects on immunity in children with AIDS. P. 6 Abstracts of the XVII International Vitamin A Consultative Group Meeting, Guatemala City, Guatemala, March.

Huupponen, M.R.H., L.H. Mäkinen, P.M. Hyvönen, C.K. Sen, T. Rankinen, S. Väisänen, and R. Rauramaa. 1995. The effect of N-acetylcysteine on exercise-induced priming of human neutrophils. Int. J. Sports Med. 16:399–403.

Ilbäck, N.G., G. Friman, D.J. Crawford, and H.A. Neufeld. 1991. Effects of training on metabolic responses and performance capacity in Streptococcus pneumoniae infected rats. Med. Sci. Sports Exerc. 23:422–427.

Inagaki, N., H. Nagai, and A. Koda. 1984. Effect of vitamin E on IgE antibody formation in mice. J. Pharmacobiodynamics 7:70–74.

Indiveri, F., I. Pierri, S. Rogna, A. Poggi, P. Montaldo, R. Romano, A. Pende, A. Morgano, A. Barabino, and S. Ferrone. 1985. Circadian variations of autologous mixed lymphocyte reactions and endogenous cortisol. J. Immunol. Meth. 82:17–24.

Inoue, T., H. Saito, R. Fukushima, T. Inaba, M.T. Lin, K. Fukatsu, and T. Muto. 1995. Growth hormone and insulin-like growth factor I enhance host defense in a murine sepsis model. Arch. Surg. 130:1115–1122.

IOM (Institute of Medicine). 1991. Fluid Replacement and Heat Stress, 3d printing., B.M. Marriott, ed. A report of the Committee on Military Nutrition Research, Food and Nutrition Board. Washington, D.C.: National Academy Press.

IOM (Institute of Medicine). 1992a. Emerging Infections: Microbial Threats to Health in the United States, J. Lederberg, R.E. Shope, and S.C. Oaks Jr., eds. Committee on

Emerging Microbial Threats Health, Division of Health Sciences Policy, Division of International Health. Washington, D.C.: National Academy Press.

IOM (Institute of Medicine). 1992b. A Nutritional Assessment of U.S. Army Ranger Training Class 11/91. A brief report of the Committee on Military Nutrition Research, Food and Nutrition Board, March 23. Washington, D.C.: National Academy Press.

IOM (Institute of Medicine). 1993a. Nutritional Needs in Hot Environments, Applications for Military Personnel in Field Operations, B.M. Marriott, ed. A report of the Committee on Military Nutrition Research, Food and Nutrition Board, Washington, D.C.: National Academy Press.

IOM (Institute of Medicine). 1993b. Review of the Results of Nutritional Intervention, Ranger Training Class 11/92 (Ranger II), B.M. Marriott, ed. A report of the Committee on Military Nutrition Research, Food and Nutrition Board. Washington, D.C.: National Academy Press.

IOM (Institute of Medicine). 1994. Fluid Replacement and Heat Stress, 3d ed., B.M. Marriott, ed. A report of the Committee on Military Nutrition Research, Food and Nutrition Board. Washington, D.C.: National Academy Press.

IOM (Institute of Medicine). 1995a. Not Eating Enough, Overcoming Underconsumption of Military Operational Rations, B.M. Marriott, ed. A report of the Committee on Military Nutrition Research, Food and Nutrition Board. Washington, D.C.: National Academy Press.

IOM (Institute of Medicine). 1995b. A Review of Issues Related to Iron Status of Women During U.S. Army Basic Combat Training [letter report]. Committee on Military Nutrition Research, Food and Nutrition Board. December 19. Washington, D.C.

IOM (Institute of Medicine). 1996. Nutritional Needs in Cold and in High-Altitude Environments, Applications for Military Personnel in Field Operations, B.M. Marriott and S.J. Carlson, eds. A report of the Committee on Military Nutrition Research, Food and Nutrition Board. Washington, D.C.: National Academy Press.

IOM (Institute of Medicine). 1997. Emerging Technologies for Nutrition Research, Potential for Assessing Military Performance Capability, S.J. Carlson-Newberry and R.B. Costello, eds. A report of the Committee on Military Nutrition Research, Food and Nutrition Board. Washington, D.C.: National Academy Press.

Irwin, M., J. McClintick, C. Costlow, M. Fortner, J. White, and J.C. Gillin. 1996. Partial night sleep deprivation reduces natural killer and cellular immune responses in humans. FASEB J. 10:643–653.

Irwin, M.T., R.L. Hauger, L. Jones, M. Provencio, and K.T. Britton. 1990. Sympathetic nervous system mediates central corticotropin-releasing factor induced suppression of natural killer cytotoxicity. J. Pharmacol. Exp. Ther. 255:101–107.

Isenberg, D.A., A.J. Guisp, W.J.W. Morrow, D. Newham, and M.L. Snaith. 1981. Variations in circulating immune complex levels with diet, exercise, and sleep: A comparison between normal controls and patients with systemic lupus erythematosis. Ann. Rheum. Dis. 40:466–469.

Israel-Biet, D., F. Labrousse, J.M. Tourani, H. Sors, J.M. Andrieu, and P. Even. 1992. Elevation of IgE in HIV-infected subjects: A marker of poor prognosis. J. Allergy Clin. Immunol. 89:68–75.

Jacob, R.A., D.S. Kelley, F.S. Pianalto, M.E. Swendseid, S.M. Henning, J.Z. Zhang, B.N. Ames, C.G. Fraga, and J.H. Peters. 1991. Immunocompetence and oxidant defense during ascorbate depletion of healthy men. Am. J. Clin. Nutr. 54:1302S–1309S.

Jacobs, D.O., D.A. Evans, K. Mealy, S.T. O'Dwyer, R.J. Smith, and D.W. Wilmore. 1988. Combined effects of glutamine and epidermal growth factor on the rat intestine. Surgery 104:358–364.

James, J.A., and M. Combes. 1960. Iron deficiency in the premature infant. Pediatrics 26:368–373.

Jeng, K-C.G., C-S. Yang, W-Y. Siu, Y-S. Tsai, W-J. Liao, and J-S. Kuo. 1996. Supplementation with vitamins C and E enhances cytokine production by peripheral blood mononuclear cells in healthy adults. Am. J. Clin. Nutr. 64:960–965.

Jepson, M.M., P.C. Bates, P. Broadbent, J.M. Pell, and D.J. Millward. 1988. Relationship between glutamine concentration and protein synthesis in rat skeletal muscle. Am. J. Physiol. 255:E166–E172.

Johnson, G., P. Jacobs, and L.R. Purves. 1983. Iron-binding proteins of iron-absorbing rat intestinal mucosa. J. Clin. Invest. 71:1467–1476.

Johnson, H.L., H.J. Krzywicki, J.E. Canham, J.H. Skala, T.A. Daws, R.A. Nelson, C.F. Consolazio, and P.P. Waring. 1976. Evaluation of calorie requirements for Ranger training at Fort Benning, Georgia. Technical Report No. 34. Presidio of San Francisco, Calif.: Letterman Army Institute of Research.

Johnson, H.M., M.O. Downs, and C.H. Pontzer. 1992. Neuroendocrine peptide hormone regulation of immunity [Review]. Chemical Immunology 52:49–83.

Johnson, H.M., E.M. Smith, B.A. Torres, and J.E. Blalock. 1982. Neuroendocrine hormone regulation of in vitro antibody production. Proc. Natl. Acad. Sci. USA 79:4171–4174.

Jones, D.G. 1984. Effects of dietary copper depletion on acute and delayed inflammatory responses in mice. Res. Vet. Sci. 37:205–210.

Jones, R.L., C.M. Peterson, R.W. Grady, T. Kumbaraci, and A. Cerami. 1977. Effects of iron chelators and iron overload on Salmonella infection. Nature 267:63–64.

Joshi, J.G., and A. Zimmerman. 1988. Ferritin: An expanded role in metabolic regulation. Toxicology 48:21–29.

Jouvet, M. 1984. Neuromediateurs et facteurs hypnogenes. Rev. Neurol. 140:389–400.

Joynson, D.H.M., A. Jacobs, D.M. Walker, and A.F. Dolby. 1972. Defect in cell-mediated immunity in patients with iron-deficiency anaemia. Lancet 2:1058–159.

Ju, G., X. Zhang, B.Q. Jin, and C.S. Huang. 1991. Activation of corticotropin-releasing factor containing neurons in the paraventricular nucleus of the hypothalamus by interleukin-1 in the rat. Neurosci. Lett. 132:151–154.

Juretic, A., G.C. Spagnoli, H. Hörig, R. Babst, K. von Bremen, F. Harder, and M. Heberer. 1994. Glutamine requirements in the generation of lymphokine-activated killer cells. Clin. Nutr. 13:42–49.

Kadiiska, M.A., P.M. Hanna, S.J. Jordan, and R.P. Mason. 1993. Electron spin resonance evidence for free radical generation in copper-treated vitamin E- and selenium-deficient rats: In vivo spin-trapping investigation. Molec. Pharmacol. 44:222–227.

Kagnoff, M.F. 1993. Immunology of the intestinal tract. Gastroenterology 105(5):1275–1280.

Kakucska, I., L.I. Romero, B.D. Clark, J.M. Rondeel, Y. Qi, S. Alex, C.H. Emerson, and R.M. Lechan. 1994. Suppression of thyrotropin-releasing hormone gene expression by interleukin-1β in the rat: Implications for nonthyroidal illness. Neuroendocrinology 59:129–137.

Kakuscska, I., Y. Qi, B.D. Clark, and R.M. Lechan. 1993. Endotoxin-induced corticotropin-releasing hormone gene expression in the hypothalamic paraventricular nucleus is mediated centrally by interleukin-1. Endocrinology 133:815–821.

Kammler, M., C. Schon, and K. Hantke. 1993. Characterization of the ferrous iron uptake system of Escherichia coli. J. Bacteriol. 175:6212–6219.

Kandil, H.M., R.A. Argenzio, W. Chen, H.M. Berschneider, A.D. Stiles, J.K. Westwick, R.A. Rippe, D.A. Brenner, and J.M. Rhoads. 1995. l-Glutamine and L-asparagine stimulate ODC activity and proliferation in a porcine jejunal enterocyte line. Am. J. Physiol. 269:G591–G599.

Kant, G.J., R.H. Pastel, R.A. Bauman, G.R. Meininger, K.R. Maughan, T.N. Robinson III, W.L. Wright, and P.S. Covington. 1995. Effects of chronic stress on sleep in rats. Physiol. Behav. 57:359–365.

Kanter, M.M., L.A. Nolte, and J.O. Holloszy. 1993. Effects of an antioxidant vitamin mixture on lipid peroxidation at rest and postexercise. J. Appl. Physiol. 74:965–969.

Kapcala, L.P., T. Chautard, and R.L. Eskay. 1995. The protective role of the hypothalamic–pituitary–adrenal axis against lethality produced by immune, infectious, and inflammatory stress. Ann. N. Y. Acad. Sci. 771:419–437.

Kapcala, L.P., J.R. He, Y. Gao, J.O. Pieper, and L.J. DeTolla. 1996. Subdiaphragmatic vagotomy inhibits intra-abdominal interleukin-1β stimulation of adrenocorticotropin secretion. Brain Res. 728:247–254.

Karter, D.L., A.J. Karter, R. Yarrish, C. Patterson, P.H. Kass, J. Nord, and J.W. Kislak. 1995. Vitamin A deficiency in non-vitamin-supplemented patients with AIDS: A cross-sectional study. J. Acquir. Immune Defic. Syndr. Hum. Retrovirol. 8:199–203.

Katila, H., K. Cantell, B. Appelberg, and R. Rimon. 1993. Is there a seasonal variation in the interferon-producing capacity of healthy subjects? J. Interferon Res. 13:233–234.

Katsuura, G., A. Arimura, K. Koves, and P.E. Gottschall. 1990. Involvement of organum vasculosum of lamina terminalis and preoptic area in interleukin 1β-induced ACTH release. Am. J. Physiol. 258:E163–E173.

Kay, J.E., and C.R. Benzie. 1986. The role of the transferrin receptor in lymphocyte activation. Immunol. Lett. 12:55–58.

Kaye, D., F.A. Gill, and E.W. Hook. 1967. Factors influencing host resistance to *Salmonella* infections: The effects of hemolysis and erythrophagocytosis. Am. J. Med. Sci. 254:205–215.

Kehrer, P., D. Turnill, J.M. Dayer, A.F. Muller, and R.C. Gaillard. 1988. Human recombinant interleukin-1β and -α, but not recombinant tumor necrosis factor-α, stimulate ACTH release from rat anterior pituitary cells in vitro in a prostaglandin E_2 and cAMP independent manner. Neuroendocrinology 48:160–166.

Kelley, D.S., and P.A. Daudu. 1993. Fat intake and immune response. Prog. Food Nutr. Sci. 17:41–63.

Kelley, D.S., L.B. Branch, and J.M. Iacono. 1989. Nutritional modulation of human status. Nutr. Res. 9:965–975.

Kelley, D.S., L.B. Branch, J.E. Love, P.C. Taylor, Y.M. Rivera, and J.M. Iacono. 1991. Dietary α-linolenic acid and immunocompetence in humans. Am. J. Clin. Nutr. 53:40–46.

Kelley, D.S., P.A. Daudu, L.B. Branch, H.L. Johnson, P.C. Taylor, and B. Mackey. 1994. Energy restriction decreases number of circulating natural killer cells and serum levels of immunoglobulins in overweight women. Eur. J. clin. Nutr. 48(1):9-18.

Kelley, D.S., P.A. Daudu, P.C. Taylor, B.E. Mackeuy, and J.R. Turnland. 1995. Effects of low-copper diets on human immune response. Am. J. Clin. Nutr. 62:412–416.

Kelley, D.S., R.M. Dougherthy, L.B. Branch, P.C. Taylor, and J.M. Iacono. 1992.a Concentration of dietary n-6 polyunsaturated fatty acids and human status. Clin. Immunol. Immunopath. 62:240–244.

Kelley, D.S., G.J. Nelson, L.B. Branch, P.C. Taylor, U.M. Rivera, and P.C. Schmidt. 1992b. Salmon diet and human immune status. Eur. J. Clin. Nutr. 46:397–404.

Kelley, D.S., G.J. Nelson, J.E. Love, L.B. Branch, P.C. Taylor, P.C. Schmidt, B.E. Mackey, and J.M. Iacono. 1993. Dietary α-linolenic acid alters tissue fatty acid composition, but not blood lipids, lipoproteins or coagulation status in humans. Lipids 28:533–537.

Kelley, D.S., P.C. Taylor, G.J. Nelson, P.C. Schmidt, and B.E. Mackey. 1996. Effects of dietary arachidonic acid on human response. FASEB J. 10:A557.

Kelley, D.S., P.C. Taylor, G.J. Nelson, P.C. Schmidt, and B.E. Mackey. 1997. Effects of dietary arachidonic acid on human response. Lipids 32:449–456.

Kelly, D.A., E. Price, V. Wright, M. Rossiter, and J.A. Walker-Smith. 1987. *Yersinia enterocolitica* in iron overload. J. Pediatr. Gastroenterol. Nutr. 6:643–645.

Kelso, A., and A. Munck. 1984. Glucocorticoid inhibition of lymphokine secretion by alloreactive T-lymphocyte clones. J. Immunol. 133:784–791.

Kemp, J.D., J.A. Thorson, T. McAlmont, M. Horowitz, J.S. Cowdery, and Z.K. Ballas. 1987. Role of the transferrin receptor in lymphocyte growth: A rat IgG monoclonal antibody against the murine transferrin receptor produces highly selective inhibition of T- and B-cell activation protocols. J. Immunol. 138:2422–2426.

Kennes, B., I. Dumont, D. Brohee, C. Hubert, and P. Neve. 1983. Effect of vitamin C supplements on cell-mediated immunity in old people. Gerontology 29:305–310.

Kern, J.A., R.J. Lamb, J.C. Reed, R.P. Daniele, and P.C. Nowell. 1988. Dexamethasone inhibition of interleukin-1β production by human monocytes. Postranscriptional Mechanisms. J. Clin. Invest. 81:237–244.

Keusch, G.T. 1994. Nutrition and infection. Pp. 1241–1258 in Modern Nutrition in Health and Diseasea, 8th ed., M.E. Shils, J.A. Olson, and M. Shike, eds. Malvern, Pa.: Lea and Febiger.

Keusch, G.T., and M.J.G. Farthing. 1986. Nutrition and infection. Annu. Rev. Nutr. 6:131–154.

Keusch, G.T., C.S. Wilson, and S.D. Waksall. 1983. Nutrition, host defenses and the lymphoid system. Arch. Host Def. Mech. 2:275–359.

Khan, A.J., C. Lee, J.A. Wolff, H. Chang, P. Khan, and H.E. Evans. 1983. Defects of neutrophil chemotaxis and random migration in thalassemia major. Pediatrics 60:349–351.

Khansari, D.N., A.J. Murgo, and R.E. Faith. 1990. Effects of stress on the immune system. Immunol. Today 11:170–175.

Khaw, K.T., P. Woodhouse. 1995. Interrelation of vitamin C, infection, haemostatic factors, and cardiovascular disease. BMJ 310(6994):1559–1563.

Kiecolt-Glaser, J.K., and R. Glaser. 1991. Stress and immune function in humans. Pp. 849–864 in Psychoneuroimmunology, R. Ader, D.L. Felten, and N. Cohen, eds. Boston: Academic Press.

Kiecolt-Glaser, J.K., R. Glaser, S. Gravenstein, W.B. Malarkey, and J. Sheridan. 1996. Chronic stress alters the immune response to influenza virus vaccine in older adults. Proc. Natl. Acad. Sci. USA 93:3042–3047.

Kiecolt-Glaser, J.K., P.T. Marucha, W.B. Malarkey, A.M. Mercado, and R. Glaser. 1995. Slowing of wound healing by psychological stress. Lancet 346:1194–1196.

Kim, Y., M. Pallansch, F. Carandente, G. Reissmann, E. Halberg, and F. Halberg. 1980. Circadian and circannual aspects of the complement cascade—new and old results, differing in specificity? Chronobiologia 7:189–204.

Kimata, H., and A. Yoshida. 1994. Differential effect of growth hormone and insulin-like growth factor-I, insulin-like growth factor-II, and insulin on Ig production and growth in human plasma cells. Blood 83:1569–1574.

Kimball, H.R., M.B. Lipsett, W.D. Odell, and S.M. Wolff. 1968. Comparison of the effects of the pyrogens, etiocholanolone and bacterial endotoxin on plasma cortisol and growth hormone in man. J. Clin. Endocrinol. Metab. 28:337–342

Kirchner, H., C. Kleinicke, and W. Digel. 1982. A whole-blood technique for testing production of human interferon by leukocytes. J. Immunol. Meth. 48:213–219.

Kiremidjian-Schumacher, L.O., and G. Stotzky. 1987. Selenium and immune responses. Environ. Res. 42:277–303.

Kirk, S.J., and A. Barbul. 1992. Arginine and immunity. Pp. 160–161 in Encyclopedia of Immunology, Book I, I.M. Roitt and P.J. Delves, eds. London: Academic Press.

Kirk, S.J., M.C. Regan, H.L. Wasserkrug, M. Sodeyama, and A. Barbul. 1992. Arginine enhances T-cell responses in athymic nude mice. J. Parenter. Enter. Nutr. 16:429–432.

Kirkpatrick, C.H. 1988. Delayed hypersensitivity. Pp. 261–277 in Immunological Diseases, M. Sampter, D.W. Talmage, M.M. Frank, K.F. Austem, and H.N. Claman, eds. Boston and Toronto: Little, Brown.

Kirkwood, B.J. 1996. Epidemiology of interventions to improve vitamin A status in order to reduce child mortality and morbidity. In Beyond Nutritional Recommendations: Implementing Science for Healthier Populations, C. Garza, J.D. Haas, J-P. Habicht, and D.L. Pelletier, eds. Proceedings from the 14th Annual Bristol-Myers Squibb/Mead Johnson Nutrition Research Symposium, June 5–7, 1995. Ithaca, N.Y.: Cornell University.

Kishida, T., M. Kita, M. Yamaji, E. Kaneta, and T. Teramatsu. 1987. Interferon-producing capacity in patients with liver diseases, diabetes mellitus, chronic diseases, and malignant diseases. Pp. 435–441 in The Biology of the Interferon System 1986, K. Cantel and H. Schellekens, eds. Dordrecht: Martinus Nijhoff Publishers.

Kjolhede, C., and W.R. Beisel. 1995. Vitamin A and the immune function: A symposium. J. Nutr. Immunol. 4:xv–143.

Klausner, R. D., T.A. Roualt, and J.B. Harford. 1993. Regulating the fate of mRNA: The control of cellular iron metabolism. Cell 72:19–28.

Klicka, M.V., D.E. Sherman, N. King, K.E. Friedl, and E.W. Askew. 1993. Nutritional assessment of cadets at the U.S. Military Academy: Part 2. Assessment of nutritional intake. Technical Report No. T94-1. Natick, Mass.: U.S. Army Research Institute of Environmental Medicine.

Knapp, M.S., N.P. Byron, R. Pownall, and P. Mayor. 1980. Time of day of taking immunosuppressive agents after renal transplantation. Br. Med. J. 281:1382–1385.

Knapp, M.S., R. Pownall, and J.R. Cove-Smith. 1981. Circadian variations in cell-mediated immunity and in the timing of human allograft rejection. Pp. 329–338 in Chronopharmacology and Chronotherapeutics, C.A. Walker, C.M. Winget, and K.F.A. Soliman, eds. Tallahassee, Fla.: A&M University Foundation.

Kniker, W.T., C.T. Anderson, and M. Roumiantzeff. 1979. The MULTITESTR system: A standardized approach to evaluation of delayed-type hypersensitivity and cell-mediated immunity. Ann. Allergy 43:73–79.

Knox, J., R. Demling, D. Wilmore, P. Sarraf, and A. Santos. 1995. Increased survival after major thermal injury: The effect of growth hormone therapy in adults. J. Trauma 39:526–530.

Knudsen, P.J., C.A. Dinarello, and T.B. Strom. 1987. Glucocorticoids inhibit transcriptional and post-transcriptional expression of IL-1 in U93F cells. J. Immunol. 139:4129–4134.

Kochanowski, B.A., and A.R. Sherman. 1985. Decreased antibody formation in iron-deficient rat pups—Effect of iron repletion. Am. J. Clin. Nutr. 41:278–284.

Koenig, J.I. 1991. Presence of cytokines in the hypothalamic-pituitary axis. Prog. Neuroendocrin. Immunol. 4:143–153.

Koenig, J.I., K. Snow, B.D. Clark, R. Toni, J.G. Cannon, A.R. Shaw, C.A. Dinarello, S. Reichlin, S.L. Lee, and R.M. Lechan. 1990. Intrinsic pituitary interleukin-1β is induced by bacterial lipopolysaccharide. Endocrinology 126(6):3053–3058.

Kojima, T., T. Terano, E. Tanabe, S. Okamoto, Y. Tamura, and S. Yoshida. 1989. Effect of highly purified eicosapentaenoic acid on psoriasis. J. Am. Acad. Dermatol. 21:150–151.

Koller, L.D., S.A. Mulhern, N.C. Frankel, M.G. Steven, and J.R. Williams. 1987. Immune dysfunction in rats fed a diet deficient in copper. Am. J. Clin. Nutr. 45:997–1006.

Kono, I., H. Kitao, M. Matsuda, S. Haga, H. Fukushima, and H. Kashiwagi. 1988. Weight reduction in athletes may adversely affect the phagocytic function of monocytes. Physician Sportsmed. 16(7):56–65.

Konopka, R.J. 1979. Genetic dissection of the *Drosophila* circadian system. Fed. Proc. 38:2602–2605.

Kontoghiorghies, G.J., and E.D. Weinberg. 1995. Iron: Mammalian defense systems, mechanisms of disease, and chelation therapy approaches. Blood Rev. 9:33–45.

Kopp, W.C., and J.T. Holmlund. 1996. Cytokines and immunological monitoring. Cancer Chemother. Biol. Response Modif. 16:189–238.

Kopp, W.C., J.T. Holmlund, and W.J. Urba. 1994. Immunologic monitoring and clinical trials of biological response modifiers. Cancer Chemother. Biol. Response Modif. 15:226–286.

Koren, S., and W.R. Fleischmann. 1993. Circadian variations in myelosuppressive activity of interferon-α in mice: Identification of an optimal treatment time associated with reduced myelosuppressive activity. Exp. Hematol. 21:552–559.

Kort, W.J., and J.M. Weijma. 1982. Effect of chronic light-dark shift stress on the immune response of the rat. Physiol. Behav. 29:1083–1087.

Koshland Jr., D.E. 1992. Science's 1992 molecule of the year [editorial]. Science 258:1861.

Kragh Jr., J.F. 1993. Use of knee and elbow pads during Ranger training. Mil Med. 158:A4.

Kramer, T.R. 1992. Support between USAMRDC and USDA for cooperative research under the Ration Sustainment Testing Program. Final report 1 July 1991–30 September 1991. Washington, D.C.: U.S. Department of Agriculture.

Kramer, T.R. 1994. Immune function I: Lymphocyte proliferation and subset analysis; Interleukin production. Chapter 9 in Nutritional and Immunological Assessment of Ranger Students with Increased Caloric Intake. Technical Report T95-5. Natick, Mass.: U.S. Army Research Institute of Environmental Medicine.

Kramer, T.R. 1996. Effects of various doses of vegetables on immune response and other health parameters in humans. USAMRMC Interagency Agreement C20M6770; ARS Agreement 60-3K47-6-060. Fredrick, Md.: U.S. Army Medical Research and Materiel Command.

Kramer, T.R., and B.J. Burri. 1997. Modulated mitogenic proliferative responsiveness of lymphocytes in whole-blood cultures by low carotene diet and mixed-carotenoid supplementation of women. Am. J. Clin. Nutr. 65:871–875.

Kramer, T.R., and M.M. Chan. 1994. Use of whole-blood cultures to monitor mitogenic responsiveness (MR) of lymphocytes in HIV+ children. FASEB J. 8:A494.

Kramer, T.R., K.E. Friedl, and R.L. Shippee. 1995. Effects of caloric restriction in high-energy demanding U.S. Army training on T-lymphocyte functions in soldiers. Presentation to the 2nd International Society of Exercise and Immunology Convention, Brussels, Belgium, November 17–18.

Kramer, T.R., M.P. Howard, and J. Chittams. In press. Mitogen-induced T-lymphocyte proliferation in whole-blood cultures: Optimization based on activity and variation. J. Nutr. Immunol.

Kramer, T.R., R.J. Moore, R.L. Shippee, K.E. Friedl, L. Martinez-Lopez, M.M. Chan, and E.W. Askew. 1997. Effects of food restriction in military training on T-lymphocyte responses. Int. J. Sports Med. 18:S84–S90.

Kramer, T.R., K. Praputpittaya, Y. Yuttabootr, R. Singkamani, and M. Trakultivakorn. 1990. The relationship between plasma zinc and cellular immunity to *Candida albicans* in young females of northern Thailand. Ann. N.Y. Acad. Sci. 587:300–302.

Kramer, T.R., N. Schoene, L.W. Douglass, J.T. Judd, R. Ballard-Barbash, P.R. Taylor, H.N. Bhagavan, and P.P. Nair. 1991. Increased vitamin E intake restores fish-oil-induced suppressed blastogenesis of mitogen-simulated T-lymphocytes. Am. J. Clin. Nutr. 54:896–902.

Kramer, T.R., E. Udomkesmalee, S. Dhanamitta, S. Sirisinha, S. Charoenkiatkul, S. Tuntipopipat, O. Banjong, N. Rojroongwasinkul, and J.C. Smith, Jr. 1993. Lymphocyte responsiveness of children supplemented with vitamin A and zinc. Am. J. Clin. Nutr. 58:566–570.

Krantman, H.J., S.R. Young, B.J. Ank, C.M. O'Donnell, G.S. Rachelefsky, and G.S.Stiehm. 1982. Immune function in pure iron deficiency. Am. J. Dis. Child. 136:840–844.

Kremer, J.M., D.A. Lawrence, G.F. Petrillo, L.L. Litts, P.M. Mullaly, R.I. Rynes, R.P. Stocker, N. Parhami, N.S. Greenstein, B.R. Fuchs, A. Mathur, D.R. Robinson, R.I. Sperling, and J. Bigaouette. 1995. Effects of high-dose fish oil on rheumatoid arthritis after stopping nonsteroidal anti-inflammatory drugs. Arthritis Rheum. 38:1107–1114.

Krishnamurti, C., and B. Alving. 1989. Effect of dengue virus on procoagulant and fibrinolytic activities of monocytes. Rev. Infect. Dis. 11(suppl. 4):S843–S846.

Krishnan, S., U.N. Bhuyan, G.P. Talwar, and V. Ramalingaswami. 1974. Effect of vitamin A and protein-calorie undernutrition on immune responses. Immunology 27:383–397.

Kronke, M., W.J. Leonard, J.M. Depper, and W.C. Greene. 1985. Sequential expression of genes involved in human T-lymphocyte growth and differentiation. J. Exp. Med. 161:1593–1598.

Krueger, J.M. 1990. Somnogenic activity of immune response modifiers. Trends Pharmacol. Sci. 11(3):122–126.

Krueger, J.M., C.A. Dinarello, and L. Chedid. 1983. Promotion of slow wave sleep (SWS) by a purified Interleukin-1(IL-1) preparation [abstract]. Fed. Proc. 42:356.

Krueger, J.M., J.R. Pappenheimer, and M.L. Karnovsky. 1982. The composition of sleep-promoting factor isolated from human urine. J. Biol. Chem. 25:1664–1669.

Krueger, J.M., L.A. Toth, R. Floyd, J. Fang, L. Kapas, S. Bredow, and F. Obal, Jr. 1994. Sleep, microbes and cytokines. Neuroimmunomodulation 1:100–109.

Krueger, J.M., E.J. Walter, C.A. Dinarello, S.M. Wolff, and L. Chedid. 1984. Sleep-promoting effects of endogenous pyrogen (Interleukin-1). Am. J. Physiol. 246:R994–R999.

Kruger, T.E., L.R. Smith, D.V. Harbour, and J.E. Blalock. 1989. Thyrotropin: An endogenous regulator of the *in vitro* immune response. J. Immunol. 142:744–747.

Kruse-Jarres, J.D. 1989. The significance of zinc for humoral and cellular immunity. J. Trace Elem. Electrolytes Health Dis. 3:1–8.

Krzystyniak, K., H. Tryphonas, and M. Fournier. 1995. Approaches to the evaluation of chemical-induced immunotoxicity. Environ. Health Perspect. 103(suppl. 9):17–22.

Kubes, P., M. Suzuki, and D.N. Granger. 1991. Nitric oxide: An endogenous modulator of leukocyte adhesion. Proc. Natl. Acad. Sci. U.S.A. 88:4651–4655.

Kubo, K., M. Hanaoka, T. Hayano, T. Miyahara, T. Hachiya, M. Hayasaka, T. Koizumi, K. Fujimoto, T. Kobayashi, and T. Honda. 1998. Inflammatory cytokines in BAL fluid and pulmonary hemodynamics in high-altitude pulmonary edema. Respir. Physiol. 111:301–310.

Kuby, J. 1994. Immunology. New York: W.H. Freeman and Company.

Kuby, J. 1997. Immunology, 3d ed. New York: WH Freeman and Company.

Kudsk, K.A., G. Minard, M.A. Croce, R.O. Brown, T.S. Lowrey, F.E. Pritchard, R.N. Dickerson, and T.C. Fabian. 1996. A randomized trial of isonitrogenous enteral diets after severe trauma. An immune-enhancing diet reduces septic complications. Ann. Surg. 224(4):531-40; discussion 540–543.

Kulapongs, P., V. Vithayasai, R. Suskind, and R.E. Olson. 1974. Cell-mediated immunity and phagocytosis and killing function in children with severe iron-deficiency anemia. Lancet 2:689–691.

Kunkel, G., and L. Jusuf. 1984. Theoretical and practical aspects of circadian rhythm for theophylline therapy. Pp. 149–155 in New Perspectives in Theophylline Therapy, M. Turner-Warwick and J. Levy, eds. London: Royal Society of Medicine.

Kusnecov, A.W., and B.S. Rabin. 1994. Stressor-induced alterations of immune function: Mechanisms and issues. Int. Arch. Allergy Immunol. 105:107–121.

Kuvibidila, S., and S. Wade. 1987. Macrophage function as studied by the clearance of ^{125}I-labeled polyvinylpyrrolidone in iron-deficient and iron replete mice. J. Nutr. 117:170–176.

Kuvibidila, S., M. Dardenne, W. Savino, and F. Lepault. 1990. Influence of iron-deficiency anemia on selected thymus functions in mice: Thymulin biological activity, T-cell subsets,.and thymocyte proliferation. Am. J. Clin. Nutr. 51:228–232.

Lacey, J.M., and D.W. Wilmore. 1990. Is glutamine a conditionally essential amino acid? Nutr. Rev. 48(8):297–309.

Lacey, J.M., J.B. Crouch, K. Benfell, S.A. Ringer, C.K. Wilmore, D. Maguire, and D.W. Wilmore. 1996. The effects of glutamine-supplemented parenteral nutrition in premature infants. JPEN J. Parenter. Enteral Nutr. 20:74–80.

Lakatua, D.J. 1994. Molecular and genetic aspects of chronobiology. Pp. 65–77 in Biologic Rhythms in Clinical and Laboratory Medicine, 2d ed., Y. Touitou and E. Haus, eds. Heidelberg: Springer-Verlag.

Lakatua, D.J., E. Haus, K. Labrosse, C. Veit, and L. Sackett-Lundeen. 1986. Circadian rhythm in mammary cytoplasmic estrogen receptor content of Balb/C female mice with and without pituitary isografts. Chronobiol. Int. 3(4):213–219.

Lakatua, D.J., M. White, L.L. Sackett-Lundeen, and E. Haus. 1983. Change in phase relations of circadian rhythms in cell proliferation induced by time-limited feeding in Balb/C x D8A/2F1 mice bearing a transplantable Harding-Passey tumor. Cancer Res. 43:4068–4072.

Lalonde, R. and T. Boetz-Marquard. 1997. The neurobiological basis of movement initiation.Rev. Neurosci. 8(1):35–54.

Lambert, M. 1994. Thyroid dysfunction in HIV infection. Baillieres Clin. Endocrinol. Metab. 8:825–835.

Landreth, K.S., R. Narayanan, and K. Dorshkind. 1992. Insulin-like growth factor I regulates pro-B-cell differentiation. Blood 80:1207–1212.

Lands, W.E. 1991. Biosynthesis of prostaglandins. Annu. Rev. Nutr. 11:41–60.

Langlois, P.H., M.H. Smolensky, W.P. Glezen, and W.A. Keitel. 1995. Diurnal variation in responses to influenza vaccine. Chronobiol. Int. 12:28–36.

Lanier, L., J.H. Phillips, J. Hackett Jr., M. Tutt, and V. Kumar. 1986. Natural killer cells: Definition of a cell type rather than a function. J. Immunol. 137: 2735–2739.

LaPerriere, A.R., M.A. Fletcher, M.H. Antoni, N.G. Klimas, G. Ironson, and N. Schneiderman. 1991. Aerobic exercise training in an AIDS risk group. Int. J. Sports Med. 12(suppl. 1):S53–S57.

Larsen, H.S. 1988. Effects of selenium on sheep lymphocyte responses to mitogens. Res. Vet. Sci. 45:11–18.

Larsen, J.H., and S. Tollersrund. 1981. Effects of dietary vitamin E and selenium on phytohaemagglutinin response and pig lymphocytes. Res. Vet. Sci. 31:301–305.

Lash, A., and A. Saleem. 1995. Iron metabolism and its regulation. A review. Ann. Clin. Lab. Sci. 25(1):20–30.

Lavie, P., and B. Weller. 1989. Timing of naps: Effects on post-nap sleepiness levels. EEG Clin. Neurophysiol. 72:218–224.

Lawless, D., C.G.R. Jackson, and J.E. Greenleaf. 1995. Exercise and human immunodeficiency virus (HIV-1) infection. Sports Med. 19:235–239.

Lawrence, R., and T. Sorrell. 1993. Eicosapentaenoic acid in cystic fibrosis. Lancet 342:465–469.

Laye, S., R.M. Bluthe, S. Kent, C. Combe, C. Medina, P. Parnet, K. Kelly, and R. Dantzer. 1995. Subdiaphragmatic vagotomy blocks induction of IL-1β mRNA in mice brain in response to peripheral LPS. Am. J. Physiol. 268:R1327–R1331.

Lechan, R.M., R. Toni, B.D. Clark, J.G. Cannon, A.R. Shaw, C.A. Dinarello, and S. Reichlin. 1990. Immunoreactive interleukin-1β localization in the rat forebrain. Brain Res. 514:135–140.

LeDuc, J.W. 1989. Epidemiology of hemorrhagic fever viruses. Rev. Infect. Dis. 11(suppl. 4):S730–S735.

Lee, C., P. Vaishali, T. Itsukaichi, B. Kiho, and I. Edery. 1996. Resetting the *Drosophila* clock by photic regulation of PER and a PER-TIM complex. Science 271:1740–1744.

Lee, D.J., R.T. Meehan, C. Robinson, T.R. Mabry, and M.L. Smith. 1992. Immune responsiveness and risk of illness in U.S. Air Force Academy cadets during basic cadet training. Aviat. Space Environ. Med. 63:517–523.

Lee, D.J., R.T. Meehan, C. Robinson, M.L. Smith, and T.R. Mabry. 1995. Psychosocial correlates of immune responsiveness and illness episodes in U.S. Air Force Academy cadets undergoing basic cadet training. J. Psychosom. Res. 39:445–457.

Lee, R.E., M.H. Smolensky, C.S. Leach, and J.P. McGovern. 1977. Circadian rhythms in the cutaneous reactivity to histamine and selected antigens, including phase relationship to urinary cortisol excretion. Ann. Allergy 38(4):231-6.

Lee, S., and C. Rivier. 1994. Hypophysiotropic role and hypothalamic gene expression of corticotropin-releasing factor and vasopressin in rats injected with interleukin-1 systemically or into the brain ventricles. Neuroendocrinology 6:217–224.

Lee, S.W., A.P. Tsou, H. Chan, J. Thomas, K. Petrie, E.M. Eugui, and A.C. Allison. 1988. Glucocorticoids selectively inhibit the transcription of the interleukin-1β gene and decrease the stability of interleukin-1β mRNA. Proc. Natl. Acad. Sci. USA 85:1204–1208.

Lee, T.H., R.L. Hoover, J.D. Williams, R.I. Sperling, J. Ravalese, B.W. Spur, D.R. Robinson, E.J. Corey, R.A. Lewis, and K.F. Austen. 1985. Effect of dietary enrichment with eicosapentaenoic acid and docosahexaenoic acids on in vitro neutrophil and monocyte leukotriene generation and neutrophil function. N. Engl. J. Med. 312:1217–1224.

Leibold, E.A., and H.N. Munro. 1988. Cytoplasmic protein binds in vitro to a highly conserved sequence in the 5' untranslated region of ferritin heavy- and light-subunit mRNAs. Proc. Natl. Acad. Sci. USA 85:2171–2175.

Lemmer, B., ed. 1989. Chronopharmacology, Cellular, and Biochemical Interactions.. New York: Marcel Dekker.

Lemmer, B., U. Schwulera, A. Thrun, and R. Lissner. 1992. Circadian rhythm of soluble interleukin-2 receptor in healthy individuals. Eur. Cytokine Netw. 3:335–336.

Leroux, M., L. Schindler, R. Braun, H.W. Doerr, H.P. Geisen, and H. Kirchner. 1985. A whole-blood lymphoproliferative assay for measuring cellular immunity against herpes viruses. J. Immunol. Meth. 79:251–262.

Leslie, K. 1989. Clinical and experimental aspects of viral myocarditis. Clin. Microbiol. Rev. 2:191–197.

Lesourd, B.M., R. Moulias, M. Favre-Beffone, and C.H. Rapin. 1992. Nutritional influences on immune responses in the elderly. Pp. 211–224 in Nutrition and Immunology, R.K. Chandra, ed. St. John's, Newfoundland: ARTS Biomedical Publishers.

Levi, F. 1994. Chronotherapy of cancer: Biological basis and clinical application. Pathol. Biol. (Paris) 42:338–341.

Levi, F. 1996a. Chronotherapy for gastrointestinal cancers. Curr. Opin. Oncol. 8:334–341.

Levi, F. 1996b. Chronopharmacologie et chronothérapie des cancers. Path. Biol. 44:631–644.

Levi, F. 1997. Chronopharmacology of Anticancer Agents. Pp. 299-332 in Physiology and Pharmacology of Biologic Rhythms. Handbook of Experimental Pharmacology. Volume 125, P.H. Redfern and B. Lemmer, eds. Heidelberg: Springer-Verlag.

Levi, F., and F. Halberg. 1982. Circaseptan (about 7 day) bioperiodicity—spontaneous and reactive—and the search for pacemakers. Ric. Clin. Lab. 12:323–370.

Levi, F., I. Blazsek, and A. Ferle-Vidovic. 1988a. Circadian and seasonal rhythms in murine bone marrow colony-forming cells affect tolerance for the anti-cancer agent 4-0-tetrahydropyranyl adriamycin (THP). Exp. Hematol. 16:696–701.

Levi, F., N.A. Boughattas, and I. Blazsek. 1986. Comparative murine chronotoxicity of anticancer agents and related mechanisms. Ann. Rev. Chronopharmacol. 4:283–331.

Levi, F., C. Canon, J.P. Blum, M. Mechkouri, A. Reinberg, and G. Mathe. 1985. Circadian and/or circahemidian rhythms in nine lymphocyte-related variables from peripheral blood of healthy subjects. J. Immunol. 134:217–222.

Levi, F., C. Canon, M. Dipalma, I. Florentin, and J.L. Misset. 1991. When should the immune clock be reset? From circadian pharmacodynamics to temporally optimized drug delivery. Ann. N.Y. Acad. Sci. 618:312–329.

Levi, F., C. Canon, Y. Touitou, A. Reinberg, and G. Mathe. 1988b. Seasonal modulation of the circadian time structure of circulating T- and natural killer lymphocyte subsets from healthy subjects. J. Clin. Invest. 81:407–413.

Levi, F.A., R. Zidani, J.M. Vannetzel, B. Perpoint, C. Focan, R. Faggiuolo, P. Chollet, C. Garufi, M. Itzhaki, and L. Dogliotti. 1994. Chronomodulated versus fixed-infusion-rate delivery of ambulatory chemotherapy with oxaliplatin, fluorouracil, and folinic acid (leucovorin) in patients with colorectal cancer metastases: a randomized multi-institutional trial. J. Natl. Cancer Inst. 86(21):1608–1617.

Levine, M., C. Conry-Cantilena, Y. Wang, R.W. Welch, P.W. Washko, K.R. Dhariwal, J.B. Park, A. Lazarev, J.F. Graumlich, J. King, and L.R. Cantilena. 1996. Vitamin C pharmacokinetics in healthy volunteers: evidence for a recommended dietary allowance. Proc. Natl. Acad. Sci. 93(8):3704–3709.

Levine, M., K.R. Dhariwal, R.W. Welch, Y. Wang, J.B. Park. 1995. Determination of optimal vitamin C requirements in humans. Am. J. Clin. Nutr. 62(suppl.):S1347–S1356.

Lewis, C.E., W.L. Jones, F. Austin, and J. Roman. 1967. Flight research program: IX. Medical monitoring of carrier pilots in combat-II. Aerospace Med. 38:581–592.

Lewis, D., M. Simmons, R. Pethybridge et al. 1991. The effect of training stress on the immune system in Royal Marine recruits. Alverstoke, GOSPORT, Hampshire: Institute of Naval Medicine.

Li, G., F. Wang, D. Kang, and C. Li. 1985. Keshan disease: An endemic cardiomyopathy in China. Hum. Pathol. 16:602–609.

Liew, F.Y., S. Millott, C. Parkinson et al. 1990. Macrophage killing of Leishmania parasite in vivo is medicated by nitric oxide from L-arginine. J. Immunol. 144:4794–4797.

Lilly, M.P., and D.S. Gann. 1992. The hypothalamic–pituitary–adrenal–immune axis. Arch. Surg. 127:1463–1474.

Linden, A., T. Art, H. Amory, A.M. Massart, C. Burvenich, and P. Lekeux. 1991. Quantitative buffy coat analysis related to adrenocortical function in horses during a three-day event competition. Zentralbl. Veterinärmed. 38:376–382.

Lipa, B.J., P.A. Sturrock, and E. Rogot. 1976. Search for correlation between geomagnetic disturbances and mortality. Nature 259:302–304.

Lissoni, P., S. Barni, C. Archili, G. Cattaneo, F. Rovelli, A. Conti, G.J.M. Maestroni, and G. Tancini. 1990. Endocrine effects of a 24-hour intravenous infusion of interleukin-2 in the immunotherapy of cancer. Anticancer Res. 10:753–758.

Lissoni, P., S. Barni, G. Tancini, A. Ardizzoia, G. Ricci, R. Aldeghi, F. Brivio, E. Tisi, R. Rescaldani, G. Quadro, and G.J.M. Maestroni. 1994. A randomized study with subcutaneous low dose interleukin-2 alone vs. interleukin-2 plus the pineal neurohormone melatonin in advanced solid neoplasms other than renal cancer and melanoma. Br. J. Cancer 69:196–199.

Lissoni, P. S. Barni, G. Tancini, A. Ardizzoia, F. Rovelli, M. Cazzaniga, F. Brivio, A. Piperno, R. Aldeghi, D. Fossati, D. Characiejus, L. Kothari, A. Conti, and G.J.M. Maestroni. 1993. Immunotherapy with subcutaneous low dose interleukin-2 and the pineal indole melatonin as a new effective therapy in advanced cancers of the digestive tract. Br. J. Cancer 67:1404–1407.

Lissoni, P., S. Barni, G. Tancini, E. Maini, F. Piglia, G.J.M. Maestroni, and A. Lewinski 1995. Immunoendocrine therapy with low-dose subcutaneous interleukin-2 plus melatonin of locally advanced or metastatic endocrine tumors. Oncology 52:163–166.

Liu, C.T., T.M. Kijek, C.A. Rossi, T.K. Bushe, C.B. Carpenter, S.D. Goodwin, A. Hail, D.A. Creasia, D.M. Walters, R.E. Dinterman, and K.A. Mereish. 1996. Staphylococcal enterotoxin B (SEB) kinetics after intratracheal instillation in Dutch rabbits. FASEB J. 10:A175.

Liu, T., M. Cavallini, F. Halberg, G. Cornélissen, J. Field, and D.E.R. Sutherland. 1986. More of the need for circadian, circaseptan, and circannual optimization of cyclosporine therapy. Experientia 42:20–22.

Longnecker, M.P., P.R. Taylor, O.A. Levander, M. Howe, C. Veillon, P.A. McAdam, K.Y. Patterson, J.M. Holden, M.J. Stampfer, J.S. Morris, et al. 1991. Selenium in diet, blood, and toenails in relation to human health in a seleniferous area. Am. J. Clin. Nutr. 53:1288–1294.

Lopez-Cabrera, M., A.G. Santis, E. Fernandez-Ruis, R. Blacher, F. Esch, P. Sanchez-Mateos, and F. Sanchez-Madrid. 1993. Molecular cloning, expression, and chromosomal localization of the human earliest lymphocyte activation antigen AIM/CD69, a new member of the C-type animal lectin superfamily of signal transmitting receptors. J. Exp. Med. 178:537–547.

Love, L.A., J.L. Rader, L.J. Crofford, R.B. Raybourne, M.A. Principato, S.W. Page, M.W. Trucksess, M.J. Smith, E.M. Dugan, and M.L. Turner. 1993. Pathological and immunological effects of ingesting L-tryptophan and 1,1'-ethylidenebis (L-tryptophan) in Lewis rats. J. Clin. Invest. 91:804–811.

Lu, M.C., M.H. Smolensky, B. Hsi, and J.P. McGovern. 1979. Seasonal changes in immunoglobulin and complement levels in atopic and non-atopic persons. Pp. 261–272 in Recent Advances in the Chronobiology of Allergy and Immunology, M.H. Smolensky, A. Reinberg, and J.P. McGovern, eds. Oxford: Pergamon Press.

Lukasewycz, O.A., and J.R. Prohaska. 1983. Lymphocytes from copper-deficient mice exhibit decreased mitogen reactivity Nutr. Res. 3:335–341.

Lukasewycz, O.A., and J.R. Prohaska. 1985. Alterations in lymphocyte subpopulations in copper-deficient mice. Infect. Immun. 48:644–647.

Lukasewycz, O.A., and J.R. Prohaska. 1990. Immune response in copper deficiency. Ann. N.Y. Acad. Sci. 587:147–159.

Lundeen, W., G.Y. Nicolau, D.J. Lakatua, L. Sackett-Lundeen, E. Petrescu, and E. Haus. 1990. Circadian periodicity of performance in athletic students. Progr. Clin. Biol. Res. 341B:337–343.

Luster, M.I., C. Portier, D.G. Pait, G.J. Rosenthal, D.R. Germolec, E. Corsini, B.L. Blaylock, P. Pollock, Y. Kouchi, and W. Craig. 1993. Risk assessment in immunotoxicology. II. Relationships between immune and host resistance tests. Fundam. Appl. Toxicol. 21(1):71–82.

Luster, M.I., C. Portier, D.G. Pait, K.L. White Jr., C. Gennings, A.E. Munson, G.J. Rosenthal. 1992. Risk assessment in immunotoxicology. I. Sensitivity and predictability of immune tests. Fundam. Appl. Toxicol. 18(2):200–210.

Lynch, E.A., C.A. Dinarello, and J.G. Cannon. 1994. Gender differences in IL-1 alpha, IL-1 beta, and IL-1 receptor antagonist secretion from mononuclear cells and urinary excretion. J. Immunol. 153(1):300-6.

Lyte, M. 1987. Generation and measurement of interleukin-1, interleukin-2, and mitogen levels in small volumes of whole blood. J. Clin. Lab. Anal. 1:83–88.

MacArthur, R.D., S.D. Levine, and T.J. Birk. 1993. Supervised exercise training improves cardiopulmonary fitness in HIV-infected persons. Med. Sci. Sports Exerc. 25:684–688.

MacBurney, M., L.S. Young, T.R. Ziegler, and D.W. Wilmore. 1994. A cost-evaluation of glutamine-supplemented parenteral nutrition in adult bone marrow transplant patients. J. Am. Diet. Assoc. 94:1263–1266.

Macdougall, L.G., R. Anderson, G.M. McNab, and J. Katz. 1975. The immune response in iron-deficient children: Impaired cellular defense mechanisms with altered humoral components. J. Pediatr. 86:833–843.

Macha, M., M. Shlafer, and M.J. Kluger. 1990. Human neutrophil hydrogen peroxide generation following physical exercise. J. Sports Med. Phys. Fit. 30:412–419.

MacKay, H.M. 1928. Anaemia in infancy: Its prevalence and prevention. Arch. Dis. Child. 3:117–147.

Mackiewicz, A., A. Kof, and P.B. Sehgal, eds. 1995. Interleukin-6-type cytokines. New York: New York Academy of Science. Pp. 1–522.

Mackinnon, L.T., and S. Hooper. 1994. Mucosal (secretory) immune system responses to exercise of varying intensity and during overtraining. Int. J. Sports Med. 15:S179–S183.

Mackinnon, L.T., T.W. Chick, A. Van As, and T.B. Tomasi. 1987. The effect of exercise on secretory and natural immunity. Adv. Exp. Med. Biol. 216A:869–876.

Mackinnon, L.T., T.W. Chick, A. Van As, and T.B. Tomasi. 1988. Effects of prolonged intense exercise on natural killer cell number and function. Exerc. Physiol.: Current Selected Research 3:77–89.

Mackinnon, L.T., E.M. Ginn, and G.J. Seymour. 1993. Temporal relationship between decreased salivary IgA and upper respiratory tract infection in elite athletes. Aust. J. Sci. Med. Sport 25:94–99.

Mackowiak, P.A., J.G. Bartlett, E.C. Borden, S.E. Goldblum, J.D. Hasday, R.S. Munford, S.A. Nasraway, P.D. Stolley, and T.E. Woodward. 1997. Concepts of fever: Recent advances and lingering dogma. Clin. Infect. Dis. 25:119–138.

MacLennan, P.A., R.A. Brown, and M.J. Rennie. 1987. A positive relationship between protein synthesis rate and intracellular glutamine concentration in perfused rat skeletal muscle. FEBS Lett. 215:187–191.

MacPhee, I.A., F.A. Antoni, and D.W. Mason. 1989. Spontaneous recovery of rats from experimental allergic encephalomyelitis is dependent on regulation of the immune system by endogenous adrenal corticosteroids. J. Exp. Med. 169:431–445.

Maestroni, G.J.M. 1993. The immunoneuroendocrine role of melatonin. J. Pineal Res. 14:1–10. 1995. T-helper-2 lymphocytes as a peripheral target of melatonin. J. Pineal Res. 18:84–89.

Maestroni, G.J.M., and A. Conti. 1993. Melatonin in relation with the immune system. Pp. 229–311 in Melatonin: Biosynthesis, Physiological Effects, and Clinical Applications, Y. Hing-Su and R.J. Reiter, eds. Boca Raton, Fla.: CRC Press.

Maestroni, G.J.M., and W. Pierpaoli. 1981. Pharmacological control of the hormonally mediated immune-response. Pp. 405–425 in Psychoneuroimmunology, R. Ader, ed. New York: Academic Press.

Maestroni, G.J.M., A. Conti, and W. Pierpaoli. 1986. Role of the pineal gland in immunity. Circadian synthesis and release of melatonin modulates the antibody response and antagonizes the immunosuppressive effect of corticosterone. J. Neuroimmunol. 13:19–30.

Maestroni, G.J.M., A. Conti, and W. Pierpaoli. 1987a. The pineal gland and the circadian opiatergic immunoregulatory role of melatonin. Ann. N.Y. Acad. Sci. 496:67–77.

Maestroni, G.J.M., A. Conti, and W. Pierpaoli. 1987b. Role of the pineal gland in immunity. II. Melatonin enhances the antibody response via an opiatergic mechanism. Clin. Exp. Immunol. 68:384–391.

Maestroni, G.J.M., A. Conti, and W. Pierpaoli. 1988. Pineal melatonin: Its fundamental immunoregulatory role in aging and cancer. Ann. N.Y. Acad. Sci. 521:140–148.

Maffulli, N., V. Testa, and G. Capasso. 1993. Post-viral fatigue syndrome. A longitudinal assessment in varsity athletes. J. Sports Med. Phys. Fitness 33:392–399.

Maier, S.F., E.P. Wiertelak, D. Martin, and L.R. Watkins. 1993. Interleukin-1 mediates the behavioral hyperalgesia produced by lithium chloride and endotoxin. Brain Res. 632:321–324.

Maini, R.N., M. Elliott, F.M. Brennan, R.O. Williams, and M. Feldmann. 1994. Targeting TNF-α for the therapy of rheumatoid arthritis. Clin. Exp. Rheumatol. 12(11):S63–S66.

Makara, G.B., E. Stark, and T. Meszaros. 1971. Corticotrophin release induced by *E. coli* endotoxin after removal of the medial hypothalamus. Endocrinology 88:412–414.

Makara, G.B., E. Stark, and M. Palkovits. 1970. Afferent pathways of stressful stimuli: Corticotrophin release after hypothalamic deafferentation. J. Endocrinol. 47:411–416.

Makinodan, T. 1995. Patterns of age-related immunologic changes. Nutr. Rev. 53:S27–S34.

Manu, P., T.J. Lane, and D.A. Matthews. 1992. The pathophysiology of chronic fatigue syndrome: Confirmations, contradictions, and conjectures. Int. J. Psychol. Med. 22:397–408.

Many, A., and R.S. Schwartz. 1971. Periodicity during recovery of the immune response after cyclophosphamide treatment. Blood 37:692–695.

Marsh, M.N., and A.G. Cummins. 1993. The interactive role of mucosal T-lymphocytes in intestinal growth, development, and enteropathy. J. Gastroenterol. Hepatol. 8:270–278.

Martin, D.W. 1985. Metabolism of purine and pyrimidine nucleotides. Pp. 357–375 in Harper's Review of Biochemistry, D.W. Martin, P.A. Mayes, V.W. Rodwell, and D.K. Granner, eds. Los Altos, Calif.: Lang Medical Publishers.

Martin, J.B., T. Easley-Shaw, and C. Collins. 1991. Use of selected vitamin and mineral supplements among individuals infected with human immunodeficiency virus. J. Am. Diet. Assoc. 91:476–478.

Martinez, F, E.R. Abril, D.L. Earnest, and R. R. Watson. 1992. Alcohol and cytokine secretion. Alcohol 9(6):455–458.

Martinez, J.L., A. Delgado Iribarren, and F. Baquero. 1990. Mechanisms of iron acquisition and bacterial virulence. FEMS Microbiol. Rev. 6:45–56.

Martinez-Lopez, L.E., K.E. Friedl, R.J. Moore, and T.R. Kramer. 1993. A prospective epidemiological study of infection rates and injuries of Ranger students. Milit. Med. 158:433–437.

Martini, E., J.Y. Muller, C. Doinel, C. Gastal, H. Roquin, L. Douay, and C. Salmon. 1988a. Disappearance of CD4 lymphocyte circadian cycles in HIV-infected patients: Early even during asymptomatic infection. AIDS 2:133–134.

Martini, E., J.Y. Muller, C. Gastal, C. Doinel, M.C. Meyohas, H. Roquin, J. Frottier, and C. Salmon. 1988b. Early anomalies of CD4 and CD20 lymphocyte cycles in human immunodeficiency virus. Presse Med. 17:2167–2168.

Martino, M., M.E. Rossi, M. Resti, C. Vullo, and A. Vierucci. 1984. Changes in superoxide anion production in neutrophils from multitransfused β-thalassemia patients: Correlation with ferritin levels and liver damage. Acta Haematol. 71:289–298.

Marucha, P.T., J.K. Kiecolt-Glaser, and M. Favagehi. 1998. Mucosal wound healing is impaired by examination stress. Psychosom. Med. 60:362–365.

Marx, J. 1995. How the glucocorticoids suppress immunity. Science 270:232–233.

Masawe, A.E.J., J.M. Muindi, and G.B.R. Swai. 1974. Infections in iron deficiency and other types of anaemia in the tropics. Lancet 2:314–317.

Masek, K., and O. Kadlec. 1983. Sleep factor, muramyl peptides, and the serotoninergic system [letter]. Lancet 2(8336):1277.

Mason, D.I., I.A. MacPhee, and F.A. Antoni. 1990. The role of the neuroendocrine system in determining genetic susceptibility to experimental allergic encephalomyelitis and implications for human inflammatory disease. Immunology 70:1–5.

Matta, S.G., J. Singh, R. Newton, and B.M. Sharp. 1990. The adrenocorticotropin response to interleukin-1β instilled into the rat median eminence depends on the local release of catecholamines. Endocrinology 127:2175–2182.

Mattson, R., I. Hannsson, and R. Holmdah. 1994. Pineal gland in autoimmunity: Melatonin-dependent exaggeration of collagen-induced arthritis in mice. Autoimmunity 17:83–86.

McDowell, E.M., K.P. Keenan, and M. Huang. 1984. Effects of vitamin A-deprivation on hamster tracheal epithelium: A quantitative morphologic study. Virchows Arch. B 45:197–219.

McKeehan, W.L. 1982. Glycolysis, glutaminolysis, and cell proliferation. Cell Biol. Int. Rep. 6:635–650.

McMurray, D.N., S.A. Loomis, L.J. Casazza, H. Rey, and R. Miranda. 1981. Development of impaired cell-mediated immunity in mild and moderate malnutrition. Am. J. Clin. Nutr. 34(1):68–77.

Meehan, R.U., U. Duncan, L. Neale, G. Taylor, H. Muchmore, N. Scott, K. Ramsey, E. Smith, P. Rock, R. Goldblum, and C. Houston. 1988. Operation Everest II: Alterations in the immune system at high altitudes. J. Clin. Immunol. 8:397–406.

Melby, K., S. Slordahl, T.J. Guttenberg, and S.A. Norbo. 1982. Septicemia due to *Yersinia enterocolitica* after oral overdoses of iron. Br. Med. J. (Clin. Res. Ed.) 285(6340):467–468.

Menzio, P., B. Morra, A. Sartoris, R. Molino, M. Bussi, and G. Cortesina. 1980. Nasal secretory IgA circadian rhythm: A single-dose suppression. Ann. Otol. 89:173–175.

Mercola, K.E., M.J. Cline, and D.W. Golde. 1981. Growth hormone stimulation of normal and leukemic human T-lymphocyte proliferation *in vitro*. Blood 58:337–340.

Meydani, M. 1995. Vitamin E. Lancet 345:170–175.

Meydani, M., W.J. Evans, G. Handelman, L. Biddle, R.A. Fielding, S.N. Meydani, J. Burrill, M.A. Fiatarone, J.B. Blumberg, and J.G. Cannon. 1993a. Protective effect of vitamin E on exercise-induced oxidative damage in young and older adults. Am. J. Physiol. 264:R992–R998.

Meydani, M., S.N. Meydani, L. Leka, J. Gong, and J.B. Blumberg. 1994a. Effect of long-term vitamin E supplementation on lipid peroxidation and immune responses of young and old subjects. FASEB J. 8:A415.

Meydani, S.N., and M. Hayek. 1992. Vitamin E and immune response. Pp. 105–128 in Nutrition and Immunology, R.K. Chandra, ed. St. John's, Newfoundland: ARTS Biomedical Publishers.

Meydani, S.N., M.P. Barklund, S. Liu, M. Meydani, R.A. Miller, J.G. Cannon, F.D. Morrow, R. Rocklin, and J.B. Blumberg. 1990. Vitamin E supplementation enhances cell-mediated immunity in healthy elderly subjects. Am. J. Clin. Nutr. 52(3):557–563.

Meydani, S.N., S. Endres, M.N. Woods, B.R. Goldin, C. Soo, A. Morrill-Labrode, C.A. Dinarello, and S.L. Gorbach. 1991. Oral n-3 fatty acid supplementation suppresses cytokine production and lymphocyte proliferation: Comparision between young and old women. J. Nutr. 121:547–555.

Meydani, S.N., A.H. Lichtenstein, S. Cornwall, M. Meydani, B.R. Goldin, H. Rasmussen, C.A. Dinarello, and E.J. Schaefer. 1993b. Immunologic effects of national cholesterol education panel step-2 diets with and without fish-derived n-3 fatty acid enrichment. J. Clin. Invest. 92:105–113.

Meydani, S.N., M. Meydani, J.B. Blumberg, L. Leka, M. Pedrosa, B.D. Stollar, and R. Diamond. 1997a. Safety assessment of long-term vitamin E supplementation in healthy elderly. FASEB J. 10:A448.

Meydani, S.N., M. Meydani, J.B. Blumberg, L.S. Leka, G. Siber, R. Loszewski, C. Thompson, M.C. Pedrosa, R.D. Diamond, and B.D. Stollar. 1997b. Vitamin E supplementation and in vivo immune response in healthy elderly subjects. A randomized controlled trial. JAMA 277(17):1380–6.

Meydani, S.N., M. Meydani, L.C. Rall, F. Morrow, and J.B. Blumberg. 1994b. Assessment of the safety of high-dose, short-term supplementation with vitamin E in healthy older adults. Am. J. Clin. Nutr. 60(5):704-9.

Meydani, S.N., M. Meydani, C.P. Verdon, A.C. Shapiro, J.B. Blumberg, and K.C. Hayes. 1986. Vitamin E supplementation suppresses prostaglandin E2 synthesis and enhances the immune response of aged mice. Mech. Aging Dev. 34:191–201.

Meydani, S.N., J.D. Ribaya-Mercado, R.M. Russell, N. Sahyoun, F.D. Morrow, and S.N. Gershoff. 1991. Vitamin B-6 deficiency impairs interleukin 2 production and lymphocyte proliferation in elderly adults. Am. J. Clin. Nutr. 53(5):1275–1280.

Meydani, S.N., D. Wu, M.S. Santos, and M.G. Hayek. 1995. Antioxidants and immune response in aged persons: Overview of present evidence. Am. J. Clin. Nutr. 62(suppl.):1462S–1476S.

Michelsen, P.A., and P.F. Sparling. 1981. Ability of *Neisseria gonorrhoeae*, *Neisseria meningitidis*, and commensal *Neisseria* species to obtain iron from transferrin and iron compounds. Infect. Immun. 33:555–564.

Michelsen, P.A., E. Blackman, and P.F. Sparling. 1982. Ability of *Neisseria gonorrhoeae*, *Neisseria meningitidis* and commensal *Neisseria* species to obtain iron from lactoferrin. Infect. Immun. 35:915–920.

Michie, H.R., J.A. Majzoub, S.T. O'Dwyer, A. Revhaug, and D.W. Wilmore. 1990. Both cyclooxygenase-dependent and cyclooxygenase-independent pathways mediate the neuroendocrine response in humans. Surgery 108:254–259.

Michie, H.R., K.R. Manogue, D.R. Spriggs, A. Revhaug, S.T. O'Dwyer, C.A. Dinnarello, A. Cerami, S.M. Wolff, and D.W. Wilmore. 1988. Detection of circulating tumor necrosis factor after endotoxin administration. N. Engl. J. Med. 318:1481–1486.

Miller, R.K., J. Brown, D. Cordero, B. Dayton, B. Hardin, and M. Greene. 1987. Teratology Society position paper: recommendations for vitamin A use during pregnancy. Teratology 35(2):269–75.

Milos, P., D. Morse, and J.W. Hastings. 1990. Circadian control over synthesis of many Gonyaulax proteins is at a translational level. Naturwissenschaften 77:87–89.

Minami, M., Y. Kuraishi, T. Yamaguchi, S. Nakai, Y. Hirai, and M. Satoh. 1991. Immobilization stress induces interleukin-1β mRNA in the rat hypothalamus. Neurosci. Lett. 123:254–256.

Minami, M., Y. Kuraishi, T. Yamaguchi, K. Yabuuchi, A. Yamazaki, and M. Satoh. 1992. Induction of interleukin-1β mRNA in rat brain after transient forebrain ischemia. J. Neurochem. 58:390–392.

Mitchell, J.P. 1933. Observations on health in relation to diet in H.M. Central Prison, Uganda. I. Prison diets and morbidity. East Afr. Med. J. 10:38–53.

Mofenson, H.C., T.R. Caraccio, and N. Sharieff. 1988. Iron sepsis: *Yersinia enterocolitica* septicemia possibly caused by an overdose of iron [letter]. N. Engl. J. Med. 316:1092–1093.

Moldawer, L.L. 1997. The validity of blood and urinary cytokine measurements for detecting the presence of inflammation. Pp. 417–430 in Emerging Technologies for Nutrition Research: Potential for Assessing Military Performance Capability, S.J. Carlson-Newberry and R.B. Costello, eds. A report of the Committee on Military Nutrition Research, Food and Nutrition Board. Washington, D.C.: National Academy Press.

Moldofsky, H. 1994. Central nervous system and peripheral immune functions and the sleep-wake system. J. Psychiatr. Neurosci. 19(5):368–374.

Moldofsky, H., F.A. Lue, J.R. Davidson, J. Jephthah-Ochola, K. Carayanniotis, and R. Gorczynski. 1989. The effect of 64 hours of wakefulness on immune functions and plasma cortisol in humans. Pp. 185–187 in Sleep '88, J. Horne, ed. New York: Gustav Fischer Verlag.

Moldofsky, H., F.A. Lue, J. Eisen, E. Keyston, and R.M. Gorczynski. 1986. The relationship of interleukin-1 and immune functions to sleep in humans. Psychosom. Med. 48:309–318.

Molvig, J., F. Pociot, H. Worssaae, L.D. Wogensen, L. Baek, P. Christensen, T. Mandrup-Poulsen, K. Anderson, P. Madsen, J. Dyerberg, and J. Nerup. 1991. Dietary supplementation with omega-3 polyunsaturated fatty acids decreases mononuclear cell proliferation and interleukin-1β content but not monokine secretion in healthy and insulin-dependent diabetic individuals. Scan. J. Immunol. 34:399–410.

Montain, S.J., R.L. Shippee, W.J. Tharion, and T.R. Kramer. 1995. Carbohydrate–electrolyte solution during military training: Effects of physical performance, mood state and immune function. Technical Report No. T95-13, AD-A297 258. Natick, Mass.: U.S. Army Research Institute of Environmental Medicine.

Mooradian, A.D., R.L. Reed, D. Osterweil, R. Schiffman, and P. Scuderi. 1990. Decreased serum triiodothyronine is associated with increased concentrations of tumor necrosis factor. J. Clin. Endocrinol. Metab. 71:1239–1242.

Moore, L.L., and J.R. Humbert. 1984. Neutrophil bactericidal dysfunction towards oxidant radical-sensitive microorganisms during experimental iron deficiency. Pediatr. Res. 18:684–689.

Moore, R.J., K.E. Friedl, T.R. Kramer, L.E. Martinez-Lopez, R.W. Hoyt, R.E. Tulley, J.P. DeLany, E.W. Askew, and J.A. Vogel. 1992. Changes in soldier nutritional status and immune function during the Ranger training course. Technical Report No. T13-92, AD-A257 437. Natick, Mass.: U.S. Army Research Institute of Environmental Medicine.

Morgan, A.P., ed. 1966. Energy Metabolism and Body Fuel Utilization, with Particular Reference to Starvation and Injury. Proceedings of the Committee on Metabolism in Trauma of the U.S. Army Research and Development Command. Cambridge, Mass.: Harvard University Printing Office.

Morikawa, K., F. Oseko, and S. Morikawa. 1995. A role for ferritin in hematopoiesis and the immune system [review]. Leuk. Lymphoma Res. 18:429–433.

Morley, A., E.A. King-Smith, and F.J. Stohlman. 1970. The oscillatory nature of hemopoiesis. Pp. 3–14 in Symposium on Hemopoietic Cellular Proliferation, F. Stohlman Jr., ed. New York: Grune and Stratton.

Mormont, M.C., R. von Roemeling, R.B. Sothern, J.S. Berestka, T.R. Langevin, M. Wick, and W.J.M. Hrushesky. 1988. Circadian rhythm and seasonal dependence in the toxicologic response of mice to epirubicin. Invest. New Drugs 6:273–283.

Morrey, M.K., J.A. McLachlan, Serkin C.D., and O. Bakouche. 1994. Activation of human monocytes by the pineal hormone melatonin. J. Immunol. 153:2671–2680.

Morris, D.M., M.M. Henry, J.N. Moore, and K. Fisher. 1989. Effect of dietary linoleid acid on indotoxin-induced thromboxane and prostacyclin production by equine peritoneal macrophages. Circ. Shock 29:311–318.

Morrissey, P.J., K. Charrier, and S.N. Vogel. 1995. Exogenous tumor necrosis factor-α and interleukin-1α increase resistance to *Salmonella typhimurium*: Efficacy is influenced by the *Ity* and *LPs* loci. Infect. Immun. 63:3196–3198.

Morse, D., P.M. Milos, E. Roux, and J.W. Hastings. 1989. Circadian regulation of bioluminescence in Gonyaulax involves translational control. Proc. Natl. Acad. Sci. USA 86:172–176.

Morse, S.S. 1997. The public health threat of emerging viral diseases. J. Nutr. 127(5 suppl.):951S–957S.

Mortin, R., and G. Courchay. 1994. Pregnenolone and dehydroepiandrosterone as precursors of native 7-hydroxylated metabolites which increase the immune response in mice. J. Steroid Biochem. Mol. Biol. 50:91–100.

Moses, H.A., and H.E. Parker. 1964. Influence of dietary zinc and age on the mineral content of rat tissues. Fed. Proc. 23:333–343.

Mossey, R.T., and J. Sondheimer. 1985. Listeriosis in patients with long-term hemodialysis and transfusional iron overload. Am. J. Med. 79:397–399.

Moynihan, J.A., R. Ader, L.J. Grota, T.R. Schachtman, and N. Cohen. 1990. The effects of stress on the development of immunological memory following low-dose antigen priming in mice. Brain Behav. Immun. 4:1–12.

Muhlbacher, F., C.R. Kapadia, M.F. Colpoys, R.J. Smith, and D.W. Wilmore. 1984. Effects of glucocorticoids on glutamine metabolism in skeletal muscle. Am. J. Physiol. 247:E75–E83.

Mukaida, N., G.L. Gussella, T. Kasahara, Y. Ko, C.O. Zachariae, T. Kawai, and K. Matsushima. 1993. Molecular analysis of the inhibition of interleukin-8 production by dexamethasone in a human fibrosarcoma cell line. Immunology 75:674–679.

Munck, A. P.M. Guyre, and N.J. Holbrook. 1984. Physiological functions of glucocorticoids in stress and their relation to pharmacological actions. Endocrinol. Rev. 5:25–44.

Munn, C.G., A.L. Markenson, A. Kapadia, and M. deSousa. 1981. Impaired T-cell mitogen responses in some patients with thalassemia intermedia. Thymus 3:119–128.

Müns, G. 1993. Effect of long-distance running on polymorphonuclear neutrophil phagocytic function of the upper airways. Int. J. Sports Med. 15:96–99.

Müns, G., H. Liesen, H. Riedel, and K-Ch. Bergmann. 1989. Einfluá von langstreckenlauf auf den IgA-gehalt in nasensekret und speichel. Deutsche Zeitschr. Sportmed. 40:63–65.

Müns, G., P. Singer, F. Wolf, and I. Rubinstein. 1995. Impaired nasal mucociliary clearance in long-distance runners. Int. J. Sports Med. 16:209–213.

Murphy, W.J., H. Rui, and D.L. Longo. 1995. Effects of growth hormone and prolactin immune development and function. Life Sci. 57:1–14.

Murray, M.J., A.B. Murray, M.B. Murray, and C.J. Murray. 1978a. The adverse effect of iron repletion on the course of certain infections. Br. Med. J. 2(6145):1113–1115.

Murray, M.J., A.B. Murray, N.J. Murray, and M.B. Murray. 1978b. Diet and cerebral malaria: The effects of famine and refeeding. Am. J. Clin. Nutr. 31:57–61.

Myers, M.P., K. Wager-Smith, A. Rothenfluh-Hilfiker, and M.W. Young. 1996. Light-induced degradation of TIMELESS and entrainment of the *Drosophila* circadian clock. Science 271:1736–1740.

Myrvik, Q.N. 1994. Immunology and nutrition. Pp. 623–662 in Modern Nutrition in Health and Diseasea, 8th ed., M.E. Shils, J.A. Olson, and M. Shike, eds. Malvern, Pa.: Lea and Febiger.

Nagy, E., I. Berczi, G.E. Wren, S.L. Asa, and K. Kovacs. 1983. Immunomodulation by bromocriptine. Immunopharmacology 6:231–243.

Naitoh, Y., J. Fukata, T. Tominaga, Y. Nakai, S. Tamai, K. Mori, and H. Imura. 1988. Interleukin-6 stimulates the secretion of adrenocorticotrophic hormone in conscious, freely moving rats. Biochem. Biophys. Res. Commun. 155:1459–1463.

Nakano, K., S. Suzuki, and C. Oh. 1987. Significance of increased secretion of glucocorticoids in mice and rats injected with bacterial endotoxin. Brain Behav. Immun. 1:159–172.

Nakano, Y., T. Miura, I. Hara, H. Aono, N. Miyano, and K. Miyajima. 1982. The effect of shift work on cellular immune function. J. Hum. Ergol. 11(suppl.):131–137.

Nakatsuru, K., S. Ohgo, Y. Oki, and S. Matsukura. 1991. Interleukin-1 (IL-1) stimulates arginine vasopressin (AVP) release from superfused rat hypothalamo-neurohypophyseal complexes independently of cholinergic mechanism. Brain Res. 554:38–45.

Nasrullah, I., and R.S. Mazzeo. 1992. Age-related immunosenescence in Fischer 344 rats: Influence of exercise training. J. Appl. Physiol. 73:1932–1938.

Natadisastra, G., J.R. Wittpenn, K.P. West Jr., Muhilal, and A. Sommer. 1987. Impression cytology for the detection of vitamin A deficiency. Arch. Ophthalmol. 105(9):1224–1228.

NATO (North Atlantic Treaty Organization). 1995. Worskhop on the Effect of Prolonged Exhaustive Military Activities on Man—Physiological and Psychological Changes—Possible Means of Rapid Recuperation. NATO AC/243 Panel VIII. April 3–5, Holmenkollen, Oslo, Norway.

Naylor, A.M., K.E. Cooper, and W.L. Veale. 1987. Vasopressin and fever: Evidence supporting the existence of an endogenous antipyretic system in the brain. Can. J. Physiol. Pharm. 65:1333–1338.

Nechaev, A., F. Halberg, A. Mittelman, and G.L. Tritsch. 1977. Circannual variation in human erythrocyte adenosine aminohydrolase. Chronobiologia 4:191–198.

Neckers, L.M., and J. Cossman. 1983. Transferrin receptor induction in mitogen-stimulated human T-lymphocytes is required for DNA synthesis and cell division and is regulated by interleukin 2. Proc. Natl. Acad. Sci. USA 89:3494–3498.

Neilands, J.B. 1995. Siderophores: Structure and function of microbial iron transport compounds. J. Biol. Chem. 270:26723–26726.

Nelson, W., L. Scheving, and F. Halberg. 1975. Circadian rhythms in mice fed a single daily "meal" at different stages of LD 12:12 lighting regimen. J. Nutr. 105:171–184.

Nelson, W., Y.L. Tong, J.K. Lee, and F. Halberg. 1979. Methods for cosinor rhythmometry. Chronobiologia 6:305–323.

Nerad, J.L., J.K. Griffiths, J.W.M. Van der Meer, S. Endres, D.D. Poutsiaka, G.T. Keusch, M. Bennish, M.A. Salam, C.A. Dinarello, and J.G. Cannon. 1992. Interleukin 1J (IL-1J), IL-1 receptor antagonist, and TNF-α production in whole blood. J. Leukoc. Biol. 52:687–692.

Neri, A., M. Brugiatelli, P. Iacopino, and F. Callea. 1984. Natural killer cell activity and T-cell subpopulations in thalassemia major. Acta Haematol. 71:263–269.

Neta, R., R. Perlstein, S.N. Vogel, G.D. Ledney, and J. Abrams. 1992. Role of interleukin 6 (IL-6) in protection from lethal irradiation and in endocrine responses to IL-1 and tumor necrosis factor. J. Exp. Med. 175:689–694.

Neta R., D. Williams, F. Selzer, and J. Abrams. 1993. Inhibition of c-kit ligand/steel factor by antibodies reduces survival of lethally irradiated mice. Blood 81(2):324–327.

Neumann, C.G., G.J. Lawlor Jr., E.R. Stiehm, M.E. Swenseid, C. Newton, J. Herbert, A.J. Ammann, and M. Jacob. 1975. Immunologic responses in malnourished children. Am. J. Clin. Nutr. 28:89–104.

Newberne, P.M., C.E. Hunt, and V.R. Young. 1968. The role of diet and reticuloendothelial system in the response of rats to Salmonella typhimurium infection. Br. J. Exp. Pathol. 49:448–457.

Newhouse, I.J., and D.B. Clement. 1988. Iron status in athletes. An update. Sports Med. 5:337–352.

Newsholme, E.A. 1994. Biochemical mechanisms to explain immunosuppression in well-trained and overtrained athletes. Int. J. Sports Med. 15(suppl. 3):S142–S147.

Newsholme, E.A., P. Newsholme, and R. Curi. 1988a. The role of the citric acid cycle in cells of the immune system and its importance in sepsis, trauma, and burns. Biochem. Soc. Symp. 54:145–162.

Newsholme, E.A., P. Newsholme, R. Curi, E. Challoner, and M.S.M. Ardawi. 1988b. A role for muscle in the immune system and its importance in surgery, trauma, sepsis, and burns. Nutrition 4:261–268.

Nguyen, T.T., D.A. Gilpin, N.A. Meyer, and D.N. Herndon. 1996. Current treatment of severely burned patients. Ann. Surg. 223:14–25.

Nicolau, G.Y. and E. Haus. 1994. Chronobiology of the hypothalamic-pituitary-thyroid axis. Pp. 330–347 in Biologic Rhythms in Clinical and Laboratory Medicine, 2nd ed., Y.Touitou and E.Haus, ed. Heidelberg: Springer-Verlag.

Nicolau, G.Y., D.J. Lakatua, L. Sackett-Lundeen, and E. Haus. 1984. Circadian and circannual rhythms of hormonal variables in elderly men and women. Chronobiol. Int. 1:301–319.

Nieman, D.C. 1994a. Exercise, infection, and immunity. Int. J. Sports Med. 15:S131–S141.

Nieman, D.C. 1994b. Exercise, upper respiratory tract infection, and the immune system. Med. Sci. Sports Exerc. 26:128–139.

Nieman, D.C., and D.A. Henson. 1994. Role of endurance exercise in immune senescence. Med. Sci. Sports Exerc. 26:172–181.

Nieman, D.C., and S.L. Nehlsen-Cannarella. 1994. The immune response to exercise. Semin. Hematol. 31(2):166–179.

Nieman, D.C., J.C. Ahle, D.A. Henson, B.J. Warren, J. Suttles, J.M. Davis, K.S. Buckley, S. Simandle, D.E. Butterworth, O.R. Fagoaga, and S.L. Nehlsen-Cannarella. 1995a. Indomethacin does not alter natural killer cell response to 2.5 hours of running. J. Appl. Physiol. 79:748–755.

Nieman, D.C., L.S. Berk, M. Simpson-Westerberg, K. Arabatzis, W. Youngberg, S.A. Tan, and W.C. Eby. 1989. Effects of long endurance running on immune system parameters and lymphocyte function in experienced marathoners. Int. J. Sports Med. 10:317–323.

Nieman, D.C., D. Brendle, D.A. Henson, J. Suttles, V.D. Cook, B.J. Warren, D.E. Butterworth, O.R. Fagoaga, and S.L. Nehlsen-Cannarella. 1995b. Immune function in athletes versus nonathletes. Int. J. Sports Med. 16:329–333.

Nieman, D.C., K.S. Buckley, D.A. Henson, B.J. Warren, J. Suttles, J.C. Ahle, S. Simandle, O.R. Fagoaga, and S.L. Nehlsen-Cannarella. 1995c. Immune function in marathon runners versus sedentary controls. Med. Sci. Sports Exerc. 27:986–992.

Nieman, D.C., D.A. Henson, D.E. Butterworth, B.J. Warren, J.M. Davis, O.R. Fagoaga, and S.L. Nehlsen-Cannarella. 1997a. Vitamin C supplementation does not alter the immune response to 2.5 hours of running. Int. J. Sport Nutr. 7:173–184.

Nieman, D.C., D.A. Henson, E.B. Garner, D.E. Butterworth, B.J. Warren, A. Utter, J.M. Davis, O.R. Fagoaga, and S.L. Nehlsen-Cannarella. 1997b. Carbohydrate affects natural killer cell redistribution but not activity after running. Med. Sci. Sports Exerc. 29:1318–1324.

Nieman, D.C., D.A. Henson, G. Gusewitch, B.J. Warren, R.C. Dotson, D.E. Butterworth, and S.L. Nehlsen-Cannarella. 1993a. Physical activity and immune function in elderly women. Med. Sci. Sports Exerc. 25:823–831.

Nieman, D.C., D.A. Henson, R. Johnson, L. Lebeck, J.M. Davis, and S.L. Nehlsen-Cannarella. 1992. Effects of brief, heavy exertion on circulating lymphocyte subpopulations and proliferative response. Med. Sci. Sports Exerc. 24:1339–1345.

Nieman, D.C., L.M. Johanssen, J.W. Lee, and K. Arabatzis. 1990a. Infectious episodes in runners before and after the Los Angeles Marathon. J. Sports Med. Phys. Fitness 30:316–328.

Nieman, D.C., A.R. Miller, D.A. Henson, B.J. Warren, G. Gusewitch, R.L. Johnson, J.M. Davis, D.E. Butterworth, J.L. Herring, and S.L. Nehlsen-Cannarella. 1994. Effect of high- versus moderate-intensity exercise on lymphocyte subpopulations and proliferative response. Int. J. Sports Med. 15:199–206.

Nieman, D.C., A.R. Miller, D.A. Henson, B.J. Warren, G. Gusewitch, R.L. Johnson, J.M. Davis, D.E. Butterworth, and S.L. Nehlsen-Cannarella. 1993b. The effects of high- versus moderate-intensity exercise on natural killer cell cytotoxic activity. Med. Sci. Sports Exerc. 25:1126–1134.

Nieman, D.C., S.L. Nehlsen-Cannarella, K.M. Donohue, D.B.W. Chritton, B.L. Haddock, R.W. Stout, and J.W. Lee. 1991. The effects of acute moderate exercise on leukocyte and lymphocyte subpopulations. Med. Sci. Sports Exerc. 23:578–585.

Nieman, D.C., S.I. Nelson-Cannarella, D.A. Henson, D.E. Butterworth, O.R. Fagoaga, B.J. Warren, and M.K. Rainwater. 1996. Immune response to obesity and moderate weight loss. Int. J. Obes. Relat. Metab. Disord. 20(4):353–360.

Nieman, D.C., S.L. Nehlsen-Cannarella, P.A. Markoff, A.J. Balk-Lamberton, H. Yang, D.B.W. Chritton, J.W. Lee, and K. Arabatzis. 1990b. The effects of moderate exercise training on natural killer cells and acute upper respiratory tract infections. Int. J. Sports Med. 11:467–473.

Nieman, D.C., S. Simandle, D.A. Henson, B.J. Warren, J. Suttles, J.M. Davis, K.S. Buckley, J.C. Ahle, D.E. Butterworth, O.R. Fagoaga, and S.L. Nehlsen-Cannarella. 1995d. Lymphocyte proliferation response to 2.5 hours of running. Int. J. Sports Med. 16:404–408.

NRC (National Research Council). 1989. Recommended Dietary Allowances, 10th ed. Subcommittee on the Tenth Edition of the RDAs, Food and Nutrition Board, Commission of Life Sciences. Washington, D.C.: National Academy Press.

Nualart, P., M.E. Estevez, I.J. Ballart, S.A. deMiani, J. Penalver, and L. Sen. 1987. Effect of α-interferon on the altered T-B-cell immunoregulation in patients with thalassemia major. Am. J. Hematol. 24:151–159.

Nye, L., T.G. Merret, J. Landon, and R.J. White. 1975. A detailed investigation of circulating IgE levels in a normal population. Clin. Allergy 5(1):13–24.

O'Connell, J., and J. Robinson. 1985. Coxsackie viral myocarditis. Postgrad. Med. J. 61:1127–1131.

O'Dorisio, M.S., C.L. Wood, and T.M. O'Dorisio. 1984. Vasoactive intestinal peptide and neuropeptide modulation of the immune response. J. Immunol. 135:792S–796S.

O'Dwyer, S.T., R.J. Smith, T.L. Hwang, and D.W. Wilmore. 1989. Maintenance of small bowel mucosa with glutamine enriched parenteral nutrition. JPEN J. Parenter. Enteral Nutr. 13:579–585.

O'Marn, C.A. 1987. Nutritional therapy in ambulatory patients. Digest. Dis. Sci. 32:95S–99S.

O'Riordain, M.G., K.C.H. Fearon, J.A. Ross, P. Rogers, J.S. Falconer, D.C. Bartolo, O.J. Gardern, and D.C. Carter. 1994. Glutamine-supplemented total parenteral nutrition enhances T-lymphocyte response in surgical patients undergoing colorectal resection. Ann. Surg. 220:212–221.

Ogle, C.K., J.D. Ogle, J-X. Mao, J. Simon, J.G. Noel, B-G. Li, and J.W. Alexander. 1994. Effect of glutamine on phagocytosis and bacterial killing by normal and pediatric burn patient neutrophils. JPEN J. Parenter. Enteral Nutr. 18:128–133.

Ohlman, S., A. Lindholm, H. Hagglund, J. Sawe, and B.D. Kahan. 1993. On the intraindividual variability and chronobiology of cyclosporine pharmacokinetics in renal transplantation. Eur. J. Clin. Pharmacol. 44:265–269.

Ohlsson, K., P. Bjork, M. Bergenfeldt, R. Hageman, and R.C. Thompson. 1990. Interleukin-1 receptor antagonist reduces mortality from endotoxin shock. Nature 348:550–552.

Ohshima, T., T. Nakaya, K. Saito, H. Maeda, and T. Nagano. 1991. Child neglect followed by marked thymic involution and fatal systemic Pseudomonas infection. Int. J. Legal Med. 104(3):167–171.

Okmole, T.A., and O.A. Onawunmi. 1979. Effect of copper on growth and serum constituents of immunized and nonimmunized rabbits infected with *Trypanosoma brucei*. Ann. Parasitol. 54:495–506.

Øktedalen, O., P.K. Opstad, J. Fahrenkrug, and F. Fonnum. 1984. Plasma concentration of vasoactive intestinal peptide during prolonged physical exercise, calorie supply deficiency and sleep deprivation. Scand. J. Gastroenterol. 19:59–64.

Oliver J.C., L.A. Bland, C.W. Oettinger, M.J. Arduino, S. K. McAllister, S.M. Aguero, and M.S. Favero. 1993. Cytokine kinetics in an in vitro whole blood model following an endotoxin challenge. Lymphokine Cytokine Res. 12:115–120.

Olsen, N.J., and W.J. Kovacs. 1996. Steroids and immunity. Endocr. Rev. 17:369–384.

Olson, B.R., T. Cartledge, N. Sebring, R. Defensor, and L. Nieman. 1995. Short-term fasting affects luteinizing hormone secretory dynamics but not reproductive function in normal-weight sedentary women. J. Clin. Endocrinol. Metab. 80:1187–1193.

Olson, J.A. 1983. Formation and function of vitamin A. Pp. 371–412 in Polyisopenoid Synthesis, vol. II, J.Q Porter, ed. New York: John Wiley & Sons.

Opp, M.R., H. Kapas, and L.A. Toth. 1992. Cytokine involvement in the regulation of sleep. Proc Soc Exp Biol Med. 201:16–27.

Oppenheimer, S.J., and R. Hendrickse. 1983. The clinical effects of iron deficiency and iron supplementation. Nutr. Abstr. Rev. 53:585–598.

Oppenheimer, S.J., F.D. Gibson, S.B. Macfarlane, J.B. Moody, C. Harrison, A. Spencer, and O. Bunari. 1986a. Iron supplementation increases prevalence and effects of malaria: Report on clinical studies in Papua New Guinea. Trans. R. Soc. Trop. Med. Hyg. 80:603–612.

Oppenheimer, S.J., S.B.J. Macfarlane, J.B. Moody, O. Bunari, and R.G. Hendrickse. 1986b. Effect of iron prophylaxis on morbidity due to infectious disease: Report on clinical studies in Papua New Guinea. Trans. R. Soc. Trop. Med. Hyg. 80:596–602.

Oppenheimer, S.J., S.B.J. Macfarlane, J.B. Moody, and C. Harrison. 1986c. Total dose iron infusion, malaria, and pregnancy in Papua New Guinea. Trans. R. Soc. Trop. Med. Hyg. 80:818–822.

Oppenheim, J.J., J.L. Rossio, and A.J.H. Gearing, eds. 1993. Clinical Applications of Cytokines: Role in Pathogenesis, Diagnosis and Therapy. New York: Oxford University Press.

Opstad, P.K. 1991. Alterations in the morning plasma levels of hormones and the endocrine responses to bicycle exercise during prolonged strain. The significance of energy and sleep deprivation. Acta Endocrinol. (Cophenh.) 125:14–22.

Opstad, P.K. 1992. Androgenic hormones during prolonged physical stress, sleep, and energy deficiency. J. Clin. Endocrinol. Metab. 74:1176–1183.

Opstad, P.K. 1994. Circadian rhythm of hormones is extinguished during prolonged physical stress, sleep, and energy deficiency in young men. Eur. J. Endocrinol. 131:56–66.

Opstad, P.K. 1995. Medical consequences in young men of prolonged physical stress with sleep and energy deficiency. NDRE Publication 95/05586. Kjeller, Norway: Forsvarets Forskningsinstituttt, Norwegian Defence Research Establishment.

Opstad, P.K., M. Bårtveit, P. Wiik, and A. Bøyum. 1994a. The dynamic response of β_2- and α_2-adrenoceptors in human blood cells to prolonged exhausting exercise, sleep and energy deficiency. Biogenic Amines 10:329–344.

Opstad, P.K., P. Wiik P, A.H. Haugen, and K.K. Skrede. 1994b. Adrenaline stimulated cyclic adenosine monophosphate response in leucocytes is reduced after prolonged physical activity combined with sleep and energy deprivation. Eur. J. Appl. Physiol. 69:371–375.

Ortaldo, J.R., and D.L. Longo. 1988. Human natural lymphocyte effector cells: Definition, analysis of activity, and clinical effectiveness. J. Natl. Cancer Inst. 80:999–1010.

Ottaway, C.A. 1991. Vasoactive intestinal peptide and immune function. Pp. 225–262 in Psychoneuroimmunology, R. Ader, D.L. Felten, and N. Cohen, eds. Boston: Academic Press.

Owen, D., and L.C. Kuhn. 1987. Noncoding 3' sequences of the transferrin receptor gene are required for mRNA regulation by iron. EMBO J. 6:1287–1293.

Owen, H.B. 1933. Observations on health in relation to diet in H.M. Central Prison, Uganda. II. The ocular manifestations of vitamin A deficiency. East Afr. Med. J. 10:53–58.

Owen, M.J., and E. Jenkinson. 1993. Ontogeny of the immune response. Pp. 3–12 in Clinical Aspects of Immunology, P.J. Lachman, D.K. Peters, F.S. Rosen, and M.J. Walport, eds. London: Blackwell Scientific.

Pace, G.W., and C.D. Leaf. 1995. The role of oxidative stress in HIV disease. Free Radical. Biol. Med. 19:523–528.

Packer, J.E., T.F. Slater, and R.L. Willson. 1979. Direct observation of a free radical interaction between vitamin E and vitamin C. Nature 278:737–738.

Palestine, A.G., C.G. Muellenberg-Coulombre, M.K. Kim, M.C. Gelato, and R.B. Nussenblatt. 1987. Bromocriptine and low dose cyclosporine in the treatment of experimental autoimmune uveitis in the rat. J. Clin. Invest. 79:1078–1081.

Palinkas, L.A. 1988. Disease and non-battle injuries among U.S. Marines in Vietnam. Milit. Med. 153:150–155.

Palmblad, J., K. Cantell, H. Strander, J. Froberg, C.G. Karlsson, L. Levi, M. Granstom, and P. Unger. 1976. Stressor exposure and immunological response in man: Interferon-producing capacity and phagocytosis. J. Psychosom. Res. 20:193–199.

Palmblad, J., B. Petrini, J. Wasserman, and T. Akerstedt. 1979. Lymphocyte and granulocyte reactions during sleep deprivation. Psychosom. Med. 41:273–278.

Palombo, J.D., S.J. DeMichele, E. Lydon, and B.R. Bistrian. 1997. Cyclic vs continuous enteral feeding with omega-3 and gamma-linolenic fatty acids: effects on modulation of phospholipid fatty acids in rat lung and liver immune cells. JPEN J. Parenter. Enteral Nutr. 21(3):123–132.

Pang, X.P., J.M. Hershman, C.J. Mirell, and A.E. Pekary. 1989. Impairment of hypothalamic–pituitary–thyroid function in rats treated with human recombinant tumor necrosis factor-α (cachectin). Endocrinology 125:76–84.

Pangerl, A., J. Remien, and E. Haen. 1986. The number of β-adrenoceptor sites on intact human lymphocytes depends on time of day, on season, and on sex. Ann. Rev. Chronopharmacol. 3:331–334.

Pappenheimer, J.R. 1983. Induction of sleep by muramyl peptides. J. Physiol. 335:1–2.

Pardalos, G., F. Kannakoudi-Tsakalidis, M. Malaka-Zafirin, H. Tsantali, and G. Papaevangelou. 1987. Iron-related disturbances of cell-mediated immunity in multitransfused children with thalassemia major. Clin. Exp. Immunol. 68:138–145.

Parry-Billings, M., J. Evans, P.C. Calder, and E.A. Newsholme. 1990. Does glutamine contribute to immunosuppression after major burns? Lancet 336:523–525.

Pati, A.K., I. Florentin, V. Chung, M. DeSousa, F. Levi, and G. Mathe. 1987. Circannual rhythm in natural killer activity and mitogen responsiveness of murine splenocytes. Cell. Immunol. 108:227–234.

Paul, W.E. 1993. Fundamental Immunology, 3d ed. New York: Bauer Press.

Paxton, H., S. Cunningham-Rundles, and M.R.G. O'Gorman. 1995. Laboratory evaluation of the cellular immune system. Pp. 887–912 in Clinical Diagnosis and Management by Laboratory Methods, J.B. Henry, ed. Philadelphia: W.B. Saunders and Company.

Payan, D.G., M.Y.S. Wong, T. Chernov-Rogan, F.H. Valone, W.C. Pickett, V.A. Blake, and W.M. Gold. 1986. Alteration in human leukocyte function induced by ingestion of eicosapentaenoic acid. J. Clin. Immunol. 6:402–410.

Payne, L.C., F. Obal, Jr., M.R. Opp, and J.M. Krueger. 1992. Stimulation and inhibition of growth hormone secretion by interleukin-1β: The involvement of growth hormone-releasing hormone. Neuroendocrinology 56:118–123.

Pedersen, B.K., and H. Bruunsgaard. 1995. How physical exercise influences the establishment of infections. Sports Med. 19:393–400.

Pedersen, B.K., and H. Ullum. 1994. NK cell response to physical activity: Possible mechanisms of action. Med. Sci. Sports Exerc. 26:140–146.

Pedersen, B.K., M. Kappel, M. Klokker, H.B. Nielsen, and N.H. Secher. 1994. The immune system during exposure to extreme physiologic conditions. Int. J. Sports Med. 15:S116–S121.

Pedersen, M., C.M. Nielsen, and H. Permin. 1991. HIV-antigen-induced release of histamine from basophils from HIV infected patients: Mechanism and relation to disease progression and immunodeficiency. J. Allergy 46:206–212.

Pedersen, B.K., N. Tvede, L.D. Christensen, K. Klarlund, S. Kragbak, and J. Halkjaer-Kristensen. 1989. Natural killer cell activity in peripheral blood of highly trained and untrained persons. Int. J. Sports Med. 10:129–131.

Pedersen, B.K., N. Tvede, K. Klarlund, L.D. Christensen, F.R. Hansen, H. Galbo, A. Kharazmi, and J. Halkjaer-Kristensen. 1990. Indomethacin in vitro and in vivo abolishes post-exercise suppression of natural killer cell activity in peripheral blood. Int. J. Sports Med. 11:127–131.

Peisen, J.N., K.J. McDonnell, S.E. Mulroney, and M.D. Lumpkin. 1995. Endotoxin-induced suppression of the somatotropic axis is mediated by interleukin-1β and corticotropin-releasing factor in the juvenile rat. Endocrinology 136:3378–3390.

Pekarek, R.S., and W.R. Beisel. 1971. Characterization of the endogenousmediator(s) of serum zinc and iron depression during infection and other stresses. Proc. Soc. Exp. Biol. Med. 138:728–732.

Peleg, L., M.N. Nesbitt, and I.E. Ashkenazi. 1989. Strain dependent response of circadian rhythms during exposure to continuous illumination. Life Sci. 44:893–900.

Penn, N.D., L. Purkins, J. Kelleher, R.V. Heatley, B.H. Mascie-Taylor, and P.W. Belfield. 1991. The effect of dietary supplementation with vitamins A, C and E on cell-mediated immune function in elderly long-stay patients: A randomized controlled trial. Age Ageing 20:169–174.

Peretz, A., J. Neve, J. Duchateau, V. Siderova, K. Huygen, J.P. Famaey, and Y.A. Carpentier. 1991. Effects of selenium supplementation on immune parameters in gut failure patients on home parenteral nutrition. Nutrition 7(3):215–221.

Perlstein R.S., M.H. Whitnall, J.S. Abrams, E.H. Mougey, and R. Neta. 1993. Synergistic roles of interleukin-6, interleukin-1, and tumor necrosis factor in adrenocorticotropin response to bacterial lipopolysaccharide in vivo. Endocrinology 132:946–952.

Perretti, M. 1994. Lipocortin-derived peptides. Biochem. Pharmacol. 47(6):931–938.

Perretti, M., C. Becherucci, G. Scapigliati, and L. Parente. 1989. The effect of adrenalectomy on interleukin-1 release in vitro and in vivo. Br. J. Pharmacol. 98:1137–1142.

Perriello, G., R. Jorde, N. Nurjhan, M. Stumvoll, G. Dailey, T. Jenssen, D.M. Bier, and J.E. Gerich. 1995. Estimation of glucose–alanine–lactate–glutamine cycles in postabsorptive humans: Role of skeletal muscle. Am. J. Physiol. 269:E443–E450.

Petering, H.G., M.A. Johnson, and J.P. Horwitz. 1971. Studies of zinc metabolism in the rat. Arch. Environ. Health 23:93–101.

Peters, E.M. 1990. Altitude fails to increase susceptibility of ultramarathon runners to post-race upper respiratory tract infections. S. Afr. J. Sports Med. 5:4–8.

Peters, E.M. 1997. Exercise, immunology, and upper respiratory tract infections. Int. J. Sports Med. 18 (suppl. 1):S69–S77.

Peters, E.M., and E.D. Bateman. 1983. Respiratory tract infections: An epidemiological survey. S. Afr. Med. J. 64:582–584.

Peters, E.M, J.M. Goetzsche, B. Grobbelaar, and T.D. Noakes. 1993. Vitamin C supplementation reduces the incidence of postrace symptoms of upper-respiratory-tract infection in ultramarathon runners. Am. J. Clin. Nutr. 57(2):170-4.

Petrovsky, N., P. McNair, and L.C. Harrison. 1994. Circadian rhythmicity of interferon-γ production in antigen-stimulated whole blood. Chronobiologia 21:293–300.

Philips, J.L., and P. Azari. 1975. Effect of iron transferrin on nucleic acid synthesis in phytohaemagglutinin-stimulated human lymphocytes. Cell Immunol. 15:94–99.

Phuapradit, W., K. Chaturachinda, S. Tannepanichskul, J. Sirivarasry, K. Khupulsup, and N. Lerdvuthisopon. 1996. Serum vitamin A and β-carotene levels in pregnant women infected with human immunodeficiency virus-1. Obstet. Gynecol. 87:564–567.

Pieniazek, N.J. and B.L. Herwald. 1997. Reevaluating the molecular taxonomy: is human-associated Cyclospora a mammalian Eimeria species? Emerg. Infect. Dis. 3(3):381–383.

Pillat, A. 1929. Does keratomalacia exist in adults? Arch. Ophthalmol. 2:256–287, 399–415.

Pinnock, C.B., and C.P. Alderman. 1992. The potential for teratogenicity of Vitamin A and its congeners. Med. J. Aust. 157:805.

Pitts, R.F., L.A. Pilkington, M.B. MacLeod, and E. Leal-Pinto. 1972. Metabolism of glutamine by the intact functioning kidney of the dog. J. Clin. Invest. 51:557–565.

Pleban, R.J., P.J. Valentine, D.M. Penetar, D.P. Redmond, and G.L. Belenky. 1990. Characterization of sleep and body composition changes during Ranger training. Milit. Psychol. 2:145–156.

Poirier, K.A. 1994. Summary of the derivation of the reference dose for selenium. Pp. 157–166 in Risk Assessment of Essential Elements, W. Mertz, C.O. Abernathy and S.S. Olin, eds. Washington, DC: ILSI Press.

Pollack, S. 1992. Receptor-mediated iron uptake and intracellular iron transport. Am. J. Hematol. 39:113–118.

Pollmacher, T., J. Mullington, C. Korth, and D. Hinze-Selch. 1995. Influence of host defense activation on sleep in humans. Adv. Neuroimmunol. 5:155–169.

Pöllman, L. and B. Pöllman. 1988. Variations of the efficiency of hepatitis B vaccination. Annual Rev. Chronopharmacol. 5:45–48.

Portaluppi, F., P. Cortelli, P. Avoni, and L. Vergnani. 1994. Progressive disruption of the circadian rhythm of melatonin in fatal familial insomnia. J. Clin. Endocrinol. Metab. 78(5):1075–1078.

Pownall, R., and M.S. Knapp. 1980. Immune responses have rhythms. Are they important? Immunol. Today 1:7–10.

Pownall, R., P.A. Kabler, and M.S. Knapp. 1979. The time of day of antigen encounter influences the magnitude of the immune response. Clin. Exp. Immunol. 36:347–354.

Pozos, R.S., D.E. Roberts, A.C. Hackney, and S.J. Feith. 1996. Military Schedules vs. Biological Clocks. Pp. 149–160 in Nutritional Needs in Cold and in High-Altitude Environments, Applications for Military Personnel in Field Operations, B.M. Marriott and S.J. Carlson, eds. A report of the Committee on Military Nutrition Research, Food and Nutrition Board, Institute of Medicine. Washington, D.C.: National Academy Press.

Prasad, A.S., ed. 1976. Deficiency of zinc in man and its toxicity. Pp. 1–20 in Trace Elements in Health and Disease, vol. 1, Zinc and Copper. New York: Academic Press.

Prasad, A.S., G.J. Brewer, E.B. Schoomaker, and P. Rabbani. 1978. Hypocupremia induced by zinc therapy in adults. J. Am. Med. Assoc. 240:2166–2168.

Prasad, A.S., S. Meftah, J. Adballah, J. Kaplan, G.J. Brewer, J.F. Bach, and M. Dardenne. 1988. Serum thymulin in human zinc deficiency. J. Clin. Invest. 82:1202–1210.

Prasad, A.S., D. Oberleas, P. Wolf, J.P. Horwitz, E.R. Miller, and R.W. Luecke. 1969. Changes in trace elements and enzyme activities in tissues of zinc-deficient pigs. Am. J. Clin. Nutr. 22:628–637.

Prasad, J.S. 1979. Leukocyte function in iron-deficiency anemia. Am. J. Clin. Nutr. 32:550–552.

Prohaska, J.R., and M.L. Failla. 1993. Copper and immunity. Pp. 309–332 in Nutrition and Immunology, D.M. Klurfeld, ed. New York: Plenum Press.

Prohaska, J.R., and O.A. Lukasewycz. 1981. Copper deficiency suppresses the immune response of mice. Science 213:559–561.

Prohaska, J.R., and O.A. Lukasewycz. 1989. Biochemical and immunological changes in mice following postweaning copper deficiency. Biol. Trace Elem. Res. 22:101–112.

Prohaska, J.R., and O.A. Lukasewycz. 1990. Effects of copper deficiency on the immune system. Adv. Exp. Med. Biol. 262:123–143.

Prohaska, J.R., S.W. Downing, O.A. Lukasewycz. 1983. Chronic dietary copper deficiency alters biochemical and morphological properties of mouse lymphoid tissues. J. Nutr. 113(8):1583–1590.

Provinciali, M., G. DiStefano, and N. Fabris. 1992. Improvement in the proliferative capacity and natural killer cell activity of murine spleen lymphocytes by thyrotropin. J. Immunopharmacol. 14:865–870.

Pruitt J.H., E.M. Copeland, and L.L. Moldawer. 1995. Interleukin-1 and interleukin-1 antagonism in sepsis, systemic inflammatory response syndrome, and septic shock. Shock 3(4):235–251.

Purasiri, P., A. Murray, S. Richardson, D. Heys, D. Horrobin, and O. Eremin. 1994. Modulation of cytokine production in vivo by dietary essential fatty acids in patients with colorectal cancer. Clin. Sci. 87:711–717.

Pyne, D.B. 1994. Regulation of neutrophil function during exercise. Sports Med. 17:245–258.

Pyne, D.B., M.S. Baker, P.A. Fricker, W.A. McDonald, and W.J. Nelson. 1995. Effects of an intensive 12-wk training program by elite swimmers on neutrophil oxidative activity. Med. Sci. Sports Exerc. 27:536–542.

Qiao, L., G. Schurmann, F. Autschbach, R. Wallich, and S.C. Meuer. 1993. Human intestinal mucosa alters T-cell reactivities. Gastroenterology 105:814–819.

Rabson, A.R., A.F. Hallett, and H.J. Koornhof. 1975. Generalized Yersinia enterocolitica infection. J. Infect. Dis. 131:447–451.

Rahmathullah, L., B.A. Underwood, R.D. Thulasiraj, and R.C. Milton. 1991. Diarrhoea, respiratory infections and growth are not affected by a weekly low dose vitamin A supplement: A masked controlled field trial in children in Southern India. Am. J. Clin. Nutr. 54:568–577.

Raine, C.S., V. Traugott, and S.H. Stone. 1978. Suppression of chronic allergic encephalomyelitis: Relevance to multiple sclerosis. Science 201:445–448.

Rall, L.C., and S.N. Meydani. 1993. Vitamin B6 and immune competence. Nutr. Rev. 51:217–25.

Rall, L.C., N.T. Lundgren, S. Reichlin, J.D. Veldhuis, and R. Roubenoff. 1996. Growth hormone (GH) kinetics in aging and chronic inflammation. FASEB J. 10:A754.

Rang, H.P., M.M. Dale, J.M. Ritter, and P. Gardner. 1995. Pharmacology. New York: Churchill Livingstone.

Rankin, E.C., E.H. Choy, D. Kassimos, and G.H. Kingsley. 1995. The therapeutic effects of an engineered human anti-tumor necrosis factor-α antibody (CDP571) in rheumatoid arthritis. Br. J. Rheumatol. 34(4):334–342.

Rasmussen, L.B., B. Kiens, B.K. Pederson, and E.A. Richter. 1994. Effect of diet and plasma fatty acid composition on immune status in elderly men. Am. J. Clin. Nutr. 59:572–577.

Rassnick, S., A.F. Sved, and B.S. Rabin. 1994. Locus coeruleus stimulation by corticotropin-releasing hormone suppresses in vitro cellular immune responses. J. Neurosci. 14:6033–6040.

Ratté, J., F. Halberg, and J.F.W. Kuhl. 1973. Circadian variation in the rejection of rat kidney allografts. Surgery 73:102–108.

Reffett, J.K., J.W. Spears, and T.T. Brown, Jr. 1988. Effect of dietary selenium and vitamin E on the primary and secondary immune response in lambs challenged with parainfluenza 3 virus. J. Anim. Sci. 66:1520–1528.

Reichlin, S. 1993. Neuroendocrine–immune interactions [review article]. New Engl. J. Med. 329(17):1246–1253.

Reichlin, S. 1994. Neuroendocrine consequences of systemic inflammation. Pp. 83–96 in Advances in Endocrinology and Metabolism, E.L. Mazzaferri, R.S. Bar, and R.A. Kreisberg, eds. St. Louis: Mosby.

Reichlin, S. 1995. Endocrine–immune interaction. Pp. 2964–3012 in Endocrinology, L.J. DeGroot, ed. Philadelphia: W.B. Saunders Company.

Reichlin, S. 1998. Neuroendocrinology. In William's Textbook of Endocrinology, 9th ed., J.D. Wilson, D. Foster, P.R. Larsen, and H. Kronenberg, eds. Philadelphia: W.B. Saunders Company.

Reichlin, S., and R.J. Glaser. 1958. Thyroid function in experimental streptococcal pneumonia in the rat. J. Exp. Med. 107:219–236.

Reinberg, A. 1967. The hours of changing responsiveness or susceptibility. Perspect. Biol. Med. 11:111–128.

Reinberg, A. 1989. Chronopharmacology of corticosteroids and ACTH. Pp. 137–167 in Chronopharmacology, Cellular, and Biochemical Interactions, B. Lemmer, ed. New York: Marcel Dekker.

Reinberg, A., and E. Sidi. 1966. Circadian changes in the inhibitory effects of an antihistaminic drug in man. J. Invest. Dermatol. 46:415–419.

Reinberg, A., and M.H. Smolensky. 1994. Night and Shift Work and Transmeridian and Space Flights. Pp. 243-255 in Biologic Rhythms in Clinical and Laboratory Medicine, 2d ed., Y. Touitou and E. Haus, eds. Heidelberg: Springer-Verlag.

Reinberg, A., P. Gervais, M. Morin, and C. Abulker. 1971. Human circadian rhythm in threshold of the bronchial response to acetylcholine. C.R. Acad. Sci. Hebd. Seances Acad. Sci. D. 272:1879–1881.

Reinberg, A., J. Ghata, and E. Sidi. 1963. Nocturnal asthma attacks: Their relationship to the circadian adrenal cycle. J. Allerg. 34:323–330.

Reinberg A., G. Labreque, and M.H. Smolensky, eds. 1991. Chronobiologie et Chronotherapeutique. Heme Optimale d'Administration des Medicamcuts. Paris: Flamarion-Medecine-Sciences.

Reinberg, A., E. Schuller, J. Clench, and M.H. Smolensky. 1979. Circadian and circannual rhythms of leukocytes, proteins, and immunoglobulins. Pp. 251–259 in Recent Advances in the Chronobiology of Allergy and Immunology, M.H. Smolensky, A. Reinberg, and J.P. McGovern, eds. Oxford: Pergamon Press.

Reinberg, A., E. Sidi, and J. Ghata. 1965. Circadian reactivity rhythms of human skin to histamine or allergen and the adrenal cycle. J. Allerg. 36:273–283.

Reinberg, A., M.H. Smolensky, G.E. D'Alonzo, and J.P. McGovern. 1988a. Chronobiology and asthma. III. Timing corticotherapy to biological rhythms to optimize treatment goals. J. Asthma 25:219–248.

Reinberg, A., Y. Touitou, M. Botbol, P. Gervais, D. Chaouat, F. Levi, and A. Bicakova-Rocher. 1988b. Oral morning dosing of corticosteroids in long term treated cortico-dependent asthmatics: Increased tolerance and preservation of the adrenocortical function. Ann. Rev. Chronopharmacol. 5:209–212.

Reinberg, A., Y. Touitou, A. Restoin, C. Migraine, F. Levi, and H. Montagner. 1985. The genetic background of circadian and ultradian rhythm patterns of 17-hydroxycorticosteroids: A cross twin study. J. Endocrinol. 105:247–253.

Reinherz, E.L., and S.F. Schlossman. 1980. The differentiation and function of human T-lymphocytes. Cell 19:821–827.

Reister, F.A. 1975. Medical Statistics in World War II. Washington, D.C.: U.S. Government Printing Office.

Rensing L. 1997. Genetics and molecular biology of circadian clocks. Pp. 55–77 in Physiology and Pharmacology of Biologic Rhythms. Handbook of Experimental Pharmacology, Volume 125, P.H. Redfern and B. Lemmer, eds. Heidelberg: Springer-Verlag.

Reynolds, J.V., J.M. Daly, S. Zhang, E. Evantash, J. Shou, R. Sigal, and M.M. Ziegler. 1988. Immunomodulatory mechanisms of arginine. Surgery 104(2):142-51.

Richmand, D.A., M.E. Molitch, and T.F. O'Donnell. 1980. Altered thyroid hormone levels in bacterial sepsis: The role of nutritional adequacy. Metab. Clin. Exp. 29:936–942.

Richtsmeier, W.S. 1985. Interferon. Present and future prospects. CRC Crit. Rev. Clin. Lab. Sci. 20:57–93.

Riedo, F.X., B. Schwartz, S. Glono, J. Hierholzer, S. Ostroff, J. Groover, D. Musher, L. Martinez-Lopez, R. Brelman, and the Pneumococcal Pneumonia Study Group. 1991. Pneumococcal pneumonia outbreak in a Ranger Training Battalion. Program and Abstracts of the Interscience Conference on Antimicrobial Agents and Chemotherapy. Abstract 48. Chicago, Ill.: American Society of Microbiology.

Rigsby, L.W., R.K. Dishman, A.W. Jackson, G.S. Maclean, and P.B. Raven. 1992. Effects of exercise training on men seropositive for the human immunodeficiency virus-1. Med. Sci. Sports Exerc. 24:6–12.

Ritchie, A.W.S., I. Oswald, H.S. Micklem, J.E. Boyd, R.A. Elton, E. Jazwinska, and K. James. 1983. Circadian variation of lymphocyte subpopulations: A study with monoclonal antibodies. Br. Med. J. 286:1773–1775.

Rivard, G.E., C. Infante-Rivard, M.F. Dresse, J.M. Leclerc, and J. Champagne. 1993. Circadian time-dependent response of childhood lymphoblastic leukemia to chemotherapy: A long-term follow-up study of survival. Chronbiol. Int. 10:201–204.

Rivest, S., and C. Rivier. 1995. The role of corticotropin-releasing factor and interleukin-1 in the regulation of neurons controlling reproductive functions. Endocr. Rev. 16:177–199.

Rivest, S., G. Torres, and C. Rivier. 1992. Differential effects of central and peripheral injection of interleukin-1β on brain c-fos expression and neuroendocrine functions. Brain Res. 587:13–23.

Rivett, A.J. 1985. The effect of mixed-function oxidation of enzymes on their susceptibility to degradation by a nonlysosomal cysteine proteinase. Arch. Biochem. Biophys. 243:624–632.

Rivier, C. 1993. Effect of peripheral and central cytokines on the hypothalamic–pituitary–adrenal axis of the rat. Ann. N.Y. Acad. Sci. 697:97–105.

Rivier, C. 1995. Influence of immune signals on the hypothalamic–pituitary axis of the rodent. Front. Neuroendocrinol. 16:151–182.

Rivier, C., and S. Rivest. 1993. Mechanisms mediating the effects of cytokines on neuroendocrine functions in the rat. Ciba Found. Symp. 172:204–220.

Rivier, C., R. Chizzonite, and W. Vale. 1989. In the mouse, the activation of the hypothalamic–pituitary–adrenal axis by a lipopolysaccharide (endotoxin) is mediated through interleukin-1. Endocrinology 125:2800–2805.

Roberts, J.A. 1985. Loss of form in young athletes due to viral infection. Br. J. Med. 290:357–358.

Roberts, J.A. 1986. Viral illnesses and sports performance. Sports Med. 3:296–303.

Robins-Browne, R.M., and J.K. Pripic. 1985. Effects of iron and desferrioxamine on infections with *Yersinia enterocolitica*. Infect. Immun. 47:774–779.

Rock, C.L., R.A. Jacob, and P.E. Bowen. 1996. Update on the biological characteristics of the antioxidant micronutrients: vitamin C, vitamin E, and the carotenoids. J. Am. Diet. Assoc. 96(7):693–702.

Rohde, T., H. Ullum, J.P. Rasmussen, J.H. Kristensen, E. Newsholme, and B.K. Pedersen. 1995. Effects of glutamine on the immune system: Influence of muscular exercise and HIV infection. J. Appl. Physiol. 79:146–150.

Roitt, I.M., and J. Brostoff. 1991. Immunology. London: Gower.

Rojanapo, W., A.J. Lamb, and J.A. Olson. 1980. The prevalence, metabolism and migration of goblet cells in rat intestine following the induction of rapid, synchronous vitamin A deficiency. J. Nutr. 110:178–188.

Romball, C.G., and W.O. Weigle. 1973. A cyclical appearance of antibody producing cells after a single injection of serum protein antigen. J. Exp. Med. 138:1426–1442.

Romball, C.G., and W.O. Weigle. 1976. Modulation of regulatory mechanisms operative in the cyclical production of antibody. J. Exp. Med. 143:497–510.

Romero, L.I., J.B. Tatro, J.A. Field, and S. Reichlin. 1996. Roles of IL-1 and TNF-α in endotoxin-induced activation of nitric oxide synthase in cultured rat brain cells. Am. J. Physiol. 270:R326–R332.

Rosado, J.L., P. Lopez, E. Munoz, H. Martinez, and L.H. Allen. 1997. Zinc supplementation reduced morbidity, but neither zinc nor iron supplementation affected growth or body composition of Mexican preschoolers. Am. J. Clin. Nutr. 1997. 65:13–29.

Rosales, F.J., S.J. Ritter, R. Zolfaghari, J.E. Smith, and A.C. Ross. 1996. Effects of acute inflammation on plasma retinol, retinol-binding protein, and its mRNA in the liver and kidneys of vitamin A-sufficient rats. J. Lipid Res. 37:962–971.

Rose, R.M., P.G. Bourne, R.O. Poe, E.H. Mougey, D.R. Collins, and J.W. Mason. 1969. Androgen responses to stress. II. Excretion of testosterone, epitestosterone, androsterone and etiocholanolone during basic combat training and under threat of attack. Psychosom. Med. 31:418–436.

Rosen, L. 1989. Disease exacerbation caused by sequential dengue infections: Myth or reality? Rev. Infect. Dis. 11(suppl. 4):S840–842.

Rosen, L.N., J.M. Teitelbaum, and D.J. Westhuis. 1993. Stressors, stress mediators, and emotional well-being among spouses of soldiers deployed to the Persian Gulf during Operation Desert Shield/Storm. J. Appl. Soc. Psychol. 23:1587–1593.

Rosenblatt, L.S., M. Shifrine, N.W. Hetherington, T. Paglierioni, and M.R. Mackenzie. 1982. A circannual rhythm in rubella antibody titers. J. Interdiscipl. Cycle Res. 13:81–88.

Røshol, H., K.K. Skrede, C.E. Ærø, and P. Wiik. 1995. Dexamethasone and methylprednisolone effect on peritoneal phagocyte chemiluminescence after administration in vivo. Eur. J. Pharmacol. 286:9–17.

Ross, A.C. 1992. Vitamin A status: Relationship to immunity and the antibody response. Proc. Soc. Exp. Biol. Med. 200:303–320.

Ross, A.C., and U.G. Hammerling. 1994. Retinoids and the immune system. Pp. 521–543 in The Retinoids: Biology, Chemistry, and Medicine, 2nd ed., M.B. Sporn, A.B. Roberts, and D.S. Goodman, eds. New York: Raven Press.

Ross, A.C., and C.B. Stephensen. 1996. Vitamin A and retinoids in antiviral responses. FASEB J. 10:979–985.

Roth, E., J. Funovics, F. Muhlbacher, P. Sporn, W. Mauritz, and A. Fritsch. 1982. Metabolic disorders in severe abdominal sepsis: Glutamine deficiency in skeletal muscle. Clin. Nutr. 1:25.

Rothman, K.J., L.L. Moore, M.R. Singer, U.S. Nguyen, S. Mannino, and A. Milunsky. 1995. Teratogenicity of high vitamin A intake. N. Engl. J. Med. 333:1369.

Roubenoff, R. 1993. Hormones, cytokines and body composition: Can lessons from illness be applied to aging? J. Nutr. 123:469–473.

Rubin, R.T., E.K. Gunderson, and R.J. Arthur. 1971. Life stress and illness patterns in the U.S. Navy: V. Prior life change and illness onset in a battleship's crew. Psychosom. Med. 15:89–94.

Rubin, R.T., R.G. Miller, R.J. Arthur, and B.R. Clark. 1970. Differential adrenocortical stress responses in naval aviators during aircraft carrier landing practice. Psychol. Rep. 26:71–74.

Russell, D.A., and K. K. Tucker. 1995. Combined inhibition of interleukin-1 and tumor necrosis factor in rodent endotoxemia: Improved survival and organ function. J. Infect. Dis. 171:1528–1538.

Russell, D.H., K.T. Mills, F.J. Talamantes, and H.A. Bern. 1988. Neonatal administration of prolactin antiserum alters the development pattern of T- and B-lymphocytes in the thymus and spleen in *Balb/C* female mice. Proc. Natl. Acad. Sci. USA 85:7404–7407.

Russell, R.C. 1998. Mosquito-borne arboviruses in Australia: the current scene and implications of climate change for human health. Int. J. Parasitol. 28:955–69.

Russo, M.F. 1992. Macrophages and the glucocorticoids. J. Neuroimmunol. 40:281–286.

Sabate, I., J.M. Grino, A.M. Castelao, B. Arranz, C. Gonzalez, E. Guillin, C. Diaz, J. Huguet, and S. Gracia. 1990. Diurnal variations of cyclosporine and metabolites in renal transplant patients. Transplant. Proc. 22:1700–1701.

Radomski, M.W., B.H. Sabiston, and P. Isoard. 1980. Development of "sport anemia" in physically fit men after daily sustained submaximal exercise. Aviat. Space Environ. Med. 51(1):41–5.

Saija, A., P. Princi, M. Lanza, M. Scalese, E. Aramnejad, and A. De Sarro. 1995. Systemic cytokine administration can affect blood–brain barrier permeability in the rat. Life Sci. 56:775–784.

Salus, R. 1957. Ophthalmology in a concentration camp. Am. J. Ophthalmol. 44:12–17.

Samuels, M.H., and P. Kramer. 1996. Differential effects of short-term fasting on pulsatile thyrotropin, gondotropin, and α-subunit secretion in healthy men—A clinical research center study. J. Clin. Endocrinol. Metab. 81:32–36.

Sanders, B.G., and K. Kline. 1995. Nutrition, immunology, and cancer: An overview. Pp. 185–194 in Nutrition and Biotechnology in Heart Disease and Cancer, J.B. Longenecker et al., eds. New York: Plenum Press.

Santos, J.I.. 1995. Nutrition, infection, and immunocompetence. Infect. Dis. Clinics North Am. 8:243–267.

Santos, M.S., S.N. Meydani, L. Leka, D. Wu, N. Fotouhi, M. Meydani, C.H. Hennekens, and J.M. Gaziano. 1996. Natural killer cell activity in elderly men is enhanced by beta-carotene supplementation. Am. J. Clin. Nutr. 64(5):772–777.

Santos, P.C., and R.P. Falcao. 1990. Decreased lymphocyte subsets and K-cell activity in iron deficiency anemia. Acta Haemtologica 84:118–121.

Saperstein, A., H. Brand, T. Audhya, D. Nabriski, B. Hutchinson, S. Rosenzweig, and C. S. Hollander. 1992. Interleukin 1β mediates stress-induced immunosuppression via corticotropin-releasing factor. Endocrinology 130:152–158.

Sapolsky, R., C. Rivier, G. Yamamoto, P. Plotsky, and W. Vale. 1987. Interleukin-1 stimulates the secretion of hypothalamic corticotropin-releasing factor. Science 238:522–524.

Sarchielli, P., and R.K. Chandra. 1991. Immunocompetence methodology. Pp. 425–545 in Nutrition Status Assessment, F. Fidanza, ed. London: Chapman and Hall.

Sauberlich, H.E. 1984. Implications of nutritional status on human biochemistry, physiology and health. Clin. Biochem. 17:132–142.

Sawchenko, P.E., E.R. Brown, R.K.W. Chan, A. Ericsson, H.-Y. Li, B.L. Roland, and K.J. Kovács. 1996. The paraventricular nucleus of the hypothalamus and the functional neuroanatomy of visceromotor responses to stress. Pp. 201–222 in The Emotional Motor System, G. Holstege, R. Bandler, and C.B. Saper, eds. Progress in Brain Research, vol. 107. Amsterdam: Elsevier.

Sawitsky, B., R. Kanter, and A. Sawitsky. 1976. Lymphocyte response to phytomitogens in iron deficiency. Am. J. Med. Sci. 272:153–160.

Sazawal, S., R. E. Black, M.K. Bhan, N. Bhandari, A. Sinha, and S. Jalla. 1995. Zinc supplementation in young children with acute diarrhea in India. N. Engl. J. Med. 333:839–844.

Sazawal, S., R.E. Black, M.K. Bhan, S. Jalla, N. Bhandari, A. Sinha, and S. Majumdar. 1996. Zinc supplementation reduces the incidence of persistent diarrhea and dysentery among low socioeconomic children in India. J. Nutr. 126(2):443–450.

Scarborough, D.E., S.L. Lee, C.A. Dinarello, and S. Reichlin. 1989. Interleukin-1 stimulates somatostatin biosynthesis in primary cultures of fetal rat brain. Endocrinology 126:3053–3058.

Schaumburg, H., J. Kaplan, A. Windebank, N. Vick, S. Rasmus, D. Pleasure, and M.J. Brown. 1983. Sensory neuropathy from pyridoxine abuse: A new megavitamin syndrome. N. Engl. J. Med. 309:445–448.

Scheibel, L.W. 1988. Plasmodial parasite biology: Carbohydrate metabolism and related organellar function during various stages of the life cycle. Pp. 171–217 in Malaria: Principles and Practice of Malariology, W. Wernsdorfer and I. McGregor, eds. Endinburgh: Churchill Livingstone.

Scheibel, L.W., and I.W. Sherman. 1988. Metabolism and organellar function during various stages of the life cycle: Proteins, lipids, nucleic acids, and vitamins. Pp. 219–252 in Malaria: Principles and Practice of Malariology, W. Wernsdorfer and I. McGregor, eds. Endinburgh: Churchill Livingstone.

Scheving, L.E., E. Burns, J.E. Pauly, S. Tsai, and F. Halberg. 1976. Meal scheduling, cellular rhythms, and the chronotherapy of cancer [abstract]. Chronobiologia 3:80.

Scheving, L.E., E.L. Kanabrocki, F. Halberg, and J.E. Pauly. 1977. Circadian variations in total and electrophoretically fractioned serum proteins of presumably healthy man. Pp. 204–214 in Chronobiology in Allergy and Immunology, J.P. McGovern, M.H. Smolensky, and A. Reinberg, eds. Springfield, Ill.: Charles C Thomas.

Scheving, L.E., J.E. Pauly, and T. Tsai. 1968. Circadian fluctuation in plasma proteins of the rat. Am. J. Physiol. 215:1096–1101.

Schlesinger, L., M. Arevalo, S. Arredondo, B. Lönnerdal, and A. Stekel. 1993. Zinc supplementation impairs monocyte function. Acta Paediatr. 82:734–738.

Schloerb, P.R., and M. Amare. 1993. Total parenteral nutrition with glutamine in bone marrow transplantation and other clinical applications (a randomized, double-blind study). JPEN J. Parenter. Enteral Nutr. 17:407–413.

Schmidt, E.B., K. Varming, J.O. Pedersen, H.H. Lervang, N. Grunnet, C. Jersild, and J. Dyerberg. 1992. Long-term supplementation with n-3 fatty acids, II: Effect on neutrophil and monocyte chemotaxis. Scand. J. Clin. Lab. Invest. 52(3):229–236.

Schöbitz, B., E.R. De Kloet, and F. Holsboer. 1994. Gene expression and function of interleukin-1, interleukin-6, and tumor necrosis factor in the brain. Prog. Neurobiol. 44:397–432.

Schotanus, K., F. Tilders, and F. Berkenbosch. 1993. Human interleukin-1 receptor antagonist prevents adrenocorticotropin, but not interleukin-6 response to bacterial endotoxin in rats. Endocrinology 132:1569–1576.

Schrauzer, G.N., and W.J. Rhead. 1973. Ascorbic acid abuse: effects on long term ingestion of excessive amounts on blood levels and urinary excretion. Int. J. Vitam. Nutr. Res. 43(2):201–211.

Schryners, A.B., and J.L. Morris. 1988. Identification and characterization of the transferrin receptor from *Neisseria meningitidis*. Mol. Microbiol. 2:281–288.

Schuurs, A.H., and H.A. Verheul. 1990. Effects of gender and sex steroids on the immune system. J. Steroid Biochem. 25:157–172.

Schwab, R., C.A. Waiters, and M.E. Weksler. 1989. Host defense mechanisms and aging. Semin. Oncol. 16:20–27.

Schwartz, J., and S.T. Weiss. 1994. Relationship between dietary vitamin C intake and pulmonary function in the First National Health and Nutrition Examination Survey (NHANES I). Am. J. Clin. Nutr. 59:110–114.

Schwartzman, W.A., M.W. Lambertus, C.A. Kennedy, and M.B. Goetz. 1991. Staphylococcal pyomyositis in patients infected by the human immunodeficiency virus. Am. J. Med. 90:595–600.

Schweiger, H.G., R. Hartwig, and M. Schweigher. 1986. Cellular aspects of circadian rhythms. J. Cell Sci. 4(suppl.):181–200.

Scrimshaw, N.S., C.E. Taylor, and J.E. Gordon. 1968. Interactions of nutrition and infection. Monograph. Geneva: World Health Organization.

Scuderi, P. 1990. Differential effects of copper and zinc on human peripheral blood monocyte cytokine secretion. Cell Immunol. 126:391–405.

Seay, W.J. 1995. Deployment medicine: Emporiatrics military style. Army Med. Dept. J. July/August:2–9.

Selmanoff, M.K., L.P. Kapcala, J.R. He, Y. Gao, D.N. Darlington, and D.E. Carlson. 1996. Adrenocorticosteroid feedback is not necessary for adrenocorticotropin stimulation by peripheral interleukin-1β. Soc. Neurosci. 21:336.4.

Semba, R.D. 1994. Vitamin A, immunity, and infection. Clin. Infect. Dis. 19:489–499.

Semba, R.D., N.M.H. Graham, W.T. Caiaffa, J.B. Margolick, L. Clement, and D. Vlahov. 1993a. Increased mortality associated with vitamin A deficiency during human immunodeficiency virus type 1 infection. Arch. Intern. Med. 153:2149–2154.

Semba, R.D., P. Miotti, J.D. Chiphangwi, G. Liomba, L.P. Yang, A. Saah, G. Dallabetta, and D.R. Hoover. 1995. Infant mortality and maternal vitamin A deficiency during HIV infection. Clin. Infect. Dis. 21:966–972.

Semba, R.D., P. Miotti, J.D. Chiphangwi, A. Saah, J. Canner, G. Dallabetta, and D.R. Hoover. 1994. Maternal vitamin A deficiency and mother-to-child transmission of HIV-1. Lancet 343:1593–1597.

Semba, R.D., Muhilal, A.L. Scott, G. Natadisastra, S. Wirasasmita, L. Mele, E. Ridwan, K.P. West Jr., and A. Sommer. 1992. Depressed immune response to tetanus in children with vitamin A deficiency. J. Nutr. 122:101–107.

Semba, R.D., Muhilal, B.J. Ward, A.L. Scott, G. Natadisastra, K.P. West, Jr., and A. Sommer. 1993b. Abnormal T-cell subset proportions in vitamin A-deficient children. Lancet 341:5–8.

Senie, R.T., P.P. Rosen, P. Rhodes, and M.L. Lesser. 1991. Timing of breast cancer excision during the menstrual cycle influences duration of disease-free survival. Ann. Intern. Med. 115:337–342.

Senkal, M., A. Mumme, U. Eickhoff, B. Geier, G. Spath, D. Wulfert, U. Joosten, A. Frei, M. Kemen. 1997. Early postoperative enteral immunonutrition: clinical outcome and cost-comparison analysis in surgical patients. Crit. Care Med. 25:1489–96.

Sensi, S., E. Haus, G.Y. Nicolau, F. Halberg, D.J. Lakatua, A. DelPonte, and M.T. Guagnano. 1984. Circannual variation of insulin secretion in clinically healthy subjects in Italy, Romania, and the U.S.A. Riv. Ital. Biol. Med. 4:1–8.

Sevinc, M.S., and W.J. Page. 1992. Generation of *Azotobacter vinlandii* strains defective in siderophore production and characterization of a strain unable to produce known siderophores. J. Gen. Microbiol. 138:587–596.

Seyberth, H.W., O. Oelz, T. Kennedy, B.J. Sweetman, A. Danon, J.C. Frolich, M. Helmberg, and J.A. Oates. 1975. Increased arachidonic acid in lipids after administration to man: Effects on prostaglandin biosynthesis. Clin. Pharmacol. Ther. 18:521–529.

Shabert, J.K., and D.W. Wilmore. 1996. Glutamine deficiency as a cause of human immunodeficiency virus wasting. Med. Hypotheses 46:252–256.

Shah, M.A., P.R. Bergethon, A.M. Boak, P.M. Gallop, and H.M. Kagan. 1992. Oxidation of peptidyl lysine by copper complexes of pyrroloquinoline quinone and other quinones: A model for oxidative pathochemistry. Biochim. Biophys. Acta. 1159(3):311–318.

Shahal, B., F.A. Lue, C.G. Jiang, A. MacLean, and H. Moldofsky. 1992. Circadian and sleep-wake related changes in immune functions. J. Sleep Res. 1(suppl.):210.

Shalaby, M.R., J. Halgunset, O.A. Haugen, H. Aarset, L. Aarden, A. Waage, K. Matsushima, H. Kvithyll, D. Boraschi, J. Lamvik, and T. Espevid. 1991. Cytokine-associated tissue injury and lethality in mice: A comparative study. Clin. Immunol. Immunopathol. 61:69–82.

Shalts, E., Y-J. Feng, and M. Ferrin. 1991. Vasopressin mediates the interleukin-1a-induced reduced decrease in luteinizing hormone secretion in the ovariectomized rhesus monkey. Endocrinology 131:153–158.

Shambaugh, G.E. and W.R. Beisel. 1966. Alterations in thyroid physiology during pneumococcal septicemia in the rat. Endocrinology. 79(3):511–723.

Shand, G.H., H. Anwar, J. Kadurugamuwa, M.R.W. Brown, S.H. Silverman, and J. Melling. 1985. In vivo evidence that bacteria in urinary tract infection grow under iron-restricted conditions. Infect. Immun. 48:35–39.

Sharp, G.W.G. 1960. Reversal of diurnal leukocyte variations in man. J. Endocrinol. 21:107–114.

Sharp, J.C.M. 1989. Viruses and the athlete. Br. J. Sports Med. 23:47–48.

Sharp, N.C., and Y. Koutedakis. 1992. Sport and the overtraining syndrome: Immunological aspects. Br. Med. Bull. 48:518–533.

Shaw, L.M., B. Kaplan, and D. Kaufman. 1996. Toxic effects of immunosuppressive drugs: Mechanisms and strategies of controlling them. Clin. Chem. 42:1316–1321.

Sheagren, J.N. 1991. Corticosteroids for the treatment of septic shock. Infect. Dis. Clin. North Am. 5:875–882.

Sheffy, B.E., and R.D. Schultz. 1979. Influence of vitamin E and selenium on immune response mechanisms. Fed. Proc. 38:2139–2143.

Shek, P.N., B.H. Sabiston, A. Buguet, and M.W. Radomski. 1995. Strenuous exercise and immunological changes: A multiple-time-point analysis of leukocyte subsets, CD4/CD8 ratio, immunoglobulin production and NK cell response. Int. J. Sports Med. 16:466–474.

Shephard, D.S., J.A. Walsh, E. Kleinau, S. Stansfield, and S. Bhalotra. 1995a. Setting priorities for the Children's Vaccine Initiative: a cost-effectiveness approach. Vaccine. 13(8):707–714.

Shephard, R.J., and P.N. Shek. 1995. Exercise, aging and immune function. Int. J. Sports Med. 16(1):1–6 .

Shephard, R.J., T. Kavanagh, D.J. Mertens, S. Qureshi, and M. Clark. 1995b. Personal health benefits of masters athletics competition. Br. J. Sport Med. 29:35–40.

Shephard, R.J., S. Rhind, and P.N. Shek. 1994a. Exercise and the immune system. Natural killer cells, interleukins and related responses. Sports Med. 18(5):340–69.

Shephard, R.J., S. Rhind, and P.N. Shek. 1994b. Exercise and training: Influences on cytotoxicity, interleukin-1, interleukin-2 and receptor structures. Int. J. Sports Med. 15(suppl. 3):S154–S166.

Shephard, R.J., S. Rhind, and P.N. Shek. 1995. The impact of exercise on the immune system: NK cells, interleukins-1 and -2, and related responses. Exerc. Sport Sci. Rev. 23:215–241.

Sheppard, B.C., and J.A. Norton. 1991. Tumor necrosis factor and interleukin-1 protection against lethal effects of tumor necrosis factor. Surgery 109:698–705.

Shifrine, M., A. Garsd, and L.S. Rosenblatt. 1982a. Seasonal variation in immunity of humans. J. Interdiscipl. Cycle Res. 12:157–165.

Shifrine, M., L.S. Rosenblatt, N. Taylor, N.W. Hetherington, F.J. Mathews, and F.D. Wilson. 1982b. Seasonal variations in lectin-induced lymphocyte transformation in Beagle dogs. J. Interdiscipl. Cycle Res. 13:151–156.

Shifrine, M., N. Taylor, L.S. Rosenblatt, and F. Wilson. 1980. Seasonal variation in cell-mediated immunity of clinically normal dogs. Exp. Hematol. 8:318–326.

Shinkai, S., H. Kohno, K. Kimura, T. Komura, H. Asai, R. Inai, K. Oka, Y. Kurokawa, and R.J. Shephard. 1995. Physical activity and immunosenescence in elderly men. Med. Sci. Sports Exerc. 27:1516–1526.

Shinkai, S., Y. Kurokawa, S. Hino, M. Hirose, J. Torii, S. Watanabe, S. Watanabe, S. Shiraishi, K. Oka, and T. Watanabe . 1993. Triathlon competition induced a transient immunosuppressive change in the peripheral blood of athletes. J. Sports Med. Phys. Fitness 33:70–78.

Shippee, R., K. Friedl, T. Kramer, M. Mays, K. Popp, E.W. Askew, B. Fairbrother, R. Hoyt, J. Vogel, L. Marchitelli, P. Frykman, L. Martinez-Lopez, E. Bernton, M. Kramer, R. Tulley, J. Rood, J. DeLany, D. Jezior, and J. Arsenault. 1994. Nutritional and immunological assessment of Ranger students with increased caloric intake. Report No. T95-5. Natick, Mass.: U.S. Army Research Institute of Environmental Medicine.

Shippee, R., S. Wood, P. Anderson, T. Kramer, M. Nieta, and K. Wolcott. 1995. Effects of glutamine supplementation on immunological responses of soldiers during the Special Forces Assessment and Selection Course. FASEB J. 9:A731.

Shoham, S., D. Davenne, A.B. Cady, C.A. Dinarello, and J.M. Krueger. 1987. Recombinant tumor necrosis factor and interleukin-1 enhance slow wave sleep. Am. J. Physiol. 253:R142–R149.

Shor-Posner, G., M.J. Miguez-Burbano, Y. Lu, D. Feaster, M. Fletcher, H. Sauberlich, and M.K. Baum. 1995. Elevated IgE level in relationship to nutritional status and immune parameters in early human immunodeficiency virus-1 disease. J. Allergy Clin. Immunol. 95:886–892.

Shronts, E.P. 1993. Basic concepts of immunology and its application to clinical nutrition. Nutr. Clin. Pract. 8(4):177–183.

Sidell, N., B. Chang., and L. Bhatti. 1993. Upregulation by retinoic acid of interleukin-2 receptor mRNA in human T-lymphocytes. Cell. Immunol. 146:28–37.

Silver, R.M., M.P. Heyes, J.C. Maize, B. Quearry, M. Vionnet-Fuasset, and E.M. Sternberg. 1990. Scleroderma, fascitis, and eosinophilia associated with the ingestion of tryptophan [see comments]. N. Engl. J. Med. 322(13):874–881.

Simon, G.A., P. Schmid, W.G. Reifenrath, T. van Ravenswaay, and B.E Stuck. 1994. Wound healing after laser injury to skin. The effect of occlusion and vitamin E. Eur. J. Pharm. Sci. 83:1101–1106.

Simon, H.B. 1984. The immunology of exercise: A brief review. J. Am. Med. Assoc. 252:2735–2738.

Simon-Schnass, I. 1996. Oxidative Stress at High Altitudes and Effects of Vitamin E. Pp. 393–418 in Nutritional Needs in Cold and in High-Altitude Environments,

Applications for Military Personnel in Field Operations, B.M. Marriott and S.J. Carlson, eds. A report of the Committee on Military Nutrition Research, Food and Nutrition Board, Institute of Medicine. Washington, D.C.: National Academy Press.

Singh, A. 1996. Micronutrient/antioxidant supplementation and immune function in women: Effects of physiological stress. Final report. Bethesda, Md.: Uniformed Services University of the Health Sciences.

Singh, A., M.L. Failla, and P.A. Deuster. 1994. Exercise-induced changes in immune function: Effects of zinc supplementation. J. Appl. Physiol. 76:2298–2303.

Singh, A., B.L. Smoak, K.Y. Patterson, L.G. LeMay, C. Veillon, and P.A. Deuster. 1991. Biochemical indices of selected trace minerals in men: Effect of stress. Am. J. Clin. Nutr. 53:126–131.

Sitar, J. 1991. Correlation of some parameters of solar wind and sudden cardiovascular deaths. Cas Lek Cesk. 130:44–47.

Slozina, N.M., and G.D. Golovachev. 1986. The frequency of sister chromatin exchanges in human lymphocytes determined at different times within 24 hours. Citologia 28:127–129.

Smith, E.M. 1992. Hormonal activities of cytokines. Chem. Immunol. 52:154–169.

Smith, E.M., W.J. Meyer, and J.E. Blalock. 1982. Virus-induced increases in corticosterone in hypophysectomized mice: A possible lymphoid adrenal axis. Science 218:1311–1313.

Smith, E.M., A.C. Morrill, W.J.I. Meyer, and J.E. Blalock. 1986. Corticotropin-releasing factor induction of lymphocyte-derived immunoreactive ACTH and endorphins. Nature 321:881–882.

Smith, J.A., R.D. Telford, I.B. Mason, and M.J. Weidemann. 1990. Exercise, training and neutrophil microbicidal activity. Int. J. Sports Med. 11:179–187.

Smith, J.C. 1980. The vitamin A-zinc connection: A review. Ann. N.Y. Acad. Sci. 355:62–74.

Smoak, B.L., A. Singh, B.A. Day, J.P. Norton, S.B. Kyle, S.J. Pepper, and P.A. Deuster. 1988. Changes in nutrient intakes of conditioned men during a 5-day period of increased physical activity and other stresses. Eur. J. Appl. Physiol. 58:245–251.

Smolensky, M.H., and G.E.D. D'Alonzo. 1994. Nocturnal asthma: mechanisms and chronotherapy. Pp. 453–469 in Biologic Rhythms in Clinical and Laboratory Medicine, 2d ed., Y. Touitou and E. Haus, eds. New York: Springer-Verlag.

Smolensky, M.H., and G.E.D. D'Alonzo. 1997. Progress in the chronotherapy of nocturnal asthma. Pp. 205-250 in Physiology and Pharmacology of Biologic Rhthyms. Handbook of Experimental Pharmacology, Volume 125, P.H. Redfern and B. Lemmer, eds. Heidelberg: Springer-Verlag.

Smolensky, M.H., P.J. Barnes, A. Reinberg, and J.P. McGovern. 1986a. Chronobiology and asthma. I. Day-night differences in bronchial patency and dyspnea and circadian rhythm dependencies. J. Asthma 23:321–343.

Smolensky, M.H., G.E. D'Alonzo, G. Kunkel, and P.J. Barnes. 1987. Circadian rhythm-adapted theophylline chronotherapy for nocturnal asthma. Chronobiol. Int. 4:301–466.

Smolensky, M.H., A. Reinberg, and J.T. Queng. 1981. The chronobiology and chronopharmacology of allergy. Ann. Allergy 47:237–252.

Smolensky, M.H., P.H. Scott, P.J. Barnes, and J.H.G. Jonkman. 1986b. The chronopharmacology and chronotherapy of asthma. Ann. Rev. Chronopharmacol. 2:229–273.

Smythe, P.M., M. Schonland, G.G. Brereton-Stiles, H.M. Coovadia, H.J. Grace, W.E.K. Loening, A. Mafoyne, M.A. Parent, and G.H. Vos. 1971. Thymolymphatic deficiency and depression of cell-mediated immunity in protein-calorie malnutrition. Lancet 2(7731):939–943.

Soiffer, R.J., C. Murray, C. Shapiro, H. Collins, S. Chartier, S. Lazo, and J. Ritz. 1996. Expansion and manipulation of natural killer cells in patients with metastatic cancer by low-dose continuous infusion and intermittent bolus administration of interleukin-2. Clin. Cancer Res. 2:493–499.

Sokol, R.J. 1996. Vitamin E. Pp. 130–136 in Present Knowledge in Nutrition, 7th ed., E. Khard, E. Ziegler, and L.J. Filer, eds. Washington, D.C.: ILSI Press.

Sommer, A. 1982. A Field Guide to the Detection and Control of Xerophthalmia. Geneva: World Health Organization.

Sommer, A., and K.P. West, Jr. 1996. Vitamin A Deficiency: Health, Survival, and Vision. New York: Oxford University Press.

Sommer, A., I. Tarwotjo, E. Djunaedi, K.P. West Jr., A.A. Loeden, R. Tilden, L. Mele. 1986. Impact of vitamin A supplementation on childhood mortality. A randomised controlled community trial. 1(8491):1169–1173.

Song, J.G., S. Nakano, S. Ohdo, and N. Ogawa. 1993. Chronotoxicity and chronopharmacokinetics of methotrexate in mice: Modification of feeding schedule. Japan J. Pharmacol. 62:373–378.

Sothern, R.B., B. Roitman-Johnson, E.L. Kanabrocki, J.G. Yager, M.M. Roodell, J.A. Weatherbee, M.R. Young, B.M. Nemchausky, L.E. Scheving. 1995. Circadian characteristics of circulating interleukin-6 in men. J. Allergy Clin. Immunol. 95:1029–1035.

Souba, W.W. 1992. Glutamine, Physiology, Biochemistry, and Nutrition in Critical Illness. Austin, Tx.: R.G. Landers Company.

Souba, W.W. 1994. Cytokine control of nutrition and metabolism in critical illness. Curr. Probl. Surg. 31(7):577–652.

Souba, W.W., R.J. Smith, and D.W. Wilmore. 1985. Glutamine metabolism by the intestinal tract. J. Parenter. Enteral Nutr. 9:608–617.

Spangelo, B.L., and W.C. Gorospe. 1995. Role of the cytokines in the neuroendocrine immune system axis. Front. Neuroendocrinol. 16:1–22.

Spence, D.W., M.L.A. Galantino, K.A. Mossberg, and S.O. Zimmerman. 1990. Progressive resistance exercise: Effect on muscle function and anthropometry of a select AIDS population. Arch. Phys. Med. Rehabil. 71:644–648.

Spittler, A., S. Winkler, P. Gotzinger, R. Oehler, M. Wilheim, C. Tempfer, G. Weigel, R. Fuggar, G. Boltz-Nitulescu, and E. Roth. 1995. Influence of glutamine on the phenotype and function of human monocytes. Blood 86:1564–1569.

Stabel, J.R., and J.W. Spears. 1993. Role of selenium in immune responsiveness and disease resistance. Pp. 331–356 in Human Nutrition: A Comprehensive Treatise, D.M. Klureld, ed. New York: Plenum Press.

Stabel, J.R., J.W. Spears, and T.T. Brown, Jr. 1993. Effect of copper deficiency on tissue, blood characteristics, and immune functions of calves challenged with infectious bovine rhinotracheitis virus and *Pasteruella hemolytica*. J. Anim. Sci. 71:1247–1255.

Stadtman, E.R. 1992. Protein oxidation and aging. Science 257:1220–1224.

Stallone, D.D., A.J. Stunkard, B. Zweiman, T.A. Wadden, and G.D. Foster. 1994. Decline in delayed-type hypersensitivity response in obese women following weight reduction. Clin Diagn Lab Immunol 1(2):202–205.

Stamler, J.S., D.J. Singel, and J. Loscalzo. 1992. Biochemistry of nitric oxide and its redox-activated form. Science 258:1898–1902.

Staruch, M.J., and D.D. Wood. 1985. Reduction of serum interleukin-1-like activity after treatment with dexamethasone. J. Leukocyte Biol. 37:193–207.

Stenson, W.F., D. Cort, J. Rogers, R. Burakoff, K. Deschyver-Kecskemeti, T.L. Gramlich, and W. Beeken. 1992. Dietary supplementation with fish oil in ulcerative colitis. Ann. Intern. Med. 116:609–614.

Sternberg, E.M. 1992. The stress response and the regulation of inflammatory disease. Ann. Int. Med. 117:854–866.

Sternberg, E.M. 1997a. Emotions and disease: From balance of humors to balance of molecules. Nat. Med. 3(3):264–267.

Sternberg, E.M. 1997b. Perspectives Series: Cytokines and the brain: Neural-Immune interactions in health and diseases. J. Clin. Invest. 100(11):107.

Sternberg, E.M., and J. Licinio. 1995. Overview of neuroimmune stress interactions: Implications for susceptibility to inflammatory disease. Ann. N.Y. Acad. Sci. 771:364–371.

Sternberg, E.M., G.P. Chrousos, R.L. Wilder, and P.W. Gold. 1992. The stress response and the regulation of inflammatory disease. Ann. Intern. Med. 11:854–866.

Sternberg, E.M., J.M. Hill, G.P. Chrousos, T. Kamilaris, S.J. Listwak, P.W. Gold, and R. Wilder. 1989. Inflammatory mediator-induced hypothalamic–pituitary–adrenal axis activation is defective in streptococcal cell wall arthritis-susceptible Lewis rats. Proc Natl. Acad. Sci. USA 86:2374–2378.

Stimpfling, J.H., and A. Richardson. 1967. Periodic variations of the hemagglutinin response in mice following immunization against sheep red blood cells and alloantigens. Transplantation 5:1496–1503.

Stimson, W.H. 1988. Oestrogen and human T-lymphocytes: Presence of specific receptors in the T-suppressor cytotoxic subset. Scand. J. Immunol. 28:345–350.

Stojiljkovic, J., M. Cobeljic, and K. Hantke. 1993. *Escherichia coli* K-12 ferrous iron uptake mutants are impaired in their ability to colonize the mouse intestine. FEMS Microbiol. Lett. 108:111–116.

Stouthard, J.M., J.A. Romijn, T. Van der Poll, E. Endert, S. Klein, P.J. Bakker, C.H. Veenhof, and H.P. Sauerwein. 1995. Endocrinological and metabolic effects of interleukin-6 in humans. Am. J. Physiol. 268:E813–819.

Straight, J.M., H.M. Kipen, R.F. Vogt, and R.W. Amler. 1994. Immune Function Test Batteries for Use in Environmental Health Studies. U.S. Department of Health and Human Services, Public Health Service. Publication Number: PB94-204328.

Strauss, R.G. 1978. Iron deficiency, infections, and immune function: A reassessment. Am. J. Clin. Nutr. 31:660–666.

Su, C., C. Gong, J. Li, L. Chen, D. Zhou, and Q. Jin. 1979. Preliminary results of viral etiology of Keshan disease. Chin. J. Med. 59:466–472.

Suda, T., F. Tozawa, T. Ushiyama, T. Sumitomo, M. Yamada, and H. Demura. 1990. Interleukin-1 stimulates corticotropin-releasing factor gene expression in rat hypothalamus. Endocrinology 126:1223–1228.

Sullivan, J.L., and H.D. Ochs. 1978. Copper deficiency and the immune system. Lancet 2(8091):686.

Sumida, S., K. Tanaka, H. Kitao, and F. Nakadomo. 1989. Exercise-induced lipid peroxidation and leakage of enzymes before and after vitamin E supplementation. Int. J. Biochem. 21:835–838.

Sumita, S., Y. Ujike, A. Namiki, H. Watanabe, M. Kawamata, A. Watanabe, and O. Satoh. 1994. Suppression of the thyrotropin response to thyrotropin-releasing hormone and its association with severity of critical illness. Crit. Care Med. 22:1603–1609.

Sundar, S.K., M.A. Cierpial, C. Kilts, J.C. Ritchie, and J.M. Weiss. 1990. Brain IL-1-induced immunosuppression occurs through activation of both pituitary–adrenal axis and sympathetic nervous system by corticotropin-releasing factor. J. Neurosci. 10:3701–3706.

Suskind, R.M., ed. 1977 Malnutrition and the Immune System. New York: Raven Press.

Suteanu, S., E. Haus, L. Dumitriu, G.Y. Nicolau, E. Petrescu, H. Berg, L. Sackett-Lundeen, I. Ionescu, R. Reilly. 1995. Circadian rhythm of pro- and anti-inflammatory factors in patients with rheumatoid arthritis - #226 [abstract]. Biological Rhythm Research 26:(4)446.

Swails, W.S., A.S. Kenler, D.F. Driscoll, S.J. DeMichele, T.J. Babineau, T. Utsunamiya, S. Chavali, R.A. Forse, and B.R. Bistrian. 1997. Effect of a fish oil structured lipid-based diet on prostaglandin release from mononuclear cells in cancer patients after surgery. J. Parenter. Enteral. Nutr. 21:266–74.

Sweet, K.L., and H.J. K'ang. 1955. Clinical and anatomic study of avitaminosis A among the Chinese. Am. J. Dis. Child. 50:699–734.

Swoyer, J., P. Irvine, L. Sackett-Lundeen, L. Conlin, D.J. Lakatua, and E. Haus. 1989. Circadian hematologic time structure in the elderly. Chronobiol. Int. 6:131–137.

Swoyer, J., F. Rhame, W. Hrushesky, L. Sackett-Lundeen, R. Sothern, H. Gale, and E. Haus. 1990. Circadian rhythm alterations in HIV infected subjects. Pp. 437–449 in Chronobiology: Its Role in Clinical Medicine, General Biology, and Agriculture, Proceedings of the XIX International Conference of the International Society for Chronobiology, Bethesda, Md., June 20–24, 1989. New York: Wiley-Liss, Inc.

Swoyer, J., L.L. Sackett, E. Haus, D.J. Lakatua, and L. Taddeini. 1975. Circadian lymphocytic rhythms in clinically healthy subjects and in patients with hematologic malignancies [abstract]. Pp. 62-63 in International Congress on Rhythmic Functions in Biological System, Vienna: Egerman.

Syed, V., N. Gérard, and A. Kaipia. 1993. Identification of an interleukin-6 like factor in rat seminiferous tubule. Endocrinology 132:293–299.

Szabo, C., C. Thiemermann, C. Wu, M. Perretti, and J.R. Vane. 1994. Attenuation of the induction of nitric oxide synthase by endogenous glucocorticoids accounts for endotoxin tolerance in vivo. Proc. Natl. Acad. Sci. USA 91:271–275.

Tachibana, K., K. Mukai, I. Haraoka, S. Moriguchi, S. Takama, and Y. Kishino. 1985. Evaluation of the effects of arginine-enriched amino acid solution on tumor growth. J. Parenter. Enter. Nutr. 9:428–434.

Takafuji, E.T., J.W. Kirkpatrick, R.N. Miller, J.J. Karwacki, P.W. Kelley, M.R. Gray, K.M. McNeill, H.L. Timboe, R.E. Kane, and J.L. Sanchez. 1984. An efficacy trial of doxycycline chemoprophylaxis against leptospirosis. N. Engl. J. Med. 310:497–500.

Takao, T., S.G. Culp, and E.B. DeSouza. 1993. Reciprocal modulation of interleukin-1β (IL-1β) and IL-1 receptors by lipopolysaccharide (endotoxin) treatment in the mouse brain–endocrine–immune axis. Endocrinology 132:1497–1504.

Tang, A.M., N.M. Graham, A.J. Kirby, L.D. McCall, W.C. Willett, and A.J. Saah. 1993. Dietary micronutrient intake and risk of progression to acquired immunodeficiency syndrome (AIDS) in human immunodeficiency virus type 1 (HIV-1)-infected homosexual men. Am. J. Epidemiol. 138:937–951.

Tang, A.M., N.M.H. Graham, and P. Saah. 1996. Effects of micronutrient intake on survival in human immunodeficiency virus 1 infection. Am. J. Epidemiol. 143:1244–1256.

Tappia, P.S., K.L. Troughton, S.C. Langley-Evans, and R.F. Grimble. 1995. Cigarette smoking influences cytokine production and antioxidant defences. Clin Sci (Colch) 88(4):485–489.

Tarquini, B. 1980. Physiopathology of peptic ulcer: A new view. Rass. di Medicina Sperimentale 27(5):279.

Tavadia, H.B., K.A. Fleming, P.D. Hume, and H.W. Simpson. 1975. Circadian rhythmicity of human plasma cortisol and PHA-induced lymphocyte transformation. Clin. Exp. Immunol. 22:190–193.

Tavo, T.A., R. Minlero, and A. Ponsono. 1977. NBT test in thalassemia [letter]. J. Pediatr. 90:666.

Taylor, G.R. 1993. Overview of spaceflight immunology studies. J. Leukocyte Biol. 54:179–188.

Taylor, P.G., A. Soyano, E. Romano, and M. Layrisse. 1988. Iron and transferrin uptake by phytohaemagglutinin-stimulated human peripheral blood lymphocytes. Microbiol. Immunol. 32:945–955.

Theil, E.C. 1987. Ferritin: Structure, gene regulation, and cellular function in animals, plants, and microorganisms. Ann. Rev. Biochem. 56:289–315.

Thisyakorn, U., and S. Nimmannitya. 1993. Nutritional status of children with dengue hemorrhagic fever. Clin. Infect. Dis. 16(2):295–297.

Thompson, H.L., and J.H. Brock. 1986. The effect of iron and agar on production of hydrogen peroxide by stimulated and activated mouse peritoneal macrophages. FEBS Lett. 200:283–286.

Thorson, J.A., K.M. Smith, F. Gomez, P.W. Naumann, and J.D. Kemp. 1991. Role of iron in T-cell activation: Th1 clones differ from Th2 clones in their sensitivity to inhibition of DNA synthesis caused by IgG Mabs against the transferrin receptor and the iron chelator desferoxamine. Cell Immunol. 134:126–137.

Tilders, F.J.H., R.H. DeRijk, A.M. vanDam, K. Schotanus, and T.H.A. Persoons. 1994. Activation of the hypothalamic–pituitary–adrenal axis by bacterial endotoxins: Routes and intermediate signals. Psychoneuroendocrinology 19:209–232.

Tilz, G.P., W. Domej, A. Diez-Ruiz, G. Weiss, R. Brezinschek, H. P. Brezinschek, E. Hüttl, H. Pristautz, H. Wachter, and D. Fuchs. 1993. Increased immune activation during and after physical exercise. Immunobiology 188:194–202.

Tobler, I., A.A. Borbely, M. Schwyzer, and A. Fontana. 1984. Interleukin-1 derived from astrocytes enhances slow wave activity in sleep EEG of rat. Eur. J. Pharmacol. 104:191–192.

Touitou, Y., A. Carayon, A. Reinberg, A. Bogdan, and H. Beck. 1983. Differences in the seasonal rhythmicity of plasma prolactin in elderly subjects. Detection in women but not in men. J. Endocrinol. 96:65-71.

Touitou, Y., and E. Haus. 1994. Aging of the human endocrine and neuroendocrine time structure. Ann. N.Y. Acad. Sci. 719:378–397.

Tomasi, T.B., F.B. Trudeau, D. Czerwinski, and S. Erredge . 1982. Immune parameters in athletes before and after strenuous exercise. J. Clin. Immunol. 2:173–178.

Tremel, H., B. Kienle, L.S. Weilemann, P. Stehle, and P. Furst. 1994. Glutamine dipeptide-supplemented parenteral nutrition maintains intestinal function in the critically ill. Gastroenterology 107:1595–1601.

Trinchieri, G. 1992. The hematopoietic system and hematopoiesis. Pp. 1–25 in Neoplastic Hematopathology, D.M. Knowles, eds. Baltimore: Williams and Wilkins.

Tritsch, G.L., A. Nechaev, and A. Mittelman. 1975. Adenosine aminohydrolase as an indicator of lymphocyte-mediated cytolysis: Possible role of cyclic adenosine monophosphate. Clin. Chem. 21:984.

Troisi, R.J., W.C. Willett, S.T. Weiss, D. Trichopoulos, B. Rosner, and F.E. Speizer. 1995. A prospective study of diet and adult-onset asthma. Am. J. Resp. Crit. Care Med. 151:1401–1408.

Turgeon-O'Brien, H., J. Amiot, L. Lemieux, and J-C. Dillon. 1985. Myeloperoxidase activity of polymorphonuclear leukocytes in iron-deficiency anaemia and anaemia of chronic disorders. Acta Haematol 74:151–154.

Turner-Warwick, M. 1988. Epidemiology of nocturnal asthma. Am. J. Med. 85(suppl. 1B):6–8.

Tvede, N., M. Kappel, J. Halkjaer-Kristensen, H. Galbo, and B.K. Pedersen. 1993. The effect of light, moderate and severe bicycle exercise on lymphocyte subsets, natural and lymphokine activated killer cells, lymphocyte proliferative response and interleukin-2 production. Int. J. Sports Med. 14:275–282.

Tvede, N., J. Steensberg, B. Baslund, J. Halkjaer-Kristensen, and B.K. Pedersen. 1991. Cellular immunity in highly-trained elite racing cyclists and controls during periods of training with high and low intensity. Scand. J. Sports Med. 1:163–166.

Udomkemsmalee, E., S. Dhanamitta, S. Sirisinha, S. Charoenkiatkul, S. Tantipopipat, O. Banjong, N. Rojroongwasinkul, T.R. Kramer, and J.C. Smith Jr. 1992. Effect of vitamin A and zinc supplementation on the nutriture of children in Northeast Thailand. Am. J. Clin. Nutr. 56:50–57.

Uezono, K., L. Sackett-Lundeen, T. Kawasaki, T. Omae, and E. Haus. 1987. Circaseptan rhythm in sodium and potassium excretion in salt sensitive and salt resistant Dahl rats. Pp. 297–307 in Advances in Chronobiology, Part A, J.E. Pauly and L.E. Scheving, eds. New York: Alan R. Liss, Inc.

Urbaschek, R., and B. Urbaschek. 1987. Tumor necrosis factor and interleukin-1 as mediators of endotoxin-induced beneficial effects. Rev. Infect. Dis. 9 (suppl. 5):S607–S615.

Urivetzky, M. D. Kessaris, and A.D. Smith. 1992. Ascorbic acid overdosing: A risk factor for calcium oxalate nephrolithiasis. J. Urol. 147:1215–1218.

USDA (U.S. Department of Agriculture Nutrition Monitoring in the United States). 1986. A progress report from the Joint Nutrition Monitoring Evaluation Committee. DHHS publ. no. 1255. Hyattsville, Md.: USDA.

U.S. Departments of the Army, the Navy, and the Air Force. 1985. Army Regulation 40-25/Navy Command Medical Instruction 10110.1/Air Force Regulation 160-95. "Nutritional Allowances, Standards, and Education." May 15. Washington, D.C.

Vadillo, M., X. Corbella, V. Pac, P. Fernandez-Viladrich, and R. Pujol. 1994. Multiple liver abscesses due to *Yersinia enterocolitica* discloses primary hemochromatosis: Three case reports and review. Clin. Infect. Dis. 18:938–941.

Vagenakis, A.G., A. Burger, G.I. Portnoy, M. Rudolph, J.R. O'Brian, F. Azzizi, R.A. Arky, P. Nicod, S.H. Ingbar, and L.E. Braverman. 1975. Diversion of peripheral thyroxine metabolism from activating to inactivating pathways during complete fasting. J. Clin. Endocrinol. Metab. 41:191–194.

Valtora, A., A. Moretta, R. Maccario, M. Bozzola, and F. Severi. 1991. Influence of growth hormone-releasing hormone (GHRH) on phytohemagglutinin-induced lymphocyte activation: comparison of two synthetic forms. Thymus 18:51–59.

Van Asbeck, B.S., J.J.M. Marx, A. Struyvenberg, J.H. van Kats, and J. Verhoef. 1984a. Effect of iron (III) in the presence of various ligands on the phagocytic and metabolic activity of human polymorphonuclear leukocytes. J. Immunol. 132:851–856.

Van Asbeck, B.S., J.J.M. Marx, A. Struyvenberg, J.H. van Kats, and J. Verhoef. 1984b. Functional defects in phagocytic cells from patients with iron overload. J. Infect. 85:232–240.

Van Cauter, E., and F.W. Turek. 1995. Endocrine and other biologic rhythms. Pp. 2487–2548 in Endocrinology, Degroot, L.J. ed. Philadelphia: W.B. Saunders Company.

van Dam, A., M. Bauer, F.J.H. Tilders, and F. Berkenbosch. 1995. Endotoxin-induced appearance of immunoreactive interleukin-1β in ramified microglia in rat brain: A light and electron microscopic study. Neuroscience 65(3):815–826.

van Dam, A., M. Brouns, S. Louisse, and F. Berkenbosch. 1992. Appearance of interleukin-1 in macrophages and in ramified microglia in the brain of endotoxin-treated rats: A pathway for the induction of non-specific symptoms of sickness? Brain Res. 588:291–296.

van Hensbroek, M.B., S. Morris-Jones, S. Meisner, S. Jaffar, L. Bayo, R. Dackour, C. Phillips, and B.M. Greenwood. 1995. Iron, but not folic acid, combined with effective antimalarial therapy promotes phaematological recovery in African children after acute falciparum malaria. Trans. Soc. Trop. Med. Hyg. 89:672–676.

Van der Hulst, R.R., B.K. van Kreel, M.F. von Meyenfeldt, R.J. Brummer, J.W. Arends, N.E. Deutz, and P.B. Soeters. 1993. Glutamine and the preservation of gut integrity. Lancet 334:1363–1365.

van der Poll, T., and S.F. Lowry. 1995. Tumor necrosis factor in sepsis: Mediator of multiple organ failure or essential part of host defense? Shock 3:1–12.

van der Poll, T., J.A. Romijn, E. Endert, and H.P. Sauerwein. 1993. Effects of tumor necrosis factor on the hypothalamic–pituitary–testicular axis in healthy men. Metabolism 42:303–307.

van der Poll, T., J.A. Romijn, W.M. Wiersinga, and H.P. Sauerwein. 1990. Tumor necrosis factor: A putative mediator of the sick euthyroid syndrome in man. J. Clin. Endocrinol. Metab. 71:1567–1572.

van der Poll, T., K.J. Van Zee, E. Endert, S.M. Coyle, D.M. Stiles, J.P. Pribble, M.A. Catalano, L.L. Moldawer, and S.F. Lowry. 1995. Interleukin-1 receptor blockade does not affect endotoxin-induced changes in plasma thyroid hormone and thyrotropin concentrations in man. J. Clin. Endocrinol. Metab. 80:1341–1346.

Van Heerden, C., R. Oosthuizen, H. Van Wyk, P. Prinsloo, and P. Anderson. 1981. Evaluation of neutrophil and lymphocyte function in subjects with iron deficiency. S. Afr. Med. J. 24:111–113.

Van Zaanen, H.C.T., H. van der Lelie, J.G. Timmer, P. Furst, and H.P. Sauerwein. 1994. Parenteral glutamine dipeptide supplementation does not ameliorate chemotherapy-induced toxicity. Cancer 74:2879–2884.

Varma, S., P. Sabharwal, J.F. Sheridan, and W.B. Malarkey. 1993. Growth hormone secretion by human peripheral blood mononuclear cells detected by an enzyme-linked immunoplaque assay. J. Clin. Endocrinol. Metab. 76:49–53.

Veening, J.G., M.J.M. van der Meer, H. Joosten, A.R.M.M. Hermus, C.E.M. Rijnnkels, L.M. Geeraedts, and C.G. Sweep. 1993. Intravenous administration of interleukin-1β induces fos-like immunoreactivity in corticotropin-releasing hormone neurons in the paraventricular hypothalamic nucleus of the rat. J. Chem. Neuroanat. 6:391–397.

Venkataramanan, R., S. Yang, G.J. Burckard, R.J. Ptachcinski, D.H. Van Thiel, and T.E. Starzl. 1986. Diurnal variation in cyclosporine pharmacokinetics. Ther. Drug Monit. 8:380–381.

Venkatraman, J.T., and G. Fernandes. 1992. Mechanisms of delayed autoimmune disease in B/W mice by omega-3 lipids and food restriction. Pp. 309–323 in Nutrition and Immunology, R.K. Chandra, ed. St. John's, Newfoundland: ARTS Biomedical Publishers.

Veterans Cooperative Group. 1987. Effect of high-dose glucocorticoid therapy on mortality in patients with clinical signs of systemic sepsis. N. Engl. J. Med. 317:659–665.

Virella, G., C. Enockson, and M. La Via. 1997. New approaches to the study of abnormal immune function. Pp. 431–450 in Emerging Technologies for Nutrition Research: Potential for Assessing Military Performance Capability, S.J. Carlson-Newberry and R.B. Costello, eds. Committee on Military Nutrition Research, Food and Nutrition Board. Washington, D.C.: National Academy Press.

Virella, G., J.M. Kilpatrick, M.R. Rugeles, B. Hayman, and R. Russell. 1989. Depression of humoral responses and phagocytic functions in vivo and in vitro by fish oil and eicosapentaenoic acid. Clin. Immunol. Immunopathol. 52:257–270.

Viteri, F.E. Prevention of iron deficiency. 1998. Pp. 45–102 in Prevention of Micronutrient Deficiencies: Tools for Policymakers and Public Health Workers. Institute of Medicine. Washington, D.C.: National Academy Press.

Voerman, H.J., A.B. Groenveld, H. de Boer, R.J. Strack van Schijndel, J.P. Nauta, E.A. van der Veen, and L.G. Thijs. 1993. Time course and variability of the endocrine and metabolic response to severe sepsis. Surgery 114:951–959.

Voerman, H.J., R.J. Strack van Scijndel, A.P. Groenevelkd, H. de Boer, J.P. Nauta, and L.G. Thijs. 1992a. Pulsatile hormone secretion during severe sepsis: Accuracy of different blood sampling regimens. Metabolism 41:934–940.

Voerman, H.J., R.J. van Schijndel, A.B. Groeneveld, H. de Boer, J.P. Nauta, E.A. van der Veen, and L.G. Thijs. 1992b. Effects of recombinant human growth hormone in patients with severe sepsis. Ann. Surg. 216:648–655

Vogel, S.N., and M.M. Hogan. 1990. Role of cytokines in endotoxin-mediated host responses. Pp. 238–258 in Immunophysiology, The Role of Cells and Cytokines in Immunity and Inflammation, J. Oppenheim and E. M. Shevach, eds. New York: Oxford University Press.

Vyas, D. and R.K. Chandra. 1983. Thymic factor activity, lymphocyte stimulation response and antibody producing cells in copper deficiency. Nutr. Res. 3:343–349.

Vyas, D. and R.K. Chandra. 1984. Functional implications of iron deficiency. In Iron Nutrition in Infancy and Childhood, A. Stekel, ed. New York: Raven Press.

Wada, T., M. Sato, M. Niimi, M. Tamaki, T. Ishida, and J. Takahara. 1995. Inhibitory effects of interleukin-1 on growth hormone secretion in conscious male rats. Endocrinology 136:3936–3941.

Wagner, H., E. Zierden, and W.H. Hauss. 1975. Effects of synthetic somatostatin on endotoxin-induced changes of growth hormone, cortisol and insulin in plasma, blood sugar and blood leukocytes in man. Klin. Wochenschr. 53:539–541.

Wagner, K.H. 1940. Die experimentelle Avitaminose A beim Menschen. Hoppe-Seyler's Zeitschr. f. physiol. Chemie 264:153–188.

Wakabayashi, G., J.A. Gelfand, J. F. Burke, R.C. Thompson, and C.A. Dinarello. 1991. A specific receptor antagonist for interleukin-1 prevents *Escherichia coli*-induced shock in rabbits. FASEB J. 5:338–343.

Walker, A.M. 1994. Phosphorylated and non-phosphorylated prolactin isoforms. Endocrinol. Metab. 5:195–200.

Walsh, C.T., H.H. Sandstead, A.S. Prasad, P.M. Newberne, and P.J. Fraker. 1994. Zinc: Health effects and research priorities for the 1990s. Environ. Health Perspect. 102:5–46.

Walter, T., S. Arredondo, M. Arevalo, and A. Stekel. 1986. Effect of iron therapy on phagocytosis and bactericidal activity in neutrophils of iron-deficient infants. Am. J. Clin. Nutr. 44:877–882.

Walton, A.J.E., M.L. Snaith, M. Locniskar, A.G. Cumberland, W.J.W. Morrow, and D.A. Isenberg. 1991. Dietary fish oil and the severity of symptoms in patients with systemic erythematosus. Ann. Rheum. Dis. 50:463–466.

Wan, W., L. Wetmore, C.M. Sorensen, A.H. Greenberg, and D.M. Nance. 1994. Neural and biochemical mediators of endotoxin and stress-induced c-fos expression in the rat brain. Brain Res. Bull. 34:7–14.

Wang, W., J.L. Napoli, and M. Ballow. 1993. The effects of retinol on in vitro immunoglobulin synthesis by cord blood and adult peripheral blood mononuclear cells. Clin. Exp. Immunol. 92:164–168.

Wang, Y., and R.R. Watson. 1993. Is vitamin E supplementation a useful agent in AIDS therapy? Prog. Food Nutr. Sci. 17:351–375.

Wang, Y., D.S. Huang, C.D. Eskelson, and R.R. Watson. 1994a. Long-term dietary vitamin E retards development of retrovirus-induced disregulation in cytokine production. Clin. Immunol. Immunopathol. 72:70–75.

Wang, Y., D.S. Huang, B. Liang, and R.R. Watson. 1994b. Nutritional status and immune responses in mice with murine AIDS are normalized by vitamin E supplementation. J. Nutr. 124:2024–2032.

Wang, Y., D.S. Huang, S. Wood, and R.R. Watson. 1995. Modulation of immune function and cytokine production by various levels of vitamin E supplementation during murine AIDS. Immunopharmacology 29:225–233.

Wannemacher Jr., R.W., H.L. DuPont, R.S. Pekarek, M.C. Powanda, A. Schwartz, R.B. Hornick, and W.R. Beisel. 1972. An endogenous mediator of depression of amino acids and trace metals during typhoid fever. J. Infect. Dis. 126:77–86.

Wartofsky, L. and K.D. Burman. 1982. Alterations in thyroid function in patients with systemic illness: the "euthyroid sick syndrome." Endocr. Rev. 3(2):164–217.

Watanobe, H., and K. Takebe. 1994. Effects of intravenous administration of interleukin-1β on the release of prostaglandin E2, corticotropin-releasing factor, and arginine vasopressin in several hypothalamic areas of freely moving rat: Estimation by push-pull perfusion. Neuroendocrinology 60:8–15.

Watanobe, T., A. Morimoto, N. Tan, T. Makisumi, S.G. Shimuda, T. Nakamori, and N. Murakami. 1994. ACTH response induced in capsaicin-desensitized rats by intravenous injection of interleukin-1 or prostaglandin. Eur. J. Physiol. 475:139–145.

Waterlot, Y., B. Cantinieaux, C. Hariga-Mulier, E. de Maertelaere-Laurant, J.L. Vanherweghmen, and P. Fondu. 1985. Impairment of neutrophil phagocytosis in haemodialysed patients—The critical role of iron overload. Br. Med. J. 291:501–504.

Watkins, L.R., L.E. Goehler, J.K. Relton, N. Tartaglia, L. Silbert, D. Martin, and S.F. Maier. 1995a. Blockade of interleukin-1 induced hyperthermia by subdiaphragmatic vagotomy: Evidence for vagal mediation of immune-brain communication. Neuroscience Lett. 183:27–31.

Watkins, L.R., S.F. Maier, and L.E. Goehler. 1995b. Cytokine-to-brain communication: A review and analysis of alternative mechanisms. Life Sciences 57:1011–1026.

Watkins, L.R., E.P. Wiertelak, L.E. Goehler, K. Mooney-Heiberger, J. Martinez, L. Furness, K.P. Smith, and S.F. Maier. 1994a. Neurocircuitry of illness-induced hyperalgesia. Brain Res. 639:283–299.

Watkins, L.R., E.P. Wiertelak, L.E. Goehler, K.P. Smith, D. Martin, and S.F. Maier. 1994b. Characterization of cytokine-induced hyperalgesia. Brain Res. 654:15–26.

Watson, R.R., ed. 1984. Nutrition, Disease Resistance, and Immune Function. New York: Marcel Decker, Inc.

Watson, R.R., and T.M. Retro. 1984. Resistance to bacterial and parasitic infections in the nutritionally compromised host. CRC Crit. Rev. Microbiol. 10:297–315.

Watters, J.M., P.Q. Bessey, C.A. Dinarello, S.M. Wolff, and D.W. Wilmore. 1986. Both inflammatory and endocrine mediators stimulate host responses to sepsis. Arch. Surg. 121:179–190.

Watzl, B., and R.R. Watson. 1992. Role of alcohol abuse in nutritional immunosuppression. J. Nutr. 122 (3 suppl.):733–737.

Weidenfeld, J., O. Abramsky, and H. Ovadia. 1989. Effect of interleukin-1 on ACTH and corticosterone secretion in dexamethasone and adrenalectomized pretreated male rats. Neuroendocrinology 50:650–654.

Weigent, D.A., and J.E. Blalock. 1995. Associations between the neuroendocrine and immune systems. J. Leukocyte Biol. 58:137–150.

Weigle, W.O. 1975. Cyclic production of antibody as a regulatory mechanism in the immune response. Adv. Immunol. 21:87–111.

Weinberg, E.D. 1984. Iron withholding: A defense against infection and neoplasia. Physiol. Rev. 64:65–102.

Weiss, G., H. Wachter, and D. Fuchs. 1995. Linkage of cell-mediated immunity to iron metabolism [review]. Immunol. Today 16:495–500.

Weiss, J.M., N. Quan, and S.K. Sundar. 1994. Widespread activation and consequences of interleukin-1 in the brain. Ann. N.Y. Acad. Sci. 741:338–357.

Welbourne, T.C. 1995. Increased plasma bicarbonate and growth hormone after an oral glutamine load. Am. J. Clin. Nutr. 61:1058–1061.

Welbourne, T.C., A.B. King, and K. Horton. 1993. Enteral glutamine supports hepatic glutathione efflux during inflammation. J. Nutr. Biochem. 4:236–242.

Wendling, D., E. Racadot, and J. Wijdeness. 1993. Treatment of severe rheumatoid arthritis by anti-interleukin-6 monoclonal antibody. J. Rheumatol. 20(2):259–262.

West, S.E.H., and P.F. Sparling. 1985. Response of *Neisseria gonorrheae* to iron limitation: Alteration in expression of membrane proteins without apparent siderophore production. Infect. Immun. 47:388–394.

Westaway, J., C.M. Atkinson, T. Davies, S.A. Petersen, and M.P. Wailoo. 1995. Urinary excretion of cortisol after immunization. Arch. Dis. Child. 72:432–434.

Wester, P.W., A.D. Vethaak, and W.B. van Muiswinkel. 1994. Fish as biomarkers in immunotoxicology. Toxicology 86:213–232.

Westphal, K.A., K.E. Friedl, M.A. Sharp, N. King, T.R. Kramer, K.L. Reynolds, and L.J. Marchitelli. 1995a. Health, performance, and nutritional status of U.S. Army women during basic combat training. Technical Report No. T96-2, AD-A32042. Natick, Mass.: U.S. Army Research Institute of Environmental Medicine.

Westphal, K.A., L.J. Marchitelli, K.E. Friedl, and M.A. Sharp. 1995b. Relationship between iron status and physical performance in female soldiers during U.S. Army basic combat training. Fed. Am. Soc. Exp. Biol. J. 9(3):A361[abstract].

Westphal K.A., A.E. Pusateri, and T.R. Kramer. 1994. Prevalence of negative iron nutriture and relationship with folate nutriture, immunocompetence, and fitness level in U.S. Army servicewomen. USARIEM Approved Protocol OPD94002-AP024-H016. Defense Women's Health Research Program 1994, Log No. W4168016. Natick, Mass.: U.S. Army Research Institute of Environmental Medicine.

Whelan, J., M.E, Surette, I. Hardardottir, G. Lu, K.A. Golemboski, E. Larsen, and J.E. Kinsella. 1993. Dietary arachidonic acid enhances tissue arachidonate levels and eicosanoid production in Syrian hamsters. J. Nutr. 123:2174–2185.

Whiteside, T.L. 1994. Cytokines and cytokine measurements in a clinical laboratory. Clin. Diagn. Lab. Immunol. 1:257–260.

Whitnall, M.H., R.S. Perlstein, E.H. Mougey, and R. Neta. 1992. Effects of interleukin-1 on the stress-responsive and -nonresponsive subtypes of corticotropin-releasing hormone neurosecretory axons. Endocrinology 131:37–44.

WHO (World Health Organization). 1993. FAO/WHO Recommendations on Fats and Oils in Human Nutrition. Geneva: WHO.

WHO (World Health Organization). 1996. Trace Elements in Human Nutrition and Health. Geneva: WHO.

Wick, G., Y. Hu, and G. Krooemer. 1993. Immunoendocrine communication via the hypothalamic–pituitary–adrenal axis in autoimmune diseases Endocr. Rev. 14:539–563.

Wiik, P. 1989. Vasoactive intestinal peptide (VIP) inhibits the respiratory burst in monocytes by a cyclic AMP mediated mechanism. Regul. Pept. 25:187–97.

Wiik, P. 1991. Glucocorticoids upregulate the high affinity receptor for VIP on human mononuclear leucocytes in vitro. Regul. Pept. 35:19–30.

Wiik, P. A.H. Haugen, D. Lovhaug, A. Bøyum, and P.K. Opstad. 1989. Effect of VIP on the respiratory burst in human monocytes ex vivo during prolonged strain and energy deficiency. Peptides 10(4):819–823.

Wiik, P., P.K. Opstad, and A. Bøyum. 1985. Binding of vasoactive intestinal polypeptide (VIP) by human blood monocytes: Demonstration of specific binding sites. Regul. Pept. 12:145–163.

Wiik, P., P.K. Opstad, and A. Bøyum. 1996. Granulocyte chemiluminescence response to serum opsonized particles ex vivo during long-term strenuous exercise, energy, and sleep deprivation in humans. Eur. J. Appl. Physiol. 73:251–258.

Wiik, P., P.K. Opstad, S. Knardahl, and A. Bøyum. 1988. Receptors for vasoactive intestinal peptide (VIP) on human mononuclear luecocytes are upregulated during prolonged strain and energy deficiency. Peptides 9(1):181–186.

Wiik, P., K.K. Skrede, S. Knardahl, A.H. Haugen, C.E. Ærø, P.K. Opstad, and A. Bøyum. 1995. Effect of in vivo corticosterone and acute food deprivation on rat resident peritoneal cell chemiluminescence after activation ex vivo. Acta. Physiol. Scand. 154:407–416.

Wilder, R.L. 1995. Neuroendocrine–immune system interactions and autoimmunity. Ann. Rev. Immunol. 13:307–338.

Williams, R.M., L.J. Kraus, D.P. Dubey, E.J. Yunis, and F. Halberg. 1979. Circadian bioperiodicity in natural killer cell activity of human blood [abstract]. Chronobiologia 6:172.

Williams, T.J., and H. Yarwood. 1990. Effect of glucocorticosteroids on microvascular permeability. Am. Rev. Resp. Dis. 141:S39–S43.

Windmueller, H.G. 1982. Glutamine utilization and the small intestine. Adv. Enzymol. 53:202.

Winget, C.M., M.R.I. Soliman, D.C. Holley, and J.S. Meylor. 1994. Chronobiology of Physical Performance and Sports Medicine. Pp. 230–242 in Biologic Rhythms in Clinical and Laboratory Medicine, 2d ed., Y. Touitou and E. Haus, eds. Heidelberg: Springer-Verlag.

Wishnok, J.S., J.A. Glogowski, S.R. Tannenbaum S.R. 1996. Quantitation of nitrate, nitrite, and nitrosating agents. Methods Enzymol. 268:130-41.

Withyachumnarnkul, B., K.O. Nonaka, C. Santana, A.M. Attia, and R.J. Reiter. 1990. Interferon-γ modulates melatonin production in rat pineal gland in organ culture. J. Interferon Res. 10:403–411.

Witt, E.H., A.Z. Reznick, C.a. Viguie, P. Starke-Reed, and L. Packer. 1992. Exercise, oxidative damage, and effects of antioxidant manipulation. J. Nutr. 122 (suppl. 3):766–773.

Wolbach, S.G., and P.R. Howe. 1925. Tissue changes following deprivation of fat-soluble A vitamin. J. Exp. Med. 42:753–777.

Wolf, R., J. Oph, and I. Yust. 1991. Atopic dermatitis provoked by AL721 in a patient with acquired immunodeficiency syndrome. Ann. Allergy 66:421–422.

Wood, P.A., and W.J.M. Hrushesky. 1994. Chronopharmacodynamics of hematopoietic growth factors and antitumor cytokines. Pp. 185–207 in Circadian Cancer Therapy, W.J.M. Hrushesky, ed. Boca Raton, Fla.: CRC Press.

Woodruff, J.F. 1980. Viral myocarditis: A review. Am. J. Pathol. 101:427–482.

Woodruff, J.F., and J.J. Woodruff. 1974. Involvement of T-lymphocytes in the pathogenesis of coxsackievirus B3 heart disease. J. Immunol. 113:17–26.

Worwood, M. 1986. Serum ferritin. Clin. Sci. 70:215–220.

Wright, A.C., L.M. Simpson, and J.D. Oliver. 1981. Role of iron in the pathogenesis of Vibrio vulnificus infections. Infect. Immun. 34:503–507.

Wright, D.N., R.P. Nelson, D.K. Ledford, E. Fernandez-Caldas, W.L. Trudeau, and R.F. Lockey. 1990. Serum IgE and human immunodeficiency virus (HIV) infection. J. Allergy Clin. Immunol. 85:445–452.

Wyler, D.J. 1992. Bark, weeds, and iron chelators—drugs for malaria. N. Engl. J. Med. 327:1519–1521.

Yamamura, M.K., R.J. Uyemura, K. Deans, T.H. Weinberg, B. Rea, B. Bloom, and R.L. Modlin. 1991. Defining protective responses to pathogens: Cytokine profiles in leprosy lesions. Science 254: 277–279.

Yan, H.Q., M.A. Banos, P. Herregodts, and E.L. Hooghe. 1992. Expression of interleukin (IL)-1β, IL-6, and their respective receptors in the normal rat brain and after injury. Eur. J. Immunol. 22:2963–2971.

Yancey, R.J., and R.A. Finkelstein. 1981. Assimilation of iron by pathogenic *Neisseria* spp. Infect. Immun. 32:592–599.

Yang, G., S. Yin, R. Zhou, L. Gu, B. Yan, Y. Liu, and Y. Liu. 1989. Studies of safe maximal daily dietary Se-intake in a seleniferous area in China. Part II. Relation between Se intake and the manifestation of clinical signs and certain biochemical alterations in blood and urine. J. Trace Elem. Electrolytes Health Dis. 3(3):123–130.

Yehuda, R., M.T. Lowy, S.M. Southwick, D. Shaffer, and E.L. Giller, Jr. 1991. Lymphocyte glucocorticoid receptor number in posttraumatic stress disorder. Am. J. Psychiatry 148:499–504.

Yehuda, R, S.M. Southwick, G. Nussbaum, V.S. Wahby, E.L. Giller, Jr., and J.W. Mason. 1990. Low urinary cortisol excretion in patients with posttraumatic stress disorder. J. Nerv. Mental Dis. 178:366–369.

Yehuda, S., B. Shredny, and Y. Kalechman. 1987. Effects of DSIP, 5-HTP, and serotonin on the lymphokine system: A preliminary study. Int. J. Neurosci. 33:185–187.

Yetgin, S., C. Altay, G. Ciliv, and Y. Laleli. 1979. Myeloperoxidase activity and bactericidal function of PMN in iron deficiency. Acta Haematol. 61:10–14.

Young, A., and R.L. Shippee. 1995. The impact of Ranger training on physiological responses and responses to thermoregulatory tolerance to cold. Human Research Protocol No. MND95009-AP027-H028, November 7. Natick, Mass.: U.S. Army Research Institute of Environmental Medicine.

Young, M.R.I., J.P. Matthews, E.L. Kanabrocki, R.B. Sothern, B. Roitman-Johnson, and L.E. Scheving. 1995. Circadian rhythmometry of serum interleukin-2, interleukin-10, tumor necrosis factor-α, and granulocyte-macrophage colony stimulating factor in men. Chronobiol. Int. 12:19–27.

Young, M.W., ed. 1993. Molecular Genetics of Biological Rhythms. New York: Dekker.

Young, M.W., F.R. Jackson, H.S. Shin, and T.A. Bargiello. 1985. A biological clock in *Drosophila*. Cold Spring Harbor Symp. Quant. Biol. 50:865–875.

Zabel, P., H. Horst, C. Kreiber, and M. Schlaak. 1990. Circadian rhythm of interleukin-1 production of monocytes and the influence of endogenous and exogenous glucocorticoids in man. Klin Wochenschr. 68:1217–1221.

Zabel, P., K. Linnemann, and M. Schlaak. 1993. Circadian rhythm in cytokines. Immun. Infekt. 20:38–40.

Zahringer, J., B.S. Baliga, and H.S. Munro. 1976. Novel mechanism for translational control in regulation of ferritin synthesis by iron. Proc. Natl. Acad. Sci. USA 81:2752–2756.

Zhang, Y.H., T.R. Kramer, P.R. Taylor, J.Y. Li, W.J. Blot, C.C. Brown, W. Guo, S.M. Dawsey, and B. Li. 1995. Possible immunologic involvement of antioxidants in cancer prevention. Am. J. Clin. Nutr. 62(suppl.):1477S–1482S.

Zhao, Z., and A.C. Ross. 1995. Retinoic acid repletion restores the number of leukocytes and their subsets and stimulates natural cytotoxicity in vitamin A-deficient rats. J. Nutr. 125:2064–2073.

Zhou, D., A.W. Kusnecov, M.R. Shurin, M. DePaoli, and B.S. Rabin. 1993. Exposure to physical and psychological stressors elevates plasma interleukin 6: Relationship to the activation of hypothalamic–pituitary–adrenal axis. Endocrinology 133:2523–2530.

Zhou, D., N. Shanks, S.E. Riechman, R. Liang, A.W. Kusnecov, and B.S. Rabin. 1996. Interleukin-6 modulates interleukin-1 and stress-induced activation of the hypothalamic-pituitary-adrenal axis in male rats. Neuroendocrinology 63:227–236.

Ziegler, T.R., K. Benfell, R.J. Smith, L.S. Young, E. Brown, E. Ferrari-Baliviera, D.K. Lowe, D.W. Wilmore. 1990. Safety and metabolic effects of L-glutamine administration in humans. JPEN J. Parenter. Enteral Nutr. 14(4 Suppl):137S–146S.

Ziegler, T.R., R.L. Bye, R.L. Persinger, L.S. Young, J.H. Antin, and D.W. Wilmore. 1994. Glutamine-enriched parenteral nutrition increases circulating lymphocytes after bone marrow transplantation. JPEN J. Parenter. Enteral Nutr. 18(suppl.):17S.

Ziegler, T.R., R.J. Smith, S.T. O'Dwyer, R.H. Demling, and D.W. Wilmore. 1988. Increased intestinal permeability associated with infection in burn patients. Arch. Surg. 123:1313–1319.

Ziegler, T.R., L.S. Young, K. Benfell, M. Scheltinga, K. Hortos, R. Bye, F.D. Morrow, D.O. Jacobs, R.J. Smith, J.H. Antin, and D.W. Wilmore. 1992. Clinical and metabolic efficacy of glutamine-supplemented parenteral nutrition after bone marrow transplantation. A randomized, double-blind, controlled study. Ann. Intern. Med. 116:821–828.

Zimmer, J., A.S. Khalifa, and J.J. Lightbody. 1975. Decreased lymphocyte adenosine deaminase activity in acute lymphocytic leukemic children and their parents. Cancer 35(1):68–70.

Zoli, M., M. Carè, C. Falco, R. Spanò, G. Bernardi, and I. Gasbarrini. 1995. Effect of oral glutamine on intestinal permeability and nutritional status in Crohn's disease. Gastroenterology 108:A766.

Zuckerman, S.H., J. Shellhaas, and L.D. Butler. 1989. Differential regulation of lipopolysaccharide-induced interleukin-1 and tumor necrosis factor synthesis: Effects of endogenous and exogenous glucocorticoids and the role of the pituitary-adrenal axis. Eur. J. Immunol. 19:301–305.

Index

immunity; Memory; Self-
limitation; Specificity; T-cells
Antioxidants, 4, 14, 117
  delayed-type hypersensitivity re-
    sponse to tetanus toxoid using
    beverage supplement, SFAS study,
    178, 179
  peripheral blood lymphocyte prolif-
    eration using supplementation,
    SFAS study, 178, 179
  See also β-carotene; Vitamin C;
    Vitamin E
Apodemis aggrarious, 546
Arachidonic acid (AA), 305, 306, 307–
    308, 312
  See also Saturated fatty acids
ARC. *See* AIDS-related complex (ARC)
Arginine, 4, 7–8, 14, 42, 51, 111, 127
  doses and toxicity, 111
  See also Amino acids (AAs); Nutri-
    ents
Arginine vasopressin (AVP), 410–411,
    412, 413–414, 415
  See also Vasopressin (VP)
Army, U.S. *See* U.S. Army
Arthus reactions
  definition, 528
  See also Allergy; Hypersensitivity
    reactions
Ascorbic acid. *See* Vitamin C
Asia
  Southeast, Vitamin A deficiency
    epidemiology, 281
  southern, Vitamin A deficiency epi-
    demiology, 281
Asthma
  allergic, children with, circadian
    rhythms in, 462
  allergic, time-dependent changes in,
    455, 456, 460–462
  bronchial, biologic rhythms role in,
    449, 461
  vitamin C and E supplementation
    effects on lung function in, studies
    review, 263, 295–296
  See also Diseases and disorders;
    Respiratory diseases and disorders

Athletes and athletics, 68
  exercise, practical guidelines for,
    377–379
  immune response, infection, and
    exercise relationship, studies of,
    365–370
  infection, effects on physical per-
    formance, studies of, 373–374
  marathon runners immune function
    effects of exertion, study findings,
    365, 366, 367, 368, 369, 371, 372
  nutrient supplements and exercise,
    review of studies, 378–379
  sports, close-contact, and transmis-
    sion of HIV, findings, 374–375
  upper respiratory tract infection sus-
    ceptibility and exercise, studies of,
    371–373
ATSDR. *See* Agency for Toxic Sub-
    stances and Disease Registry
    (ATSDR)
Autoimmune disease
  definition, 528
  linolenic acid (n-3 PUFA) manage-
    ment of, clinical trials findings,
    310–311
  See also Diseases and disorders;
    Immune function
AVP. *See* Arginine vasopressin (AVP)

Bacillus Calmette-Guirin (BCG) vaccina-
    tion, 241, 459
  See also Vaccines and vaccination
Bacteria. *See* Microbes; Microbial viru-
    lence
Bangkok, Thailand
  infectious disease risk in, 545
Basophil, 443
  definition, 528
  See also White blood cells (WBC)
β-carotene, 7, 14, 109, 127, 134
  See also Antioxidants
B-cell growth factors, 224–225
  See also Cytokines; Interleukin-4
    (IL-4); Interleukin-6 (IL-6); Inter-
    leukin-14 (IL-14)

Laboratories
  interleukin-6 and acute stress re-
    sponse, laboratory-based studies,
    future research recommendations,
    133
  military nutrition laboratory research
    methods, 17, 20, 102–105
  See also Research
Lactation. *See* Breastfeeding
Lactobacillus spp., 320
Lagos, Nigeria
  infectious disease risk in, 545
Land use
  changes in, infectious disease intro-
    duction/dissemination factor, 544
  See also Environment
Lean body mass, 2, 9, 18, 20
  cytokines (proinflammatory) effects
    on, 105
  military personnel loss and deploy-
    ment, recommendations, 130
Legionella pneumophila, 320
Lethality. *See* Mortality
Leukocytes. *See* White blood cells
  (WBC)
Leukocytic endogenous mediator. *See*
  Interleukin-1 (IL-1)
Leukotrines. *See* Eicosanoids
Light-dark changes
  biologic rhythms and, 362, 438, 440,
    459, 473
Linoleic acid (n-6 PUFA), 305–306
  immune function and, 55, 118
  intake amount and immune function,
    57–58
  intake amount and immune response,
    307–308
  See also Fatty acids; Polyunsaturated
    fatty acids (PUFAs)
Linolenic acid (n-3 PUFA), 305–306
  autoimmune/inflammatory diseases
    management with, clinical trials
    findings, 310–311
  immune function and, 55, 118
  intake amount and immune function,
    58–59

intake amount and immune response,
    308–310
  See also Fatty acids; Polyunsaturated
    fatty acids (PUFAs)
Lipocortins, 422
  See also Proteins
Lipopolysaccharides (LPS), 392, 399,
    413, 417–418, 421, 422–423, 424
  hypophysectomized rats, effects on
    survival of, 419, 420
  interleukin-1 effects elucidation, use
    of, 415–416
Lipoproteins. *See* Serum lipoproteins
Listeria, 327
Listeria monocytogenes, 104, 214
Liver
  function and systemic inflammation,
    361, 391–392, 398
  See also Acute-phase response
Long-Life Ration Packet (LLRP), 5, 30,
    171
  See also Military food and rations;
    Operational rations
Louisiana State University, 5, 20
LPS. *See* Lipopolysaccharides (LPS)
Lung function
  vitamin C and E supplementation
    effects on asthma and lung func-
    tion, 295–296
Lymphocyte activating substance. *See*
  Interleukin-1 (IL-1)
Lymphocyte repertoire
  definition, 533
  See also Diversity; Epitopes
Lymphocytes, 209, 361, 392
  antigens and mitogens response,
    nutritional status indicator, 209
  biologic rhythms and, 438, 443,
    444–446, 447, 448, 449, 450, 465,
    466, 467
  blood volume and proliferation in
    whole-blood cultures, methods,
    251, 253
  glutamine and, 263, 268, 269
  ^{3}H-thymidine labeling duration, for
    proliferation in whole-blood cul-

Manchuria
Hantavirus illness in, 37
See also China
Marasmus. *See* Protein-energy malnutri-
tion (PEM)
Martek Biosciences Corporation
(ARASCO Oil), 308
Mason, John, 144
Mast-cell growth-enhancing factor. *See*
Interleukin-9 (IL-9)
Maternity
Vitamin A deficiency risks for preg-
nant women, 263, 280–281, 282
See also Women
Meal, Ready-to-Eat (MRE), 5, 29, 30,
163, 166, 171, 174
See also Military food and rations;
Operational rations
Measles
Africa outbreak, unusual manifesta-
tions, 547
See also Diseases and disorders;
Infectious diseases and disorders
Medical procedures. *See* Surgical proce-
dures
Medicine. *See* Antibiotics; Drugs; Vac-
cines and vaccination
Membrane fluidity
fat, dietary, and, immune response
effects of, 312
Memory, 517
definition, 534
See also Antigen-specific immunity;
Immune response (IR)
Memory cells
definition, 534
See also Lymphocytes
Menkes syndrome, 65, 339
See also Diseases and disorders
Menstrual cycle
immune system variables, changes
during, 465–466
See also Women
Merieux multitine tests, 148
Merrill's Marauders
World War II troops infectious dis-
ease exposure, 23, 140

Metabolism, 2, 18, 20
acute-phase reaction effects on, 361,
391–392
cytokines (proinflammatory) effects
on, 105
iron metabolism, overview, 318–319
See also Catabolism; Health; Nutrition
Methodology, 2, 11–13
cytokine, circulating, assays, issues
concerning, 540
cytokine production *in vitro*, use of
whole-blood cultures, experiment
methods, 257–259
effector cell response development,
in vitro assessment, 243
field measures, 11–13, 102–105,
132–133
flow cytometry *in vitro* assessment
of cell types, 243–244
immune function and nutrition, future research recommendations,
133–134
immune function assessment, issues
in, 102–105, 132–133
immune response assessment, methodologies review, 233, 242–244
in vitro assessment of immune response, 240, 242–244
in vivo assessment of immune response, 241–242
lymphocyte proliferation *in vitro*
measurement, whole-blood cultures use, experiment methods,
251–257
military awareness of civilian research, recommendations, 133
military nutrition laboratory research
methods, 102–105
proliferative response, *in vitro* assessment, 242–243
research protocols design, recommendations, 133
soluble interleukin receptors release
in vitro, measurement use of
whole-blood cultures, experiment
methods, 258–259

cytokine production in response to,
whole-blood cultures experiments,
257–259
definition, 535
energy deficit and, military operations studies, 28, 147
lymphocyte proliferation in response
to, whole-blood cultures experiments, 251–257
soluble interleukin receptors release
in response to, whole-blood cultures experiments, 258–259
Pituitary gland. *See* Hypothalamic-
pituitary-adrenal axis (HPAA);
Hypothalamic-pituitary-adrenal
system; Hypothalamic-pituitary-
thyroid system; Pituitary stalk section (PSS)
Pituitary-gonadal system
inflammation, systemic, and regulation, 73, 398–399
See also Neuroendocrine function
Pituitary stalk section (PSS), 420, 421
Plasma cells, 540
definition, 535
See also Blood
Plasmodia, 328
Plasmodium berghei, 328
Platelets, 443, 450
See also Blood
Pleiotropy
definition, 535
Pneumonia, 5
lobar, syndrome of inappropriate
antidiuretic hormone secretion
and, 396–397
See also Diseases and disorders;
Infectious diseases and disorders
Pollution. *See* Environmental pollution
Polymerase chain reaction (PCR), 347
Polymorphonuclear leukocytes. *See* Neu-
trophils
Polymorphonuclear neutrophils (PMNs).
See Neutrophils
Polypeptide molecules. *See* Inflammatory
cytokines

Polyunsaturated fatty acids (PUFAs), 4,
7, 38, 41, 42, 305–306
doses and toxicity of, 110, 111
immune function role of, 55–56,
105, 110, 111, 118, 127
intake amount and immune function,
57–59
military situations, special concerns
in, 110, 111
military supplementation, conclusions, 128
See also Essential fatty acids
(EFAs); Fatty acids; Linoleic acid
(n-6 PUFA); Linolenic acid (n-3
PUFA); Nutrients
Population. *See* Age and aging; Adults;
Children; Demographics; Infants;
Population density; Population
migration; Women
Population density
high-density locations, infectious
disease introduction/dissemination
factor, 545
See also Demographics
Population migration
rural to urban, infectious disease
introduction/dissemination factor,
544–545
See also Demographics
Post-viral fatigue syndrome (PVFS),
373–374
See also Diseases and disorders
Pre-B-cell growth factor. *See* Interleukin-
7 (IL-7)
Pregnancy. *See* Maternity
Proinflammatory cytokines, 2, 18, 20, 41
definition, 536
disease (infectious) resistance, effects of, 105
lean body mass effects of, 105
metabolic activity and, effects of,
105
thermoregulatory mechanisms, effects of, 105
See also Cytokines; Interferon-
gamma (INF-γ); Interferons; In-
terleukin-1 (IL-1); Interleukin-6